Jason 2

W9-AQU-020

3rd edition

pediatrics

National Medical Series

In the basic sciences

anatomy, 2nd edition
the behavioral sciences
   in psychiatry, 3rd edition
biochemistry, 3rd edition
clinical epidemiology and
   biostatistics
genetics
hematology
histology and cell biology,
   2nd edition

human developmental anatomy
immunology, 3rd edition
introduction to clinical medicine
microbiology, 2nd edition
neuroanatomy
pathology, 3rd edition
pharmacology, 3rd edition
physiology, 3rd edition
radiographic anatomy

In the clinical sciences

medicine, 2nd edition
obstetrics and gynecology,
   3rd edition
pediatrics, 3rd edition
preventive medicine and
   public health, 2nd edition
psychiatry, 3rd edition
surgery, 3rd edition

In the exam series

review for USMLE Step 1,
   3rd edition
review for USMLE Step 2
geriatrics

The National Medical Series for Independent Study

3rd edition
pediatrics

EDITOR

Paul H. Dworkin, M.D.

Professor and Associate Chairman of Pediatrics
Head, Division of General Pediatrics
University of Connecticut
School of Medicine
Farmington, Connecticut
Director and Chairman
Department of Pediatrics
St. Francis Hospital and Medical Center
Hartford, Connecticut

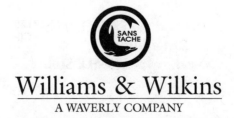

Williams & Wilkins
A WAVERLY COMPANY

BALTIMORE • PHILADELPHIA • LONDON • PARIS • BANGKOK
BUENOS AIRES • HONG KONG • MUNICH • SYDNEY • TOKYO • WROCLAW

**Williams
& Wilkins**

Senior Acquisitions Editor: Elizabeth A. Nieginski
Associate Development Editor: Beth Goldner
Managing Editor: Amy G. Dinkel
Production Manager: Laurie Forsyth
Illustrator: Patricia MacAllen

Copyright © 1996
Williams & Wilkins
Suite 5025
Rose Tree Corporate Center
Building Two
1400 N. Providence Road
Media, PA 19063 USA

All rights reserved. This book is protected by copyright. No part of this book may be reproduced in any form or by any means, including photocopying, or utilized by any information retrieval system without written permission of the copyright owner.

Printed in the United States of America

Library of Congress Cataloging-in-Publication Data
Pediatrics / editor, Paul H. Dworkin. — 3rd ed.
    p. cm. — (The National medical series for independent study)
  Includes index.
  ISBN 0-683-06245-X
  1. Pediatrics—Outlines, syllabi, etc. 2. Pediatrics—
Examinations, questions, etc. I. Dworkin, Paul H. II. Series.
  [DNLM: 1. Pediatrics—examination questions. 2. Pediatrics—
outlines. WS 18.2 P3705 1996]
RJ48.3.P44 1996
618.92—dc20
DNLM/DLC
for Library of Congress   95-37175
                                    CIP

96 97 98
10 9 8 7 6 5 4 3 2

Acknowledgments

The editor and contributing authors thank Debra Dreger, former Medical Acquisitions Editor at Harwal Publishing, for soliciting the reviews of the second edition of *NMS Pediatrics*. We are grateful for the comprehensive critiques offered by medical students and pediatric faculty members. I am personally indebted to Carol Ann Webb for her invaluable administrative and secretarial assistance in the preparation of this third edition.

Paul H. Dworkin, M.D.

Contents

Contributors

Paula S. Algranati, M.D.
Associate Professor of Pediatrics
University of Connecticut School of Medicine
Farmington, Connecticut

Arnold J. Altman, M.D.
Hartford Whalers Professor of
    Childhood Cancer
Head, Division of Pediatric
    Hematology/Oncology
University of Connecticut School of Medicine
Farmington, Connecticut

Mark Ballow, M.D.
Professor of Pediatrics
State University of New York at Buffalo
School of Medicine and Biological Sciences
Chief, Division of Allergy, Immunology,
    and Pediatric Rheumatology
The Children's Hospital of Buffalo
Buffalo, New York

Leonard I. Banco, M.D.
Associate Professor of Pediatrics
University of Connecticut School of Medicine
Farmington, Connecticut
Director, Connecticut Childhood Injury
    Prevention Center
Director, Department of Pediatrics
Director, Pediatric Ambulatory Services
Hartford Hospital
Hartford, Connecticut

Suzanne B. Cassidy, M.D.
Professor of Genetics and Pediatrics
Case Western Reserve University
Clinical Director
Center for Human Genetics
University Hospitals of Cleveland
Cleveland, Ohio

Leon Chameides, M.D.
Clinical Professor of Pediatrics
Head, Division of Pediatric Cardiology
University of Connecticut School of Medicine
Farmington, Connecticut
Director, Pediatric Cardiology
Hartford Hospital
Hartford, Connecticut

Michelle M. Cloutier, M.D.
Professor of Pediatrics
Head, Division of Pediatric Pulmonology
University of Connecticut School of Medicine
Farmington, Connecticut

Daniel J. Diana, M.D.
Assistant Clinical Professor of Pediatrics
University of Connecticut School of Medicine
Farmington, Connecticut
Pediatric Cardiologist
Hartford Hospital
Hartford, Connecticut

Paul H. Dworkin, M.D.
Professor and Associate Chairman
    of Pediatrics
Head, Division of General Pediatrics
University of Connecticut School of Medicine
Farmington, Connecticut
Director and Chairman
Department of Pediatrics
St. Francis Hospital and Medical Center
Hartford, Connecticut

Henry M. Feder, Jr., M.D.
Professor of Pediatrics and Family Medicine
University of Connecticut School of Medicine
Farmington, Connecticut

M. Alex Geertsma, M.D.
Associate Professor of Pediatrics
University of Connecticut School of Medicine
Farmington, Connecticut
Director, Pediatric Primary Care Program
Director, Early Childhood Development
    Program
Hartford Hospital
Hartford, Connecticut

Michael A. Gerber, M.D.
Professor of Pediatrics
Head, Division of Pediatric Infectious Diseases
University of Connecticut School of Medicine
Farmington, Connecticut

Jeffrey S. Hyams, M.D.
Professor of Pediatrics
Head, Division of Pediatric
    Gastroenterology and Nutrition
University of Connecticut School of Medicine
Farmington, Connecticut
Chief, Division of Pediatric
    Gastroenterology and Nutrition
Hartford Hospital
Hartford, Connecticut

Thomas L. Kennedy, III, M.D.
Associate Clinical Professor of Pediatrics
Yale School of Medicine
New Haven, Connecticut
Associate Clinical Professor of Pediatrics
University of Connecticut School of Medicine
Farmington, Connecticut
Chairman, Department of Pediatrics
Bridgeport Hospital
Bridgeport, Connecticut

Peter J. Krause, M.D.
Professor of Pediatrics
University of Connecticut School of Medicine
Farmington, Connecticut
Chief, Division of Pediatric Infectious
    Diseases
Hartford Hospital
Hartford, Connecticut

Carol R. Leicher, M.D.
Associate Professor of Pediatrics
University of Connecticut School of Medicine
Farmington, Connecticut
Pediatric Neurologist
Hartford Hospital
Hartford, Connecticut

Harris B. Leopold, M.D.
Assistant Clinical Professor of Pediatrics
University of Connecticut School of Medicine
Farmington, Connecticut
Pediatric Cardiologist
Hartford Hospital
Hartford, Connecticut

Milton Markowitz, M.D.
Emeritus Professor of Pediatrics
Former Chairman, Department of Pediatrics
University of Connecticut
School of Medicine
Farmington, Connecticut

John J. Quinn, M.D.
Professor of Pediatrics
Pediatric Clerkship Director
University of Connecticut School of Medicine
Farmington, Connecticut

Susan K. Ratzan, M.D.
Chase/Freedman Associate Professor
    of Pediatrics
Head, Division of Pediatric Endocrinology
University of Connecticut School of Medicine
Farmington, Connecticut

James Edmund Robinson, M.D.
Professor of Pediatrics
Director, Pediatric HIV Program
University of Connecticut School
    of Medicine
Farmington, Connecticut

Ted S. Rosenkrantz, M.D.
Associate Professor of Pediatrics
    and Obstetrics and Gynecology
Associate Director of Newborn Services
University of Connecticut School of Medicine
Farmington, Connecticut

Barry S. Russman, M.D.
Professor of Pediatrics and Neurology
Head, Division of Pediatric Neurology
University of Connecticut School of Medicine
Farmington, Connecticut
Chief, Pediatric Neurology
Newington Children's Hospital
Newington, Connecticut

Neil L. Schechter, M.D.
Professor of Pediatrics
Head, Division of Developmental
   and Behavioral Pediatrics
University of Connecticut School of Medicine
Farmington, Connecticut
Director, Section of Developmental
   and Behavioral Pediatrics
Saint Francis Hospital and Medical Center
Hartford, Connecticut

Aric Schichor, M.D.
Associate Professor of Pediatrics
Head, Division of Adolescent Medicine
University of Connecticut School of Medicine
Farmington, Connecticut
Director, Section of Adolescent Medicine
Saint Francis Hospital and Medical Center
Hartford, Connecticut

Betty S. Spivack, M.D.
Assistant Professor of Pediatrics
Head, Division of Pediatric Critical Care
University of Connecticut School of Medicine
Farmington, Connecticut
Director, Pediatric Intensive Care Unit
Hartford Hospital
Hartford, Connecticut

William R. Treem, M.D.
Professor of Pediatrics
Duke University School of Medicine
Chief, Division of Pediatric
   Gastroenterology and Nutrition
Duke University Medical Center
Durham, North Carolina

David A. H. Whiteman, M.D.
Director, Medical Genetics Service
Children's Hospital
Boston, Massachusetts

Preface

The popularity of the first two editions of *NMS Pediatrics* has been most gratifying. Our intent with this third edition is to ensure that the text remains useful as an in-depth review of pediatrics for students preparing for the USMLE examination, as well as a helpful supplement during the pediatric clerkship.

Reviews solicited from medical students and pediatric faculty members have greatly influenced the preparation of this edition. All chapters have been updated to include new information. In particular, sections on topics such as AIDS, immunizations, and genetic disorders have been extensively revised. A new chapter by Dr. M. Alex Geertsma addresses critical psychosocial issues of paramount importance in pediatric practice. Case-based questions have been selected to emphasize practical and important clinical information. Case studies illustrate how information is applied to clinical decision making.

As with previous editions, this text reflects the commitment to medical education of the Department of Pediatrics of the University of Connecticut School of Medicine. All authors are current or former members of this department. Our hope is that this text remains a useful tool for trainees in the rapidly evolving field of children's health care.

Paul H. Dworkin, M.D.

To the Reader

Since 1984, the *National Medical Series for Independent Study (NMS)* has been helping medical students meet the challenge of education and clinical training. In this climate of burgeoning knowledge and complex clinical issues, a medical career is more demanding than ever. Increasingly, medical training must prepare physicians to seek and synthesize necessary information and to apply that information successfully.

The *National Medical Series* is designed to provide a logical framework for organizing, learning, reviewing, and applying the conceptual and factual information covered in basic and clinical studies. Each book includes a concise but comprehensive outline of the essential content of a discipline, with up to 500 study questions. The combination of an outlined text and tools for self-evaluation allows easy retrieval of salient information.

All study questions are accompanied by the correct answer, a paragraph-length explanation, and specific reference to the text where the topic is discussed. Study questions that follow each chapter use current USMLE format to reinforce the chapter content. Study questions appearing at the end of the text in the Comprehensive Exam vary in format depending on the book. Wherever possible, Comprehensive Exam questions are presented as a clinical case or scenario intended to simulate real-life application of medical knowledge. The goal of this exam is to challenge the student to draw from information presented throughout the book.

All of the books in the *National Medical Series* are constantly being updated and revised. The authors and editors devote considerable time and effort to ensure that the information required by all medical school curricula is included. Strict editorial attention is given to accuracy, organization, and consistency. Further shaping of the series occurs in response to biannual discussions held with a panel of medical student advisors drawn from schools throughout the United States. At these meetings, the editorial staff considers the complicated needs of medical students to learn how the *National Medical Series* can better serve them. In this regard, the staff at Williams & Wilkins welcomes all comments and suggestions.

Chapter 1

Child Health Supervision

Paula S. Algranati
Paul H. Dworkin

I. **GOAL AND SCOPE OF PEDIATRIC PRACTICE.** The goal of child health supervision is promotion of optimal growth and development of children. A long-term partnership established during sequential visits between clinician and the patient and family provides the vehicle for meeting this challenge. Currently, most pediatric encounters occur in the ambulatory setting with practice time divided as follows.

A. **Child health supervision** (i.e., well-child "check-ups") accounts for about 30% of practice time.

B. **Infectious diseases** occupy about 50% of practice time, and the most common problems are upper respiratory tract illnesses and otitis media.

C. **Other disorders** that account for the remainder of practice time include injuries and trauma, skin disorders, and behavioral and developmental disorders.

D. **Recent trends.** The scope of pediatric practice has changed significantly over the past decade. Time spent caring for hospitalized children and life-threatening problems has diminished. Areas that receive increased attention from pediatricians include asthma and allergies, effects of environmental pollutants such as lead, school functioning, child behavior, substance abuse, family functioning, and child health supervision.

II. **THE PRENATAL VISIT.** Optimally, this visit establishes an exchange of information between parents and physician, which serves to diminish parental anxiety and enhance infant care during the neonatal period. It also sets the stage for future visits that emphasize mutual participation and anticipatory guidance.

A. **History.** Information to be reviewed is presented in Table 1-1.

B. **Anticipatory guidance**

1. **Physician–parent relationship.** Information to be discussed may include the pediatrician's schedule of availability, provisions for after-hours coverage, telephone arrangements (e.g., call hours), appointment procedures, and the schedule for health supervision visits.

2. **Parental readiness** for the arrival of the infant may be suggested by parental expectations concerning changes in home life, paternal involvement, and attendance at prenatal classes.

3. **Delivery room and nursery procedures.** Routine procedures and personnel should be reviewed as well as issues such as rooming-in, natural childbirth, and circumcision.

4. **Infant feeding.** Does the mother plan to breast-feed or bottle-feed?

TABLE 1-1. Prenatal Visit: Patient History

Maternal health history
Age, general health, nutritional status
Previous illnesses and chronic disorders
Previous pregnancies and childbirth experiences

Current pregnancy
Reaction to pregnancy and fears, prenatal care, due date
Complications (e.g., bleeding, diabetes, hypertension) and medicines
Exposure to infectious diseases
Use of drugs, alcohol, tobacco

Family health history
Risk factors, including familial and inherited disorders

Family psychosocial history
Proposed household situation, available support for parents
(e.g., extended family, financial resources)

5. **Care arrangements.** Parents may have questions regarding equipment, clothing, and sleeping arrangements. Parents must have access to an approved infant car seat.

6. **Economics.** The cost of medical care for delivery and the postpartum period should be reviewed. Do parents have adequate medical insurance?

7. **Newborn behavior.** The pediatrician's interest in infant development and behavior should be stressed from the beginning. A preliminary discussion of newborn behavior, with an explanation of state organization (see III F 6 a) and synchrony (see III F 6 b), sets the stage for future discussions.

III. NEWBORN NURSERY HEALTH SUPERVISION (see Chapter 6)

A. Goals

1. Assess wellness of the newborn, screening for congenital anomalies, birth trauma, or acquired medical problems.

2. Assess the newborn for gestational age and appropriateness of size for gestational age.

3. When appropriate, confirm infant's normality to parents.

4. When appropriate, demystify and reassure parents about common, benign variations in newborn physical examination or behavior.

5. Foster early infant–parent bonding and parental self-confidence.

B. History.
Maternal health and current pregnancy history, family health history, and family psychosocial history are reviewed (see Table 1-1). Details about labor, delivery, and neonatal condition are added (Table 1-2).

C. Physical examination
of the newborn should seek to identify major and minor congenital anomalies, sequelae of birth trauma, and neonatal medical problems, and determine gestational age and appropriateness of size for gestational age.

1. **General appearance.** Important observations include body proportions, activity, quality of cry, skin color, gross abnormalities, unusual features, and signs of respiratory distress. Weight, length, and head circumference measurements are obtained and recorded.

2. **Skin. Color** may suggest cyanosis, pallor, or jaundice.

TABLE 1-2. Newborn Nursery Health Supervision: Patient History

Review maternal history, prenatal history, family health, and psychosocial history (see Table 1-1)

Labor and delivery
  Length of gestation, onset of labor, spontaneous or induced
  Reason for induction
  Duration of labor, rupture of membranes, spontaneous or induced, meconium staining
  Medication during labor and delivery
  Fetal presentation vertex, breech, or other
  Delivery vaginal, cesarean, reason for cesarean
  Maternal reaction to experience of labor and delivery

Neonatal
  Birth date, weight, estimated gestational age
  Apgar score (see Chapter 6), condition of newborn in delivery room, intervention or resuscitation required
  Blood type and Coombs
  Infant feeding, breast or formula
  Problems in nursery such as jaundice, poor feeding

  a. Manifestations of **normal peripheral vascular instability** include skin mottling, perioral cyanosis, and cyanosis of the hands and feet, with lips, mucous membranes, and nailbeds remaining pink.
  b. **Cracking or desquamation** of the skin is normal in the term and postmature infant. In the term infant, fine downy hair known as lanugo covers the skin, particularly the shoulders and upper back.
  c. **Jaundice** in the neonate is first visible on the face, and as the serum bilirubin level rises it progresses caudally to include the rest of the body and the sclerae. Natural sunlight should be used to inspect the skin for the extent of jaundice.
  d. Common **birthmarks** that are visible at birth include flat vascular nevi (i.e., salmon patch nevus and port wine stains) and mongolian spots. Raised vascular nevi usually become apparent several weeks after birth (i.e., a capillary or strawberry hemangioma, cavernous hemangioma).
  e. Benign **rashes** are common.
    (1) **Erythema toxicum** has a "flea-bite" appearance with scattered erythematous macules that may contain papulopustular centers filled with eosinophils. This rash typically changes distribution from day to day.
    (2) **Milia** are fine, pinpoint, yellow-white papules caused by retained sebum that typically cover the bridge of the nose, chin, and cheeks. These are transient.
    (3) **Neonatal pustular melanosis** consists of small vesiculopustules that are present at birth and rupture within a few days, leaving transient pigmented macules with scaly borders.

3. Head and neck. The head and face frequently exhibit sequelae of the birth process, including bruises and asymmetries. Most resolve spontaneously. Facial features should be carefully inspected for size, placement, and symmetry.
  a. Palpation of the skull determines contour, extent of separation or overriding of sutures, and the size of the fontanelles.
    (1) **Molding** of the head shape into an elongated or asymmetric contour occurs secondary to intrauterine pressure or forces during delivery.
    (2) **Cephalhematoma** is a subperiosteal hemorrhage manifested by a unilateral scalp swelling.
    (3) **Caput succedaneum** is edema of the scalp due to the pressure caused during labor and delivery. In contrast to cephalhematomas, these swellings extend beyond suture lines.

b. Eyes. Dimming the room lights, talking to the baby, or cradling the occiput in the examiner's hand to lift the baby's head off the mattress may stimulate the baby to open her eyes.
  (1) Conjunctival or scleral hemorrhages resolve spontaneously and usually are of no clinical significance.
  (2) The presence of a **red reflex** excludes the presence of lens opacities (e.g., cataracts) and retinoblastoma.
  (3) Up to the age of 3 months, the eyes normally may appear to cross intermittently. A fixed eye misalignment is always abnormal.
c. Ears. Patency of the canal should be determined. Malformed or low-set ears may be associated with auditory or renal abnormalities. A tympanic membrane examination is unnecessary in a healthy newborn.
d. Nose. Newborns are nose-breathers. Obstruction of the nasal passages results in respiratory distress.
e. The **mouth** should be examined by inspection and palpation. Common minor anomalies include small, white **epithelial pearls** along the gum margins; small, white cysts termed **Epstein's pearls** along the median raphe of the hard palate; and small, hard tumors within the gingiva, termed **epulis**. Palpation may reveal a submucosal bony cleft of the palate.
f. The **neck** must be hyperextended to inspect adequately for masses. Congenital masses include **goiter, cystic hygroma, branchial cleft cysts,** and **thyroglossal duct cysts**. A webbing of the neck is seen in a variety of syndromes, the most common of which is Turner syndrome.

4. Chest
  a. The **clavicles** are palpated for signs of fracture, including irregularities or crepitations, most often resulting from a difficult delivery.
  b. Respiratory rate, pattern, and the presence of **chest asymmetry, retractions, grunting,** and **nasal flaring** must be determined. In some healthy infants, transient crackles may be auscultated during the first few hours after birth, unaccompanied by signs of respiratory distress. A normal pattern of periodic breathing, with pauses up to 10–15 seconds, unaccompanied by bradycardia or changes in color and tone, may be observed.
  c. An abnormality in **cardiac location** is screened for by determining that the heart sounds are loudest in the left chest. Soft systolic heart murmurs are commonly heard in the first 24 hours of life, probably because of a closing ductus arteriosus or normal changes in pulmonary vascular resistance. These murmurs usually disappear within 48 hours after birth.

5. The **abdomen** is convex and moves prominently with respiration.
  a. A normal **liver edge** may be palpated 1–2 cm below the right costal margin, and the tip of the normal spleen may be palpated at the left costal margin.
  b. Because the most common **abdominal masses** in the newborn involve the genitourinary tract, palpation of the kidneys is especially important. The kidney may be palpated with fingertips pressing deeply onto the lower lateral aspect of the abdomen, with the opposite hand resting under the baby's back at a level just superior to the iliac crest.

6. Inguinal region and genitalia
  a. Femoral pulses must always be palpated because diminished pulses suggest coarctation of the aorta.
  b. Examination of **male genitalia** should include location of the urethral meatus, palpation of the testes, and a search for a bulge in the groin or scrotum suggesting a hernia or hydrocele.
  c. Examination of the **female genitalia** should ascertain the presence of urethral and vaginal openings as well as a normal-sized clitoris to exclude ambiguous genitalia, imperforate hymen, and vaginal atresia. In normal infants, a transient swelling of the labia minora or a vaginal discharge that is mucoid or bloody results from the influence of maternal hormones.
  d. The **anus** is inspected for patency and placement.

7. **Extremities.** Temporary flexion contractures at the elbows, hips, and knees are seen in the term newborn as a result of intrauterine pressure effects. Approximately 5% of all newborns have more significant limb deformities, either deformations caused by positional abnormalities and intrauterine posture, or true malformations.

   a. **Developmental dysplasia** of the hip occurs in 1 in 1000 live births and is much more common in girls and breech deliveries. Asymmetries in lower limb length, placement of medial thigh and gluteal folds, or degree of hip flexion should raise suspicion for unilateral hip dislocation. When the hips are flexed to 90 degrees, the legs normally can be abducted fully to touch the examining table. "Telescoping" of the femoral head with the subluxation (Barlow) maneuver or a palpable "thump" with the Ortolani maneuver suggests dislocation.

   b. Trauma to the cervical nerves during delivery may result in asymmetric or diminished arm movements, indicating **Erb palsy** (C5 and C6 nerve roots) or **Klumpke palsy** (C8–T2 nerve roots).

   c. **Metatarsus adductus** is a condition in which the fore part of the foot is adducted and usually supinated. It may result from intrauterine positional compression.

8. **Back.** The spine is inspected and palpated for sinus tracts or overlying lesions such as lipomas, hairy tufts, or hemangiomas, any of which may be signs of a covert neural tube defect.

9. **Neurologic examination.** Overall state of consciousness and the ease with which the infant makes transitions from waking to sleeping or fussing to calming, as well as strength of cry, should be noted. Cranial nerves, primitive reflexes, and tone should also be assessed (Figure 1-1).

10. **Gestational age** and appropriateness of **size** for gestational age

    a. Gestational age may be determined by assessing certain physical and neurologic characteristics that evolve in a predictable and progressive fashion during the latter part of gestation. Findings are assigned numerical values when compared to standard rating scales, and summed totals are correlated to specific gestational ages (see Figure 1-1).

    b. After determining gestational age, **weight, length,** and **head circumference** values are plotted on graphs that classify newborns according to appropriateness of size for gestational age.

D. | **Procedures**

1. **Prophylaxis of gonococcal ophthalmia** is mandated for all newborns. Either a 1% silver nitrate solution in single-dose ampules or a sterile ophthalmic ointment containing 1% tetracycline or 0.5% erythromycin in single-use tubes is an acceptable regimen.

2. Every newborn should receive a single parenteral dose of 0.5–1.0 mg of natural **vitamin K_1 oxide** (phytonadione) within 1 hour of birth to prevent vitamin K-dependent hemorrhagic disease and coagulation disorders.

3. **Metabolic screening.** Before discharge, a blood sample should be obtained from every neonate for screening for the presence of the **hyperphenylalaninemias,** including **phenylketonuria (PKU),** and for congenital **hypothyroidism**. In many states, screening is also performed for other inborn errors or diseases such as **homocystinuria, maple syrup urine disease, histidinemia, galactosemia, cystic fibrosis,** and **sickle cell anemia**. Cost effectiveness is greatly improved by a screening program that encompasses multiple disorders (e.g., the PKU and hypothyroidism screening performed through state laboratories). This screening must be part of a comprehensive program ensuring effective treatment for problems that are disclosed.

   a. Blood should be drawn from the heel to screen for PKU and the hyperphenylalaninemias as close as possible to the time of discharge. If an infant is discharged early, and, as a result, is screened before 24 hours of age, he must be rescreened before the third week of life. Cases may be missed if screening is done too soon after delivery—before there is adequate protein input. Many states require repeat screening at 2 weeks of age.

Neuromuscular maturity

Sign	Score							Record score here
	-1	0	1	2	3	4	5	
Posture								
Square window (wrist)	>90°	90°	60°	45°	30°	0°		
Arm recoil		180°	140-180°	110-140°	90-110°	<90°		
Popliteal angle	180°	160°	140°	120°	100°	90°	<90°	
Scarf sign								
Heel to ear								

NEUROMUSCULAR MATURITY SCORE

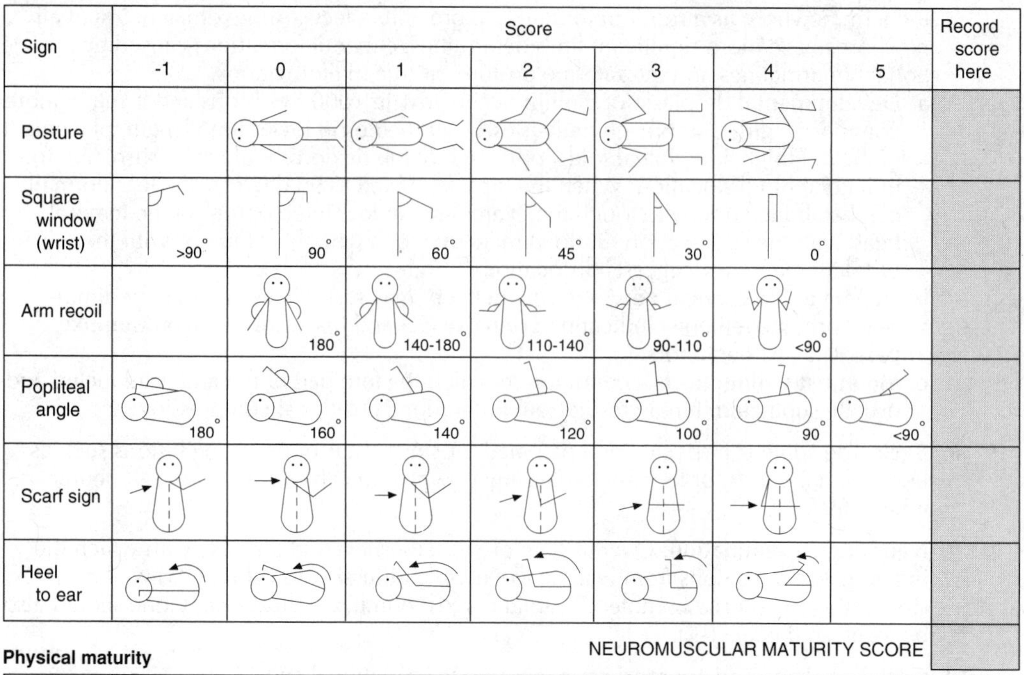

Physical maturity

Sign	Score							Record score here
	-1	0	1	2	3	4	5	
Skin	sticky friable transparent	gelatinous red translucent	smooth pink visible veins	superficial peeling &/or rash, few veins	cracking pale areas rare veins	parchment deep cracking no vessels	leathery cracked wrinkled	
Lanugo	none	sparse	abundant	thinning	bald areas	mostly bald		
Plantar surface	heel-toe 40-50mm:-1 <40mm:-2	>50 mm no crease	faint red marks	anterior transverse crease only	creases ant. 2/3	creases over entire sole		
Breast	imper-ceptible	barely perceptible	flat areola no bud	stippled areola 1-2mm bud	raised areola 3-4 mm bud	full areola 5-10 mm bud		
Eye/ear	lids fused loosely: -1 tightly: -2	lids open pinna flat stays folded	sl. curved pinna; soft; slow recoil	well-curved pinna; soft but ready recoil	formed & firm instant recoil	thick car-tilage ear stiff		
Genitals (male)	scrotum flat, smooth	scrotum empty faint rugae	testes in upper canal rare rugae	testes descending few rugae	testes down good rugae	testes pendulous deep rugae		
Genitals (female)	clitoris prominent & labia flat	prominent clitoris & sm. labia minora	prominent clitoris & enlarging minora	majora & minora equally prominent	majora large minora small	majora cover clitoris & minora		

PHYSICAL MATURITY SCORE

Maturity rating

Score	-10	-5	0	5	10	15	20	25	30	35	40	45	50
Weeks	20	22	24	26	28	30	32	34	36	38	40	42	44

TOTAL NEUROMUSCULAR AND PHYSICAL MATURITY SCORE

Gestational age (weeks)

By age _____ By ultrasound _____ By exam _____

FIGURE 1-1. Maturational assessment of gestational age (New Ballard Score). (Reproduced with permission from: Ballard JL, Khoury JC, Wedig K, et al: New Ballard Score, expanded to include extremely premature infants. *J Pediatr* 119:417–423, 1991; and Ross Laboratories, Columbus, Ohio, 43216, 1991.)

    b. Cord blood at birth or heel blood at discharge may be used to screen for congenital hypothyroidism, and many states require rescreening for this disorder at 2 weeks of age.

4. Newborn circumcision has potential medical benefits and advantages, but also has risks and disadvantages. If parents are considering this procedure, benefits and risks should be carefully explained.

    a. Benefits and advantages. Properly performed circumcision prevents inflammation of the glans and prepuce of the penis and decreases the incidence of cancer of the penis among adults. It may reduce the incidence of urinary tract infections in male infants.

    b. Risks and disadvantages. The most common complications are local infection and bleeding. Because the newborn experiences pain with the procedure, some centers use local anesthesia.

5. All newborns should be vaccinated with the first dose of **hepatitis B recombinant vaccine** (Tables 1-3, 1-4, and 1-5).

    a. The actual volume of vaccine administered varies according to the specific product and according to the mother's hepatitis B status.

    b. Infants at high risk for perinatally acquired hepatitis B infection (e.g., the mother is hepatitis B surface antigen-positive) should also receive a dose of **hepatitis B immunoglobulin** as soon as possible after birth.

TABLE 1-3. Recommended Childhood Immunization Schedule

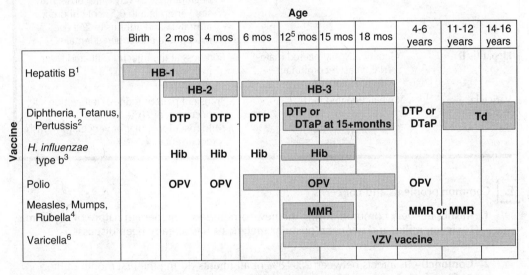

	Birth	2 mos	4 mos	6 mos	12^5 mos	15 mos	18 mos	4-6 years	11-12 years	14-16 years
Hepatitis B^1	HB-1	HB-1								
		HB-2	HB-2		HB-3	HB-3	HB-3			
Diphtheria, Tetanus, Pertussis^2		DTP	DTP	DTP	DTP or DTaP at 15+months			DTP or DTaP	Td	
H. influenzae type b^3		Hib	Hib	Hib	Hib	Hib				
Polio		OPV	OPV		OPV	OPV		OPV		
Measles, Mumps, Rubella^4					MMR	MMR		MMR or MMR		
Varicella^6					VZV vaccine	VZV vaccine	VZV vaccine	VZV vaccine	VZV vaccine	

Vaccines are listed under the routinely recommended ages. Shaded bars indicate range of acceptable ages for vaccination.

[1]Infants born to HBsAg-negative mothers should receive the second dose of Hepatitis B vaccine between 1 and 4 months of age, provided at least 1 month has elapsed since receipt of the first dose. The third dose is recommended between 6 and 18 months of age. Infants born to HBsAg-positive mothers should receive immunoprophylaxis for hepatitis B with 0.5 ml Hepatitis B immune globulin (HBIG) within 12 hours of birth, and 0.5 ml of either Merck Sharp & Dohme vaccine (Recombivax HB) or of SmithKline Beecham vaccine (Engerix-B) at a separate site. In these infants, the second dose of vaccine is recommended at 1 month of age and the third dose at 6 months of age. All pregnant women should be screened for HBsAg in an early prenatal visit.

[2]The fourth dose of DTP may be administered as early as 12 months of age, provided at least 6 months have elapsed since DTP3. Combined DTP-Hib products may be used when these two vaccines are to be administered simultaneously. DTaP (diphtheria and tetanus toxoids and acellular pertussis vaccine) is licensed for use for the 4th and/or 5th dose of DTP vaccine in children 15 months of age or older and may be preferred for these doses in children in this age group.

[3]Three H. influenzae type b conjugate vaccines are available for use in infants: HbOC [HibTITER] (Lederle Praxis); PRP-T [ActHIB; OmniHIB] (Pasteur Mérieux, distributed by SmithKline Beecham; Connaught); and PRP-OMP [PedvaxHIB] (Merck Sharp & Dohme). Children who have received PRP-OMP at 2 and 4 months of age do not require a dose at 6 months of age. After the primary infant Hib conjugate vaccine series is completed, any licensed Hib conjugate vaccine may be used as a booster dose at age 12 to 15 months.

[4]The second dose of MMR vaccine should be administered EITHER at 4 to 6 years of age OR at 11 to 12 years of age.

[5]Vaccines recommended in the second year of life (12 to 15 months of age) may be given at either one or two visits.

Approved by the Advisory Committee on Immunization Practices (ACIP), the American Academy of Pediatrics (AAP), and the American Academy of Family Physicians (AAFP).

(Adapted with permission from Hall CB: The recommended childhood immunization schedule of the United States. *Pediatrics* 95:136, 1995.)

[6]One dose of varicella (VZV) vaccine is recommended for children 18 months to 12 years of age. If vaccination occurs after the 13th birthday, two doses should be administered 4–8 weeks apart.

TABLE 1-4. Routine Immunizations

Immunization	Type	Usual Reactions
DTP		
Diphtheria	Bacterial toxoid	Transient local redness, pain or swelling
Tetanus	Bacterial toxoid	at injection site, occurrence: 33%–50%
Pertussis	Bacterial killed whole organism	Mild–moderate systemic (fever, drowsy or fretful), occurrence: 33%–50%
Hib		
Haemophilus influenzae type b	Bacterial conjugate vaccine, capsular polysaccharide or oligosaccharide covalently linked to carrier protein	Transient local inflammation at injection site or mild fever within 24 hours and rapidly subside, occurrence: 25%
TOPV		
Poliovirus types 1, 2, 3	Live attenuated virus	None
MMR		
Measles	Live attenuated virus	Beginning 5 days after dose, 5%–15%
Mumps	Live attenuated virus	with fever lasting 1–2 days, transient
Rubella	Live attenuated virus	rash and/or lymphadenopathy in 5%; beginning 7–21 days after dose, transient arthralgia in 0.5% of children, arthralgia and arthritis in 25% of susceptible postpubertal females
Hepatitis B	Genetically engineered material, yeast recombinant-derived antigen	Soreness at the injection site and fever in 1%–6%
Varicella	Live attenuated virus	Transient pain or redness at injection site, occurrence: 20%–35% Mild maculopapular or varicelliform rash, occurrence: 7%–8%

E. | **Common problems and concerns**

1. **Rashes** are very common during the newborn period. The benign nature of **erythema toxicum, milia,** and **neonatal pustular melanosis** has already been discussed (see III C 2 e).

2. **Conjunctivitis** affects between 2%–8% of all infants during the first month of life.
   a. **Chemical conjunctivitis** that is secondary to administration of silver nitrate drops usually appears within the first day of life and disappears within 3–4 days.
   b. *Chlamydia trachomatis* is the most prevalent identifiable infectious cause of neonatal conjunctivitis, accounting for 20%–30% of cases. The incubation period is 5–14 days.
   c. **Gonococcal ophthalmia** has decreased in frequency as a result of neonatal prophylaxis, with an annual incidence of 2–3 cases in 10,000 live births. The mean incubation period is about 6 days, with a range of 1–21 days.

3. **Weight loss.** A normal newborn may lose 5%–8% of her birth weight during the first 3 days of life. A weight loss of up to 10% is acceptable if the infant's examination and behavior are normal.

4. **Jaundice** is very common among newborns, with 50% having serum bilirubin levels of at least 5–7 mg/dl.
   a. **Physiologic jaundice**—as opposed to pathologic jaundice—is characterized in term newborns by
      (1) Clinical jaundice appearing after 24 hours
      (2) An increase in the total serum bilirubin concentration of less than 5 mg/dl/day

TABLE 1-5. Contraindications to Immunizations

Contraindications to All Vaccines
  Acute febrile illness
  Prior allergic or severe reaction to same or related vaccine component

Contraindications to Live Virus Vaccines
  Immune-suppressed patient:
    Immunosuppressive therapy
    Immunodeficiency disorder (exception: people with HIV infection may receive MMR)
    Malignancy
    Recent (within 8 weeks) recipient of gamma globulin or plasma or blood transfusion

Additional Contraindications to TOPV
  Household member or close contact of vaccine recipient who is immune suppressed
  Immunization during pregnancy generally should be avoided because of theoretical risk

Additional Contraindications to MMR
  History of anaphylactic reaction to eggs: vaccinate with extreme caution after skin testing
  History of anaphylactic reaction to neomycin
  Administer at least 2 weeks before or at least 3 months after administration of immune globulin
    or blood transfusion (substantially longer intervals are indicated after administration of large
    doses of immune globulin).
  Known pregnancy because of theoretical risk

Additional Contraindications to Pertussis Vaccine
  Encephalopathy within 7 days, defined as severe, acute, central nervous system disorder unexplained
    by another cause, which may be manifested by major alterations of consciousness or by general-
    ized or focal seizures that persist for more than a few hours without recovery within 24 hours.
  If the following adverse events occur in temporal relation to DTP or acellular pertussis, the decision
    to administer additional doses of pertussis vaccine should be carefully considered. These events
    are now considered precautions, not contraindications, because of circumstances such as a pertus-
    sis outbreak in which the potential benefits of pertussis immunization outweigh the possible risks,
    and particularly because the following events have not been proven to cause permanent sequelae:

  • A convulsion, with or without fever, occurring within 3 days of DTP or acellular pertussis
    vaccination
  • Persistent, severe, inconsolable screaming or crying for 3 or more hours within 48 hours
  • Collapse or shock-like state (hypotonic–hyporesponsive episode) within 48 hours
  • Temperature of 40.5°C (104.9°F) or higher, unexplained by another cause within 48 hours
  • For infants and children with underlying neurologic disorders, the decision to give pertussis
    vaccine should be made on an individual, case-by-case basis

  Children with a progressive neurologic disorder characterized by developmental delay or neuro-
    logic findings should have pertussis immunization deferred.
  Children with a personal history of convulsions have an increased likelihood of having a post-
    vaccination seizure. In children with a recent seizure, immunization should be deferred until
    a progressive neurologic disorder has been excluded or the child's diagnosis has been estab-
    lished. This decision should be reassessed at each medical visit, weighing the potential risks of
    the vaccine against the potential risks of pertussis and its complications.
  Children known to have, or suspected of having, neurologic conditions that predispose them
    either to seizures or neurologic deterioration should be considered for deferral of immuniza-
    tion. Pertussis immunization should be reconsidered at each visit. Children whose condition is
    resolved, corrected, or controlled can be vaccinated.

Additional Contraindication to Hib Vaccine
  Patient with Hodgkin disease undergoing chemotherapy:
  Administer either 2 or more weeks before initiating chemotherapy or defer until 3 or more
    months after cessation of chemotherapy.

Additional Contraindications to Varicella Vaccine
  Allergy to neomycin; administration of salicylates within 6 weeks following vaccination (theo-
    retical risk of Reye syndrome). Known pregnancy (theoretical risk). Pregnancy should be
    avoided for 1 month following vaccination

Adapted from Peter G: *1994 Red Book, 23rd ed: Report of the Committee on Infectious Diseases.* Elk Grove Village, IL, American
Academy of Pediatrics, 1994.
DTP = diphtheria–tetanus–pertussis; Hib = *Haemophilus influenzae* type B; HIV = human immunodeficiency virus;
MMR = measles–mumps–rubella; TOPV = trivalent oral polio vaccine.

      (3) A total serum bilirubin concentration of less than 13 mg/dl and direct serum bilirubin concentration of less than 1.5–2.0 mg/dl

      (4) Persistence of clinical jaundice for less than 1 week

  b. Breast-feeding jaundice may have either an early onset (i.e., within 3–4 days of birth) or a late onset (i.e., within 4–5 days of birth, with a peak at 10–15 days). Peak bilirubin levels may reach 20–30 mg/dl, although kernicterus has never been reported. Temporarily discontinuing breast-feeding for 24–48 hours typically lowers bilirubin levels; this is diagnostic for breast-feeding jaundice.

5. Breast-feeding problems

  a. Cracked and painful nipples may be helped by altering the nursing position of the infant to ensure that the baby is not pulling down on the nipple during feeding, by airing the nipples after nursing, and by using a lanolin-based cream.

  b. Plugged milk ducts may be caused by improper breast emptying, a tight-fitting brassiere, or by sleeping prone.

6. Effects of maternal hormones. As previously mentioned, transient labial swelling, vaginal discharge, or vaginal bleeding may result from the influence of maternal hormones. For the same reason, breasts of both sexes may demonstrate transient swelling, reddening, and discharge of a milky substance.

F. **Anticipatory guidance.** Areas for discussion with parents during the postpartum period include the following:

1. Physical status. During the immediate postpartum period, concerns for the baby's well-being are of highest priority for parents.

2. General care. Issues include bathing, dressing, skin care, and cord care.

3. Feeding

  a. Breast-feeding is facilitated by a hospital rooming-in policy, which permits a demand-feeding schedule of every 2–4 hours. Routine dietary supplementation with either formula or water should be discouraged for breast-fed babies. Nursing and medical staff must provide consistent, accurate advice about breast-feeding.

  b. Commercial **infant formula** is a satisfactory substitute for human milk. For most newborns, a lactose-containing modified cow's milk formula is well tolerated. Rarely, infants who are intolerant of lactose or of cow's milk protein may require a formula containing alternative carbohydrates (e.g., sucrose, dextrose, maltose, dextrins) or an alternative protein source (e.g., soy isolate, casein hydrolysate). Commercial infant formulas for normal infants contain 20 calories/ounce liquid. After the first few days of life, the normal infant usually requires approximately 100–110 kcal/kg/day, or 150 ml/kg/day, of formula for adequate growth.

4. Safety and injury prevention

  a. Crib safety. Crib bars should be no further than 2 inches apart. Bumpers should be used to avoid suffocation from mattresses and to prevent injury from head banging. To avoid suffocation, objects such as pacifiers and mobiles should not be hung within the crib. Based on data indicating an association between sudden infant death syndrome (SIDS) and prone sleeping position, it is recommended that healthy infants, when being put down for sleep, be positioned on their side or back.

  b. Setting the water-heater temperature below 120°F (49°C) helps to prevent accidental scalding.

  c. An approved car seat should be used to transport infants in automobiles.

  d. Toys should be soft and washable, without sharp edges or removable parts, and should be too large to fit within the infant's mouth.

  e. Parents must be alerted to the danger of the infant rolling off elevated surfaces.

5. Elimination. Infants vary considerably in their patterns of elimination. A pattern of urinating six times within 24 hours suggests adequate fluid intake. Infants may have a bowel movement as frequently as after every feeding or as infrequently as once every 4–5 days. Breast-fed babies tend to have loose stools with small curds, and the bowel movements may be explosive.

6. **Behavioral and developmental issues**
   a. **State organization.** The normal variability in infant behavior is vividly demonstrated by the newborn's frequent changes in state of consciousness. The newborn is able to shut out disturbing aspects of the new environment and has the capacity to choose to respond to certain stimuli.
   b. **Synchrony.** From the outset, the nature of the parent–infant relationship is one of mutual awareness, with parents and newborn each responding to one another via cues.
   c. **Attachment.** The unique relationship between parent and child is being established as early as the postpartum period.
   d. **Temperament.** Individual differences in behavior style are evident as early as the newborn period.

IV. HEALTH SUPERVISION VISITS

A. **Goals.** Priority is given to parents' agendas and an emphasis is placed on longitudinal surveillance.

1. Assess the child's current biopsychosocial functioning.

2. Address parents' concerns.

3. Identify, diagnose, and manage current problems.

4. Prevent or diminish future problems.

B. **Schedule and content** for child health supervision

1. Recommendations for the timing of routine child health supervision visits have evolved through consensus on the part of pediatricians. Factors that contribute most significantly to these guidelines include immunization schedules, timing of pivotal physical and developmental issues, and pediatricians' own perceptions of appropriate scheduling. Recommendations for routine postnatal visits are
   a. **Early infancy:** 2–4 weeks, 2, 4, and 6 months
   b. **Late infancy:** 9, 12, 15, 18 months, and 2 years
   c. **Preschool:** 3, 4, and 5 years
   d. **School age:** 6, 8, 10, and 12 years
   e. **Adolescent:** Every 2 years beginning at 14 years of age. Yearly visits are currently being considered.

2. Recommendations for the **content** of individual routine health supervision visits have also evolved through pediatrician consensus. Factors that contribute most significantly to these guidelines include immunization schedules, data about the efficacy of certain procedures and screening tests, expectations of parents and patients, and pediatricians' own experience with delivering well-child care. Specific recommendations for content are discussed within each age-related section that follows.

C. **History.** Seeks to determine the child's current functioning in biopsychosocial spheres. Parents' overall assessment of their child's functioning is requested, in addition to specific information. Parents and children are encouraged to ask questions and discuss concerns. Initial visits should include a comprehensive review of past medical history, family health history, and family psychosocial history. Interval visits require an update in each of these areas, providing current data within the context of longitudinal surveillance.

D. **Physical examination.** A complete physical examination is performed during each visit. Particular areas should receive emphasis depending on the age of the child. Priority is given to systems undergoing rapid change (e.g., head growth in the infant, pubertal manifestations in the adolescent), areas with a high incidence of pathology (e.g., tympanic membranes in the toddler), and areas most responsive to early intervention (e.g., hearing and vision deficits in the infant).

1. Examination **sequence** is determined by the child's age and developmental stage, state of health, previous experiences, and individual temperament.

2. Measurements should ideally be obtained and plotted on the appropriate **growth charts** at the onset of the visit so that problems may be pursued via relevant history and physical examination. Current measurements are assessed by comparison to age-related norms as well as to the child's own previous values.

E. **Developmental monitoring** is performed during each well-child visit through a combination of history and examination. As with other aspects of child health supervision, monitoring occurs within the context of longitudinal surveillance. Developmental surveillance includes:

1. **History** that elicits parents' assessment of their child's developmental progress, explores concerns, and reviews specific relevant developmental milestones.

2. **Observations** to confirm developmental history and reveal actual levels of functioning. Accurate and informative observations may be obtained through a variety of techniques, including either an informal collection of age-appropriate tasks or the administration of a specific screening instrument (e.g., Denver II developmental screening test; Figure 1-2).
   a. The well-recognized limitations of such tools must be considered when interpreting results. Whenever possible, efforts should be made to compare findings with the opinions of the child's parents, day care provider, preschool teacher, social worker, or public health nurse.
   b. A developmental screening test must not be considered equivalent to intelligence quotient testing or as a definite predictor of current or future abilities. Screening merely identifies children at risk for possible developmental problems and confirms subjective suspicions of delay.

F. **Procedures**

1. **Sensory screening.** Objective vision and hearing screening is performed in preschool and school-age children when they are able to cooperate. During infancy, sensory screening is accomplished via relevant history from parents and observations during physical examination.

2. **Laboratory screening**
   a. **Metabolic screening** is performed during the newborn period (see III D 3).
   b. Beyond the newborn period, laboratory procedures should be performed selectively. The individual needs of the child and the prevalence of disorders being screened for should determine the frequency of such tests. Problems the clinician may choose to consider for screening include iron deficiency anemia, lead poisoning, sickle cell disease, and tuberculosis.

3. **Immunizations.** At present, children are routinely immunized against diphtheria, pertussis, tetanus, polio, measles, mumps, rubella, varicella, and infections due to *Haemophilus influenzae* type b (Hib). Universal immunization against hepatitis B has recently been recommended. Other vaccines (e.g., pneumococcal and influenza vaccines) are administered to certain high-risk groups (see Tables 1-3, 1-4, and 1-5). Parents must have the opportunity to give their informed consent prior to immunization. Benefits and risks should be reviewed with the parent at the time of each immunization, and any previous reactions or side effects should be documented.

   a. **Factors determining the usefulness of a vaccine** include:
   (1) Current risk of the disease
   (2) Benefit of disease prevention to the individual and society
   (3) Efficacy, safety, cost, and availability
   (4) Alternatives regarding prevention
   (5) Special needs and characteristics of the individual or group to be immunized
   b. **Combination and spacing recommendations** are empiric. Antigenic combinations are recommended for general use when investigation has shown that they are effective and safe. An adequate immune response to each antigen must develop, and there must be no enhancement of side effects from any component (i.e., from the interaction of one antigen with another).

G. **Anticipatory guidance** is the process by which pediatric health care providers offer counseling during child health supervision (e.g., on such topics as nutrition, safety, child behavior and development, parent–child interaction, various medical issues). Through such counseling, the pediatrician helps parents foresee normal deviations in children's behavior, thereby alleviating undue parental anxiety and concern.

V. EARLY INFANCY HEALTH SUPERVISION (2 weeks to 6 months)

A. **Goals**

1. Assess infant's and mother's recovery from the birth process.

2. Assess the infant's progress during this period of rapid growth and intense developmental progress.

3. Assess the family's adjustment to the new infant and quality of initial parent–child interactions.

4. Administer the primary series of important immunizations.

5. Foster new parents' sense of competency.

B. **Interval history.** Parents' agendas, questions, and concerns are explored.

1. **Daily functioning.** Inquire about patterns and adequacy of breast- or formula-feeding and solid foods, sleep location and schedule, bowel and bladder functioning, measures taken for injury prevention, and toys provided.

2. **Health concerns.** Inquiry may focus on parents' assessment of the infant's growth rate and physical appearance. Consider specific inquiry about healing of umbilicus and circumcision sites, rashes, first illnesses such as colds or fevers, teething, use of medicines and vitamins, reactions to immunizations, and assessment of infant's vision and hearing.

3. **Development**
   a. **Affective.** Parents are encouraged to discuss their assessment of the infant's temperament (e.g., easy vs. difficult, predictability of behaviors) and their response to typical behaviors (e.g., to crying or fussing). Other topics include evidence for increasing mutual attachment between infant and caretakers, and after the first few months of life evidence for increasing regularity of schedules. Toward the latter end of this period, evidence for emergence of stranger and separation anxiety may be pursued.
   b. **Milestones.** This begins with a general question such as "What's he doing lately?" Topics may also include emerging motor skills ("What's he doing with his head or his body?"), social skills ("What does he do when he sees you?"), and language ("Does he make any sounds?"). [See Figure 1-2 for age-related milestones.]

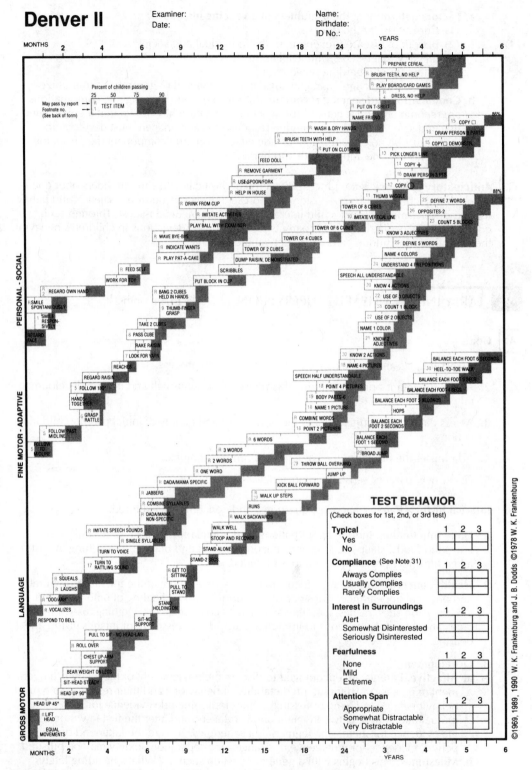

FIGURE 1-2. Denver II. (Reprinted with permission from Frankenburg WK, Dodds J, Archer P, et al: The Denver II: A major revision and restandardization of the Denver Developmental Screening Test. *Pediatrics* 89:91–97, 1992.)

DIRECTIONS FOR ADMINISTRATION

1. Try to get child to smile by smiling, talking or waving. Do not touch him/her.
2. Child must stare at hand several seconds.
3. Parent may help guide toothbrush and put toothpaste on brush.
4. Child does not have to be able to tie shoes or button/zip in the back.
5. Move yarn slowly in an arc from one side to the other, about 8" above child's face.
6. Pass if child grasps rattle when it is touched to the backs or tips of fingers.
7. Pass if child tries to see where yarn went. Yarn should be dropped quickly from sight from tester's hand without arm movement.
8. Child must transfer cube from hand to hand without help of body, mouth, or table.
9. Pass if child picks up raisin with any part of thumb and finger.
10. Line can vary only 30 degrees or less from tester's line. ⟋
11. Make a fist with thumb pointing upward and wiggle only the thumb. Pass if child imitates and does not move any fingers other than the thumb.

      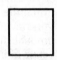

12. Pass any enclosed form. Fail continuous round motions.

13. Which line is longer? (Not bigger.) Turn paper upside down and repeat. (pass 3 of 3 or 5 of 6)

14. Pass any lines crossing near midpoint.

15. Have child copy first. If failed, demonstrate.

When giving items 12, 14, and 15, do not name the forms. Do not demonstrate 12 and 14.

16. When scoring, each pair (2 arms, 2 legs, etc.) counts as one part.
17. Place one cube in cup and shake gently near child's ear, but out of sight. Repeat for other ear.
18. Point to picture and have child name it. (No credit is given for sounds only.)
    If less than 4 pictures are named correctly, have child point to picture as each is named by tester.

  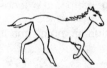

19. Using doll, tell child: Show me the nose, eyes, ears, mouth, hands, feet, tummy, hair. Pass 6 of 8.
20. Using pictures, ask child: Which one flies?... says meow?... talks?... barks?... gallops? Pass 2 of 5, 4 of 5.
21. Ask child: What do you do when you are cold?... tired?... hungry? Pass 2 of 3, 3 of 3.
22. Ask child: What do you do with a cup? What is a chair used for? What is a pencil used for?
    Action words must be included in answers.
23. Pass if child correctly places <u>and</u> says how many blocks are on paper. (1, 5).
24. Tell child: Put block **on** table; **under** table; **in front of** me, **behind** me. Pass 4 of 4.
    (Do not help child by pointing, moving head or eyes.)
25. Ask child: What is a ball?... lake?... desk?... house?... banana?... curtain?... fence?... ceiling? Pass if defined in terms of use, shape, what it is made of, or general category (such as banana is fruit, not just yellow). Pass 5 of 8, 7 of 8.
26. Ask child: If a horse is big, a mouse is __? If fire is hot, ice is __? If the sun shines during the day, the moon shines during the __? Pass 2 of 3.
27. Child may use wall or rail only, not person. May not crawl.
28. Child must throw ball overhand 3 feet to within arm's reach of tester.
29. Child must perform standing broad jump over width of test sheet (8 1/2 inches).
30. Tell child to walk forward, ⌒⌒⌒➤ heel within 1 inch of toe. Tester may demonstrate.
    Child must walk 4 consecutive steps.
31. In the second year, half of normal children are non-compliant.

OBSERVATIONS:

FIGURE 1-2. *See legend facing page.*

4. Family health and family psychosocial histories. Topics may include family's adjustment to the new baby, spouse involvement in child care, parent returning to work, day care arrangements, sibling rivalry, and presence of smokers in the household.

C. **Physical examination.** Physical examination of the young infant should focus on recovery from birth trauma, continued surveillance for congenital anomalies, evidence of rapid progress in physical growth and motor development, confirmation of intact senses, and assessment of parent–child attachment and interactions. The following areas are emphasized:

1. **General appearance and measurements.** General appearance and state of hygiene are observed. Weight, length, and head circumference are measured and plotted on the appropriate charts.

2. **Skin.** Rashes are particularly common in this age group. Their presence, appearance, and distribution are noted.
   a. **Infantile acne** resembles the adolescent form of acne vulgaris. It appears during the first few months of life and resolves spontaneously. It probably results from the hormonal stimulation of sebaceous glands that have not yet involuted to their childhood state of immaturity.
   b. **Miliaria rubra.** This is also known as heat rash. These are red papulovesicular lesions that may be found anywhere on the body but typically predominate in clothed areas.
   c. **Infantile seborrheic dermatitis.** This appears during the first few months of life as a greasy, yellow-tinged, scaly rash on the face, eyebrows, skin folds, and scalp (cradle cap).
   d. **Atopic dermatitis.** The infantile form usually begins when the infant is 2–6 months of age and is characterized by erythema, papules, vesicles, crusting, and pruritus. The rash usually begins on the cheek, forehead, or scalp and extends to the trunk or extremities.
   e. If **jaundice** persists, its presence and distribution are noted and measurement of serum bilirubin is considered.

3. **Head and neck**
   a. **Sutures** usually are palpable as ridges until the infant is about 6 months of age. The **posterior fontanelle** closes by the second month of age, but the anterior fontanelle is patent for 1–2 years.
   b. **Vision** may be assessed grossly by noting the infant's response to a light or bright object, and by noting fixation on faces and inanimate objects. By the age of 2 months, infants follow an object past the midline and by age 4 months to a full arc of 180 degrees. Routine screening for strabismus should begin at approximately 3–4 months of age. Screening consists of querying parents for presence of crossed eyes or lazy eye and examination for symmetry of the corneal light reflex.
   c. **Hearing** may be assessed grossly by noting the infant's response to sound and at 2 months observing for a turning of the head and eyes. Examination of the **tympanic membranes** in infants is facilitated by pulling the auricle down, because the canal is directed upward. Mobility of the drum should be evaluated by pneumatic otoscopy.
   d. Small white patches on the buccal mucosa that cannot be scraped off indicate **candidal infection (thrush).**
   e. **Congenital muscular torticollis** results from a shortening of one side of the sternocleidomastoid muscle. It is manifested by lateral head flexion to one side and chin rotation toward the opposite side of the body. Abnormalities of the cervical spine and cranial nerves must be ruled out. This condition usually resolves during the first year, and responds to physical therapy.

4. **Chest.** Cardiac auscultation during the first 6 months of life may reveal **functional murmurs** (i.e., physiologic sounds of turbulence) or murmurs of such disorders as patent ductus arteriosus, atrial septal defect, and ventricular septal defect (see also Chapter 12).

5. **Abdomen.** The **umbilical site** heals by 1 month of age. Once the cord has separated and healed, fluid drainage suggests an abnormal connection between the surface of the abdomen and underlying structures, such as a patent urachus. **Umbilical hernias** are commonly noted in infants, often with **diastasis** of the rectus muscles. Most umbilical hernias resolve by school age.

6. A **hydrocele** is frequently evident, manifested by a swollen, nontender scrotum that easily transilluminates. The presence of an accompanying hernia may be difficult to ascertain. Many hydroceles spontaneously resolve by the end of the first year. Spontaneous voiding is observed for forcefulness and straightness.

7. The **hips** of all infants must be carefully examined for **dislocation,** even if the newborn examination was reported to be negative. After the first few weeks of life, the principal screening maneuver for developmental hip dysplasia consists of observing for symmetric and full, 90-degree abduction of hips when they are positioned in 90 degrees of flexion.

8. **Neurologic examination.** After approximately 2 months of age, the healthy infant should be alert, make eye contact with the clinician, and display some evidence of interest in the examiner. Primitive reflexes elicited during the first months of life include Moro, grasping, and tonic neck reflexes. By the time the infant is 4–6 months of age, these reflexes diminish.
   a. **Developmental assessment.** History is confirmed by direct observation. Wide variations in normal development are the rule. The significance of an infant's failure to achieve a milestone must be interpreted with caution.
   b. Specific assessments should include **vision, hearing, vocalization,** and **gross and fine motor skills**. By 2 months of age, many infants smile responsively. (For specific milestones, see Denver II, Figure 1-2.)

D. | Procedures

1. **Metabolic screening.** Some states require repeat screening at 2 weeks of age for PKU and hyperphenylalaninemias as well as congenital hypothyroidism (see III D 3).

2. **Immunizations** (see Tables 1-3, 1-4, and 1-5)

3. **Lead screening.** Identifying infants who are at high risk for environmental lead intoxication may be enhanced by the use of a series of screening questions. Current Centers for Disease Control and Prevention recommendations suggest that a blood lead level be obtained on infants beginning at 6 months of age if answers to any of the following questions are positive. Does your child . . .
   a. Live in or regularly visit a house with peeling or chipping paint built before 1960? This includes day care centers, preschool areas, babysitters' homes, and so forth.
   b. Live in or regularly visit a pre-1960 house being renovated or having been renovated, or with renovation ongoing or planned?
   c. Have a sibling, housemate, or playmate with blood lead levels greater than 15 µg/dl?
   d. Live with an adult whose job or hobby involves lead exposure?
   e. Live near a lead smelter, battery recycling plant, or other industry likely to release lead?

E. | Anticipatory guidance

1. **Feeding.** Breast milk is the optimal source of infant nutrition, and commercially prepared formula is an acceptable alternative. Whole cow's milk is inappropriate for use during the first 6 months of life. During the first 6 months of life, normal healthy infants require approximately 100–110 kcal/kg/day of breast milk or formula for adequate growth. The introduction of solid food should be deferred until the infant is 4–6 months of age.
   a. Infants receiving commercially prepared formula fortified with iron require no vitamin and mineral supplementation.

    b. Breast-fed infants may benefit from receiving 400 IU of **vitamin D** per day. **Iron supplementation** is probably not required during this time because of the increased bioavailability of iron in breast milk. **Fluoride supplementation** for breast-fed infants or those receiving formula prepared with water from a nonfluorinated source is not recommended during the first 6 months of life owing to concerns with fluorosis. Beginning at 6 months of age up to 3 years of age, fluoride in a dose of 0.25 mg daily is recommended for those children requiring supplementation.

2. Safety and injury prevention. Crib safety, the use of a car seat, water temperature, toy safety, and danger of falls should be reviewed (see III F 4).

3. Elimination. Breast-fed infants tend to have thin, yellow, seedy stools with almost every feeding, whereas formula-fed infants tend to have stools with more form but less frequency. There is, however, considerable variation in elimination patterns.

4. Sleep habits. Most infants sleep through the night by 4 months of age. Problematic night waking later in infancy may potentially be avoided if parents routinely place the baby in bed sleepy but awake, thus encouraging a habit of self-soothing at bedtime. The danger of a nighttime bottle causing milk-bottle caries should be stressed.

5. Immunization (see IV F 3; Tables 1-3, 1-4, and 1-5).

6. Developmental issues
    a. Affective
        (1) State organization. The "predictable unpredictability" of the newborn is followed by increasing regularity in demands when the infant is approximately 2 months of age. By this time, feeding and sleep schedules may be established.
        (2) Synchrony. Parent–infant interaction is reciprocal in nature, and a sense of mutual awareness and expectations evolves during the first months of the infant's life.
        (3) Attachment becomes the main affective issue by 2–3 months of age. By this time, the infant both recognizes and uniquely responds to parents.
        (4) Temperament. The infant's behavioral style becomes increasingly evident during this time. The regular patterns, adaptability, and positive mood of the "easy" infant contrast with the irregularity, unpredictability, and intensely negative mood of the "difficult" infant. The wide range of normal behavior should be stressed.
    b. Motor skills. The infant's increasing mobility is usually evident by 4–6 months of age, as the infant rolls over, sits with support, grasps a rattle, and places objects within her mouth.

F. | **Common problems and concerns in young infants**

1. Eye drainage, typically from one eye, may indicate a blocked tear duct, or **dacryostenosis.** Swelling, erythema, and induration around the lacrimal sac may indicate an acquired infection, or **dacryocystitis.**

2. Conjunctivitis. Ophthalmia neonatorum is conjunctivitis occurring within the first 4 weeks of life (see III E 2).

3. Diaper rash. Common varieties of diaper dermatitis include the following:
    a. Generic diaper rash is erythematous, spares the skin folds, and produces dry, wrinkled skin.
    b. Candidal rash involves the deep skin folds and is characterized by satellite lesions and bright red erosions.
    c. Infantile seborrheic dermatitis starts as erythema and satellite lesions in the diaper area and typically spreads to involve the face, scalp, and flexural areas (see V C 2 c).
    d. Staphylococcal diaper rash is characterized by superficial erythematous pustules and bullae.

      e. Intertrigo is a poorly understood dermatitis that is characterized by a white or yellow exudate involving the deep skin folds.

4. **Colic.** Fussing is normal infant behavior. Many infants exhibit intermittent, unexplained crying, usually beginning in the first month and typically occurring in the late afternoon and evening hours. During this time, the infant is difficult to console. Formula intolerance, constipation, teething, illness, and so forth usually do not explain episodes of colic. Spontaneous resolution usually occurs by the age of 3 months.

5. **Constipation.** Infants commonly may have a bowel movement only once every several days. Unless stools are hard and pellet-like, accompanied by significant infant distress, parents should be reassured. Few infants become constipated owing to an iron-containing formula. True constipation in an otherwise healthy infant may be treated by offering water or prune juice between feedings.

6. **Teething.** Infants may begin teething by 6 months of age. Excessive drooling, rhinorrhea, mild diarrhea, irritability, and decreased appetite may be associated with teething. High fevers should not be attributed to teething.

VI. LATE INFANCY HEALTH SUPERVISION (6 months to 2 years)

A. Goals

1. Assess the infant's progress during this period of changing nutritional requirements and frequently diminishing appetite.

2. Assess the infant's progress in becoming a mobile, verbal, and autonomously functioning individual.

3. Assess the "goodness of fit" between the family's expectations and the infant's increasingly visible behavioral style and emerging abilities.

4. Administer booster doses of important immunizations and primary measles-mumps-rubella (MMR) and varicella vaccines.

B. Interval history. Parents' agenda, questions, and concerns are explored.

1. **Daily functioning.** Feeding questions center around quantity and type of milk, other liquids and solids consumed, weaning from breast or bottle, use of a cup, spoon, finger foods, and number of meals offered per day. Beginning around 1 year of age, conflicts during mealtimes and diminishing appetite are inquired about. Other topics include sleep patterns and concerns, especially disturbing night awakening, bowel and bladder functioning (including attempts at toilet training), care of newly emerging teeth, age-appropriate toys, and injury prevention measures.

2. **Health concerns.** Inquiry may include parents' assessment of the infant's overall health, with particular focus on frequency of common infections such as upper respiratory tract infections and otitis media. Other topics may include reaction to diminishing growth rate, appearance of extremities as gait emerges, hearing ability and speech development, presence of crossed or lazy eye, use of medicines, risk of lead poisoning and iron deficiency anemia, and reactions to immunizations.

3. **Development**
   a. **Affective.** Parents are encouraged to discuss reactions to their infant's emerging struggle to achieve autonomy and independence as evidenced by resistance to passive feeding, bedtime struggles or disturbing night awakening, and the appearance of temper tantrums. "Goodness of fit" between parents' expectations and the infant's abilities and behavioral style is assessed by exploring parents' management of problem behaviors and overall expressions of approval, flexibility, and satisfaction with respect to their child.

    b. Milestones. Topics include emergence and content of language, evidence of independent sitting, cruising, and walking, manipulation of small objects, ability to indicate want without crying, and enjoyment of simple games such as peek-a-boo (see Denver II, Figure 1-2).

  4. Family health and family psychosocial histories. Stage-related inquiry may include adjustment to day care, parent return to work, and the family's response to the infant's struggle between dependence and independence.

C. **Physical examination.** Physical examination of the older infant emphasizes evaluation of the sensory systems (hearing, vision, and language), which are frequently objects of concern (e.g., frequent episodes of acute otitis media), motoric functioning, the appearance of the extremities, and dentition. The examination also offers the clinician the opportunity to observe for evidence of attachment between parent and child, and the parents' management of the child's negative responses to the examination maneuvers. The following areas are emphasized:

  1. General appearance is assessed with attention to both physical and behavioral characteristics such as motoric activity and verbal expression, general hygiene, affection between infant and caretaker, and overall mood. Weight, length, and head circumference (1 year of age or younger) are measured and plotted on the appropriate charts.

  2. Skin. The benign phenomenon known as **carotenemia** may be confused with jaundice. This is an orange discoloration of the skin seen in infants who consume large quantities of orange and yellow vegetables and fruits. The absence of scleral discoloration and the relevant dietary history confirm the diagnosis of this spontaneously resolving phenomenon.

  3. Head and neck
    a. Eyes. Strabismus screening with observation for conjugate movement of eyes and a symmetric corneal reflex may be supplemented by the alternate cover test. Vision is subjectively evaluated as the child reaches out for and manipulates objects. **Pseudo-strabismus,** a phenomenon in which the child appears to have strabismus, but in fact is normal, is seen in children with epicanthal folds. In these children, the corneal light reflex is symmetric.
    b. Ears. Given the high incidence of middle ear disease that occurs during this age period, careful inspection of the **tympanic membranes** must include color, landmarks, and mobility as assessed by pneumatic otoscopy. Distraction with whispered noises during insertion of the otoscope may enhance cooperation during this examination. The child's response to sound is observed. Tympanometry may be used to detect middle ear effusions (see Chapter 10).
    c. Teeth. Teeth are inspected and counted. Timing of tooth eruption is somewhat variable, but the order of eruption is relatively uniform. The first teeth to erupt are usually the lower central incisors at approximately 6–8 months. By 2 to 2½ years of age, most children have acquired the full set of 20 primary teeth. Decay, particularly involving the upper central and lateral incisors, suggests milk-bottle caries resulting from inappropriate bedtime practices. Mottled, pitted teeth may suggest excessive fluoride ingestion.

  4. Genitalia
    a. Boys. Surgical referral at 1 year of age is indicated if either a hydrocele has not resolved or a testicle cannot be manipulated into the scrotum.
    b. Girls. Labial adhesions, which form postnatally, may be observed without treatment as long as there is no obstruction to flow of urine. Most of these disappear spontaneously either with repeated minor trauma of diaper changes or later, during puberty, under the influence of estrogen.

  5. Extremities
    a. The novice walker demonstrates a wide-based gait, and, normally, the feet point outward secondary to external rotation of the hips. With increased confidence in

walking, the legs come together. With further development, the feet point straight ahead, as the extent of external and internal rotation of the hip joints becomes equal. During the first few years of life, this predictable sequence is commonly altered by the appearance of **intoeing**. Intoeing is usually caused by torsional deformities. The three most common torsional deformities are femoral anteversion, internal tibial torsion, and metatarsus adductus.

    (1) Increased femoral anteversion results when the degree of internal rotation of the femoral head exceeds external rotation. This typically improves with age.

    (2) Internal tibial torsion produces intoeing, which also typically improves with age. In this condition, the tibia is rotated inward on its longitudinal axis.

    (3) Metatarsus adductus may be overlooked at birth and may not be detected until later infancy. When the foot is flexible, spontaneous resolution is the rule. A rigid varus deformity may require casting.

  b. During late infancy and early toddler years, the feet appear to be **flat**. This impression is caused by fat pads that normally are present under the arch of the foot.

6. Neurologic and developmental assessment. Neurologic examination seeks evidence of intact cranial nerves, with special attention toward assessing vision and hearing. Gross and fine motor functioning are assessed by observing the child's age-related "accomplishments" in sitting, standing, and walking, as well as manipulation of small objects. In a nonambulatory child, the degree of head control when pulled from supine to sitting is also observed. Deep tendon reflexes may be assessed with either a reflex hammer or with the examiner's fingers tapping directly on the tendon.

  a. Most **primitive reflexes** of early infancy disappear during the middle of the first year (e.g., Moro, suck, root, tonic neck). Significant delay in timing of disappearance of early reflexes or failure to demonstrate full and symmetric reflexes normally present later during the first year (e.g., lateral prop, parachute) is a nonspecific sign of neurologic abnormality (see Chapter 18).

  b. Developmental assessment is completed by observing for age-appropriate vocalization and language, gross and fine motor activities, and interactions between infant, parent, and examiner (see Denver II, Figure 1-2).

D. **Procedures**

1. Immunizations (see Tables 1-3, 1-4, and 1-5)

2. Anemia. In certain high-risk populations (e.g., poor growth or nutritional status, infants who have not received iron-supplemented formulas or iron-fortified cereals, infants weaned to whole milk before 9 months of age), screening for iron deficiency anemia should be performed near the end of the first year when depletion of iron stores is maximum. Hemoglobin, hematocrit, red blood cell indices, or free erythrocyte protoporphyrin may be measured.

3. Lead poisoning. For children at environmental risk for lead intoxication, screening should be performed by fingerstick blood lead levels at 1 and 2 years of age (see V D 3 and Chapter 2).

4. Tuberculosis. Owing to a recent increase in the incidence of tuberculosis within the United States and the changing epidemiology of this disease, the current status of screening recommendations is in flux. The incidence of tuberculosis in most areas of the United States is still quite low, but in certain geographic areas and in certain population groups, the prevalence has risen dramatically. For these reasons, routine screening of all low-risk children does not currently appear to be cost effective. If performed, screening should use the **intracutaneous (Mantoux) test,** which contains purified protein derivative (PPD).

  a. Children at high risk (Table 1-6) should be tested annually using Mantoux tuberculin tests. All results should be interpreted by qualified medical personnel.

TABLE 1-6. Infants, Children, and Adolescents at High Risk for Tuberculosis Infection

Contacts of adults with infectious tuberculosis
Those who are from or have parents who are from regions of the world with a high prevalence of tuberculosis
Those with abnormalities on chest roentgenogram suggestive of tuberculosis
Those with clinical evidence of tuberculosis
HIV-seropositive children
Those with immunosuppressive conditions
Those with other medical risk factors: Hodgkin disease, lymphoma, diabetes mellitus, chronic renal failure, malnutrition
Incarcerated adolescents
Children frequently exposed to the following adults: HIV-infected individuals, homeless persons, users of intravenous and other street drugs, poor and medically indigent city dwellers, residents of nursing homes, migrant farm workers

From the AAP Committee on Infectious Diseases, 1993–1994. *Pediatrics* 93:131–136, 1994.
HIV = human immunodeficiency virus.

  b. Children who have no risk factors but who reside in high-prevalence regions, and children whose history for risk factors is incomplete or unreliable, may be candidates for periodic Mantoux skin tests, such as at the ages of 1, 4–6, and 11–16 years. Decisions should be based on local epidemiology of tuberculosis.

E. Anticipatory guidance

 1. Feeding
   a. By the end of the first year, a schedule of three meals per day is feasible.
   b. Table foods should be introduced slowly, adding one new food every several days while observing for any adverse reactions. With increasing fine motor control, finger foods should be encouraged. Foods should be prepared without added salt.
   c. Weaning from bottle to cup should commence by the end of the first year. Beginning use of a spoon is possible by the age of 15 months.
   d. Whole cow's milk may replace iron-fortified formula or breast milk beginning at 9–12 months of age. The use of low-fat or skimmed milk is not recommended until after 2 years of age.
   e. With physical growth slowing by the end of the first year of life, a normal decrease in appetite occurs.

 2. Safety and injury prevention
   a. With increasing mobility, potential dangers for the child include stairways, open windows, electric sockets, hanging tablecloths, and electric cords. Proper use of a playpen, high chair, expandable gates, and covers for wall sockets reduces dangers. The use of infant walkers is highly discouraged (see Chapter 2).
   b. When the infant reaches 18–20 pounds, use of a forward-facing toddler car seat is appropriate.
   c. Owing to the possible danger of accidental ingestion of poisonous substances, parents should obtain syrup of ipecac and the phone number of the poison control center. Household plants and common remedies (e.g., acetaminophen) are potential toxins (see Chapter 2).

 3. Sleep habits. If night awakening occurs, it is recommended that the child not be brought into the parents' bed nor offered a nighttime bottle. Rather, after the child's safety is ensured, he should be put back in bed in a loving but firm manner and allowed to fall back asleep without assistance (see V E 4).

4. **Toilet training** should be child oriented and deferred until at least 18 months of age. Signs of readiness include:
   a. A desire to please the parents
   b. Pleasure in imitating adults
   c. A desire to develop autonomy and to master primitive impulses
   d. Adequate motor development, including the ability to sit and walk

5. **Dental care.** After eruption, teeth should be cleaned. Initially, gauze or a soft cloth may be used, with the substitution of a soft brush during the second year of life. For those children between the ages of 6 months and 3 years who require supplementation, new recommendations call for fluoride to be administered in a dose of 0.25 mg/day.

6. **Immunization** (see IV F 3; Tables 1-3, 1-4, and 1-5)

7. **Developmental issues**
   a. Autonomy. The struggle between dependence and independence now becomes the main affective issue. Manifestations may include the infant's refusal of passive spoon feedings and the appearance of temper tantrums. The toddler continually explores the limits of the environment. By 15–18 months of age, the child's negativism and resistant behavior dramatically reflect the struggle for autonomy.
   b. Temperament remains highly discernible and may allow parents to predict the child's responses to certain circumstances.
   c. Attachment. Behaviors reflecting the continued importance of attachment include clinging to parents, night awakening, and stranger and separation anxiety.
   d. Motor skills. Further refinement of motor skills parallels the development of autonomy. Increased motor development renders the environment a potentially greater threat to the child's safety.
   e. Cognitive development
      (1) Object permanence is reflected by the infant's ability that develops around 9–10 months of age to uncover a hidden toy.
      (2) Also around 9–10 months of age, the infant's interest in a wind-up toy relates to **an understanding of causality**.
      (3) Around 18 months of age, the toddler is able to represent mentally an object or action that is not perceptually present. Symbolic play is now possible, as the child is capable of **thought**.

F. **Common problems and concerns**

1. **Temper tantrums** are a normal manifestation of the toddler's struggle for autonomy while she is still dependent on adults. Attempting to distract the child or ignoring her behavior after ensuring the child's safety are reasonable approaches to a temper tantrum.

2. **Night crying.** Many infants 6–12 months of age abruptly awaken at night and cry, despite a previously good sleep pattern. Such awakening typically resolves within 1–4 weeks if parents provide brief positive interactions and avoid reinforcing the crying by picking up or feeding the child.

3. **Stranger and separation anxiety** are typical manifestations of attachment during the latter half of the first year of life.

4. Parents are frequently concerned about their child's **poor appetite**. In actuality, a decrease in appetite should be anticipated because the child's slower physical growth demands fewer calories; in addition, the child may refuse passive spoon feedings with increasing independence. The child's basic needs are met by a daily intake of a pint of milk, an ounce of fruit juice or a piece of fruit, 2 ounces of iron-containing protein, and possibly a multivitamin for the "picky" eater.

5. **Teething** (see V F 6)

6. The incidence of acute **otitis media** is highest in this age group. Recurrent infection and persistent middle ear effusion (serous otitis media) are extremely common problems that may be associated with poor growth, behavior problems, diminished hearing, and interference with normal language development. Avoiding recumbent milk feeding (e.g., bottle in bed) and exposure to cigarette smoke may diminish the risk of infection.

VII. THE PRESCHOOL YEARS HEALTH SUPERVISION (2–5 years)

A. Goals

1. Assess the younger preschool-age child's progress through this rough-and-tumble period of high motor activity and rapid emergence of speech and language abilities.

2. Assess the older preschool-age child's readiness for school.

3. Assess the "goodness of fit" between child's readily visible personal style and the family.

4. Administer formal sensory screenings.

5. Administer important booster immunizations.

6. Lay foundation for future independent relationship between child and physician.

B. Interval history. Parents' agenda, questions, and concerns are explored. By the time that the child is 3–4 years of age, a separate dialogue should be established with him during the visit.

1. **Daily functioning.** Feeding questions center around participation in family meal schedule, typical diet consumed, snacking patterns, food refusal, and management of conflicts. Other topics include sleep patterns and concerns, especially disturbing night awakening, progress and problems in toilet training, dental care, and injury prevention measures.

2. **Health concerns.** Inquiry may include parents' assessment of the preschooler's overall health, with particular focus on frequency of common infections, issues related to motor activity and gait, and occurrence of accidents and unintentional ingestions. Other important topics include speech intelligibility, hearing and vision concerns, use of medicines, risk of lead poisoning, and reactions to immunizations.

3. **Development**
   a. **Affective.** Parents are encouraged to discuss reactions to their preschooler's continuing struggles between dependence and independence as manifested by behaviors such as negativism, separation anxiety, and absence of impulse control. Additional topics include peer interactions, play preferences, and overall "goodness of fit" between preschooler and other family members.
   b. **Cognitive development.** A major focus of inquiry centers around the content and complexity of language. Other topics include evidence for emerging curiosity and interest in objects or people not actually present (representation). Parents' and child's perceptions of school readiness become paramount concerns as the child prepares to begin formal schooling.
   c. **Milestones** (see Denver II, Figure 1-2).

4. **Family health and family psychosocial histories.** Stage-related inquiry may include adjustment to nursery school, sibling rivalry, and anticipated changes to family life on school entry.

C. Physical examination. Physical examination of the preschool-age child emphasizes observations of overall motoric activity (active vs. quiet), appearance of teeth, tympanic membranes, and extremities, and speech content and intelligibility. The older preschooler is

also assessed for degree of cooperation and resistance to examination, and ability to separate from parent and engage in independent interaction with the physician. The following areas are emphasized:

1. **General appearance** is assessed with attention to both physical and behavioral characteristics such as motoric activity, general hygiene, interest and curiosity, overall mood, and ease of separation from parent. Weight and length (supine measurement) or height (standing measurements) are obtained and plotted on the appropriate charts. When plotting measurements for the child between 2 and 3 years of age, care should be taken to plot the child on the chart appropriate to the method used to obtain length ("0–36 months") or height ("2–18 years").

2. **Ears** (see VI C 3 b)

3. **Teeth.** The number and condition of the primary teeth and the type of occlusion should be noted.

4. **Speech.** By 2 years of age, approximately 50% of the child's speech should be intelligible, and by 3 years of age, 75% should be intelligible. By age 4, almost all of the child's speech should be intelligible. Articulation errors, such as substituting "w" for "r" in rabbit, or "d" for "th," are common and normal in the toddler age group.

5. **Chest. Innocent heart murmurs** are most commonly discovered in this age group. The explanation for this phenomenon may be the child's improved ability to cooperate for auscultation, combined with the thinner, less rounded thorax compared to infants. Some investigators believe that with careful scrutiny, every child may demonstrate an innocent heart murmur at some time during childhood. Innocent heart murmurs reflect sounds of blood flowing through normal cardiac and great vessel architecture. The most common innocent heart murmur of childhood is the Still's murmur. This murmur is a systolic ejection murmur that is low-pitched, musical, or vibratory in quality, and loudest at the lower left sternal border or midway between the lower left sternal border and cardiac apex. Its intensity is increased in the supine position and in states of increased cardiac output such as fever or after exercise. By definition, there are no associated symptoms or signs of cardiac disease.

6. **Blood pressure.** With the increasing cooperation of the child, blood pressure measurements become routine around the age of 3 years.

7. **Back.** The normal toddler displays an exaggerated lower lumbar lordosis or forward curvature of the spine. The combination of the lordosis and abdominal musculature, which is not yet fully developed, explains the classic pot-bellied appearance in this age group.

8. **Extremities.** With ambulation, torsional deformities of the legs and flatfeet may be noted (see VI C 5).
    a. **Increased femoral anteversion** is a relatively common cause of intoeing in children 3–7 years of age.
    b. **Flatfeet.** Children who have a flatfoot when standing but an arch when sitting may benefit from an arch support. Constitutional flatfeet, which are flat whether or not they are bearing weight, do not benefit from correction.

9. **Developmental assessment.** The 3-year-old child begins to share playthings and begins to play interactive games. By the time of school entry, the child should easily separate from the mother. (For milestones see Denver II, Figure 1-2.)

D. Procedures

1. **Immunizations** (see Tables 1-3, 1-4, and 1-5)

2. **Vision screening.** By the age of 3–4 years, objective screening of visual acuity is possible using pictures, the "E" test, or other measures. Children's acuity should be 20/40 or better by the age of 3–4 years and 20/30 by the age of 5 years.

3. **Hearing** can be screened objectively at about the age of 4 years using a pure tone stimulus. Screening should be repeated every 2 years. If the examiner judges cooperation to be adequate, failure of audiometric screening is defined as inability to hear sounds of 1000 Hz or 2000 Hz at 20 dB or 4000 Hz at 25 dB in either ear. Formal audiologic testing should be requested when a child fails audiometric screening.

4. Periodic routine **urinalysis** screening is probably not cost effective. Nevertheless, some school systems continue to require this test on school entry and periodically thereafter. If required, it is relatively inexpensive and easy to perform.

5. **Tuberculosis screening** (see VI D 4 and Table 1-6).

6. **Screening for anemia** is typically performed before school entry (see VI D 2).

7. **Screening for lead poisoning.** For children at environmental risk for lead intoxication, screening should be performed by fingerstick blood lead levels at 3 and 4 years of age (see V D 3 and Chapter 2).

8. **Cholesterol testing.** The role of universal cholesterol screening is controversial. At present, screening of all children is not recommended. Rather, testing of children older than 2 years of age who have a family history of hyperlipidemia or early myocardial infarction is suggested (see Chapter 17). Such a strategy will not identify all children at risk.

E. | **Anticipatory guidance**

1. **Safety and injury prevention.** Topics for discussion include traffic and playground safety, the danger of serious bites from pets, fire, and water safety. The effectiveness of helmets in reducing head injuries from bicycle falls has been demonstrated. Therefore, urging children always to wear an approved helmet while riding is important.

2. **Toilet training.** Maintaining a child-oriented approach is important (see VI E 4). Allowing the child to sit undressed on a potty-chair and dropping soiled diapers into the chair's bowl are helpful.

3. **Dental care.** The child should be instructed in the use of a toothbrush with a thin ribbon of toothpaste. Two-year-olds requiring supplementation should receive fluoride in a dose of 0.25 mg/day. The recommended dosage increases to 0.5 mg/day at 3 to 6 years of age. By the age of 3 years, a referral for a dental check-up is indicated.

4. **Immunizations** (see IV F 3; Tables 1-3, 1-4, and 1-5).

5. **Play.** The 2-year-old child is not capable of sharing and engages in solitary, parallel play. During successive years, an interest in and the ability to engage in interactive play with peers emerge.

6. **Television.** Observing violence on television is believed to cause children to be more willing to harm others and to play more aggressively. Thus, monitoring a child's television viewing is appropriate.

7. **School readiness.** Attitudes concerning separation and readiness for school should be discussed with the parents and child.

8. **Developmental issues**
   a. **Autonomy.** Problematic behavior reflects the child's continuing negativism and may be encountered during such activities as eating, toilet training, and tooth care, as well as in play groups.
   b. **Attachment.** The toddler's problems with separation continue to reflect the importance of attachment. As school entry approaches, the child's ability to separate is increasingly important.
   c. **Temperament.** The consistency of a child's behavior allows parents to predict the child's responses to certain situations. For example, responses to school entry may differ greatly for the "slow-to-warm-up" child as opposed to the "difficult" child.

    d. Impulse control. Wide variability in impulse control among children is apparent. Increasing demands are placed on the child as school entry approaches.

    e. Motor skills. The "motor-minded" toddler enjoys rough-and-tumble play, whereas more passive activities are enjoyed by the calm child.

    f. Cognitive development. This age period is the preoperational period of cognitive development, and mastery of language is the major cognitive issue. The 2-year-old's incessant asking of "what's this?" and "what's that?" is followed by "why do I have to?" at the age of 4 years. Rational thinking is not yet possible.

    g. Gender identity. The concept of gender as fixed and stable emerges around 4–5 years of age, reflecting the child's ability to establish a stable definition of physical concepts.

    h. Peer interactions. At 3–4 years of age, sharing and interactive play emerge. Sibling rivalry is typical at this age. As school entry nears, values and attitudes of those outside the family, particularly a child's peers, become increasingly important.

F. | **Common problems and concerns**

    1. Separation anxiety (see VII E 8 b)

    2. Sibling rivalry (see VII E 8 h)

    3. Night awakening (see VI F 2). Parents must be careful not to reinforce the child's night awakening and crying by feeding the child or allowing the child to sleep in their bed.

    4. Stuttering. Intermittent difficulty in producing a smooth flow of speech may begin 1 or 2 years after a child learns to speak. Between 2 and 5 years of age, many children experience normal disfluency, which is characterized by repetitions of whole words and phrases. In contrast, stuttering is characterized by partial-word repetitions, multiple rather than single repetitions, irregular, rapid, or abrupt repetitions, and a high frequency of nonfluency. By late childhood, many children have recovered from stuttering.

VIII. THE SCHOOL-AGE YEARS (5–12 years)

A. | **Goals**

    1. Assess the school-age child's overall health status through this period of relatively slow, steady growth and diminishing frequency of intercurrent illness.

    2. Assess the child's adjustment and progress in school.

    3. Assess the child's social functioning, with particular attention to peer interactions and extracurricular activities.

    4. Assess the older school-age child for signs of puberty and evidence of early adolescence and discuss upcoming changes with both child and family.

    5. Administer booster immunization for MMR.

    6. Nurture an independent relationship between child and physician and foster the child's self-monitoring of healthy habits.

B. | **Interval history.** The greater portion of the interview should now be conducted directly with the child. Parents' agenda, questions, and concerns are explored as well.

    1. Daily functioning. Potential topics include typical diet, concerns about body image, sleep patterns, independence in toileting, regularity of dental care, sports and exercise participation, leisure activities, and safety habits.

    2. Health concerns. Inquiry may include recent illnesses, recurrent pains and aches, sports injuries, speech, hearing, or vision problems, questions about upcoming puberty, use of medicines, and reactions to immunizations.

3. **Development**
    a. **Affective.** For the younger school-age child, questions center around descriptions of behavioral style (e.g., outgoing, shy), adaptation to the rhythm of a formal school year, and peer interactions. For the older school-age child, attention focuses on evidence of increased involvement with peers and peer values, conflicts with authority figures, increasing responsibilities at home, and increasing evidence of self-reliance for personal needs and school responsibilities.
    b. **Cognitive development.** The major focus of inquiry centers around school adjustment and, thereafter, school functioning. Areas to explore include the child's likes and dislikes about school, actual grades, absenteeism, and retention. Inquire about areas of difficulty and plans for remediation.
    c. **Milestones.** Inquiries about school performance and athletic ability constitute major areas of focus.

4. **Family health and family psychosocial histories.** Stage-related inquiry may include family's adjustment to the child's school entrance, after-school supervision, activities shared by family members, and rules and conflicts at home.

C. **Physical examination.** Height, weight, and blood pressure should be recorded. Areas deserving special emphasis during the complete examination include the following:

1. **General appearance.** The overall mood, facial appearance, degree of eye contact with the examiner, and relationship to the parent are observed. For the older child, a "weather report" assessment may be requested (e.g., "In general, if you were to give me a weather report to describe your life, what would you say? For example, would you say things for you are generally sunny, cloudy, stormy?").

2. **Skin.** With the onset of puberty, acne may develop (see Chapter 5).

3. **Teeth.** The secondary teeth begin to erupt when the child is about 7–8 years of age. The top teeth should overlap the bottom teeth all the way around the mouth and the child should bite down on the back teeth.

4. **Pharynx.** Relative to adults, the tonsils in this age group frequently appear enlarged. This is the result of normal, age-related lymphoid hyperplasia that is often exacerbated by upper respiratory tract infections. If swallowing or breathing functions are not affected, no intervention is required.

5. **Genitalia and breast development.** Documenting pubertal changes is important (see Chapter 5).

6. **Back.** Screening for scoliosis is necessary during the rapid growth of puberty (see Chapter 5).

7. **Developmental assessment.** School performance, classroom behavior, relationship to peers, and athletic activities are important indicators of developmental status.

D. **Procedures**

1. **Vision screening** (see VII D 2). Objective screening every 2 years is recommended.

2. **Hearing screening** (see VII D 3). Objective screening using a pure tone stimulus is recommended at the beginning and end of the school-age years and whenever history suggests a possible problem.

3. **Urinalysis** (see VII D 4)

4. **Tuberculosis screening** (see VI D 4 and Table 1-6)

5. **Immunizations** (see Tables 1-3, 1-4, and 1-5)

6. **Cholesterol testing** (see VII D 8)

E. **Anticipatory guidance**

1. **School progress.** Asking both parent and child about school performance is important.

2. **Safety and injury prevention.** Topics for review include the proper use of seat belts in the car, bicycle safety, pedestrian safety, protective equipment for sports, adequacy of supervision during nonschool hours, and water safety.

3. **Immunizations** (see IV F 3; Tables 1-3, 1-4, and 1-5)

4. **Sex education.** With puberty approaching, topics to be discussed with parents include their attitudes toward sex education and plans for discussing sexuality with their children.

5. **Health habits.** With increasing autonomy and separation, the child is making decisions and developing her own health habits. The child should be encouraged to make wise decisions about diet, exercise, safety, and so forth.

6. **Developmental issues**
   a. **Autonomy.** The challenging of limits precedes the ability to make wise decisions, and thus requires parental limit setting. By around 8 years of age, the child declares her independence by transferring allegiance to a peer group. Allowing the child to assume increasing responsibility may lessen family conflict. By early adolescence, the drive for autonomy culminates in the child's challenging of long-standing beliefs.
   b. **Peer interaction.** Growing peer influence may represent a challenge to family values. Increasing segregation among peers occurs. The development of a "best friend" is a milestone in interpersonal growth.
   c. **Cognitive development**
      (1) **Concrete operations.** Around the age of 8 years, the child is able to focus on multiple aspects of a problem, establish hierarchies, use logic, and see the viewpoints of others.
      (2) **Formal operations.** By 12 years of age, the ability to use hypothetical and abstract reasoning emerges.
   d. **Physical development.** The physical changes heralding the onset of puberty may cause concern on the part of the parents or the child.

F. **Common problems and concerns**

1. **Acting-out behavior.** With the child striving for independence, some challenging of limits is likely. With increasing peer influence, confrontations with authority figures (i.e., teachers, parents) occur.

2. **Separation anxiety.** If the child is unsuccessful in securely achieving independence from home and family, school avoidance and school phobia may become problems (see Chapter 4).

3. **Recurrent pains.** During the middle childhood years, children may have recurrent somatic complaints such as headache, abdominal pain, and limb pain. Pains of this sort typically have no clear-cut organic etiology. They are usually the consequence of environmental, temperamental, and constitutional factors (see Chapter 4).

4. **Poor school performance.** School-related problems often are brought to the attention of the pediatric health care provider. The role of the provider includes helping the parents understand special education programs and services, and the law requiring that school systems evaluate children experiencing difficulties in both learning and behavior. The pediatrician should also provide the names of local resources for help (see Chapter 4).

IX. **ADOLESCENCE** (see Chapter 5). The pediatric health care provider must encourage the adolescent to express any concerns and to ask any questions, particularly those that he does not feel comfortable asking parents or friends. The pediatrician must be non-judgmental to allow the adolescent to discuss emotion-laden topics.

BIBLIOGRAPHY

Algranati PS: Pediatric clinical encounter. In: *Introduction to Clinical Medicine.* Edited by Willms JL, Lewis J. Baltimore, Williams & Wilkins, 1991, pp 121–153.

Algranati PS: *The Pediatric Patient: An Approach to History and Physical Examination.* Baltimore, Williams & Wilkins, 1992.

American Academy of Pediatrics Committee on Psychosocial Aspects of Child and Family Health: *Guidelines for Health Supervision,* 2nd ed. Elk Grove Village, IL, American Academy of Pediatrics, 1988.

Brazelton TB: Anticipatory guidance. *Pediatr Clin North Am* 22:533–544, 1975.

Casey P, Sharp M, Loda F: Child-health supervision for children under 2 years of age: a review of its content and effectiveness. *J Pediatr* 95:1–9, 1979.

Telzrow RW: Anticipatory guidance in pediatric practice. *J Cont Ed Pediatr* 20:14–27, 1978.

Willms JL, Schneiderman H, Algranati PS: *Physical Diagnosis: Bedside Evaluation of Diagnosis and Function.* Baltimore, Williams & Wilkins, 1994.

STUDY QUESTIONS

DIRECTIONS: Each of the numbered items or incomplete statements in this section is followed by answers or by completions of the statement. Select the ONE lettered answer or completion that is BEST in each case.

1. While examining a 2-day-old infant, small vesicles on an erythematous base are noted on the infant's face and chest. Wright's stain of the lesions reveals sheets of eosinophils. The diagnosis of this rash is

(A) miliaria rubra
(B) milia
(C) neonatal acne
(D) erythema toxicum
(E) neonatal pustular melanosis

2. The mother of a 2-year-old boy is concerned about the child's speech. He began speaking single words at 12 months of age and now has a speaking vocabulary of at least 20–30 words. He even is combining words into simple sentences. However, for the past month he has begun to repeat words while speaking, which results in an uneven speech pattern. His complete history and physical examination are otherwise normal. Based on this information, what is the most appropriate management plan?

(A) Refer the child for a hearing evaluation
(B) Refer the child for a speech and language evaluation
(C) Recommend a language-oriented preschool program
(D) Encourage the mother to correct the child's speech gently
(E) Reassure the mother and observe the child during later visits

Questions 3 and 4

During a health maintenance visit, the mother of a 12-year-old boy mentions that she and her husband are concerned about their son's reluctance to try out for the local swim team. Despite the boy's ability to compete effectively, he becomes upset whenever his parents raise the topic. The results of his physical examination are entirely normal, although he is prepubertal. A review of the boy's early health records reveals concerns about past behavior (his parents were initially reluctant to leave him with sitters because of his difficulties with separation; he adapts slowly to new situations such as school and camp).

3. Anticipatory guidance in this case should consider each of the following developmental issues EXCEPT

(A) gender identity
(B) temperament
(C) puberty
(D) autonomy/independence
(E) peer interaction

4. On the basis of this information, which of the following is the most developmentally appropriate advice to offer the boy's parents?

(A) Ask about the possibility of the boy competing with a younger group of children
(B) Allow the boy to make up his own mind about trying out for the team
(C) Request that the boy's friends encourage him to try out for the team
(D) Urge the boy to attend the try-out sessions
(E) Arrange for mental health counseling for the boy

DIRECTIONS: Each of the numbered items or incomplete statements in this section is negatively phrased, as indicated by a capitalized word such as NOT, LEAST, or EXCEPT. Select the ONE lettered answer or completion that is BEST in each case.

5. Healthy children are routinely immunized against all of the following EXCEPT

(A) pertussis
(B) pneumococcal infections
(C) mumps
(D) *Haemophilus influenzae* type b (Hib) infections
(E) diphtheria

6. Of the following signs and symptoms, the one that should NOT be attributed to teething is

(A) rhinorrhea
(B) diarrhea
(C) decreased appetite
(D) irritability
(E) a fever of 39°C (102.2°F)

DIRECTIONS: Each set of matching questions in this section consists of a list of four to twenty-six lettered options (some of which may be in figures) followed by several items. For each numbered item, select the ONE lettered option that is most closely associated with it. To avoid spending too much time on matching sets with large numbers of options, it is generally advisable to begin each set by reading the list of options. Then, for each item in the set, try to generate the correct answer and locate it in the option list, rather than evaluating each option individually. Each lettered option may be selected once, more than once, or not at all.

Questions 7–10

For each aspect of physical examination, select the age period during which it should be emphasized.

(A) Newborn
(B) Early infancy (2 weeks to 6 months)
(C) Late infancy (6 months to 2 years)
(D) Preschool years (2–5 years)
(E) School-age years (5–12 years)

7. Examination of the back for scoliosis

8. Elicitation of the tonic neck reflex

9. Examination of the permanent dentition for decay and occlusion

10. Fundoscopic determination of a bilateral red reflex

ANSWERS AND EXPLANATIONS

1. The answer is D *[III C 2 e (1)]*. Benign rashes often are noted during the newborn period. Common rashes include milia, miliaria rubra, erythema toxicum, neonatal acne, and transient neonatal pustular melanosis. The finding of eosinophils when the drainage from small vesicles is stained is diagnostic for erythema toxicum. These lesions are not of infectious etiology and require no treatment.

2. The answer is E *[VII F 4]*. One or two years after learning to speak, many children experience an intermittent difficulty in producing a smooth flow of speech. Such normal speech disfluency is typically characterized by the repetition of whole words and phrases, and thus differs from stuttering. Normal disfluency spontaneously resolves between 2 and 5 years of age and requires no treatment.

3 and 4. The answers are: 3-A *[VII E 8 g; VIII E 6]*, **4-B** *[VIII E 6]*. At 12 years of age, important developmental issues to consider during anticipatory guidance include autonomy/independence, temperament, peer interaction, and puberty. The concept of gender identity as fixed and stable emerges around 4–5 years of age and is unlikely to be a major issue at age 12 years for most children.

The drive for autonomy typically is characterized by the child's strong desire to assume increasing responsibility for his own actions and resist parental suggestions and limit setting. A further manifestation of this drive for independence is the transferring of allegiance from the family to a peer group. A relative delay compared to peers in the onset of physical changes of puberty may cause concern on the part of the child or parents. The consistency of a child's "slow-to-warm-up" temperament or behavioral style should suggest his likely response to a new situation.

During the school-age years, allowing the child to assume increasing responsibility for his actions may lessen family conflict and promote autonomy and positive self-regard. Competing with younger children would be unacceptable because it would be likely to lead to segregation among peers at a time when allegiance to a peer group is normal and important. Parental attempts to coerce the boy into participation, either directly or indirectly through friends, would likely be met with resistance. Neither the boy's "slow-to-warm-up" temperament nor his stage-related behavior indicate the need for a mental health refer-

ral, although pediatric counseling for parents and child is indicated.

5. The answer is B *[Tables 1-3 and 1-4]*. Vaccines routinely recommended for all children include diphtheria, pertussis, tetanus, polio, measles, mumps, rubella, *Haemophilus influenzae* type b (Hib), varicella, and hepatitis B. Other vaccines, such as those for pneumococcal infections, are administered only to certain high-risk groups. Factors determining the usefulness of a vaccine include the risk of the disease, benefits of prevention, efficacy, safety, cost, availability, alternatives to prevention, and the special needs of certain groups of individuals.

6. The answer is E *[V F 6]*. Teething may begin by the age of 6 months and may be associated with excessive drooling, rhinorrhea, mild diarrhea, irritability, and decreased appetite. Whether teething may also be accompanied by fever is controversial. However, high fevers should not be attributed to teething.

7–10. The answers are: 7-E *[VIII C 6]*, **8-B** *[V C 8]*, **9-E** *[VIII C 3]*, **10-A** *[III C 3 b (2)]*. As the child enters puberty, screening for scoliosis becomes an important part of the routine screening examination. Although scoliosis may become apparent at any age, idiopathic scoliosis, the most common type of scoliosis, progresses most rapidly during the pubertal growth spurt. Primitive reflexes (e.g., the Moro, grasp, and tonic neck reflexes) indicate the integrity of the central nervous system. In a term infant, such reflexes may be elicited within the first months of life, and they disappear around the age of 6 months. The absence or distortion of these reflexes may suggest prematurity or damage to the central nervous system. Similarly, persistence of such primitive reflexes beyond early infancy suggests neurologic dysfunction. From the time of the initial eruption of the primary dentition, the teeth should be examined for decay and occlusion. Children should be referred for their initial dental examination around the age of 3 years. Secondary (permanent) dentition typically erupts around the age of 7–8 years. Detailed fundoscopic examination typically is not performed during childhood unless it is specifically indicated. However, the determination of a red reflex bilaterally is an important part of the newborn examination because the presence of a red reflex excludes the presence of significant lens opacities or retinoblastoma.

Chapter 2

Injuries and Poisonings
Leonard I. Banco

I. GENERAL CONSIDERATIONS

A. Nomenclature

1. **Injury.** There are no basic scientific distinctions between injury and disease; therefore, injuries and poisonings should be viewed as being no more random or unexpected than disease. Use of the term **accident**—which implies unpredictability or fate—is gradually being replaced by the use of the term **injury,** which more accurately reflects the nature of the problem. Most childhood injuries are unintentional; however, intentional (inflicted) causes (e.g., abuse, homicide, and suicide) are increasingly being recognized as a major problem, particularly among adolescents (see I E).

2. The **agent–host–environment model,** which is often used in reference to the epidemiology of infectious disease, can also be used to describe childhood injuries.
   a. The **agent** is the type of energy that causes damage, including:
      (1) **Kinetic energy** in collisions or falls
      (2) **Thermal energy** in burns
      (3) **Chemical energy** in poisonings
   b. The **host** is the injured child, who has particular attributes that can be used for description and categorization, such as:
      (1) **Age**
      (2) **Sex**
      (3) **Developmental level**
   c. The **environment** is the situation in which the injury occurs, and comprises the:
      (1) **Physical environment,** such as the playground, automobile, or medicine cabinet
      (2) **Social environment,** such as familial stress and disorganization or parental absence

3. **Prevention** is the ultimate goal of understanding how injuries occur. Four basic principles should be used in developing prevention strategies.
   a. **Passive strategies** are more effective than those requiring repeated actions.
   b. **Specific advice** is more effective than general information.
   c. Injury control includes **posttraumatic care and rehabilitation**.
   d. Particular attention should be focused on **common problems with effective prevention strategies**.

B. Epidemiology

1. **Injuries** are recognized as the **leading cause of death** in childhood over the past 40 years.
   a. In the United States, more than 20,000 children, ranging in age from birth to 19 years, die each year from injuries, for a death rate of 30.3 in 100,000.
   b. The number of childhood deaths from injuries is four times the number of childhood deaths due to any other cause.

2. **Death and morbidity** are two criteria by which the significance of childhood injuries can be measured. Although death is the worst outcome, injuries cause widespread morbidity, which results in the need for medical care as well as in the inability to perform normal daily activities.

    a. It is estimated that for each child who dies because of injury, 40 children are admitted to the hospital.

      (1) Each year in the United States, an estimated 600,000 children are hospitalized for injuries.

      (2) Injuries account for 17% of all hospitalizations of children, compared to 8% of hospitalizations of adults.

    b. For each death, 1100 children are seen in hospital emergency rooms and are released. In the United States, more than 16 million children per year are treated.

    c. For each death, many thousands of children are treated at home and many of them miss 1 or more days of school.

3. Loss of potential years of life is a more powerful measure of outcome than death or morbidity because it places loss to society in perspective. As a consequence, the earlier in life one is debilitated or killed, the greater is the loss of working years of life. Pediatric injuries are shown by this measure to be a very significant problem to society at large.

4. Cost, both direct and indirect, was estimated to be 7.5 billion dollars in 1989.

C. | **Relationship of child development to injuries.** The types of injuries that children experience at different ages can be explained and even predicted by age-specific development and the mismatch between developmental level and the child's environment. Both motor and cognitive development play major roles (Table 2-1).

1. Infant: birth to 1 year

    a. Motor development is key. In the first 6 months, infants squirm and can fall from a changing table or adult bed even before they can roll over. The crib or playpen offers the safest environment.

    b. In the second half of the year, infants become more mobile and an increasing challenge to their parents. They can reach out for objects that they want and place them in their mouths with increasing efficiency. As a result, mechanical suffocation is a leading cause of death. Child abuse also becomes common in this age-group.

2. Toddler: 1–2 years

    a. First walking and then climbing allow toddlers mobility, reach, and speed. Fine motor control improves so that containers and closets previously inaccessible can now be investigated. Ingestions occur frequently.

    b. Toddlers have no sense of danger; therefore, their motor activity is limited only by their physical ability. Falls, burns, and drowning are common.

    c. Toys must be safe; play must be supervised.

3. Preschooler: 2–5 years

    a. Running, climbing, and jumping are the mainstays of activity. Preschoolers can throw objects, ride tricycles, and interact with each other and their environment.

    b. Their thinking, however, remains illogical and egocentric. They are unable to appreciate cause and effect, and, as a result, injury to themselves or others may not prevent similar episodes in the future. However, children can be taught in a way that can develop their skills and alter their behavior.

4. School-age child: 5–10 years

    a. Fine and gross motor skills are refined. Organized games and rules are incorporated into play. Adventure and daring, including risk-taking without appreciation of the consequences, become the hallmarks of activity.

    b. Riding a bicycle becomes commonplace, as do its associated injuries.

    c. Children begin to assume increasing responsibility for their own safety, often out of the sight of their parents and teachers; pedestrian injuries result.

5. Preteenage and early teenage child: 10–14 years

    a. Strenuous physical activity becomes common, and the incidence of sports-related injuries increases markedly.

TABLE 2-1. Common Classes of Injury by Age

Age	Falls	Foreign Body	Ingestion of Poison	Burn	Bicycle	Pedestrian	Sports	Violence	Automobile Passenger	Work	Suicide	Drowning
1 Year	X	X						X	X			
1–2 Years	X		X	X					X			
2–5 Years	X		X	X		X						X
5–10 Years	X				X	X	X		X			X
10–14 Years	X				X	X	X			X		
> 14 Years			X		X			X	X		X	

     b. Hobbies and scientific activities are begun.

     c. Values and judgment become factors in decision-making and risk-taking. Firearm-related injuries occur.

  6. Adolescent: older than 14 years

     a. Physical prowess is refined. Organized sports and part-time jobs make adolescents prone to sports- and work-related injuries.

     b. Decision-making becomes more logical but more abstract. Although there is knowledge of potential consequence, denial and a feeling of invulnerability often predominate in evaluating risks. Adolescents become drivers and auto passenger injuries rise.

     c. Peer pressure and a need to feel comfortable in and accepted by a group may lead to substance- or alcohol-related injury, as well as assault and homicide.

     d. Difficulty in finding one's role in peer groups, family, school, and society in general may lead to depression or acting out, which sometimes culminates in suicide gestures or attempts.

D. **The "injury-prone" child.** A subject of much discussion and some research is the attempt to define the characteristics of children at increased risk for recurrent injury. Characteristics include the following.

  1. Motor skills. There is one group of children with immature or deficient skills. Another group of children with advanced skills attempt things that most children would not.

  2. Perception. Deficits in visual–perceptual scanning exist such that attention is deployed differently than it is by children without these deficits.

  3. Behavior. Increased impulsiveness, increased activity level, and emotional lability can lead to recurrent injury.

  4. Environment. Some studies show that environment plays the major role in an increased risk for injury.

     a. Parents may need to be advised to monitor and modify the physical environment of the child.

     b. Factors such as family stress and disorganization also may contribute to more injuries in the home.

     c. The possibility that recurring injuries actually indicate child abuse must be considered.

E. **Recognition of intentional injury**

  1. Child abuse. Physically abused children usually present to physicians with an acute injury or a history of recurrent injury. A detailed history of the circumstances surrounding each episode of injury is essential to screen for the possibility of abuse or neglect. Red flags that should arouse suspicions of abuse are discussed in Chapter 3 III D.

  2. Suicide primarily is an adolescent phenomenon (see Chapter 5 VI B); it is the third leading cause of death for male adolescents and the fourth leading cause for female adolescents. Both injuries and poisonings are methods of suicide. Some episodes are straightforward (e.g., medication overdose, self-inflicted gunshot wound); others are less obvious (e.g., single-passenger automobile crashes, many of which are thought to be suicide attempts).

  3. Homicide rates for children of all age-groups have doubled over the past 25 years. In some communities, homicide among children and youth younger than 20 years of age exceeds deaths caused by vehicular injuries. If current trends continue, this will be the case nationwide by 2001.

     a. In **children younger than 3 years of age,** homicide is primarily the result of child abuse perpetrated by a parent or relative. The injury is often the result of blunt force, usually hitting or shaking.

    b. In **children age 4–12 years,** the pattern of homicide is mixed. Causes include injury inflicted by a parent or relative, risk-taking behaviors (e.g., playing with guns), and violence related to substance abuse.

    c. In **adolescents,** the injury is primarily inflicted by a friend or acquaintance after an argument and often is related to alcohol or drug abuse. The instrument usually is a handgun.

II. MOTOR VEHICLE INJURIES

A. **Epidemiology.** Trauma to child passengers in motor vehicles is the **leading cause of death** between the ages of 6 months and 19 years.

1. There are 7500 deaths per year in child passenger-related events.
    a. The age-specific death rate peaks at 12 per 100,000 infants at 2 months, drops to 3 per 100,000 school-age children, and rises again in the teenage years to 16–31 per 100,000.
    b. Nonfatal trauma is underestimated. Based on police reports, nonfatal trauma occurs at an annual rate of 186 per 100,000 children aged 1–14 years, but many more incidents probably go unreported. There are more than 133,000 hospitalizations and 1.1 million emergency department visits yearly.

2. The epidemiology of motor vehicle injuries involving young children is different from that involving adult passengers and adolescent drivers.
    a. The most likely situation in adolescent/adult injury involves a young, inebriated male driver at night on a wet road.
    b. An injury involving a child passenger is most likely to occur with a sober female driver during the day on a dry road.

3. Adolescent drivers, as a group, are more likely than older drivers to be involved in a fatal automobile crash and are more likely to kill others in a collision. Both youth and lack of experience play a role.
    a. Drivers who are 16–18 years of age have a fatality rate per miles driven that is 8–10 times that of 30-year-old drivers.
    b. A study of Connecticut communities after state funding for public school driver education was ended revealed that the licensure, crash rate, and death rate for 16- to 17-year-old drivers declined significantly in towns that ended driver education programs compared to communities that continued them. This implies that the number of adolescents able to drive is directly proportional to their involvement in crashes, regardless of level of education.
    c. Alcohol plays a significant role in adolescent vehicle-related death and morbidity.

B. **Most motor vehicle injuries are caused by kinetic energy** resulting from movement of occupants either against the automobile, against other passengers, or against the outside environment, as in ejection. A much smaller number of injuries result from thermal energy (i.e., burns).

1. The **nature and extent of injuries** depend on the:
    a. Mass of the victim
    b. Speed of travel
    c. Tolerance of impacted tissue to injury
    d. Degree of energy absorbed by impacting surfaces

2. An **unrestrained passenger becomes a projectile** during rapid deceleration.
    a. Because force of impact = mass × deceleration, a 20-lb infant involved in the crash of a car going 30 mph would generate 600 pounds of force in kinetic energy imparted or required for restraint.

b. A child who is held on the lap of an unrestrained passenger may be crushed by the force of the passenger, which is much greater than the force imparted by the unrestrained child alone.

C. | **Prevention of injury**

1. Restraints. Use of **car seats** and **seat belts** is the most important strategy to prevent injury and death to children in automobile crashes.

  a. Data in the United States, Canada, and the Scandinavian countries demonstrate a potential reduction of 90% in fatality rate and 50% in morbidity rate through use of restraints.

  b. All states in the United States now have laws that mandate the use of car seats or seat belts for children in the first 5 years of life. Although many of these laws are not optimum and are being revised, data demonstrate increased use of car seats.

  c. Numerous studies show that car seat availability for newborns, patient–consumer education programs, and reinforcement at health care visits all increase car seat use significantly.

  d. Improper installation and use of car seats is a problem. A seat that is easy to attach to the car with a seat belt and that allows easy seating and removal of the child is likely to yield the greatest success in correct, regular use.

   (1) In one study of child restraint use, over 75% of seats were improperly anchored.

   (2) Of seats with tether attachments, 68% were not attached and 16% were attached incorrectly. As a result, car seats with tether straps are not recommended.

   (3) In cars with a passenger-side airbag, rear-facing infant car seats should be used only in the back seat. Inflation of the airbag could cause compression and collapse of the rear-facing seat, with potential severe injury to the infant.

  e. It is likely that it will take a full generation of use before car seat restraint is the norm rather than the exception.

2. Other safety factors

  a. Safer cars. Over the past two decades, federal law has mandated that new cars be equipped with seat belts, a padded dashboard, a padded steering wheel, and passive restraints, such as air bags or auto-locking belts and shoulder harnesses.

  b. Safer roads

   (1) Dangerous roads should be identified and modified by changes in width, curve, and bank.

   (2) Breakaway signs and posts should be installed.

III. | **PEDESTRIAN INJURIES**

A. | **Epidemiology.** Pedestrian injuries are the major cause of death to children between 5 and 9 years of age.

1. More than 1700 children younger than 20 years of age die each year.

2. Police report approximately 51,000 nonfatal pediatric pedestrian injuries each year, and there are 18,000 hospital admissions annually.

3. The case–fatality rate is estimated to be 3.6% (motor vehicle occupant ratios average 0.5%–1.0%).

4. Pedestrian collisions most commonly involve younger school-aged children who dart across the street at midblock.

  a. These injuries are more likely to occur in urban areas.

  b. Geographic and demographic analysis identifies neighborhoods with a high density of at-risk children as having the highest injury rates.

  c. Drivers are most often men younger than 30 years of age.

B. **Prevention**

1. Pedestrians should walk on sidewalks, or, if sidewalks are not present, against the flow of traffic.

2. Adequate lighting should be provided at night.

3. Bright, reflective clothing should be worn at night.

4. Supervision of small children should be increased, especially in congested areas.

5. Legal speed limits and observance of stop signs and traffic lights should be enforced, particularly in congested areas.

6. School bus stops should be moved to minimize the need for children to cross streets after exiting.

7. The effects of educational strategies on the frequency of pedestrian injuries have demonstrated mixed results.

IV. BICYCLE INJURIES

A. **Epidemiology.** Bicycles are associated with significant injuries because they are used on streets and roads in competition with other motor vehicles.

1. Each year approximately 600 children die.

2. The rate of nonfatal injuries is 235 per 100,000 annually.

3. The age of highest risk is between 4 and 13 years.

4. Most serious injuries are related to head trauma, and most deaths (93%) are a result of crashes with motor vehicles. Most of these injuries and deaths involve traffic violations by the cyclist or driver.

B. **Prevention**

1. **Bicycle helmets** can prevent an estimated 85% of head injuries.
   a. Active community-based helmet programs have increased use from 5% to almost 50% in some communities.
   b. An increasing number of states and localities mandate use of helmets for children.

2. **Education** regarding safe cycling and traffic regulations decreases the incidence of bicycle-related injuries.

3. **Cycling on protected bike paths,** as opposed to shoulders and roads, minimizes the risk of collisions with motor vehicles.

V. FALLS are the most common injury requiring an emergency department visit. They also are the most common cause of injury in the home. Although a much greater cause of morbidity than mortality, falls are the fourth leading cause of death from injury among children.

A. **Epidemiology**

1. The **peak incidence** of falls occurs in the toddler period, with a relative decline throughout childhood. **Death resulting from falls** has two peaks, one in the toddler period and another in adolescence.

2. Falls are more common in boys than in girls. They occur twice as frequently in urban areas as in suburban and rural areas, and are most prevalent in low socioeconomic groups.

B. Sites of falls

1. **The home** is the major site of falls for toddlers and preschoolers. Causes of falls in the home include:
   a. **Structures,** such as:
      (1) Stairs and steps (related to the use of walkers in infancy and to poor footing in the toddler period)
      (2) Floors, porches, and windows
      (3) Bathtubs
   b. **Furniture,** such as:
      (1) Beds
      (2) Chairs and stools
      (3) Tables, especially coffee tables, which children fall against
      (4) Baby furniture
   c. **Toys,** such as:
      (1) Riding toys
      (2) Falls over toys
      (3) Broken toys

2. **Nonhome sites** of falls include:
   a. Playground equipment and surfaces, which play a major role (grass, sand, and rubber are most desirable; concrete and asphalt, least)
   b. Baby carriages
   c. Bicycles
   d. Grocery carts

C. Morbidity and mortality.

Morbidity and mortality. Only 3.3% of all injuries from falls seen at medical facilities require admission to the hospital. Death as the result of falls is infrequent, and in 56% of cases is caused by head and neck trauma.

1. **Head-related injuries** involve contusion, laceration, and fracture.
   a. Contusion is most common.
   b. Laceration is particularly common in toddlers.
   c. The fracture rate in children younger than 1 year of age is five times that in older children.

2. **Nonfatal, non–head-related falls** are associated with laceration in 38% of cases, sprains in 38%, and fractures (usually involving the extremities or clavicles) in 14%.

D. Prevention of injury

1. **Legislation and regulation.** Laws regarding safe housing standards should be created and strictly enforced. Strict regulation in Canada has led to infant walkers no longer being sold there.

2. **Barriers**
   a. Gates on stairways should be used at both the top and bottom. These should be pressure gates, not the accordion type, which can cause head entrapment.
   b. Window guards should be used, and laws mandate their use in many urban localities.

3. **Behavior modification for parents**
   a. The mattress and side rails of the crib should be appropriately adjusted.
   b. Infants should not be left unattended, even briefly, on adult beds or changing tables.
   c. Tables with sharp edges and pointed corners should be removed.
   d. Doors to the basement should be kept closed.
   e. Use of infant walkers should be abandoned, as recommended by the American Academy of Pediatrics.

VI. DROWNING (SUBMERSION INJURY)

A. **Epidemiology.** Drowning is the third most common cause of accidental death in children; it is second only to motor vehicle injury as a cause of unintentional death in adolescents.

1. The male-to-female ratio is 5:1; the black-to-white ratio is 3:1. The **peak incidence** occurs at 1–5 years of age for both sexes; the incidence peaks again at 10–19 years of age for boys only.

2. Freshwater drownings outnumber saltwater drownings, even along the coast and in Hawaii. **Major sites of drowning** for children include:
   a. Pools and lakes, especially for toddlers who fall in and are unable to swim
   b. Streams, rivers, quarries, and oceans
   c. Bathtubs, which are the most common site of drowning in the first year of life

3. There is a **high mortality-to-morbidity ratio;** however, many minor incidents are never brought to medical attention.
   a. In one survey, of 132 drownings and near-drownings reported in individuals ranging in age from newborn to 21 years, 65 people died; among the 58 cases involving 1- to 3-year-olds, there were 20 deaths.
   b. In another study, 25% of patients presenting to an emergency room with submersion injury were admitted.

B. **Pathophysiology**

1. **Hypoxemia** is the principal problem in submersion injuries.
   a. Aspiration occurs in 90% of cases, but less than 2.2 ml of fluid/kg of body weight is involved.
   b. There is no significant clinical difference between saltwater and freshwater drowning, and chlorine in the water is not a special problem in that it causes no injury beyond the submersion damage.

2. **Major organ system involvement**
   a. **Brain. Hypoxic brain injury** is most serious and life-threatening as well as being most likely to cause long-term damage. Full impact may not be known for days or weeks if the patient survives.
   b. **Lung. Pulmonary edema** results from decreased surfactant and resulting atelectasis.
   c. **Kidney. Acute renal failure** occurs in most lengthy drownings and near-drownings, but 80% of patients recover in 10 days.

C. **Prediction of outcome.** Certain variables can predict the likelihood of a good outcome after a submersion injury.

1. **Water temperature.** The outcome is better when the water temperature is greater than 40°F (4°C) and less than 70°F (21°C).

2. **Duration of submersion.** Submersion for more than 5 minutes in warm water leads to a major risk of damage.

3. **Fixed, dilated pupils and coma** result in a 100% incidence of serious deficit, damage, or fatal outcome.

4. **Need for cardiopulmonary resuscitation (CPR)** among normothermic patients on arrival in the emergency room is the **major determinant of outcome.** In one study, of 21 patients requiring CPR on arrival at the hospital, 17 had a poor outcome; of 29 patients with spontaneous pulse and respiratory effort, all had a good outcome.

D. **Prevention of injury**

1. All children younger than 4 years of age should be supervised while in the bathtub.

2. A fence with a gate that closes should be used around in-ground pools, and a gate should be used at stairs or entries to above-ground pools.

3. All children should be supervised closely while swimming, especially those with known medical problems.

4. The depth of the water should be checked before children and adolescents are allowed to dive.

5. A basic CPR course should be provided for all parents who own or live near pools or other bodies of water.

6. Children should be taught how to swim. This does not, however, negate the need for supervision.

VII. **BURNS** rank third behind motor vehicle accidents and drownings as a cause of injury to children. They cause more than 1300 childhood deaths per year in the United States and account for more than 21,000 hospital admissions.

A. **Types of burns**

1. Flame burns most frequently result from house fires.
   a. Etiology
      (1) Smoking causes 30%–45% of all house fires.
      (2) Heating equipment (space heaters and woodstoves) and electrical malfunction (e.g., faulty extension cords, frayed wires) are the next most common cause.
      (3) Matches and fire-setting account for less than 5% of house-fire deaths, but still cause 120 childhood deaths/year.
   b. Epidemiology
      (1) House fires in the United States occur most frequently in the East and Southeast.
      (2) They occur most frequently at night, in December through March.
      (3) Children are often alone when the event occurs.
   c. Prevention of injury
      (1) **Smoke detectors** provide early warning of house fires and can prevent 85%–90% of house-fire–related deaths. Their use has increased from 5% in 1970 to 70% in 1989. They are particularly useful because:
         (a) Fatal residential fires more frequently occur when occupants are asleep.
         (b) Residential fires burn for a long time before detection.
         (c) Most deaths result from smoke inhalation.
      (2) **Sprinklers.** The use of sprinklers is mandated in commercial high-rise buildings. They are neither required nor widely used in residential settings.
      (3) Increasingly **stringent sleepwear standards** have been implemented since 1967, and these have been responsible for a dramatic decrease in deaths.
      (4) Prototypical **fire-safe cigarettes** have been produced, but are not widely available.

2. Scald burns are the most common cause of inpatient hospitalization.
   a. The **kitchen** is the major site of burns from water, beverages, and grease. Hot liquid in a cup or pot turned over in the kitchen is the most common scenario.
      (1) Of scald burns, 60% occur in the kitchen.
      (2) Hot liquids caused 44% of burn admissions to a children's hospital in one study.
      (3) In a study conducted in New Zealand in 1970, hot liquids accounted for 78% of burn injuries to children.
   b. Tap water causes one-fourth of all scald burns.
      (1) Half of all tap water burns occur in children younger than 5 years of age.

      (2) Tap water burns are most likely to occur in bathroom sinks and bathtubs.

      (3) Tap water burns may result when older siblings turn on hot water for younger children.

      (4) This type of burn is a possible result of abuse.

  c. Prevention of injury

      (1) A child should not be held by an adult who is drinking a hot liquid.

      (2) Pot handles on the stove should be turned to the side. The back burner should be used when possible.

      (3) Stable cups and coffee-making apparatus should be used.

      (4) Children should be in a safe area during food preparation.

      (5) Placemats should be used rather than tablecloths.

      (6) Children should be supervised in the bath and at the sink.

      (7) The temperature of the water heater should be reduced to 120°F (most water heaters are kept at approximately 150°F).

3. Electrical burns. Each year, more than 4000 extension and appliance cord injuries require emergency room treatment. Most occur in children younger than 5 years of age. Such injuries can result in disfiguring mouth burns, other skin burns, and electrocution.

  a. Major causes of electrical burns

      (1) Injuries are principally caused by a child sucking on the plug-receptor connection of an extension wire.

      (2) Another cause is a child inserting conducting objects into live wall sockets.

      (3) A less common cause is a child chewing on poorly insulated wire.

  b. Prevention of injury

      (1) Extension cords should be unplugged from wall sockets after use.

      (2) Safety plugs or caps should be used on unused wall sockets.

      (3) Appliance wires should be inspected for fraying.

4. Contact burns are the most common cause of emergency department visits in many urban areas. Most injuries involve the extremities.

  a. Sources include:

      (1) Hot appliances, such as irons, hair curlers, toasters, and broilers (hands)

      (2) Wood-burning stoves (hands)

      (3) Heating register grates (feet)

  b. Prevention of injury

      (1) Hot appliances should be kept away from children, and vice versa. Irons should be cooled in a location inaccessible to small children. Ironing should not be performed on the bed or floor.

      (2) Toddlers should be kept away from a wood-burning stove.

      (3) Slippers or shoes should be worn in homes with floor heating grates.

5. Chemical burns in children often are related to ingestion of caustic agents.

6. Ultraviolet radiation primarily results from sun exposure.

B. **Acute therapy for fires and burns**

1. For an active flame burn, the victim should "drop and roll." Running only fans the flames that are already active.

2. For skin burns, cool water should be applied immediately to minimize active tissue damage.

3. In case of house fires, occupants should be instructed to know the evacuation route and to crawl under smoke.

4. For electrocution, the victim should be removed from contact by use of a nonconducting material such as wood or plastic. CPR should be initiated as needed.

VIII. **CHOKING AND FOREIGN BODY INJURY.** A foreign body is any substance that is not natural to the body passage in which it is found. The reasons why children ingest foreign objects range from the normal infant behavior of putting everything into the mouth to a child trying to eat, run, and breathe at the same time. In addition, parents often have unrealistic expectations of what their children should be able to eat or do at a given age.

A. **Epidemiology.** Foreign body injury is the most common cause of injury-related death in children younger than 1 year of age. Twenty percent of all foreign body aspiration deaths in the United States occur in children younger than 4 years of age.

B. **Clinical findings.** Symptoms may be minimal, especially if the foreign body is small. Many (approximately 50%) of the episodes are unwitnessed.

1. **Factors involved in foreign body injury include:**
   a. **Size** and **composition** of the foreign body
   b. **Location.** The younger the child, in general, the higher the involved anatomic site, which is directly a result of the relative size of the airway.
      (1) The **larynx** is the most common site in children younger than 1 year of age.
      (2) The **trachea** and **bronchi** are most commonly involved in children 1–4 years of age.
   c. **Degree** and **duration** of obstruction

2. **Upper airway obstruction** may cause asphyxiation and pose an immediate threat to life. It is manifested by gagging, choking, wheezing, cyanosis, and dysphonia or aphonia.

3. **Lower tract obstruction** may be tolerated for longer periods of time, especially the more distal the obstruction. It is usually manifested by wheezing or asymmetric or absent breath sounds.

C. **Acute management** of choking and foreign body ingestion consists of **nonintervention if the child can cough, breathe, or speak**. A natural cough is more effective than an artificial one.

1. Fingers should not be thrust blindly into the mouth to search for a foreign body. This might lodge the object in the airway.

2. Intervention for **upper airway asphyxiation** has been the subject of much controversy (see Chapter 7).
   a. The American Heart Association recommends abdominal thrusts (Heimlich maneuver) for children older than 1 year of age.
   b. Back blows and chest thrusts are recommended for children younger than 1 year because of the theoretical risk of abdominal viscus perforation with the Heimlich maneuver.
   c. As a general rule, if three or four attempts at one maneuver fail, the other should be tried.

3. If necessary, **rigid bronchoscopy** should be performed under general anesthesia. Occasionally, **thoracotomy** and **bronchotomy** may be required.

D. **Prevention of injury**

1. **Toys.** Infants should not have access to toys meant for older children (e.g., dolls with button eyes, beanbag toys).

2. **Food**
   a. Food should be cut, broken, or mashed into bite-sized pieces. Conversation and motor activity should be discouraged during eating.
   b. Nuts, hard beans, pretzels, gumballs, raw vegetables, and so forth should not be given to young children.

3. **Chewable pills** should not be given to children younger than 3 years of age.

4. **Small objects** (e.g., uninflated balloons, diaper pins, coins) should not be given to or left near small children. Children should be taught not to place these objects in their mouths.

IX. **TOYS.** More than 150,000 different toys are produced worldwide by 1500 toy manu-
facturers. Understanding the hazards peculiar to each developmental stage in childhood
aids in choosing appropriate toys and preventing injury.

A. **Aspiration and ingestion dangers**

1. Toys should be large enough so that they cannot be swallowed, nor should they come
apart or be easily shattered.

2. Toys for small children should not have easily removable buttons or fillings (e.g., beans).

3. Small children should not be given uninflated balloons. They can be aspirated, and
they have caused death.

4. Small plastic toys and parts of toys are not radiopaque and are rarely visualized in
radiographs of the trachea, chest, and abdomen.

B. **Burns and electric shock** can be caused by toys. Battery-operated toys are preferable to
those with electric cords. Plug-in toys should not be used by children younger than 8 years
of age. Children should be taught how to use the toys and should be supervised when
playing with them.

C. **Lacerations**

1. Toys with sharp or poorly finished edges can cause lacerations.

2. Glass toys should not be used by small children.

3. Sharp points on toys should have protective covers.

D. **Projectile injuries.** The major site of projectile injury is the eye. BB guns, archery sets, and
boomerangs should be restricted to use by older children with adult supervision.

E. **Skateboards** are associated with a high rate of injury because of the high speed attained
(up to 35 mph) and the need for a high level of coordination.

1. **Epidemiology.** The major group at risk is boys 10–14 years of age. Injuries include fractures, contusions and abrasions, and sprains and muscle injuries.

2. **Recommendations for use** include:
   a. Use of protective equipment (e.g., helmets, gloves, elbow and knee pads)
   b. Prohibition of use on public streets
   c. Smooth skating surfaces free of traffic
   d. Skateboarding parks
   e. Safety rules

X. **SPORTS INJURIES.** As children get older, participation in organized sports increases.
Team and individual sports are commonplace for both boys and girls either in school or
through organized leagues. In adolescence, physical maturity allows high proficiency at
sports but also increases the risk of serious injury.

A. **Epidemiology**

1. In a statewide study of accidents in Massachusetts, 1 in 7 school-age children visited an
emergency department each year for sports-related injuries.

2. In another study of high school students in Seattle, Washington, injury rates for different sports were monitored. Over 2 years, 82% of participants in football and 75% of

participants in wrestling suffered injuries. Between 30% and 60% of all students in gym class were injured. Sports least likely to be associated with injury were tennis, swimming, and volleyball, each of which had no more than a 10% injury rate (Table 2-2).

3. **Most injuries occur during practice,** not competition.
   a. Most injuries are minor, primarily sprains, strains, and bruises.
      (1) Of injured children, 70% miss less than 1 week of participation, and 29% miss only 1 day.
      (2) Most children are treated initially by the coach, who must determine the general status of the child and if CPR is required (all coaches should be certified in CPR). If the injury is determined not to be severe, ice, compression, and elevation should be used as necessary, as well as referral to a physician as appropriate.
   b. The use of medical resources is prevalent, however.
      (1) Of those injured, 42% are referred to a physician for care.
      (2) Of those seen by a physician, 91% have a radiograph and 2% are hospitalized, most of whom require surgical procedures.

B. **Types of injury.** Potentially life-threatening injuries include:

1. Severe head or neck injury

2. Cardiac or respiratory arrest

3. Severe hemorrhage and shock

4. Heat exposure

C. **Reinjury is a major problem,** both at the site of the original injury and at other sites. Causes of reinjury include resumption of sports too soon after the initial injury and inadequate rehabilitation.

TABLE 2-2. Sports-Related Injuries (1980) and Deaths (1973–1980)

Sport	Estimated Number of Injuries Treated in Hospital Emergency Rooms, 1980		Number of Deaths, 1973–1980	
	All Ages	5–14 Years	All Ages	5–14 Years
Football	463,800	173,100	260	19
Baseball	442,900	121,700	183	40
Basketball	421,000	92,800	37	6
Soccer	94,200	37,800	11	6
Racquet sports	74,700	5400	3	1
Volleyball	73,700	13,900	4	0
Wrestling*	67,500	20,000	23	2
Gymnastics	61,400	38,200	8	0
Ice hockey	36,400	10,800	10	2
Track and field	31,600	8800	10	2
Golf†	18,800	4600	28	14
Trampoline	6100	2900	13	6

Injuries were estimated from the U.S. Consumer Product Safety Commission's National Electronic Injury Surveillance System (NEISS). Deaths were identifed from death certificates, newspaper clippings, consumer complaints, medical examiner reports, and NEISS data. Adapted from Baker SP, O'Neill B, Ginsburg MJ, Li G: *The Injury Fact Book,* 2nd ed. New York, Oxford University Press, 1992, p 92; original data from Rutherford GW, Miles RB, Brown VR, MacDonald B: *Overview of Sports-Related Injuries to Persons 5–14 Years of Age.* Washington, DC, U.S. Consumer Product Safety Commission, 1981.
*Includes injuries from "roughhousing."
†Includes spectators and children playing with golf clubs.

XI. POISONING

A. Epidemiology

1. Poisoning involves 2 million children younger than 5 years of age each year. It is the third most common injury treated in emergency departments for all children younger than 16 years of age.

2. There are two peak ages for poisonings: 1–5 years and adolescence. The former group is involved in involuntary, inadvertent poisonings. The latter group most often is involved in suicide gestures or attempts. Although the developmental basis may be different, the initial treatment for a given agent remains the same regardless of the age and motivation of the victim.

B. Environmental factors

1. **Circumstances that increase the risk of ingestion**
   a. Storing dangerous chemicals (e.g., cleaning agents, motor oil, pesticides) in drinking glasses, soda bottles, or unlabeled, open containers
   b. Changes in normal home routines (overall, 80% of ingestions occur at home)
      (1) These can occur during moving, preparation for vacation, spring cleaning, or periods of family stress.
      (2) Visiting friends and relatives may not be careful with their medications around children.
   c. Over-reliance on childproof caps on medicine containers
   d. Storing different medications in the same container

2. **Common sources of poisoning** are depicted in Figure 2-1.

C. Examination

1. A child who is behaving strangely or who is unresponsive must be considered to have ingested something, and a cause should be sought by taking a careful history and by screening blood and urine for toxic substances.

2. The level of consciousness should be documented and monitored frequently. Size and reactivity of pupils, odor of breath, cardiorespiratory status, and a careful neurologic examination are key points.

D. Principles of therapy

1. **Removal of gastric contents.** In general, removal of toxic agents from the stomach as soon after ingestion as possible is the first step in therapy. Some experts prefer adsorption of poison as the first step, especially if treatment is delayed or symptoms develop (see XI D 2). Removal may be accomplished by induction of emesis or by gastric lavage.

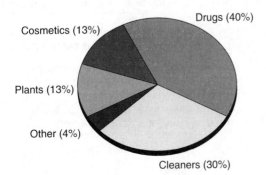

Cosmetics (13%)
Drugs (40%)
Plants (13%)
Other (4%)
Cleaners (30%)

FIGURE 2-1. Common sources of poisoning in children younger than 5 years of age.

a. Emesis. In children, emesis is more effective and less traumatic than gastric lavage for most ingestions.

  (1) Some toxic agents cause **spontaneous vomiting**. Vomiting may occur before consultation with a poison control center or physician has taken place.

  (2) Emesis may be induced by ingestion of **syrup of ipecac,** a mixture of plant alkaloids. Ipecac induces vomiting by local gastric irritation as well as by central activity through the chemoreceptor trigger zone of the floor of the fourth ventricle of the brain.

    (a) Ipecac can be given at home before transport to an emergency facility after telephone contact with a health care provider or poison control center.

    (b) Dose. Children between 6 and 12 months of age should be administered 10 ml; children older than 1 year of age should be given 15 ml. Either dose should be followed by fluids. Emesis results within 20 minutes in 90%–100% of children. The dose may be repeated once if no vomiting occurs.

    (c) Contraindications

      (i) Most authorities advise against use of ipecac in children younger than 6 months of age.

      (ii) A depressed level of consciousness may result in lung aspiration.

      (iii) Emesis is contraindicated when volatile hydrocarbons have been ingested, because aspiration into the lungs is possible owing to the nature of the compound.

      (iv) Corrosive substances cause an increased risk of esophageal burn if vomited.

      (v) Emetics may not be effective if antiemetics or major tranquilizers of the chlorpromazine group are ingested.

b. Gastric lavage should be reserved for use in children who cannot take ipecac, in whom the level of consciousness is depressed, and in whom there is no response to ipecac.

  (1) For children with severe depression of mental state, intubation with a cuffed endotracheal tube is required to prevent aspiration.

  (2) The largest bore tube that can be passed should be used because it will allow the removal of larger pill fragments. Lavage with normal saline should be continued until the return fluid is clear for two or three passes.

2. **Adsorption of poison.** The next step in therapy after the removal of poison from the stomach is binding the poison to inhibit gastrointestinal absorption. **Activated charcoal** adsorbs a variety of materials in the gastrointestinal tract. Adsorption occurs within the first few minutes and may be inhibited by food. Most toxins are adsorbed by activated charcoal; however, some agents [i.e., iron salts, boric acid, cyanide, mineral acids, strong bases (caustics), lithium, other small ionized molecules] are not.

  a. Dose. The completeness of adsorption depends on the amount of activated charcoal relative to toxin. Ideally, the amount of charcoal should be 5–12 times that of the ingested material. This often cannot be estimated accurately. The recommended pediatric dose is 15–30 g for children younger than 12 years of age and 50–100 g for children older than 12 years. It is administered as a slurry in cold water. Poor palatability is a major drawback in its use in the pediatric population. Use of a nasogastric tube may be required.

  b. Contraindications. Because activated charcoal can bind with and render ipecac ineffective, charcoal should not be used until vomiting induced by ipecac is complete.

3. **Intestinal cleansing. Cathartics** are routinely recommended after gastric emptying and adsorption. Cathartics decrease the transit time of toxins through the gastrointestinal tract, thus making them less available for absorption into the circulation.

  a. Magnesium sulfate administered at 250 mg/kg, sodium sulfate administered at 250 mg/kg, and magnesium citrate administered at 4 ml/kg are the most frequently used cathartics.

  b. The cathartic may be added to the activated charcoal for ease of administration without loss of efficacy for either substance.

E. Specific poisonings

1. **Aspirin** is widely consumed by adults and children, and it is the **most common cause of drug poisoning** in children. It generally is not perceived as "medicine." Although the incidence has been decreasing over the past 20 years, aspirin poisoning remains a problem.
   a. **Pharmacology**
      (1) Aspirin is a weak acid that is absorbed rapidly from the stomach and small bowel into the circulation, and is both freely ionized and protein bound.
      (2) The drug is metabolized by the liver and excreted through the kidney.
      (3) The half-life is prolonged in overdoses to 18–36 hours, compared to 4–6 hours in therapeutic doses. When urine pH is greater than 7.4, most of the drug is ionized in the urine and not reabsorbed, thus shortening plasma half-life to 6–8 hours.
   b. **Pathogenesis**
      (1) There is increased sensitivity of the respiratory centers of the brain to changes in carbon dioxide and oxygen concentrations, leading to increased rate and depth of respiration, and resultant respiratory alkalosis. To compensate, hydrogen ions move from cells to the extracellular space.
      (2) Oxidative phosphorylation is uncoupled, increasing the metabolic rate and causing increased metabolism of glucose and oxygen, resulting in excess heat production. This causes tachycardia, tachypnea, fever, and hypoglycemia. Aspirin also inhibits the Krebs cycle, causing metabolic acidosis.
      (3) Aspirin damages hepatocytes, causing liver toxicity and prolonged prothrombin time. It also inhibits platelet organization, causing prolonged bleeding time.
   c. **Clinical features**
      (1) Clinical features include tinnitus and vomiting (the vomitus may be heme-positive); hyperpnea; fever, lethargy, and confusion; and convulsions, coma, and respiratory or cardiac failure.
      (2) In an acute overdose at 6 hours past ingestion, the serum level is predictive of the clinical course.
         (a) At less than 35 mg/L, there are no symptoms.
         (b) At 35–70 mg/L, symptoms are mild to moderate.
         (c) At 70–100 mg/L, symptoms are severe.
         (d) At over 120 mg/L, the outcome is potentially fatal.
   d. **Therapy** includes:
      (1) Ipecac-induced emesis, followed by administration of activated charcoal and cathartics
      (2) Alkalization with sodium bicarbonate given intravenously (a urinary pH of 8 is desired)
      (3) Adequate fluids to correct loss; colloid (as albumin or plasma) given to correct shock
      (4) Dialysis or hemofiltration, which should be considered in severe cases or when there is renal, hepatic, or cardiac failure
   e. **Prevention**
      (1) The number of baby aspirin is limited by regulation to thirty-six 75-mg tablets per bottle.
      (2) Safety closures (childproof caps) should be used on bottles.
      (3) The association of Reye syndrome with aspirin further curtails aspirin use in children and, as a result, likely decreases the number of poisonings.

2. **Acetaminophen** has replaced aspirin as an antipyretic–analgesic for use in children and is also widely used by adults. Consequently, the incidence of poisoning by this agent has markedly risen in recent years. In general, children younger than 5 years of age seem relatively resistant to severe toxic sequelae compared to adults, but still should be evaluated and managed aggressively.
   a. **Clinical features.** There are three main phases of acetaminophen poisoning.
      (1) **Phase I** usually begins 30–60 minutes after ingestion and may last for 12–24 hours.

        (a) Most patients with mild poisoning never progress beyond this stage and are asymptomatic.

        (b) In moderate to severe poisoning, gastrointestinal signs—anorexia, nausea, and vomiting—as well as pallor and diaphoresis predominate.

        (c) Changes in level of consciousness do not occur at this stage and, if present, suggest the ingestion of a different agent, perhaps in addition to acetaminophen.

  (2) Phase II occurs 24–48 hours after ingestion and may persist up to 4 days.

        (a) During this phase, the patient usually is clinically asymptomatic, although mild right upper quadrant tenderness relative to hepatic enlargement may occur.

        (b) Liver function test results—hepatic enzymes, serum bilirubin, and prothrombin time—rise as hepatic necrosis progresses.

        (c) Patients who are moderately poisoned do not progress beyond this point and gradually recover.

  (3) Phase III occurs 3–5 days after ingestion. Symptoms are related to hepatotoxicity.

        (a) Symptoms may be limited to anorexia, nausea, malaise, and abdominal pain.

        (b) More severe cases may progress to confusion and stupor as well as sequelae related to hepatic toxicity, including jaundice, coagulation defects, hypoglycemia, and encephalopathy. Renal failure and myocardiopathy also may occur.

        (c) Death occurs from irreversible hepatotoxicity.

b. Therapy

  (1) Assessment

        (a) Maximum number of tablets or liquid missing from the container should be presumed ingested.

        (b) If the presumed ingested dose is less than 100 mg/kg of body weight, the ingestion is mild and need not be treated.

        (c) If the presumed dose is unknown or above 100 mg/kg, the child requires clinical evaluation and intervention.

  (2) Intervention

        (a) Syrup of ipecac should be given to empty the stomach; if there is a change in the level of consciousness because of ingestion of another substance, gastric lavage should be performed.

        (b) Activated charcoal usually has not been advised because it binds and inactivates *N*-acetylcysteine, the antidote for acetaminophen. Recent data suggest that a higher dose of *N*-acetylcysteine might overcome residual activated charcoal.

        (c) A loading dose of *N*-acetylcysteine (140 mg/kg body weight) should be given, followed by a maintenance dose (70 mg/kg) every 4 hours for 17 doses.

        (d) A serum sample for acetaminophen assay should be obtained 4 hours or more after ingestion and results compared to a published nomogram. Use of the nomogram will determine whether the full treatment course is needed or whether treatment can be stopped (Figure 2-2).

        (e) If the serum acetaminophen level is in the toxic range, the patient should be hospitalized, liver function tests performed, and electrolyte, glucose, and creatinine concentrations obtained. Laboratory tests should be repeated daily while treatment is underway, until 4 days after ingestion.

        (f) Supportive care should be provided, depending on clinical observation and laboratory data.

3. Iron. Iron-containing products, such as ferrous salts alone or iron as part of multivitamin tablets, are a significant toxicologic hazard. More than 4000 cases of acute iron ingestion are reported to regional poison control centers annually, and iron is among the top 10 substances ingested by children younger than 5 years of age. Iron is widely available without prescription. It is formulated in large tablets that look like candy and is sold in containers of as many as 250 tablets. In addition, iron is commonly not appreciated by parents as potentially dangerous to their children.

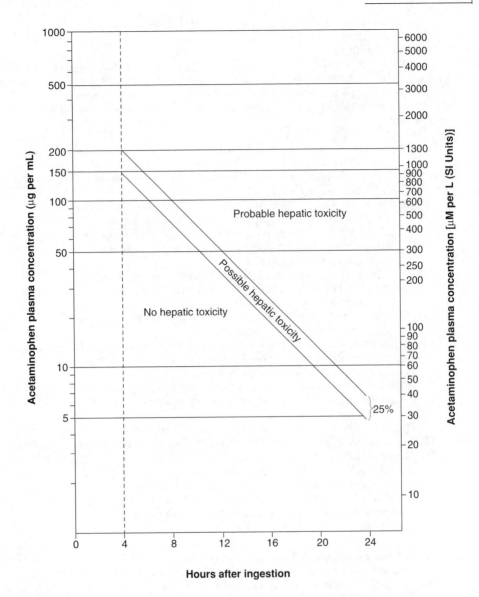

FIGURE 2-2. Semilogarithmic plot of plasma acetaminophen levels versus time, for use after single ingestions of acetaminophen. (Adapted with permission from *Pediatrics* 55:871, 1975; and Micromedex, Inc.)

  a. Clinical features. There are four main phases of iron poisoning.
    (1) Gastrointestinal symptoms. Within 30–60 minutes, vomiting, colicky abdominal pain, gastrointestinal hemorrhage, and diarrhea occur. Iron acutely and directly damages the gastrointestinal tract, especially the gastric and small intestinal mucosa.
    (2) There is a period of **relative stability** from 3–4 hours until 48 hours. It is marked by subtle changes and failure to recognize them. There is no evidence of change in the central nervous system (CNS).
    (3) Circulatory shock occurs after 48 hours. It is caused by a combination of gastrointestinal fluid and blood loss, increased capillary permeability, and loss of vascular tone, all of which are direct effects of excess iron. A secondary

coagulopathy may result. Shock results from absolute hypovolemia and the inability of the body to respond to it.

(4) Late manifestations

(a) Gastric scarring occurs within 2–6 weeks. Because iron acts directly on the gastrointestinal tract as a corrosive, the healing process may result in areas of scarring and stenosis at both the pylorus and the small bowel.

(b) Rarely, hepatic necrosis may result from direct liver damage by iron.

b. Therapy

(1) Potential risk must be determined.

(a) It should be assumed that the maximum number of tablets missing was ingested by the child.

(b) The weight of elemental iron in each preparation should be used to calculate the toxic dose ingested.

(c) The toxic dose ingested (mg/kg) should be calculated, based on the child's weight. In general, less than 20 mg/kg of elemental iron poses little risk; 20–60 mg/kg requires syrup of ipecac–induced emesis and reevaluation if gastrointestinal pain or bleeding occurs; greater than 60 mg/kg requires examination by a physician.

(2) Any patient with gastrointestinal or CNS symptoms must be evaluated, even if the calculated dose is nontoxic. Not only may the calculation be incorrect, but multiple ingestions may have occurred.

(3) All adolescents with iron overdose should be seen by a physician because the ingestions must be regarded as intentional.

(4) Serum iron levels should be measured 4–6 hours after ingestion. By that time, emesis and cathartics will have been given (activated charcoal has no effect).

(a) If the concentration is less than 300 μg/dl, it is not significant.

(b) If the iron concentration is 300–500 μg/dl, if it is greater than the total iron-binding capacity, or if the patient is symptomatic, the serum iron levels are considered to be significant.

(c) If the concentration is greater than 500 μg/dl, it is toxic.

(5) An abdominal radiograph might be helpful because iron pills are radiopaque.

(6) Deferoxamine, a chelating agent specific for iron, is recommended for intravenous use in patients with the significant or toxic levels noted earlier. It is given by slow continuous infusion at 15 mg/kg/hour. Its positive effect is noted when the urine turns pink, because the iron–chelate complex is excreted in the urine. Treatment is discontinued when the serum iron level is less than 300 μg/dl.

4. Hydrocarbons–petroleum distillates. Hydrocarbons are derivatives of crude petroleum and are mixtures of aromatic and aliphatic hydrocarbons. Naturally occurring derivatives extracted from plants, such as turpentine and pine oil, have similar properties and are included in this discussion. Common hydrocarbons include gasoline, kerosene, lighter fluid, paint thinner, turpentine, mineral seal oil (the major ingredient in furniture polish), and pine oil.

a. Toxic effects

(1) Aspiration of the substance into the respiratory tract is the major danger. The more highly volatile the hydrocarbon, the more likely is aspiration. The major effect of aspiration is chemical irritation, which damages the alveolar lining and the capillaries, causing pneumonitis, atelectasis, or pulmonary edema. The degree of lung involvement is parallel to the degree of clinical compromise. Results are severe hypoxemia and ventilation–perfusion abnormalities, causing respiratory acidosis. Because of this risk, **emesis should not be induced** in management of volatile hydrocarbon ingestion.

(2) CNS depression. All hydrocarbons are absorbed to some degree. The amount absorbed determines the degree of CNS depression. Aromatic distillates (e.g., toluene or xylene, turpentine, gasoline, mineral spirits) are most likely to cause a depressed sensorium.

b. Clinical features
   (1) Early on, there is burning in the mouth and throat, choking and gagging, coughing, nausea, vomiting, and hemoptysis.
   (2) Tachycardia and tachypnea reflect the degree of pulmonary insult. Often, a chest radiograph shows changes before the onset of significant clinical findings. The radiograph may reveal punctate, mottled densities of pneumonitis, atelectasis, or both, with findings tending to be more prominent in the dependent portion of the lung. Radiographic findings peak at 72 hours and then begin to clear.
   (3) One hour after ingestion, symptoms of CNS depression occur (e.g., general weakness, hypotonia, dizziness, mental confusion, lethargy). Irritability, agitation, or convulsions may be seen.
   (4) There is a poor correlation among clinical symptoms, physical findings, and radiographic abnormalities.
c. Therapy
   (1) When a small amount—a mouthful or two—has been ingested, the child is best left without attempts at removal, in an upright position.
   (2) In large ingestions, spontaneous vomiting usually occurs. Comatose patients should be intubated with a cuffed endotracheal tube and lavaged.
   (3) All patients with respiratory or CNS symptoms should be admitted to the hospital, observed closely, and treated to support respiratory and fluid status. Oxygen, bronchodilators, and constant distending airway pressure should be used.

5. Lead poisoning (plumbism), in contrast to the other acute poisonings discussed in this section, actually is a chronic disorder that may be punctuated by acute episodes. Studies indicate that 5%–15% of children in the United States have increased lead absorption. Most are asymptomatic, but many children may have decreased school performance associated with chronic lead exposure.
   a. Sources of increased lead absorption among children include:
      (1) Ingestion of paint and plaster chips in old, dilapidated buildings
         (a) The eating of nonfood items (pica) is common among infants and toddlers.
         (b) The combination of pica and living in old housing accounts for most cases of symptomatic poisoning.
      (2) Exposure to household dust in old houses
      (3) Living in close proximity to a lead smelter
      (4) Exposure to contaminated workclothes of parents
      (5) Lead-contaminated soil
      (6) Other, less common sources (e.g., contamination of acidic beverages and foods in lead-lined containers and lead-glazed ceramic pots, lead-painted furniture and toys, the burning of battery casings in fireplaces)
   b. Clinical features. The clinical diagnosis tends not to be suspected until the onset of CNS symptoms. The insidious nature of lead poisoning emphasizes the importance of screening for increased lead absorption during child health maintenance visits (see Chapter 1).
      (1) General symptoms include apathy, decreased play, clumsiness, and intermittent vomiting.
      (2) Acute encephalopathy is manifested by vomiting, lethargy, stupor, and ataxia, followed by coma and seizures.
      (3) Chronic lead poisoning may present as nonspecific developmental delay, behavioral and attention disorders (see Chapter 4), seizures, or a peripheral neuropathy (see Chapter 18). Follow-up studies suggest that developmental abnormalities persist over a 10-year period and may manifest as poor school performance.
   c. Laboratory findings
      (1) Biochemical evidence of lead toxicity includes elevations of blood lead and signs of interference with hemoglobin synthesis, such as an increase in free erythrocyte protoporphyrin as well as increased lead excretion in the urine after

administration of a chelating agent, such as calcium ethylenediaminetetraacetic acid (CaEDTA).

(2) There may be evidence of a **sideroblastic anemia** (see Chapter 15 III B 4).

(3) Radiographic findings may include lead lines at the metaphyses of the long bones and radiopaque foreign material within the small bowel.

d. Therapy

(1) For children with symptomatic lead poisoning, the **source of lead must be identified** and the child's intake immediately interrupted. This may require temporary housing for the child until the home is lead-free.

(2) For such children, chelation therapy with agents such as CaEDTA, dimercaprol, succimer, or D-penicillamine is indicated.

(a) After an initial course of parenteral CaEDTA or CaEDTA–dimercaprol or oral succimer, oral D-penicillamine can be given for 2–6 months to prevent rebound increases in blood lead.

(b) Supportive treatment may include control of increased intracranial pressure and seizure control, as well as monitoring urine output.

(c) Careful, long-term follow-up is essential because learning and behavioral problems are late sequelae.

(3) The approach to asymptomatic children with evidence of increased lead absorption is still controversial.

(a) The Centers for Disease Control and Prevention recommends aggressive screening for all children every 6 months in the first 5 years of life, with more frequent screening of children with mildly elevated blood lead levels (> 15 μg/dl) that do not require chelation (see Chapter 1 V D 3).

(b) Prompt identification of environment hazards is critical.

(c) Parents should be counseled routinely to encourage frequent handwashing in children and to damp-mop house dust.

(d) CaEDTA or succimer may be administered to children with persistent elevations of blood lead who also have biochemical evidence of adverse effects, such as marked elevation of free erythrocyte protoporphyrin or a positive CaEDTA challenge test.

e. Prevention is the key in eliminating this important source of morbidity.

(1) Replacing or renovating old, substandard housing is the ultimate solution.

(2) Avoidance of paints with lead additives is critical.

(3) Screening of children decreases the incidence of frank lead poisoning, although this will not in itself eliminate increased lead absorption among children.

(4) Decreased lead in gasoline will help reduce environmental exposure.

(5) Pilot studies on decreasing other environmental sources (e.g., soil) are of some small benefit, but extremely costly and logistically difficult.

F. Prevention of poisonings

1. Preschool children. Because developmental factors are the major issue, parents play the primary preventive role. Actions are aimed at physically preventing small children from ingesting toxic substances through:

a. Use of childproof caps

b. Dispensing a limited amount of medication

c. Locking medicine cabinets

d. Not combining different medications in the same container

e. Not misrepresenting medications as "candy"

2. Adolescents. Because the etiology of poisoning in this age-group may be experimentation or suicide related, methods of passive prevention are not helpful. An attempt to identify adolescents with problems and to deal with them before they act out those problems is the best approach in suicide-related cases. Education about the hazards of drug and alcohol abuse may be helpful in avoiding the serious consequences of experimentation.

G. **Poison control centers.** Because the number of potential poisons is immense and because gathering the necessary information about them is so time consuming, statewide and regional poison control centers have been established.

1. These centers may be accessed by the public as well as by health professionals.

2. They serve not only to assist in recognition and management of potentially serious ingestions, but to provide reassurance regarding ingestion of or exposure to benign substances.
   a. One study found that inappropriate use of the emergency department could be reduced by up to 95% as a result of prior consultation by a parent with a poison control center.
   b. In another survey of poison control centers, 75% of calls concerned poisons with relatively low toxicity and required only reassurance, 20% required rapid removal of the ingested poison, and fewer than 5% required more intensive medical management.

H. **Telephone calls** may come directly to health care providers or emergency departments instead of poison control centers. The person calling often is agitated, and it may be difficult to interpret the exact situation.

1. **Basic information** obtained over the telephone must include the:
   a. Patient's name, address, and telephone number (this information should be obtained first, because a hysterical person may hang up the phone prematurely)
   b. Patient's age and weight
   c. Type and amount of exposure or ingestion
   d. Clinical status and change in condition of the patient

2. Unfortunately, **telephone data are inaccurate half of the time,** and often a worst-case scenario must be invoked until it can be disproved or the patient can be examined.

BIBLIOGRAPHY

Baker SP, O'Neill B, Ginsburg MJ, Li G: *The Injury Fact Book,* 2nd ed. New York, Oxford University Press, 1992.

McIntire MS (ed): *Injury Control for Children and Youth.* Elk Grove Village, IL, American Academy of Pediatrics, 1987.

Rosenberg M, Jenley MA (eds): *Violence in America: A Public Health Approach.* New York, Oxford University Press, 1991.

Wilson M, Baker SP, Teret S, et al: *Saving Children: A Guide to Injury Prevention.* New York, Oxford University Press, 1991.

STUDY QUESTIONS

DIRECTIONS: Each of the numbered items or incomplete statements in this section is followed by answers or by completions of the statement. Select the ONE numbered answer or completion that is BEST in each case.

Questions 1 and 2

A 2-year-old boy is brought to the emergency department 30 minutes after having ingested his mother's 325-mg ferrous sulfate tablets. An open bottle was found on the floor and the child had a pill in his hand. His mother reports that 20 tablets are missing from the bottle. Each tablet contains 65 mg of elemental iron. He has vomited once, but his behavior is otherwise normal. The child's physical examination is unremarkable. He weighs 13 kg.

1. Which of the following statements about this child's status is correct?

(A) The dose of iron that this child ingested should cause no clinical sequelae
(B) His single episode of vomiting is probably unrelated to the ingestion
(C) Although he has vomited once, ipecac should be administered
(D) Activated charcoal should be given to adsorb excess iron in the stomach
(E) Cathartics are ineffective in iron poisonings

2. With respect to further treatment and outcome, which of the following statements about this case is correct?

(A) The child should be observed over the next 4–6 hours, and if no further symptoms occur, he may be sent home and be followed-up the next day
(B) A serum iron level should be drawn 4–6 hours after the ingestion, and if it exceeds 500 μg/dl, the child should be admitted and treated
(C) Treatment with deferoxamine will alter the outcome and should be begun immediately after vomiting has stopped
(D) A radiograph of the abdomen would be of no help in this case because pills generally are not radiopaque
(E) Had the parent of this child called a poison control center immediately after ingestion, an unnecessary emergency department visit could have been avoided

3. The most serious acute medical outcome of drowning is

(A) pulmonary edema
(B) acute renal failure
(C) hypoxic brain injury
(D) blood loss
(E) cardiac arrhythmia

4. According to the "agent–host–environment model," the agent most often responsible for motor vehicle injuries is

(A) chemical energy
(B) kinetic energy
(C) thermal energy
(D) electrical energy

5. Disfiguring mouth burns are most likely to occur as a result of

(A) an electrical burn
(B) a scald burn
(C) a contact burn
(D) ingestion of a caustic substance
(E) child abuse

6. Which statement about sports injuries is correct?

(A) Most injuries occur during competition
(B) Most injuries require hospital-based care
(C) Football is the school sport most highly associated with risk of injury
(D) Reinjury is rarely a problem

7. Which of the following injuries accounts for the greatest number of emergency ward visits?

(A) An injury caused by a motor vehicle accident
(B) A burn
(C) An injury caused by a fall
(D) Poisoning
(E) Drowning

8. Which of the following signs and symptoms may be associated with foreign body aspiration?

(A) Cyanosis
(B) Wheezing
(C) Absent breath sounds
(D) Aphonia
(E) All of the above

9. Predictors of a good overall outcome in drowning include

(A) water temperature above 70°F
(B) submersion less than 10 minutes
(C) fresh water rather than salt water
(D) spontaneous pulse and respiratory effort on arrival in the emergency room

---

DIRECTIONS: Each of the numbered items or incomplete statements in this section is negatively phrased, as indicated by a capitalized word such as NOT, LEAST, or EXCEPT. Select the ONE lettered answer or completion that is BEST in each case.

---

10. Each of the following statements about adolescent drivers is true EXCEPT

(A) they are more likely than older drivers to be involved in a fatal automobile crash
(B) they are more likely than older drivers to kill others in a collision
(C) when corrected for miles driven, the adolescent death rate in automobile crashes is the same as that for older drivers
(D) in communities with driver education, the death rate for adolescents in collisions is higher than that in communities without driver education
(E) alcohol plays a significant role in adolescent vehicle-related death and morbidity

11. Contraindications to induction of emesis in childhood poisoning include all of the following EXCEPT

(A) ingestion of turpentine
(B) rapidly increasing drowsiness
(C) ingestion of drain cleaner
(D) ingestion of acetaminophen
(E) ingestion by a child younger than 6 months

1–2. The answers are: 1-C *[XI E 3]*, **2-B** *[XI E 3 b (4)]*. In situations when an ingestion is unwitnessed, the "worst-case scenario" must be assumed at the outset to estimate potential toxicity. The maximum dose of iron ingested by this child is 65 mg elemental iron × 20 pills/13 kg = 100 mg/kg, which is a potentially serious dose. Among the symptoms caused by serious iron ingestion is vomiting; therefore, in this case, the vomiting must be considered related to the ingestion. This implies potential serious sequelae. Over-all, the ingestion must be regarded as clinically significant.

Because a single episode of vomiting does not empty the stomach sufficiently, either ipecac should be administered or gastric lavage performed. Activated charcoal does not adsorb iron and need not be given. Cathartics are helpful, once the stomach has been emptied. Serum iron and iron-binding capacity levels always should be drawn under such circumstances. A radiograph of the abdomen would be helpful because iron pills are radiopaque, and would give some indication of pills remaining in the gastrointestinal tract after initial treatment.

3. The answer is C *[VI B 2 a]*. Brain injury resulting from drowning may be severe, resistant to therapy or support, and is often permanent. The degree of hypoxia as part of the initial episode is probably the major determination with respect to outcome. Blood loss is rare in drownings. Arrhythmias are sometimes a secondary and possibly terminal event as a result of hypoxia, but the brain is severely damaged by the time an arrhythmia occurs. Pulmonary edema and acute renal failure, frequently associated with drowning, can be treated and supported during acute intensive therapy. Both usually resolve.

4. The answer is B *[I A 2; II B]*. The rapid deceleration that occurs as a result of motor vehicle collisions is responsible for massive changes in kinetic energy, and the transmission of kinetic energy to the human body is responsible for the severe tissue injuries that can be sustained. Thermal injury, such as that caused by a fire occurring as a result of a crash, is a much less common mode of injury. Electrocution can occur, although rarely, when a car hits a high-voltage pole.

5. The answer is A *[VII A 3 a]*. Electrical burns most often occur when a child chews on extension cord receptacles or frayed wires. As a result, severe burns to the corner of the mouth may require extensive plastic surgery. Scald burns are more likely to be external. Caustic substances can cause mouth burns, but these usually heal spontaneously. Esophageal scarring, which leads to stricture, is the most serious outcome from ingestion of caustics. Although burns on a child with no access to hot liquids or faucets can indicate child abuse, disfiguring mouth burns are not a common indicator of abuse.

6. The answer is C *[X A 2]*. Not surprisingly, football is the school sport most likely to result in injury. In most cases, however, sports injuries are minor and treated at school or at home. In school-related sports injuries, hospital care is sought infrequently. However, when a physician is consulted, radiographs or other tests are frequently obtained. Most sports injuries occur during practice and recreation. Reinjury is a significant problem and is usually caused by full exertion too soon after the initial injury, or by inadequate rehabilitation.

7. The answer is C *[V]*. Falls are responsible for the highest number of injury-related emergency ward visits. Head injuries and fractures are the most common serious diagnoses beyond bruises and sprains. Although relatively few emergency ward visits are the result of drowning, a large percentage of these patients (25% in one study) are admitted to the hospital. Since the establishment of poison control centers with telephone hotlines, there has been a decrease in the number of poisonings seen in emergency wards.

8. The answer is E *[VIII B 2, 3]*. Cyanosis, aphonia, absence of breath sounds, and wheezing all may be associated with foreign body aspiration. The site at which the object lodges determines the specific signs or symptoms noted. Cyanosis is associated with major airway obstruction at the level of the glottis. Aphonia (absence of speech) is associated with either esophageal obstruction with external pressure on the larynx or direct obstruction of that area of the airway. Absence of breath sounds results from obstruction of an entire lobe or lobar segment of the lung. Wheezing is caused by partial obstruction of the lower airway (bronchi and bronchioles), leading to a ball-valve effect that results in air trapping.

9. The answer is D *[VI B, C]*. Spontaneous pulse and respiratory effort are favorable predictors of either complete recovery or minimal sequelae after a submersion injury. Conversely, absence of these factors (i.e., the necessity for complete cardiopulmonary resuscitation in the emergency room) is a predictor of very poor outcome (over 90% death rate or severe sequelae). Submersion for less than 5 minutes and water temperature under 70°F (40°–60°F is optimum) are associated with better overall outcome. The salinity of water is not a determinant of recovery.

10. The answer is C *[II A 3]*. Adolescents are much more likely to die as a result of an automobile accident than adults, even when the rate is corrected for miles driven. Drivers who are 16–18 years of age have a fatality rate per miles driven that is 8–10 times that of 30-year-old drivers. Driver education has been shown to be associated with an increased incidence of motor vehicle-related death in communities where it is offered. This probably results from the increased number of licensed adolescent drivers as a consequence of the program. Alcohol plays a major role in both adolescent and adult vehicular death, but is a much less significant factor in child passenger deaths.

11. The answer is D *[XI D 1 a (2), E 2 b (2)]*. Acetaminophen can be removed by emesis without danger to the patient. Turpentine, which behaves as a volatile hydrocarbon, should not be removed by emesis because of the risk of lung aspiration. Drain cleaner, a corrosive, should not be removed owing to risk of repeated burning of the esophagus, which increases the risk of scarring. Emesis should not be induced in a child with a rapidly changing mental state because, in the 15–20 minutes it takes for ipecac to work, the child's alertness may become severely depressed, which can result in lung aspiration. Ipecac is safe for use in children older than 6 months of age.

Chapter 3

Psychosocial Pediatrics
M. Alex Geertsma

I. GENERAL CONSIDERATIONS

A. **Scope.** The topics outlined in this chapter involve a spectrum of issues and disorders that the pediatric practitioner will increasingly face owing to **changes in society and shifts in child-rearing philosophies**. The topics are largely psychosocial in nature but they may interact with various medical conditions, thereby affecting the overall health and well-being of children and their families.

B. **Practitioner's role.** The practitioner's role with these issues needs to be **multifaceted**. Each issue requires **a comprehensive, coordinated, and continuous approach**. Prior knowledge concerning factors such as the developmental status of the child, the emotional environment of the home, and the child's intrinsic temperament is invaluable in approaching these problems. The primary care pediatric practitioner who is committed to broad and thorough child health supervision will have that knowledge readily available.

1. In some cases, the practitioner's role may be primarily to diagnose and to help devise a treatment plan.

2. In other cases, it may be solely to consult individuals or the community concerning approaches to child-rearing or public agency guidelines (e.g., custody in divorce, guidelines for medical screening of adoptees).

3. In still other cases, the practitioner's role may be limited to practical advice and empathetic support (e.g., death of a family member).

II. FAILURE TO THRIVE

A. **Definition.** Failure to thrive is a term typically used to describe infants and young children whose weight is persistently below the third percentile for age on an appropriate standardized growth chart, or less than 80% of ideal weight for age. It may also present as an acute weight loss or failure to gain weight at an expected rate.

B. **Etiology.** Failure to thrive is viewed as the final **common pathway** for multiple problems that result in an **inadequate caloric intake or utilization**.

C. **Assessment**

1. A detailed **history and physical examination** often identify the etiology of failure to thrive. Observations of the mother–infant interaction may suggest a disordered relationship. In particular, the physician should gather:
   a. A detailed history of the child's **caloric intake** (i.e., a 48-hour dietary recall)
   b. Information about a typical mealtime experience
   c. Information about poor feeding, drooling, distractibility, and bowel habits

2. **Laboratory data** usually are not significant without positive findings in the history and physical examination.
   a. **Routine laboratory tests** should include complete blood count, urine culture, urinalysis, blood urea nitrogen, and examination of stool for ova and parasites and for reducing substances. A sweat test and chest radiograph may be considered.
   b. **Additional laboratory investigation** should be conducted based on information gathered in the history and physical examination.

D. **Therapy**

1. If any organic illness is identified, treatment specific for that disorder should be undertaken.

2. If the initial history and physical and laboratory data do not suggest an organic explanation for the failure to thrive, a **high-calorie diet** consisting of one and one-half to two times the child's daily caloric requirements should be devised.

3. Parents should keep a **detailed diary** of the child's caloric intake. If they are unable to get the child to take the high-calorie diet, consultation with a dietitian may be helpful in creating a diet with increased calories but without increased volume.

4. If the parents cannot enforce the high-calorie diet and if no weight gain occurs, **hospitalization** should be considered so that intake and weight gain can be carefully monitored and further evaluation can take place. Parental involvement in feeding the child during the hospitalization is crucial.

5. **Interactive issues must be addressed.**
   a. An **interdisciplinary team** including social workers, psychiatrists/psychologists, nurses, and developmental specialists is very helpful.
   b. In 80% of cases of failure to thrive in which an initial detailed history, physical examination, and routine laboratory tests are negative, an interactive etiology will eventually be discovered. Treatment must be directed to remediation of the interactive problem.

E. **Outcome.** When an organic etiology is discovered, prognosis depends on the severity of the disease process.

1. Outcome for **interactional failure to thrive** is more variable and dependent on the effectiveness of remediation of the interactive problem.

2. These children usually **remain at risk** for growth problems, developmental delays, and various patterns of psychosocial maladaptation. This is especially true when the interactional problem and failure to thrive have been of long standing.

III. **CHILD ABUSE**

A. **Definitions**

1. **Physical abuse** is the nonaccidental injury of a child.

2. **Sexual abuse** is any sexual activity between an adult and a child (assaultive or nonassaultive; see Chapter 5 VI E).

3. **Physical neglect** is failure to provide the necessities of life for a child (i.e., nourishment, clothing, shelter, supervision, and medical care).

4. **Emotional neglect** involves parental failure to provide an environment in which the child can thrive and develop.

5. **Munchausen syndrome by proxy** is defined as a syndrome in which the child becomes a victim of parentally induced or parentally fabricated illness, which often causes the child to undergo unnecessary diagnostic and sometimes therapeutic interventions.

B. **Incidence.** Seven hundred new cases of child abuse occur per million people per year in the United States. The mortality rate is 3%, or 2000 deaths per year. In children aged 1–6 months, child abuse is second only to sudden infant death syndrome as a cause of child mortality. In the group aged 1–5 years, it is second to accidental injuries as a killer of children. One third of child abuse victims are younger than 1 year of age, one third are aged 1–6 years, and one third are older than 6 years. Premature infants have a risk of abuse three times higher than full-term infants.

C. **Etiology.** The abuser is a related adult in 90% of cases of child abuse. Only 10% of abusers are seriously emotionally ill. The overwhelming majority are isolated and stressed individuals with limited social support.

D. **When to suspect child abuse.** Physically abused children usually present to physicians with an acute injury or a history of recurrent injury. A detailed history of the circumstances surrounding each episode of injury is essential to screen for the possibility of abuse or neglect. Red flags that should arouse suspicions of abuse include:

1. **Recurrent injuries or ingestions.** Some "accident-prone" children are really abused children.

2. **Injuries that are out of proportion to or atypical for a child's developmental stage:**
   a. Head contusion in a child who cannot yet stand or walk
   b. Back bruises in a child who cannot yet climb
   c. Burns in a child who has no access to hot liquids or faucets

3. **Evidence or marks of inflicted injury** (e.g., from a belt buckle)

4. **Injuries that are known to have a high association with abuse:**
   a. Scald burns of the buttocks
   b. Cigarette burns
   c. Spiral fracture of the femur
   d. Retinal hemorrhage due to shaken baby syndrome
   e. Subdural hematoma

5. **Parental supervision that is inadequate** for the child's age

6. **Parental psychiatric disease,** including psychosis and depression

7. **A history of the events surrounding the incident that is inconsistent** with the observed injury

E. **Obtaining confirmatory information and a further detailed history.** Before the physical examination, it is critical to obtain as accurate and detailed a history as possible. However, discussion with the child should be developmentally appropriate and nonthreatening. Repeated questioning or badgering is both inhumane and nonproductive. The parents should be interviewed in a nonconfrontational, nonjudgmental manner that is culturally sensitive. The pediatric provider should seek answers to the following questions.

1. Are the **circumstances** surrounding the injury as documented by the parents consistent with the physical findings?

2. Is the **explanation** of the injury plausible, given the child's age and developmental capabilities?

3. Is there a **history of previous trauma?**

4. Was there a **delay** in seeking care?

F. **Physical examination.** Photographs of the trauma should be obtained, if possible.

1. **Cutaneous lesions frequently seen in abuse** and a **guide to dating bruises** are presented in Table 3-1.

TABLE 3-1. Cutaneous Lesions Often Seen in Abused Children

Lesion	Likely Cause
Linear bruising	Striking with a stick or rod
Loop marks	Striking with a belt or cord
Circumferential bruises	Binding injury (e.g., hands tied with rope)
Scald injuries in a "stocking/ glove" distribution	Submersion in hot water

Time Since Injury	Appearance
0–2 days	Area swollen and tender
0–5 days	Area red or blue in color
5–7 days	Area green in color
7–10 days	Area yellow in color
10–14 days	Area brown in color
2–4 weeks	Discoloration gone

2. If **sexual abuse** is a concern, careful examination of the external genitalia and rectum is imperative. If available, colposcopic examination should be performed. However, with younger children, the need for accurate and rapid documentation of findings must be carefully weighed against the potential psychological trauma of an invasive genital examination performed by inexperienced staff. If time and resources allow, it may be advisable to defer the more invasive aspects of the examination to more experienced staff in a more developmentally appropriate and supportive setting (e.g., sexual abuse specialty program).

G. **Laboratory data**

1. Coagulation studies (to determine if there is a bleeding disorder present), urinalysis, and a long bone survey should be performed.

2. If sexual abuse is considered, cultures of the mouth, rectum, vagina, and urethra should be obtained (see III F 2). A Venereal Disease Research Laboratory test should be performed, and vaginal fluid should be aspirated to check for semen.

H. **Therapy and outcome**

1. **Notification** of the appropriate **state protective agency** is vital. **Physicians and other providers are mandated to report** abuse in every state and are protected from liability. Failure to report abuse can lead to further harm to the child and prosecution of the non-reporting provider.

2. Children who are physically or sexually abused or neglected and who have serious physical injuries or acute psychological symptoms (e.g., suicidal behavior or ideation) may require **acute hospitalization**.

3. For otherwise stable children, it is the combined responsibility of the pediatric provider and the state protective agency to identify and provide **a safe place of protection for the child** until more formal temporary placement can be arranged. This may require hospitalization.

4. Hospitalization may also be required if the case for or against abuse is confusing and further reliable evaluation is necessary.

5. If not involved from the beginning, the **primary care provider should be contacted** as soon as possible and be afforded the opportunity to be involved directly or, at least, to provide helpful background information. The primary care provider can also serve as a valuable liaison with the family.

6. The current trend is to **provide services to the family** to allow them to care for the child more adequately. Removal of the child from the home, or termination of parental rights, is usually a last resort and occurs only after serious abuse has occurred without response to treatment. This philosophy is **controversial,** especially when interventional services to families are limited because of resource restrictions and the risk for recurrent abuse is accordingly high.

7. With treatment, most abusing families can provide adequate care for their children. **Without effective intervention, 25%** of these children will be **repeatedly abused, and 5% will be killed**.

IV. FOSTER CARE

A. **Purpose of foster care.** The overall purpose of foster care is to provide a **safe, temporary placement for a child who is at social, emotional, or physical risk**.

1. Remediation of the factors that led to the child's placement, usually related to family dysfunction, is to be accomplished successfully and rapidly to minimize disruption of the child–family relationship.

2. The complexities of family dysfunction, in addition to limitations in available resources and coordination of services, often make this goal difficult to achieve.

3. Therefore, children in foster care are frequently **at risk of remaining out of the home too long or of being returned to a home that remains disrupted or even dangerous**.

B. **Relevant statistics and changing characteristics.** It is estimated that **4 of every 1000 children in the United States (i.e., approximately 300,000 total)** are in foster care. Over the last two decades, foster children have come from increasingly more difficult social situations than in the past.

1. The most common reasons for placement had been extreme poverty, absence or death of the parents, and severe chronic disease or mental retardation.

2. Now, the most common reasons for placement are neglect, physical or sexual abuse, and acquired immune deficiency syndrome (AIDS). Foster placements for child abuse or neglect increased 82% between 1982 and 1988.

C. **Structure of the foster care system**

1. Individual **states are responsible** to set up foster systems, usually via state departments of social service. The state systems are regulated by state and federal statutes.

2. Because of the federal program called Aid to Families of Dependent Children, children in foster care are eligible for basic health services via Medicaid and the Early Periodic Screening, Diagnosis, and Treatment Program. Therefore, **coordination between state departments** of social service and public health agencies is important.

3. Title IV-E of the federal Social Security Act provides for **remediation services for parents,** administered by state social service departments.

D. **Referral and placement pattern**

1. Increasing numbers of children remain in foster care for prolonged periods and later in life. Nearly 50% are adolescents.

2. Among foster children, minorities are highly overrepresented.

3. **More boys than girls** are in foster care. **Girls** are more likely to be placed in foster care because of **sexual abuse,** whereas boys are more likely to be placed because of physical abuse. **Boys are more likely to be physically or cognitively impaired** at the time of placement.

    4. Between 20% and 30% of foster children who go back to their families are **returned to foster care**. Although 50% return within 30 days, 25% take 2 years or more. Approximately 25% of children in foster care have three or more placements in their lives before permanent resolution.

    5. Placement may be:
      a. Voluntary by a stressed parent
      b. Voluntary with court ratification
      c. Involuntary via court order

    6. Once the case is adjudicated, a foster case worker who must collect, transmit, and coordinate information to referral agencies is assigned to the case to coordinate placement, remediation, and reunion with the family.

    7. The main potential problem often stems from too few trained case workers.

E. | **Characteristics of foster homes**

    1. Types of foster arrangements are listed in Table 3-2.

    2. Problems with foster arrangements include the following.
      a. The **reimbursement is often low,** usually only covering the foster family's costs, attracting either the very altruistic or the economically impoverished.
      b. As a result, there may be **shortages of qualified foster families** in a given area.
      c. Siblings may be placed in separate foster homes, leading to **possible dissolution of the sibling relationship**.

F. | **Characteristics of the birth family and risk for recurrent foster placement or loss of custody**

    1. Lower socioeconomic status families are more likely to have their children placed in foster care, even when controlling for severity of family dysfunction.

    2. These families often have **histories of continuing multigenerational dysfunction,** abuse, neglect, psychiatric problems, and substance abuse.

    3. However, funding for rehabilitation of the birth family is often inadequate.

    4. With the tendency to favor reunification with the birth family in the face of poor rehabilitation funding, foster children can be returned to the birth home prematurely, which may lead to further abuse or neglect, and reentry into foster placement.

    5. Minimal instruction for foster families on how to interact with and support the birth family can lead to an adversarial relationship and avoidance of visitation. This may lead to abandonment or permanent loss of custody.

G. | **Problems of children in foster care**

    1. Development and emotional risk
      a. Children placed in foster care have a **high incidence of failure to thrive** and growth problems.

TABLE 3-2. Types of Foster Arrangement

Type of Foster Home	Advantages	Disadvantages
Extended family (kinship care)	Familiarity to child	Risk for similar pathology as parents
Group homes	Highly specialized for special-needs children or adolescents	Expense and availability
Private foster homes	Often highly dedicated	Availability; depends on adequacy of screening

b. They are at risk for **developmental delay, behavioral problems, and psychiatric disorders**.

c. Contributing factors include maternal substance use during pregnancy, prematurity, and emotional and cognitive deprivation, in addition to sexual and physical abuse.

d. One study suggests that 23% of children younger than 5 years of age who are placed in foster care will have abnormal or suspect development.

2. **Physical health and health care of foster children**

   a. Foster children are **less likely** to have a defined, constant source of **primary health care**. This makes preplacement and postplacement documentation of health status difficult.

   b. Between 40% and 76% of foster children have **chronic medical problems** that are often inadequately addressed.

   c. Dental, visual, and hearing problems are the most common. Also frequent are preventable or treatable diseases such as allergy and asthma, which may be worsened by noncontinuous, episodic (e.g., emergency department) medical contacts rather than regular care.

3. **The special problem of AIDS** (see Chapter 9)

   a. Increasing numbers of children whose parents have AIDS are being placed in foster care. Currently, 27% of children whose parents are actively infected with human immunodeficiency virus (HIV) are in foster care. The numbers and percentages are likely to rise.

   b. Permanent placement or adoption may occur as a result of parental psychosocial issues and prognosis or the death of the parents.

H. Outcome

1. Foster **placement** in a stable home **decreases abuse** and maltreatment.

2. **Improved school attendance** is observed in placed foster children versus similar-risk children who remain with their biologic families. School performance differences are less often noted.

3. Foster children are **more likely to receive special education and psychiatric services** when needed than if they remain in their unstable home situations.

4. Previous fears of foster care leading to further abuse by foster families are unfounded **if the foster families are adequately screened and prepared**.

5. There is a higher incidence of **conduct problems and assault** by children placed in foster care versus other children once they reach adolescence and adulthood. This is reflective of the degree of preplacement abuse and psychological disturbance rather than a result of foster care.

I. **Role of the pediatric provider.** The pediatric provider who chooses to care for and advocate for foster children should:

1. **Screen and evaluate** children for foster care placement, concentrating on developmental, behavioral, and medical issues

2. Serve as **a source of continuous, coordinated primary medical care** when possible

   a. As an alternative, the provider should seek out comprehensive data on the child from previous multiple sources of care, summarize it, and devise an **overall medical plan** for use by other designated providers. **Foster care clinics** exist to assist with medical care of these children.

   b. The **"medical passport,"** which is a continuously updated medical record that accompanies the foster child from placement to placement, can provide shifting providers a degree of consistent medical information.

3. Serve as **consultant** to state and local foster care agencies

4. **Advocate for** consistently applied **standards** for the assessment of foster families

5. **Advocate for training for foster families,** especially to support the developmental, behavioral, and emotional needs of the child; also, to supportively communicate and cooperate with the biologic family

6. If the goal is to reunite families, advocate for more extensive remediation services for the biologic family

V. ADOPTION

A. Scope and incidence

1. Approximately 2%–3% of children in the United States younger than 18 years of age (i.e., approximately 2.5 million children) are adopted.

2. Two thirds of all adopted children are adopted by related family, and the remaining one third by people outside the family.

B. Changing patterns of adoption

1. The peak number of adoptions per year in the United States was 175,000 in 1970. It fell to 142,000 per year in 1982, where it has leveled.

2. For adoptees younger than 2 years of age, the number of yearly adoptions fell from 89,000 in 1970 to approximately half that in 1975, and has leveled.

3. The **decreasingly available number of adoptees,** especially younger children, **is the result of:**
   a. The greater use of **contraception** and **abortion**
   b. Changes in societal **attitudes about illegitimacy:** more children born out of wedlock are kept by the biologic parents
   c. Improved financial and nutritional **support for single mothers and lower socioeconomic status mothers** with young children
   d. The birth rate growth is highest in inner-city, lower socioeconomic status groups. However, **inner-city families** tend to maintain and support children of single mothers within an **extended family system** rather than give up children to adoption.

4. Because of the increased divorce rate, increasing numbers of children are being adopted by a step-parent spouse of the biologic parent who has sole custody.

5. A greater proportion of available adoptees are older, have special developmental or emotional needs, are of mixed racial backgrounds, are from foreign countries, or are at high medical risk.

C. Laws and regulations

1. The Adoption Assistance and Child Welfare Act of 1980 (PL 96-272) established **standards for adoption procedures;** it also provided for subsidies for adopted children with special needs.

2. The states, usually via departments of social service, actually implement the standards and fund subsidies.

D. Methods of adoption

1. **Screening of adoptive parents** occurs via a process of in-depth **"home study,"** which is an extensive formal review of the adoptive family, household, and past history.

2. **Types of placement.** There are three types of adoption placement—**private, agency, and international**.

E. **Problems and controversies involving adoption.** As a result of decreasing numbers of young infants for adoption, the pool of children considered available for adoption has expanded.

1. **Increasing numbers of "at-risk" children for adoption.** With increasing numbers of "at-risk" children, more of these children are available for adoption (see V B 5), which causes problems with having enough available homes and support resources for adoptive families.

2. **Increasing numbers of interracial adoptions** have occurred. Recent concerns have been raised about possible racial identity problems.
   a. Early in childhood, there are no such problems for most interracially adopted children. Most children are raised in the same culture as the adoptive parents.
   b. The overall success of interracial adoptions is better with a stable adoptive family with a high socioeconomic status, as well as when a younger child is adopted.
   c. Exaggerated identity issues may arise at adolescence.

3. **International adoption** has increased sporadically as a result of economic downturns, war, and political upheaval in certain countries.
   a. Whereas these situations provide a source of adoptees, they have raised **ethical and legal questions** internationally, and have led to **instability and irregularities in the adoption process**.
   b. In some extreme circumstances, this may lead to adoptive parents traveling great distances at great expense only to be disappointed or to receive a different child than promised.
   c. **Special health issues** exist for these children, **largely involving infectious diseases**. A study of infectious disease screening of 293 adoptees from 15 countries has shown that:
      (1) **Hepatitis B** is present in approximately 5% of adoptees, most of whom are Asian, and many of whom have histories of transfusion.
      (2) **Tuberculosis** is present in approximately 3% of adoptees, 40% of whom have evidence of pulmonary tuberculosis.
      (3) **Pathogenic intestinal parasites** are present in approximately 14% of adoptees.

4. **Increasing numbers of older and single adults** have begun to seek children for adoption. These people often receive children who are older, handicapped, emotionally at risk, and generally more difficult to place.
   a. Financial and general child-rearing demands of the single parent are magnified by adoption. Children with handicaps or emotional problems also may be difficult for single parents to handle alone.
   b. Some agencies, therefore, refuse to place children with single parents. However, when controlling for child risk factors and economics, the outcome with single-parent placements can be very good.
   c. The older adoptive parent may be relatively set in lifestyle and have a greater need for adjustment to the demands of child-rearing. Overall, they are highly motivated and more economically stable, which leads to a better outcome.

F. **Outcome for adoptive children**

1. Limited retrospective studies have suggested **greater than expected risk** histories of adoption **among children referred for mental health services**.

2. Early prospective studies have suggested **special risk for adopted boys**.
   a. The odds for adopted boys having psychiatric problems at 8 to 20 years of age are 2.28 times higher than for boys who are not adopted.
   b. The most frequent diagnoses are **conduct disorders, affective disorders, attention-deficit hyperactivity disorders,** and **obsessive-compulsive disorders**.
   c. The odds of negative outcome are further increased for adopted boys if they have associated performance problems early in their school years.
   d. **No such differences** are noted **for adopted girls**.

3. The **origins** of increased psychiatric problems for adopted boys **are unclear**.
   a. Adoptive family issues appear not to play a role.
   b. Factors implicated include adoption later in childhood, identity and developmental stage issues, and biologic family mental health history.

4. Overall, although there is a higher incidence of psychiatric problems, **more recent prospective work** shows there is **less risk than previously feared** for adoptive children.

5. **Intelligence quotient scores and school attainment** appear to be **as good** as for nonadopted children and actually higher than expected from the biologic parents' profile.

6. **Factors** that are associated with **unsuccessful adoptions** include:
   a. Previous unsuccessful adoptions involving the child
   b. Older age at placement
   c. Antecedent behavioral or emotional problems
   d. Borderline socioeconomic status of the adoptive family without subsidy
   e. Adoptive family with multiple other children
   f. Inadequate preparation of the adoptive family for an "at-risk" child

G. | **Role of the pediatric health care provider**

1. **Information on the medical status** of the child should be compiled and discussed with the adoptive family. Histories may be incomplete. A thorough initial health assessment, including behavioral and developmental status, is essential.

2. **Screens for various diseases,** including **hepatitis B** [especially if the child is Asian or at infection risk (i.e., biologic mother's history)], **tuberculosis,** and **intestinal parasites** should be performed. Routine screening for **HIV is usually not indicated**.

3. The adoptee's identity and attachment issues should be assessed, especially for older children. Evidence of other historical **behavioral, emotional, or developmental risk factors** should be considered. If needed, possible referrals should be discussed at a later date.

4. The family structure and expectations of the adoptive family should be reviewed.

5. The family should be aided with the dilemma of **"when to tell"** the child of her or his adoptive status.
   a. The **common wisdom** has been **between 2 and 3 years** of age, despite limited understanding during the preoperational period (see Chapter 1). Being told the child was "chosen" is usually taken positively by the child and may allow for better adjustment during the next period.
   b. At **school age** (concrete operations period, see Chapter 1), the child is better **able to comprehend "being given up."** With growing identity concerns, supportive ongoing discussion is required. A school-age adoptee is at risk of having feelings of being unworthy or different, along with being worried about change, disruption, and intrusion by the biologic parents.
   c. During both **late school age and adolescence,** learning of the adoption for the first time may magnify normal adolescent issues of ambivalence toward and relative alienation from the adoptive parents.

VI. CHILD CARE

A. | **Definition.** A child is receiving child care when he or she is regularly being cared for **part of the day or night by someone other than his or her parent**. Other common popular terms used are "day care," preschool, early childhood care program, nursery school, and babysitting.

B. Relevance and scope

1. **By the late 1980s** in the United States, **59% of women** with children younger than 15 years of age (approximately 30.6 million children) **were employed**.

2. The fastest-growing group of families is those in which both parents work and have an infant younger than 1 year of age.

3. Two thirds of mothers with children between 3 and 5 years of age are employed.

4. Approximately 40% of marriages end in divorce. The number of families headed by a never-married mother has increased fourfold since 1970. Both of these situations have contributed to the need for more out-of-home care for children.

5. Yet, the United States is the only one of 75 industrialized countries without a formal government-sponsored plan that subsidizes or regulates child care.

C. Types of child care

1. **Intrafamilial arrangements,** in which other members of the immediate or extended family care for the child, cannot be accurately assessed. In some cases, older school-age children may care for younger siblings during part of the day.

2. **Care in the child's own home** is provided by a nonfamily employee (e.g., a babysitter, a nanny).

3. **Family-run child care homes** are where six or more children are cared for in a **private caregiver's home**.

4. **Center-based child care** is provided in relatively large centers where professional staff care for 13 or more children.

D. Impact of child care on the child

1. **Emotional development.** The **hotly debated issue** of whether early child care (i.e., for infants younger than 1 year of age) adversely affects the child has been a mix of science, politics, religion, and child-rearing philosophy.
   a. The **case against early day care** has been based on **studies of "attachment"** of children placed in day care early in their lives. They have suggested poor attachment to the mother and possible later emotional problems.
   b. There is **no clear evidence of actual emotional damage** referable to early day care in controlled, longitudinal studies; that is, emotional outcome is no worse than home care with an at-home mother.
   c. However, the lack of detrimental effects **depends on high-quality child care** (see VI E).

2. **Apparent beneficial social effects**
   a. Children who are in day care early in their lives are often **more socially competent**. They are more peer oriented and somewhat more assertive and aggressive.
   b. With an emphasis by caretakers on verbal interaction and cognitive learning experiences, assertiveness is usually expressed in positive ways.
   c. There are apparent **additional social and emotional benefits** to children from deprived, **at-risk** environments. Therefore, day care is often used as a diagnostic and therapeutic placement for at-risk children.

3. **Potential cognitive benefits**
   a. There are overall cognitive gains from day care early in life, and they are most marked in deprived and socially at-risk children.
   b. **Improvements are seen primarily with high-quality child care,** where there is an emphasis on a structured learning curriculum, the best large-scale example being the federally funded Head Start program.
   c. Parallel effects on emotional development and positive attitudes toward learning make academic achievement more likely.

      d. The persistence of effects, including intelligence, **depends on continued enrichment** during the school-age years, in addition to improvement in the home social environment.

  4. Other effects and benefits of child care

      a. High-quality child care can provide general **support to parents** by:

         (1) Relieving stress and guilt

         (2) Providing reassurance about the child's well-being and safety

         (3) Decreasing the risk for child abuse/neglect by providing day care respite for an at-risk parent and child

      b. Improved parental job attendance and performance

      c. High-quality programs can be a vehicle for **promotion of optimal health behaviors**. They can:

         (1) Provide a means of monitoring immunization status and encouraging parental compliance

         (2) Promote health maintenance visits

         (3) Teach preventive health and present a child development perspective to young or at-risk parents

E. Assessing the quality of child care

  1. Regulation and standards. At present, there are no federal guidelines for child care. Regulation is at the discretion of each state.

      a. Most states focus on the physical setting and health and safety issues only. Little emphasis is placed on other measures of quality.

      b. Of the 50 states, 34 states have hand-washing and staff hygiene requirements. All but three states have basic immunization verification requirements.

      c. Requirements for curricula in larger centers exist in 34 states, but do not address small or family-run child care programs.

      d. The dilemma facing regulators and state legislators is **maintaining quality while not putting already scarce child care providers out of business**.

  2. Determinants of child care quality. Standards for assessing the quality of child care have been established and published by nongovernmental agencies. These should be made available to parents by pediatric providers, early educators, and social service and community agencies.

F. **Infectious illnesses in child care.** Common, acute, non–life-threatening infectious diseases are a major problem for working parents and their employers.

  1. Between **80% and 85% of working parents miss time from work because of their children's illnesses**. Most center-based and many family-based child care programs do not allow ill children to be present.

  2. In the United States, mothers miss 5.6 to 28.8 days per year from work because of their children's illnesses. Approximately 40% of parental work absences are the result of children's illness.

  3. Children in group day care are significantly more likely to experience six or more limited infectious illnesses per year and four or more prolonged illnesses. There is a decline in illnesses by 3 and 4 years of age, but the overall rate is significantly greater than in children cared for at home by nonworking mothers (Figures 3-1 and 3-2).

G. **Role of the pediatric provider.** The pediatric provider can **help support families in selecting** high-quality child care by:

  1. Reviewing with parents **plans for work** and child care as early as the prenatal visit

  2. Providing **information and resources for parents** such as:

      a. How to assess the quality of child care (see VI E)

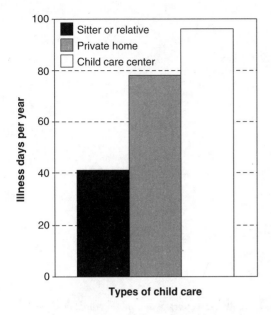

FIGURE 3-1. Days per year a child is sick in various types of child care situations.

Legend:
- Sitter or relative
- Private home
- Child care center

Y-axis: Illness days per year
X-axis: **Types of child care**

    b. Sources for potential financial subsidy; centers with governmental funding, "sliding scales," or scholarships

    c. Lists of local and state accreditation agencies

    d. Lists of local centers and nanny services, including their accreditation status and payment arrangements

  3. Sharing **knowledge on the effects of child care,** stressing positive aspects and emphasizing quality issues

  4. **Advocating** at the local and state level **for support and funding** for the development of high-quality child care

  5. **Consulting** to child care agencies and local and state governments on health and safety standards and measures of quality

  6. **Communicating** specific health, developmental, and behavioral concerns to the child care facility **via the required admissions forms** after appropriate parental consent is documented, including:
    a. Special medical instructions
    b. How to be contacted for specific concerns or emergencies involving the child

  7. Considering alternative or **extended office hours** to support working parents' needs

VII. DIVORCE

A. Incidence, patterns, and trends

  1. The **rate of divorce** in the United States has **doubled** between the 1960s and the 1980s.

  2. Approximately 38% of children born in the mid-1980s will experience divorce by 18 years of age.

  3. Approximately 1.2–1.5 million children (i.e., 5%) face divorce in their families each year.

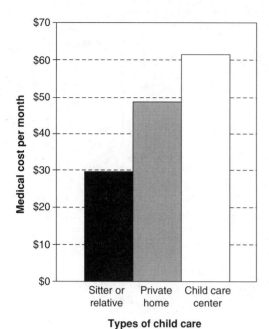

Types of child care

FIGURE 3-2. Average monthly medical cost per child versus the type of child care situation.

B. **Characteristic issues facing divorcing families**

1. **Major life changes,** and physical and emotional disruptions for children **are the rule** rather than the exception. Depending on family or extrafamilial resources (e.g., friends, relatives), major life changes may or may not adversely interact with sensitive age-related and developmental stage-related issues (e.g., separation anxiety, adolescent "rebellion") to magnify **problems of adjustment for child and family**.

2. **Parental hostility,** which frequently is present before and after divorce, may not resolve for years.

3. **Custody may be contentious,** and final arrangements may not always be made in the best interest of the child.

C. **Custody**

1. **Definition.** Custody is defined as the formal or legal living arrangement for the child of divorced parents in addition to the pattern of contact and the legal responsibilities of the parents.

2. Table 3-3 summarizes patterns of custody.

3. The dilemma of custody is how to balance several important issues:
   a. Financial security for the child
   b. The need to minimize changes in the child's life routine (i.e., school, friends) and to promote extended family support
   c. Maintenance of as much contact as possible with each parent
   d. The need to avoid hostile contacts between divorced parents, especially in the presence of the child

D. **Short-term effects**

1. The **acute stage** lasts from 6 months to 2 years after the divorce is initiated. It is characterized by **emotional and daily functional disruptions** for the child and family. **Anger and preoccupation of the parents** can result in ineffective parenting. The two **most**

TABLE 3-3. Patterns of Custody in Divorce Settlements

Type	Description	Advantages	Disadvantages	Comments
Sole	One parent has exclusive legal responsibility and physical custody; visitation and some financial child support may be ordered by the courts	Less potential contact between parents; less emotional entrapment for child	Higher risk of fewer financial resources for child and custody parent (mother); high risk for lost contact with other parent (father)	Sole custodian is mother 75%–90% of time; boys do less well if mother is sole custodian; decreased contact with other parent may lead to long-term emotional problems for child
Joint legal	Both parents share legal responsibility; one parent often has primary physical custody (mother); other parent has more contact than in sole custody	Less risk of financial deterioration for child; more contact with other parent (father)	More contact between parents; more risk for emotional entrapment of the child	Works best when there is an "amiable" divorce
Joint physical	Both parents (in principle) share 50–50 physical custody	Less risk of financial deterioration; continued contact with both parents	Maximal contact between parents; possible disruption of child's daily or weekly routine	Requires significant cooperation between parents

stressful events are learning about the divorce and the actual departure of one of the parents. Table 3-4 summarizes acute age-related manifestations of divorce for the child.

2. The **transition stage** begins once acute adjustment issues are resolved. There are fewer actual changes or challenges for the child. The real issues are related more to the custodial parent's life adjustments and their indirect effects on the child (e.g., new job or career pursuits, beginning new adult relationships).

3. The **postdivorce stage** is marked by "final" changes (e.g., adjustment to a new neighborhood and home for the child; a new job or marriage for the custodial parent).
   a. Approximately 75% of women and 80% of men remarry. However, 50% of children of divorce whose parents remarry will experience a second divorce.
   b. Significant potential problems can occur with adaptation to and acceptance of the step-parent and any family the step-parent may bring. These problems may reoccur.

E. | **Long-term outcome**

1. **Most children of divorce do reasonably well** compared to nondivorced children of the same age.

2. However, **the incidence of poor adaptation is greater in children of divorce**.

3. **Negative long-term findings (5–10-year follow-up):**
   a. The older the child at the time of divorce, the greater the chance of negative outcome. Those who were preschoolers at the time of divorce did best.
   b. In one sample, 41% of children of divorce showed continued depression, feelings of rejection, and alienation from their parents 10 years after the divorce.
   c. Approximately 25% of children of divorce had experienced severe and lasting deterioration in their standard of living, which affected their overall adjustment.
   d. **Boys** showed a significantly **greater incidence and number of problems** than girls. Problems were largely externalizing disorders (e.g., impulse control, conduct disorders, peer relationship difficulties, and aggression).
   e. More of a delayed onset was noted for girls, involving problems in relationships **with men in adulthood**.
   f. To a lesser degree, internalizing disorders also were present for boys and girls, including depression, anxiety disorders, social withdrawal, and increased need for mental health services.

4. **Factors contributing to long-term outcome**
   a. **Predivorce and postdivorce functioning of parents. Continued parental hostility** has been shown to be the single strongest predictor of long-term maladjustment for children of divorce.

TABLE 3-4. Acute Age-Related Manifestations of Divorce

Age Period	Manifestations
Preschool (2–4 years)	Regressive behaviors: sleep instability, tantrums, separation resistance, bowel/bladder problems, increased need for attention Egocentric sense of guilt/responsibility
Early–mid school-aged (5–8 years)	Overt depressive behavior, open grieving, fear of being replaced, deterioration of peer relationships, phobias
Late school-aged, early adolescence (9–13 years)	Anger directed at parents, blame and recrimination about parents "not having done enough" to avoid divorce, school and peer problems
Adolescence (14–18 years)	Exaggeration of adolescent issues: insecurity, loneliness, social isolation, depression Magnified acting out: school failure, truancy, criminal behavior, substance abuse, pregnancy

b. Other factors negatively influencing outcome include:
   (1) Limited access to the noncustodial parent
   (2) Past and continued exposure of children to physical violence
   (3) Poor, inconsistent patterns of parenting (e.g., inconsistent limits, lack of warmth and emotional support when needed, poor parental skills in conflict resolution)
   (4) Lack of siblings
   (5) Unstable school and peer situations
   (6) Difficult temperament profile
   (7) Older age at the time of divorce
   (8) Male gender
   (9) Unstable economic situation with inadequate child support provisions

F. **Role of the pediatric provider**

1. Pediatricians are viewed by divorcing parents as a valuable source of help and advice. However, relatively few parents actually turn to their pediatricians. Most pediatricians learn of the divorce after it is final.

2. The pediatric provider can be a helpful resource.
   a. It is important to be aware of signs of family crisis (e.g., a change in mood while in the office, increased use of services for minor medical problems, agitated or depressed affect of parent or child).
   b. The pediatric provider should try to "leave the door open" by giving attention to behavioral and developmental issues during well-child visits.
   c. The pediatric provider's being a supportive source of information to both parents without taking sides can be very helpful.
   d. Scheduled appointments to discuss openly the divorce plans and to provide information on the effects of divorce and how to go about avoiding a negative outcome should be offered to divorcing parents.
   e. The pediatric provider's being available to discuss effective approaches to specific behavioral and adjustment problems and to consider referral for more involved problems is also helpful.
   f. When considering to whom to refer parents, it appears that a combination of both child- and family-centered intervention plus attention to the issues of home and environmental change, economic stability, and social support for the child (i.e., a multidimensional approach) may be most effective.

3. **Advice to parents** about informing the child of the impending divorce includes:
   a. Consider the developmental stage of the child when choosing words to explain the situation.
   b. Reinforce and reassure the child that all that could be done to keep the marriage together has been done.
   c. Repeatedly assure the child that he or she will be safe and will not be alone, and that everything possible will be done to keep familiar, reassuring things unchanged.
   d. Avoid undermining the other parent in the child's mind.

VIII. CHILDHOOD BEREAVEMENT: DEATH OF A PARENT

A. **Incidence.** Approximately **5%** of children in the United States (i.e., 1.5 million children) will experience the **death of a parent by 15 years of age**.

B. The **impact** on the child varies.

1. Although similarities to adult grieving exist in children, there are differences related to:
   a. Developmental stage
   b. Different behavioral manifestations of grief versus adults
   c. Temperamental variation

2. Typical stages of bereavement include:
   a. Understanding and coming to terms with the death
   b. True mourning, a true sense of loss
   c. Resumption of normal living

C. Short-term outcome

1. Retrospective studies of children whose parents die when the children are young have suggested **increased risk for early behavior problems and depression**.

2. A poor outcome may be avoided if the surviving parent, family, schoolteachers, and peers provide support and allow the child to resume normal routines.

3. **Factors** associated with **relatively greater risk** for behavioral and emotional problems include:
   a. The mother is the survivor and the sole source of economic support
   b. A preexisting, untreated child psychiatric disorder
   c. Family history of depression
   d. Overall problems of family adjustment to the death
   e. Previous troubled relationship with dead parent
   f. Violent or suicidal death of the parent

4. **Adolescents** may not necessarily do better simply because they are older and understand better.
   a. There is a relatively high degree of school dysfunction and depressive symptoms in adolescents who lose a parent.
   b. Although the adolescent is better able to understand death, the issues of adolescent independence and identity confusion may adversely affect adjustment to the loss of a parent.

D. Long-term outcome. The adult psychiatric literature implicates early parental loss in **adult depression**.

1. As with short-term adjustment, the surviving parent and family environment play important roles. The risk factors are similar to those for short-term adjustment (see VIII C 3).

2. **Protective factors against** the long-term development of **depression** include:
   a. Physical and emotional support and constancy
   b. Allowing the child to express distress, conflict, and anger, which requires adult emotional stability
   c. Judicious maintenance of limits balanced by emotional support, especially for adolescents

3. The development of a **chronic sense of vulnerability** to loss can be a predictor of later depression. This may be associated with multiple previous losses or tragedies, but also with an emotionally distant and nonsupportive surviving family.

E. The role of the pediatric provider

1. **Advice and consultation** should be provided to surviving adults **concerning the child's adjustment;** for example, how to tell the child about the death or pending death should be discussed:
   a. The surviving family should discuss the meaning of death with the child. The pediatric provider should advise the family to be aware of the limits of the child's developmental stage.
   b. The pediatric provider should advise the family how to discuss the cause of death, without using anxiety-provoking analogies (e.g., death as sleep).
   c. The family should be advised to assure the younger child about his or her well-being and safety.

2. Factors influencing short-term and long-term adjustment (see VIII C, D) should be discussed.

3. The pediatric provider should be ready to discuss practical issues, such as whether to have the child attend the viewing, funeral, or wake.

   a. Differences exist from the adult mourning process, especially for the younger child (i.e., younger than 6 or 7 years of age). Whereas attending the viewing and funeral may aid the grieving process of an older child, viewing the body may be disturbing for the young child.

   b. The actual reaction may be affected by the child's temperament, intrinsic fearfulness, and the emotional state of the surviving family members.

   c. A reasonable marker is what the child says he or she wants to do.

   d. The surviving family members should be advised to provide for an emotionally less involved but trusted adult who can support the child or take the child home if necessary.

   e. Family members should be warned of the potential apparent indifference in a 2- to 4-year-old, which is stage related.

4. The pediatric provider should allow for frequent early follow-up or, at least, telephone contact.

   a. Pediatric providers should be available for further behavioral advice and general support.

   b. The family should be made aware of concerning signs, such as greater than 4–6 months of persistent mourning in the older child, or behavioral difficulties affecting normal functioning.

   c. The family should be alerted to specific signs and symptoms, such as regressive behavior, depressive symptoms, school and social dysfunction, heightened adolescent acting-out, and phobias.

F. | **Treatment of prolonged mourning**

1. Children who experience a prolonged state of mourning should be referred to a child psychiatrist or clinical child psychologist.

2. The use of bereavement groups for children should be considered, if recommended by a child psychiatrist or psychologist.

BIBLIOGRAPHY

American Academy of Pediatrics Committee on Psychosocial Aspects of Child and Family Health: The pediatrician and childhood bereavement. *Pediatrics* 89(3):516–518, 1992.

Bithoney WG, Dubowitz H, Egan H: Failure to thrive/growth deficiency. *Pediatr Rev* 13(12):453–459, 1992.

Caldwell BM: Impact of day care on the child. *Pediatrics* 91(1):225–228, 1993.

Caring For Our Children. National Health and Safety Performance Standards: Guidelines for Out-of-Home Child Care Programs. Washington, DC, and Elk Grove Village, IL, American Public Health Association and American Academy of Pediatrics, 1992.

Wallerstein JS, Johnston JR: Children of divorce: Recent findings regarding long-term affects and recent studies of joint and sole custody. *Pediatr Rev* 11(7):197–203, 1990.

DIRECTIONS: Each of the numbered items or incomplete statements in this section is followed by answers or by completions of the statement. Select the ONE lettered answer or completion that is BEST in each case.

1. A 4-month-old male infant brought to the emergency department with prolonged seizure activity is noted to have multiple old bruises over his body. Child abuse and "shaken baby syndrome" are later confirmed. Which one of the following statements about the perpetrator is most likely true?

(A) The abuser is likely to be seriously mentally ill
(B) The story behind the injuries given by the perpetrator will be consistent with the injuries
(C) The abuser is likely to be outside of the family, such as a babysitter
(D) The abuser is likely to be socially isolated with minimal social support

2. A 15-month-old girl who had been growing steadily was not brought in for her 9-month or 12-month visits. At her 15-month visit, a significant weight loss is noted. No specific organic cause is indicated by history or physical examination. Of the following, which would be the best next step?

(A) Hospital admission for observation and medical evaluation
(B) Extensive outpatient laboratory investigation, including diagnostic imaging
(C) A high-calorie diet with close outpatient follow-up
(D) Referral to a pediatric gastroenterologist
(E) Referral of the family for psychological and social service evaluation

3. A grandmother brings her 5-year-old, frightened granddaughter to the pediatrician's office 10 days after her first overnight visitation with her newly divorced father. She is concerned about her granddaughter's vaginal irritation and discharge. To investigate the possibility of sexual abuse, the best first step would be

(A) Immediately notify the police so that a police officer can take over the investigation
(B) Advise the mother and grandmother to look into termination of visitation rights
(C) Separately interview the child and both parents to obtain more information
(D) Avoid interviewing the child to limit psychological trauma
(E) Arrange for colposcopy as quickly as possible, while obtaining cultures of the mouth, rectum, vagina, and urethra

4. A 15-year-old female patient is hospitalized for acute depression. The divorced parents ask the pediatrician to share with the hospital psychiatrist any relevant medical, developmental, or social issues. Of the following, which is most likely to be a significant contributing factor to psychological problems?

(A) The parents were divorced when the child was 3 years of age
(B) The noncustodial parent (father) has had frequent contact with the child
(C) The child is a girl
(D) The divorced parents, when in contact with the pediatrician about the child, have continued to express anger and hostility toward each other
(E) The child has always presented a "slow-to-warm-up" temperament in the pediatrician's office

5. As a result of the pediatrician's report to the local child protection agency, a 4-year-old male patient is to be placed in foster care. Knowing the family and foster system, which of the following best characterizes the situation?

(A) Now that the child has been placed, the family will receive effective remediation, allowing the safe return of the child to his home

(B) Because of inadequate regulations nationally, the child is unlikely to be eligible to receive basic health services while in foster care

(C) There is a 20%–30% chance that this child, if returned to his family, will be returned to foster care

(D) Owing to generous funding of the foster care system in most states, there will be no shortage of qualified foster homes

(E) Because of the relatively early removal of this child from his home environment, the risk for problems during adolescence will be no more than for children not placed in foster homes

DIRECTIONS: Each of the numbered items or incomplete statements in this section is negatively phrased, as indicated by a capitalized word such as NOT, LEAST, or EXCEPT. Select the ONE lettered answer or completion that is BEST in each case.

6. A young married couple has had their adopted child since shortly after his birth. At his 3-year office visit, the adoptive parents describe the common triad of temper tantrums, sleep resistance, and eating avoidance. This raises unfounded fears for the adoptive parents that this may be an early sign of major psychiatric difficulties. Of the following statements about adoptive children's long-term outcome, which one is LEAST likely to be true?

(A) The age of adoption plays no significant role in poor psychological outcome

(B) Adopted boys have a greater risk for psychiatric problems than adopted girls

(C) Intelligence and success in school are the same as in children who are raised with their biologic parents

(D) Lower socioeconomic status and multiple other children in the adoptive home may play a role in emotional difficulties

7. The mother of a 16-year-old female patient calls to tell the pediatrician that her husband died 2 months ago of a sudden intracranial hemorrhage. The mother is concerned about her daughter's continued depressed behavior. In trying to predict potential long-term negative psychological outcome, which of the following is LEAST likely to be relevant?

(A) A history of depression on both sides of the family

(B) The sudden nature and cause of the father's death

(C) Continued past arguments between the father and daughter about her boyfriends and her late hours

(D) Minimal death benefits for the mother along with no immediate prospects for the mother's employment

(E) Problems of limit setting by the mother due to her own relative depression

DIRECTIONS: Each set of matching questions in this section consists of a list of lettered options followed by several numbered items. For each numbered item, select the ONE lettered option that is most closely associated with it. To avoid spending too much time on matching sets with large numbers of options, it is generally advisable to begin each set by reading the list of options. Then, for each item in the set, try to generate the correct answer and locate it in the option list, rather than evaluating each option individually. Each lettered option may be selected once, more than once, or not at all.

Questions 8–10

For each of the types of foster care listed below, match the one advantage or disadvantage that best fits the foster care type.

(A) Best suited for special-needs children or adolescents
(B) Possible similar pathology as the biologic parents
(C) More likely to split up siblings
(D) Dedication and success depend on the adequacy of screening
(E) More likely to lead to a lack of a consistent source of primary health care

8. Extended family (kinship care)

9. Group homes

10. Private foster family

Questions 11–13

For each of the three types of custody listed below, match the statement that best fits the specific type of custody.

(A) Maximal contact between parents and potentially the greatest risk for disruption of the child's daily routines
(B) Least likely to disrupt contacts with other supportive family members
(C) Less potential contact between parents, less possibility of emotional entrapment of the child
(D) Best suited when the child is younger (i.e., younger than 5 years of age)
(E) One parent has primary physical custody, both share legal responsibility for the child's needs

11. Sole custody

12. Joint legal custody

13. Joint physical custody

ANSWERS AND EXPLANATIONS

1. The answer is D *[III C]*. Perpetrators of child abuse rarely suffer from serious mental illness. However, they are often socially isolated and often face major life and personal stresses without social support. Also, they are most often family members of the child. In attempting to explain the child's injury, the history they give will often be inconsistent with the actual injury, or not plausible given the child's developmental age and capabilities.

2. The answer is C *[II D 2]*. Provision of a high-calorie diet is the first step in treating failure to thrive. It is also a diagnostic trial in that failure to gain weight when on a prescribed high-calorie diet may necessitate hospital admission for further formal evaluation of the child and family. Extensive laboratory testing is rarely fruitful without indications from the patient's history or physical examination of specific organic causes. Similarly, referral for extensive subspecialty or agency involvement before hospital observation and evaluation is also not advisable unless there are specific history or physical examination findings to justify it.

3. The answer is C *[III E, F 2]*. A high index of suspicion for child physical or sexual abuse is necessary for all pediatric care providers. However, actual investigation must be conducted sensitively and objectively. In most states, child protection agencies rather than police are involved in cases of physical or sexual abuse thought to be perpetrated by a family member. Abuse by a person outside of the family is usually reported to the police in addition to the state or local child protection agency. In either case, pediatric providers should not relinquish total responsibility for further information gathering. It is important to start with nonjudgmental, nonaccusatory interviews of the family and the child. Genital examination and cultures are important for confirmation and documentation of sexual abuse, but should not be rushed before sensitive history taking and assessment of the child's coping ability.

4. The answer is D *[VII E 3, 4]*. Children of divorce, as a general rule, adjust reasonably well over time. They are, however, at higher risk than children of intact families for long-term emotional maladjustment. Certain other factors may contribute to the deleterious effects of divorce to increase the likelihood of negative outcome, such as depression. These include the divorce occurring when the child is older, minimal or no contact with the noncustodial parent, and the child having evidence of "difficult child" temperament. However, the single strongest predictor of poor outcome is when the divorced parents continue to express anger and hostility toward each other in the child's presence.

5. The answer is C *[IV C 2, D 4, E 2, F 3, G 1]*. Children in foster care, regardless of age, have a higher incidence of long-term psychological adjustment problems. Resources for the rehabilitation of families who have given their children up to foster care are often inadequate, which makes effective remediation problematic. Similarly, inadequate funding at a state level often leads to inadequate numbers of qualified foster families. All of this contributes to a 25% chance that any child returned from foster care to his or her home, will return to foster care. Nevertheless, federal and local laws do provide for certain services for foster children (e.g., basic medical care).

6. The answer is A *[V F 2, 5, 6]*. Adopted children are at greater risk for long-term psychological problems than are children raised with their biologic parents. Factors that apparently contribute include gender (boys have a worse outcome than girls), lower socioeconomic status, greater numbers of children in the adoptive home, and older age of the child at the time of adoption. Intelligence and school success are not significantly different from matched nonadopted controls.

7. The answer is B *[VIII C 3, D 2 c]*. A number of factors may contribute to an increased likelihood of poor long-term psychological adjustment of a child to the death of a parent. They include a family history of depression, a previously troubled relationship between the child and the deceased parent, poor financial support for the child, and problems for the surviving parent in setting firm and consistent behavior limits.

8–10. The answers are: 8-B *[Table 3-2]*, **9-A** *[Table 3-2]*, **10-D** *[Table 3-2]*. Although foster placement of a child with other family members is often conveniently available and provides a potentially familiar environment for the child, the risk is that close relatives may share similar psychosocial pathology with the parents. Group homes provide more diversity of providers and therefore greater breadth of skills, which is very useful for special-needs or handicapped children. The group environment is often more conducive to adolescent adjustment than foster parents in a private home. Private foster homes can provide a nurturing and helpful haven for at-risk children, as long as the foster parents have been well screened and prepared.

11–13. The answers are: 11-C *[Table 3-3],* **12-E** *[Table 3-3],* **13-A** *[Table 3-3].* Sole custody limits contact with the noncustodial parent at the expense of erosion of the relationship between that parent and the child. It also often diminishes the financial resources for the child because the custodial parent is often a mother who has not drawn a salary sufficient to maintain the family's previous standard of living. On the other hand, joint legal custody provides for shared legal and financial responsibility, although the child lives primarily with one parent. Joint physical custody diminishes the possibility of deterioration of the relationship between the child and one of the parents by ensuring relatively balanced contact with each parent. However, this balanced contact may also lead to more contact between the divorced parents and potentially more opportunity for expressed anger and hostility.

Chapter 4

Developmental Disabilities and Behavioral Disorders
Neil L. Schechter

I. **INTRODUCTION.** This chapter reviews disorders that represent deviations from the broad range of normative development and individual human variation. These problems have been categorized as either high incidence, low severity (e.g., recurrent abdominal pain, enuresis, learning disabilities) or low incidence, high severity (e.g., autism, blindness, mental retardation). Even the more common, less severe problems should not be trivialized, however, because they still may have a significant impact on the child's self-esteem. The problems reviewed in this chapter often have multifactorial etiologies that may involve the interaction of biologic, psychological, and social factors. As a result, the evaluation and treatment of these disorders are often multidisciplinary.

II. **CONTINENCE DISORDERS**

A. **Enuresis**

1. **Definition.** Enuresis is the involuntary discharge of urine at an age after continence has been reached by most children. Typically, this is age 5 years in girls and 6 years in boys. Approximately 5%–8% of school-age children are enuretic. The incidence decreases with age to 1% of 18-year-olds. Two subclassifications of enuresis are important.
   a. **Primary versus secondary**
      (1) Children with **primary** enuresis have never been continent for a period of time lasting at least 3–6 months.
      (2) Children with **secondary** enuresis have had a prolonged period of bladder control but have resumed enuretic behavior.
   b. **Nocturnal versus diurnal**
      (1) **Nocturnal** enuresis occurs only at night and affects about 85% of all enuretic children.
      (2) **Diurnal** enuresis occurs during the day and affects about 5% of enuretic children.
      (3) Approximately 10% of enuretic children have a **mixed type** (nocturnal and diurnal) enuresis.

2. **Etiology.** Enuresis is a symptom for which varying underlying causes have been implicated.
   a. **Maturation.** Because of high spontaneous remission rate (in approximately 10% of the enuretic population per year) and increased frequency in boys, the level of physiologic maturity has been implicated as a cause of enuresis.
   b. **Sleep disorder.** Many enuretics are incontinent during stages 3 and 4 of the first sleep cycle, suggesting that enuresis is a non–rapid-eye-movement dyssomnia, like sleepwalking and night terrors.
   c. **Genetics.** In 70% of families with an enuretic child, the symptom has occurred in at least one other family member.
   d. **Organic causes.** Urinary tract infections, obstructions of the outflow tract, lumbosacral disorders that affect bladder innervation (e.g., meningomyelocele), diabetes mellitus, diabetes insipidus, and sickle cell disease are all possible causes of incontinence, but represent only 1%–5% of the causes of enuresis. Chronic stool retention also is a cause of enuresis.

    e. Psychological factors have been implicated in some children with enuresis. Stressors such as the birth of a sibling or a move may precipitate bed-wetting in the suscepti- ble child.

    f. Abnormal antidiuretic hormone cycles have been suggested.

3. Assessment

    a. History. Essential elements of the history include:

      (1) The family history of enuresis

      (2) The pattern of enuresis (primary versus secondary; nocturnal versus diurnal)

      (3) Defining urinary habits (frequency, urgency, dysuria, dribbling)

      (4) Identifying psychological stressors

    b. Physical examination. Essential elements include:

      (1) Height and weight

      (2) Blood pressure

      (3) A thorough **neurologic examination** emphasizing lower spinal vertebral function

      (4) Examination of the **external genitalia** for abnormalities such as hypospadias

    c. Laboratory and radiographic investigation

      (1) A **urinalysis** should be obtained and should include specific gravity as well as determinations of glucose, protein, blood, and white cells. A **urine culture** should also be obtained.

      (2) Routine radiographic studies are not indicated for enuretic children with normal urinalysis results, a negative physical examination, and no evidence of neurologic disease. Children with diurnal enuresis may require more extensive evaluation.

4. Therapy

    a. Behavioral approaches include counseling, charting, hypnosis, bladder stretching exercises, night awakening by parents 1 hour after sleep onset, and use of a buzzer alarm, which is the most successful treatment currently available.

    b. Pharmacologic management

      (1) Tricyclic antidepressants (e.g., imipramine) have a success rate of approximately 50% in reducing enuretic episodes, but the relapse rate on discontinuation is high. In addition, there are potentially serious side effects and marked toxicity in overdosage. Antidepressants are indicated only for rapid, short-term relief of symptoms (e.g., use before summer camp or vacation).

      (2) Desmopressin may have a role in a subgroup of children with enuresis, but it has a high relapse rate on discontinuation, and there are limited long-term follow-up data to support its safety or efficacy.

B. | Encopresis

1. Definition. Encopresis is involuntary fecal soiling at an age beyond which continence should have been achieved, which in most children is age 4 years. Approximately 1.5% of 7-year-old children have encopresis.

    a. Primary versus secondary

      (1) Primary encopresis occurs in children who have never been totally toilet trained.

      (2) Secondary encopresis occurs in children who have had at least 3–6 months of fecal continence.

    b. Retentive versus nonretentive

      (1) Most encopretic children suffer from chronic stool retention, with subsequent overflow incontinence.

      (2) Nonretentive encopretic children (i.e., nonconstipated children with encopresis) tend to have neurogenic sphincters or severe psychiatric illness.

2. Etiology

    a. Developmental and behavioral factors. Slower transit time, hyperactivity, the lack of school bathroom facilities, harsh toilet training, sexual abuse, and negative defeca- tion experiences (e.g., those associated with prior gastroenteritis) have all been impli- cated as causing chronic stool retention, which can lead to encopresis.

    b. Anatomic factors. Hirschsprung disease, anal stenosis, and anal fissures also are potential causes of chronic stool retention.

    c. Metabolic factors. Hypothyroidism, various endocrine neoplasms, and various drugs (e.g., opiates, phenothiazines) also can cause chronic constipation.

    d. Occasionally, no underlying pathology or predisposition to constipation is identified.

3. Assessment

  a. History

    (1) A detailed bowel history, including the age of the child at toilet training, the frequency of bowel movements, the history of constipation, and a description of the stools, is necessary to assess encopresis.

    (2) Also, gaining insight into the child's and the family's functioning can help determine if there are predisposing factors for encopresis.

  b. Physical examination. Essentials include:

    (1) Assessing **growth patterns**

    (2) A **neurologic examination** evaluating lower extremity deep tendon reflexes

    (3) An **abdominal examination**

    (4) A **rectal examination,** which should reveal stool in the rectal ampulla within the reach of the examiner

  c. Laboratory and radiographic investigation

    (1) Thyroid testing should take place if deemed necessary from physical findings.

    (2) An abdominal radiograph to determine the extent of fecal retention may be helpful if there is no response to initial therapy.

    (3) If Hirschsprung disease is suspected, anal manometry or rectal biopsy is indicated.

4. Therapy

  a. Initial treatment

    (1) Discussion should remove blame from the child and parent and demystify the origins of the problem.

    (2) Initial catharsis with a series of enemas and laxatives or stool softeners will remove retained stool.

  b. Maintenance therapy

    (1) Mineral oil (the typical course is a gradual decrease of mineral oil with discontinuation after approximately 4–6 months)

    (2) Bowel retraining by sitting on the toilet after meals to take advantage of the gastrocolic reflex

    (3) Dietary changes, which should emphasize increased roughage and liquid and decreased milk and milk products

III. SCHOOL-RELATED PROBLEMS

A. Specific learning disabilities

1. Definition

  a. As defined by federal legislation, learning disabilities is

> a generic term that refers to a heterogenous group of disorders manifested by significant difficulties in the acquisition and use of listening, speaking, reading, writing, reasoning, or mathematical abilities. These disorders are intrinsic to the individual and presumed to be due to central nervous system dysfunction. Even though a learning disability may occur concomitantly with other handicapping conditions or environmental influences, it is not the direct result of these conditions or influences.

  b. This definition is based on a recognized discrepancy between a child's academic performance and potential. This discrepancy is presumed to be secondary to subtle central nervous system dysfunction or subtle human variation.

    c. These disabilities occasionally are described by reference to the academic function they affect (e.g., dyslexia for difficulty in reading, dyscalculia for difficulty in mathematics) or by the psychological process that is weak (e.g., deficits in auditory processing, visual-motor integration, sequential memory, or executive functioning).

    d. Learning disabilities are found in 1%–10% of school-age children.

2. Etiology. No specific cause for learning disabilities is commonly accepted. Most likely, a number of subgroups of children with specific learning disabilities will be identified. Etiologic hypotheses include central nervous system damage, individual human variation, toxins, diet, and environmental factors.

3. Assessment

    a. History. Elements of the history should include:

      (1) A review of the perinatal course

      (2) Evidence of medical problems (e.g., persistent otitis media, seizure disorders)

      (3) The early developmental history, with an emphasis on language acquisition (there is often an uneven profile in the development of children with learning disabilities)

      (4) The history of other family members with learning problems

      (5) A review of school functioning

    b. Physical examination usually is negative.

      (1) An emphasis often is placed on a search for minor **neurologic indicators,** or "soft signs," which have been reported more frequently in learning-disabled children than in controls [e.g., synkinesis (mirror movements), dysdiadochokinesia (difficulty with rapid, alternating movements), choreiform movements of the fingers]. The implications of these signs remain controversial.

      (2) Hearing and vision should be screened.

    c. Laboratory investigation is not called for unless it is suggested by the history or physical examination. Computed tomography (CT) scan and electroencephalography are not helpful.

    d. Psychoeducational assessment includes a battery of tests of intellectual functioning (IQ tests) as well as specific academic tests to profile a child's strengths and weaknesses. Usually these are performed by the public schools, which are mandated to test the child under the Individuals with Disabilities Education Act [Public Law 101-476 (IDEA, 1990)]. The psychoeducational profile is the basis on which an individualized educational program is constructed. Amendments to IDEA extend the mandate for special education assessment to the 3- to 5-year-old age-group.

4. Therapy. Many unorthodox therapies have been offered for children with learning problems, including dietary therapies, perceptual training, optometric training, and sensory integration training. None of these therapies has documented efficacy at this time.

    a. Educational intervention is the mainstay of treatment for learning disabilities. Typically, this occurs through a modification of the child's regular classroom experience or by varying degrees of special education, ranging from resource room support to a separate classroom. Educational intervention should identify specific goals (i.e., should be **individualized**) and should be monitored carefully.

    b. Psychological counseling is indicated for children with learning disabilities who suffer from diminished self-esteem that is not improved by a special education program. School phobia and avoidance can develop in children with learning disabilities (see III C), and this can be addressed in counseling.

    c. Various **support organizations** are helpful in providing parents and teachers with a forum to address the complex issues associated with these disabilities. Examples include the Association for Children and Adults with Learning Disabilities and the Council for Exceptional Children.

B. **Attention-deficit hyperactivity disorder (ADHD)**

1. **Definition.** ADHD involves an inadequate attention span, impulsiveness, and hyperactivity. The syndrome in general is marked by a lack of task performance, and easy distractibility (Table 4-1).

   a. This disorder has been plagued by vague and changing diagnostic criteria. This confusion is reflected in the numerous diagnostic labels for ADHD (minimal brain damage, minimal brain dysfunction, hyperkinetic impulse disorder, and, most recently, attention deficit disorder with or without hyperactivity), which reflect varying conceptual frameworks. The most recent categorization (*Diagnostic and Statistical Manual of Mental Disorders,* 4th ed. [DSM-IV]) offers three subtypes: ADHD predominantly inattentive type, ADHD predominantly hyperactive–impulsive type, and ADHD combined type.

   b. Incidence figures suggest that 2%–4% of children may be affected, making ADHD the most common behavioral disorder of school-age children. Boys are affected 10 times more frequently than girls.

2. **Etiology.** No single etiology is currently accepted, and the cause of ADHD is thought to be multifactorial. The following may have a role:

   a. Genetic–temperamental factors
   b. Neurologic immaturity
   c. Biochemical aberration of dopamine production
   d. Toxins, such as lead, food dyes, and salicylates
   e. Psychological factors
   f. Perinatal adversity
   g. Inappropriate societal and teacher expectations

3. **Assessment**

   a. **History.** Essentials of the history include:
      (1) The perinatal history
      (2) The child's early temperament
      (3) A detailed preschool and school history
      (4) The family history of inattention or school problems

   b. **Physical examination.** Behavioral observations of the child during the physical examination should be cautiously interpreted, because anxiety may increase or decrease inattention. Elements of the physical examination that deserve emphasis are:
      (1) Evidence of minor physical anomalies that occasionally correlate with ADHD, such as:
         (a) Epicanthal folds and hypertelorism of the eyes

TABLE 4-1. Selected Symptoms Associated With Attention-Deficit Hyperactivity Disorder

Symptoms Associated With Inattention
Often makes careless mistakes
Problems sustaining attention in school and at play
Problems with organization and forgetfulness
Lack of follow-through on schoolwork and chores
Easily distracted
Symptoms Associated With Hyperactivity–Impulsivity
Often fidgets, squirms, or is out of seat
Often "on the go" and frequently running
Excessive talking
Often blurts out answers or interrupts others
Problems awaiting a turn

Adapted from the *Diagnostic and Statistical Manual of Mental Disorders,* 4th ed. Washington, DC, American Psychiatric Association, 1994.

          (b) Low-set or malformed ears
          (c) High-arched palate
          (d) Clinodactyly (inward curvature) of the fifth finger
      (2) Head circumference
      (3) Neurologic examination, including soft signs [see III A 3 b (1)]
      (4) Hearing and vision assessment
   c. Laboratory studies. No single test establishes the diagnosis of ADHD. Hematocrit or hemoglobin concentration may be obtained to screen for anemia, blood lead testing may be performed to look for evidence of lead toxicity, and thyroid studies may be obtained if suggested by the history and physical. Electroencephalography and CT scan appear to have no role in diagnosis.
   d. Behavioral observation (e.g., teacher questionnaires). It is essential that communication with teachers, special educators, and psychologists take place because the child's behavior may differ depending on the setting.

  4. Therapy
   a. Behavioral management is the mainstay of treatment. Strategies include increasing structure in the environment, positive reinforcement, counseling, and a number of cognitive approaches that emphasize relaxation and self-control.
   b. Special education. Children with attention deficits often require highly structured classrooms with low student–teacher ratios to maximize their educational experience. Coexisting learning disabilities may require educational interventions (see III A 4 a).
   c. Medication may have an adjuvant role in treatment by increasing attention span and decreasing distractibility, but should be considered only after behavioral and educational interventions have been tried.
      (1) Stimulants (e.g., methylphenidate, dextroamphetamine, pemoline) are the drugs most commonly used to treat ADHD and should be the initial choice.
          (a) Stimulants primarily are intended to help with school performance, so they usually are given on school days rather than on vacation days.
          (b) Side effects of stimulants include anorexia, headache, sleep disturbances, and possible growth retardation. **Tourette syndrome** (see Chapter 18) has been reported as a possible complication of stimulant therapy, so any child with tics or a family history of tics probably should not receive stimulants.
      (2) Tricyclic antidepressants (e.g., desipramine, imipramine), **clonidine,** and **fluoxetine** have also been helpful in treating ADHD.
   d. Alternative therapies. Dietary restrictions, megavitamin therapy, and sensorimotor integration training have all been suggested as treatment, but there is little evidence that they can alter hyperactive or inattentive behavior in most of the affected children.

C. | School phobia

  1. Definition. School phobia in a child is manifested by **poor school attendance** caused by unwarranted fear or by inappropriate anxiety about leaving home, or, in particular, the child's mother. The school-phobic child prefers to remain at home and avoid school. School phobia is seen in approximately 1.7% of school-age children per year. Typically, the phobic child has problems beginning school in the fall and returning to school after vacations.

  2. Etiology. The reason for the development of school phobia in any given child depends on a variety of factors within the child and within the family. The typical scenario involves a passive and dependent child who encounters an additional stressor (e.g., illness, school problems, the death of a loved one).

  3. Assessment
   a. School phobia has been described as "the great imitator." Typical findings are:
      (1) Vague physical symptoms
      (2) Negative physical examination and laboratory findings
      (3) Poor school attendance attributed to the somatic symptoms

b. A thorough history and physical examination, in addition to select laboratory tests (e.g., complete blood count, erythrocyte sedimentation rate, urinalysis) often are necessary to assure parents that the child's symptoms are not secondary to organic disease. A symptom diary also is often helpful in this regard.

4. **Therapy**
   a. After the parents are assured that their child is well, the physician should insist on the **immediate return of the child to school**. The physician should then review with the parents what approach to use if the child reports that he or she is sick the next day.
   b. **Psychotherapy** may be indicated for the parents and child. Behavioral management techniques, such as desensitization, may be helpful.
   c. The short-term use of **antianxiety medications** may be necessary if the child's anxiety is overwhelming.

IV. PROFOUND DEVELOPMENTAL DISORDERS

A. Autistic spectrum disorders

1. **Definition**
   a. Autistic spectrum disorders are characterized by profound impairment in social interaction (e.g., lack of eye contact, poor peer relationships) and by restricted, repetitive, and stereotyped patterns of behavior (e.g., unusual preoccupations, inflexibility, stereotyped motor movements).
   b. **Clinical subtypes**
      (1) **Autism** (autistic disorder, per DSM IV): In addition to social impairments and stereotyped patterns of behavior, children with autism have profound impairments in communication. They demonstrate delays in the acquisition of language, the ability to sustain conversation, and the capacity for play. Onset of some of the symptoms occurs at less than 3 years of age. Seventy-five percent of this group functions in the retarded range on intellectual testing.
      (2) **Asperger syndrome** (Asperger's disorder, per DSM IV): Children with this syndrome meet criteria for autistic spectrum disorders but are intellectually normal and have no language delays, although they may have abnormalities of spoken language.
      (3) **Pervasive developmental disorder** [PDD, NOS (not otherwise specified), per DSM IV]: Children are given this diagnosis if they meet many of the criteria for autism but not all (i.e., later onset of symptoms or subthreshold symptoms).

2. **Etiology.** Autistic spectrum disorders are believed to be caused by an as yet **unidentified constellation of brain dysfunctions**. Prenatal complications, fragile X syndrome and other nonspecific chromosomal rearrangements, other genetic conditions, maternal rubella, phenylketonuria, and, rarely, encephalitis are thought to be contributing factors. Many children with these disorders have no known predisposing factors, however.

3. **Assessment**
   a. No specific biochemical or anatomic aberration has been consistently associated with autism, although abnormalities of serotonin and at the neocerebellum have been reported in some children with the disorder. In particular, children with motor dysfunction may have rare metabolic disorders.
   b. Retarded children with autism are more prone to development of seizures in adolescence than the nonretarded group.
   c. Assessment of the child with an autistic spectrum disorder should rule out other conditions that may present similarly, such as mental retardation, childhood schizophrenia, hearing impairment, developmental language disorders, genetic disorders, and the results of profound isolation and neglect.
   d. Routine chromosome analysis for unexpected rearrangements and DNA testing for fragile X syndrome should be considered.

4. Therapy

a. **Medical management.** There is no proven medical treatment for autistic spectrum disorders, although experimental treatment with drugs such as fenfluramine has been tried. If seizures are present, anticonvulsant agents should be used appropriately. Many nonstandard therapies are in use.

b. **Special education.** The child should be in an educational program designed to address the complex needs of these children, with a strong emphasis on communication and appropriate social interaction.

c. **Psychological management.** The rearing of a child with these disorders is frustrating and emotionally draining, and parents should be offered professional support and exposure to other parents facing similar issues.

B. Mental retardation

1. **Definition.** Mental retardation is defined as significantly subaverage intellectual functioning existing concurrently with deficits in adaptive behavior (e.g., communication, self-care, self-direction) and manifested during the developmental period (i.e., before age 18 years).

2. **Incidence.** Between 1.5% and 3% of the population is affected.

3. **Classification.** Four subgroups of retardation have been designated.

a. **Mild—IQ levels of 55–70.** This group represents 80% of the retarded population. As adults, these people are able to live independently, marry, and be employed, and they have functional reading and writing skills. Their major deficits are in judgment.

b. **Moderate—IQ levels of 40–55.** This group represents 12% of the retarded population. These people do not necessarily require custodial care, but they do require continuous supervision and economic support. They are capable of self-care and employment in a sheltered setting.

c. **Severe—IQ levels of 20–40.** This group represents about 7% of the retarded population. These people are totally economically dependent and require close supervision. They may acquire language and can be trained in elementary self-care skills.

d. **Profound—IQ levels of less than 20.** This group represents 1% of the retarded population. These people have limited communication and self-care skills and often have associated complex medical needs. They require a highly structured environment, with continuous care and supervision.

4. **Etiology.** The causes of mental retardation are varied and represent a wide variety of biologic and environmental factors. They are summarized in Table 4-2. Only a minority of cases of mental retardation can be attributed to known biologic factors. Mild retardation is more prevalent among lower socioeconomic groups, and is rarely explained by biologic causes. Moderate and severe retardation are more evenly distributed throughout all socioeconomic groups and more frequently tend to have a biologic explanation.

5. **Assessment**

a. **History.** The family's pedigree and details of the pregnancy, delivery, and the immediate postnatal period are critical.

b. **Physical examination.** Attention should be given to the head circumference, to dysmorphic features and associated anomalies that might suggest a syndrome, and to the neurologic examination. As mentioned, children in the mildly retarded range rarely have evidence of biologic abnormalities.

c. **Developmental testing**

(1) Diagnosis of mental retardation can be made only with the use of standardized psychometric testing administered by a trained professional. It cannot be made with screening instruments, and it rarely is made in young children because of the lack of stability of the test scores of children younger than age 5 years. Children younger than 5 years with cognitive difficulties are considered to be developmentally delayed.

TABLE 4-2. Conditions Associated With Mental Retardation

Period of Development	Type of Condition	Examples
Pre- and periconceptual	Metabolic disorders	Mucopolysaccharidoses Tay-Sachs disease
	Brain malformation	Encephalocele Hydranencephaly
	Neurocutaneous disorders	Tuberous sclerosis Neurofibromatosis
	Chromosomal abnormalities	Down syndrome Cri du chat (5p-) syndrome
Prenatal	Teratogen exposure	Chemicals Radiation Alcohol
	Infection	Rubella Cytomegalovirus
	Fetal malnutrition	Mother with high blood pressure or kidney disease
Perinatal	Prematurity	Complications such as poor oxygenation of the brain and intracranial hemorrhage
	Metabolic abnormalities	Asphyxia at birth Hypoglycemia
	Infection	Herpes simplex encephalitis
Postnatal	Infection	Meningitis
	Trauma	Automobile accident Child abuse
	Lack of oxygen	Near-drowning Strangulation
	Severe nutritional deficiency	Kwashiorkor
	Environmental toxin exposure	Lead
	Environmental and social problems	Psychosocial deprivation Parental psychiatric disorders

Reprinted from Blackman J (ed): *Medical Aspects of Developmental Disabilities in Children.* Rockville, MD, Aspen Publishers, 1984, p 148.

(2) Developmental delay is a less specific term than mental retardation, because it implies only that the child's performance at the present time is delayed compared to peers of the same age. It does not predict future performance.

V. SENSORY IMPAIRMENT

A. Hearing impairment

1. **Definitions**
   a. **Degree of impairment.** The designation **hearing-impaired** applies to any hearing disability within the mild to profound range.
   (1) **Mild** loss refers to a 20–40-dB loss.
   (2) **Moderate** (40–60 dB) or **severe** (60–80 dB) loss has significant impact on speech acquisition.

(3) Profound loss (deafness) refers to a more than 80-dB loss in the speech frequency. A deaf child is unable to process language through audition, even with a hearing aid.

b. **Functional subtypes of hearing loss**

(1) Conductive hearing loss is defined as interference in the transmission of sound from the external auditory canal to the inner ear, most commonly due to otitis media or its sequelae. Most conductive loss can be corrected by medical treatment or surgery.

(2) Sensorineural hearing loss is hearing loss secondary to damage to the inner ear or auditory nerve. This type of hearing loss is nearly always irreversible, and treatment is usually amplification.

(3) A **mixed-type** of hearing loss involves both sensorineural and conductive loss simultaneously.

2. **Etiology.** Table 4-3 lists the causes of conductive and sensorineural hearing loss.

3. **Assessment**

a. **History.** Table 4-4 lists the situations and conditions that should alert the physician to possible hearing loss.

b. **Physical examination**

(1) Abnormalities of and around the pinna, ear canal, or tympanic membrane should be noted. Pneumatic otoscopy should be performed.

(2) Other abnormalities that may suggest a genetic explanation for hearing impairment should be identified.

c. **Audiologic evaluation.** Depending on the age and cognitive abilities of the child, various audiologic evaluations are appropriate. These include behavioral and observational hearing assessments, pure tone audiometry, and evoked response audiometry.

4. **Therapy**

a. **Medical management** may involve the antibiotic treatment of otitis media and the placement of tympanostomy tubes for chronic middle ear effusions (see Chapter 10). Surgical techniques (e.g., cochlear implants) are available for some children. Amplification may be necessary for sensorineural hearing loss.

b. **Education.** The hearing-impaired child requires educational intervention to allow for maximal development.

(1) Alternate methods of communication. Depending on the degree of impairment, signing may be required for effective education.

TABLE 4-3. Causes of Conductive and Sensorineural Hearing Loss

Conductive Hearing Loss
Abnormalities of the external auditory canal or ossicles
Otitis media
Trauma
Foreign bodies
Otosclerosis
Cerumen in the ear canal

Sensorineural Hearing Loss
Rubella or another congenital infection
Mumps, meningitis, or another postnatal infection
Perinatal asphyxia or prematurity
Trauma
Kernicterus
Ototoxic drugs (e.g., aminoglycosides)
Genetic causes (e.g., Waardenburg syndrome, Alport syndrome, Usher syndrome, mucopolysaccharidosis, Pendred syndrome)
Environmental (noise-induced)

TABLE 4-4. Risk Factors and Conditions That Should Alert the Physician to Possible Hearing Loss in Newborns and Young Children

High-Risk Situations Affecting Newborns
Familial hearing loss
Congenital rubella, cytomegalovirus, toxoplasmosis, or herpes
Low birth weight (less than 1500 g)
Hyperbilirubinemia
Congenital malformation of the pinna, skull, lip, or palate
Meningitis
Ototoxic drugs (e.g., aminoglycosides)
Significant perinatal asphyxia

Conditions in Infants and Young Children Indicative of Possible Hearing Loss
Parental concern
A history of otitis media occurring before 6 months of age or recurrent otitis occurring before 2 years of age
Chronic serous otitis media
Failure on a school hearing test
Speech problems and language delay

    (2) Modification of curriculum ranges from preferential seating in the front of the classroom to placement in a residential school. The degree of intervention is determined by the degree of hearing loss.
  c. Genetic counseling may be indicated, depending on the etiology of the hearing loss.

B. **Visual impairment**

1. Definitions
  a. Visual impairment is an educational term that implies that vision is impaired sufficiently to affect school functioning.
  b. A **partially sighted** person has vision in the better eye between 20/70 and 20/200.
  c. Blindness is defined as vision of not more than 20/200 in the better eye, after correction, or as a defect in the visual field such that the widest diameter of vision subtends an angle of 10° or less.

2. Etiology
  a. Congenital etiologic factors include developmental malformations, perinatal infections (e.g., rubella, cytomegalovirus, toxoplasmosis), and genetic syndromes (e.g., albinism).
  b. Neonatal etiologic factors include birth asphyxia, prematurity, and infections.
  c. Postnatal etiologic factors include trauma, retinitis pigmentosa, demyelinating disease, neurodegenerative disease, tumor, and increased intracranial pressure.
  d. Functional causes also are possible. For example, in cortical blindness the eye is structurally sound, but the cortex is unable to process visual information.

3. Assessment
  a. History. A number of risk factors should increase the suspicion of possible visual impairment in infants and young children, including:
    (1) A family history of visual defects
    (2) A history of congenital infections
    (3) A history of premature delivery or prolonged labor
    (4) Evidence of mental retardation, cerebral palsy, or hearing difficulty (40%–50% of partially sighted children have additional handicaps)
  b. Physical examination
    (1) In the **neonatal period,** the physical examination should assess the gross appearance of the eyes, the alignment of the eyes, brightness and clarity of the red reflex, and some funduscopic details.

    (2) In **older children,** the visual field should be assessed and more detailed fundu-scopic examinations should be performed. If more complicated assessments are required, or if there is a history of oxygen therapy or a family history of major visual defects, referral to an ophthalmologist is appropriate.

  c. Visual assessment

    (1) Infancy. By age 3 months, the child should be able to follow familiar objects. Optokinetic nystagmus should be assessed. **Visual evoked response testing** is a technique available for the assessment of vision in an infant.

    (2) Preschool period. Modified charts, such as the Stycar and the Random Dot E, can be used to assess visual acuity.

    (3) School years. Visual acuity is typically estimated using the Snellen E chart.

4. Therapy

  a. Management of visual impairment includes the correction of refraction errors with lenses, eye patching, as well as surgery for strabismus.

  b. Developmental factors should be considered when dealing with a visually impaired child.

    (1) Blind children require an extremely rich sensory environment to maximize the use of their other senses. Referral to an **early intervention** program is essential.

    (2) Blind children have a tendency to acquire unusual movement patterns (**blindisms**), which can potentially isolate these children even further. Some of these behaviors can be easily extinguished using **behavior modification** techniques.

  c. Education. Many educational techniques are available to visually impaired children, including Optacon, which converts words to tactile print, as well as print-to-speech converters. Talking books, laser-guided canes, and other low-vision aids enable visually impaired people to function more independently in society.

  d. Genetic counseling is also necessary in many cases of visual impairment.

VI. COMMON RECURRENT PAIN SYNDROMES

A. **Introduction and definition.** Recurrent pain occurs frequently in children. The emphasis in this section is on those entities that are not caused by organic disease—**recurrent abdominal pain syndrome, "psychogenic" headache,** and **limb pain**. These are pains that occur at least monthly for a 3-month period, in which no organic pathology is found; during the interval between episodes, the child is well. Because of similarities in the approach to assessing and treating these entities, they are discussed here as a group.

B. **Incidence.** Recurrent abdominal pain occurs in 10%–15% of school-age children, with a peak incidence at age 9 years. Growing pains occur in 15% of school-age children, with a peak incidence at age 11. Headache occurs in 15%–20% of school children, with a peak incidence at age 12.

C. **Etiology.** Purely organic or purely emotional etiologic explanations account for only a minor percentage of recurrent pain. Current thinking regarding recurrent pain refutes the previous dichotomy of either an organic or a psychological explanation for these problems, and substitutes a new category—**dysfunctional pain**. The pain is neither the result of pathophysiology nor obvious psychopathology, but is the result of mild individual differences in physiology, which make the child vulnerable to pain and which may be exacerbated by stress. For example, in children with recurrent abdominal pain, there may be slower transit time, resulting in constipation, lactose intolerance, or increased autonomic nervous system activity. The **differential diagnosis** for recurrent pain other than dysfunctional pain includes:

1. Recurrent abdominal pain

  a. Genitourinary problems (e.g., recurrent infections, lower tract obstruction, vulvo-vaginitis)

      b. Gastrointestinal disorders (e.g., inflammatory bowel disease, ulcer disease, hepatitis)
      c. Psychological causes (e.g., conversion reactions, somatoform disorders)
      d. Other disorders, including porphyria and trauma

  2. Headache
      a. Medical causes (e.g., infection, increased blood pressure)
      b. Neurologic causes (e.g., migraine, increased intracranial pressure; see Chapter 18)
      c. Vascular abnormalities
      d. Psychological causes (e.g., anxiety)

  3. Limb pain (growing pains)
      a. Orthopedic disorders (e.g., Osgood-Schlatter disease, Legg-Calvé-Perthes disease, trauma)
      b. Collagen vascular disease
      c. Infection
      d. Neoplastic disease

D. **Assessment**

  1. History. Essentials include the following:
      a. Characteristics of the pain must be noted, such as onset, frequency, duration, and associated symptoms. Continuous pain, localized pain, pain that awakens the child from sleep, and pain associated with other symptoms (e.g., vomiting, fever, changes in stool color) suggest organic disease.
      b. Evidence of obvious psychopathology must be sought in the parents and in the child, and major stressors on the family should be identified. It is also important to identify whether other family members have symptoms similar to those of the patient.

  2. Physical examination to rule out obvious organic explanations for the symptoms is essential. Normal growth and development are unlikely in the face of chronic organic disease.
      a. Recurrent abdominal pain. The further the pain is from the umbilicus, the more likely it is to be organic. A rectal examination is imperative.
      b. Headache. The more localized the pain, the less likely it is to be "psychogenic." Blood pressure determination, assessment of the visual field, and a thorough fundu-scopic examination are essential.
      c. Limb pain. The more localized the pain, the less likely it is to be growing pains. The physical examination should include assessment of the affected limb for evidence of atrophy, swelling, weakness, and effusion.

  3. Laboratory investigation. Complete blood count, erythrocyte sedimentation rate, and urinalysis comprise a good screen. Further investigation should take place only if suggested by the history and physical examination.

E. **Therapy**

  1. If **organic disease** is identified, it should be treated appropriately.

  2. If there is a strong indication that **psychological factors** are responsible for the symptoms, the physician should provide appropriate counsel or referral to a mental health agency.

  3. Most often, neither organic nor psychological factors appear responsible. If this is the case, and if the characteristics fit the definition of **dysfunctional pain,** this type of pain should be explained to the family (see VI C). The long-term outlook for recurrent pain during childhood is promising.
      a. For dysfunctional pain, **normal activity should be encouraged,** and the pain should not be allowed to restrict the child significantly.
      b. A **symptom diary** should be kept by the parents and the child, detailing information regarding episodes of pain. Frequent visits to the physician with review of this diary are helpful.
      c. Symptomatic relief should be offered. Mild analgesics (e.g., acetaminophen) for pain episodes, dietary changes, exercise, and stress reduction all may be helpful.

VII. EMOTIONAL DISORDERS

A. Depression

1. Definition. Depression is a clinical syndrome characterized by a persistent mood disorder and dysfunctional behavior. Although findings may differ at the various developmental stages, they usually include sadness or unhappiness, social withdrawal, eating problems, sleeping disorders, loss of interest in usual activities, and a decreased ability to concentrate. The incidence of childhood depression in the general population is 2%, and depression accounts for 30% of childhood psychiatric disorders.

2. Etiology is multifactorial. Genetic causes, chronic illness, as well as psychosocial stress have been implicated. Certain specific disease states are associated with depression (e.g., epilepsy, hypothyroidism, adrenal insufficiency, migraine), and a number of medical problems can mimic it (e.g., neuromuscular disease that affects facial expression, degenerative disease that causes psychomotor retardation).

3. Assessment
  a. History
    (1) Details from home and school regarding the cause of the symptoms and the degree of dysfunction should be elicited. Learning disabilities should be ruled out by administration of the appropriate testing.
    (2) Information about social withdrawal, mood, appetite, sleep patterns, and irritability should be obtained.
    (3) A history of family members with possible depressive illnesses who were hospitalized, who required electroconvulsive therapy, or who committed suicide is important to a complete assessment.
  b. Physical examination
    (1) In addition to the routine physical examination, funduscopic examination for evidence of increased intracranial pressure should be done.
    (2) Deep tendon reflexes should be carefully reviewed for evidence of hypothyroidism.
  c. Laboratory and radiographic investigation
    (1) If the cause of depression is not obviously psychosocial, complete blood count, erythrocyte sedimentation rate, and thyroid studies are helpful.
    (2) Evidence of drug abuse should be sought.
    (3) A CT scan is indicated if intracranial pathology is suspected.
    (4) A dexamethasone suppression test might be considered. Among adults with endogenous depression, hypersecretion of cortisol and failure to suppress cortisol secretion with dexamethasone have been reported in two thirds of patients. The extent of such findings among depressed children is unclear.

4. Therapy
  a. Psychotherapy for the child and family is indicated.
  b. Antidepressant medication—typically a tricyclic antidepressant—may be considered.

B. Schizophrenia

1. Definition
  a. Schizophrenia is a syndrome of grossly impaired behavior that is characterized by:
    (1) Characteristic disturbances of thought, perception, and relationship to the external world
    (2) Deterioration from a previous level of functioning
    (3) A duration of at least 6 months
    (4) Often loose associations, delusions, and hallucinations
  b. Episodes of childhood schizophrenia typically occur after the age of 7 years and increase in frequency to adolescence. Nevertheless, they are rare in children younger than 12 years.

2. Etiology
   a. Many authorities suggest that the development of childhood schizophrenia is a multifactorial process involving **social and emotional stressors** in a child with a **genetic predisposition** or a **biologic vulnerability,** or both.
   b. A number of **medical conditions** have been associated with childhood psychosis, including:
      (1) Wilson disease
      (2) Thyroid disease
      (3) Systemic lupus erythematosus
      (4) Homocystinuria
      (5) Leukodystrophy
   c. Factors in the **differential diagnosis** include:
      (1) Brief reactive psychoses
      (2) Overwhelming anxiety
      (3) Depression
      (4) Imaginary friends and other normal developmental occurrences in childhood

3. Assessment
   a. History. The essential aspects of the patient's history to be determined include:
      (1) Whether the child's current problem represents a deterioration from a previous level of functioning or merely the continuation of a previous delay in development
      (2) Evidence of delusions and hallucinations
      (3) A family history with evidence of mental illness
   b. Physical examination. The focus of the physical examination should be on evidence of an organic explanation for the psychosis (e.g., drug ingestion, thyroid disease, Wilson disease, increased intracranial pressure).
   c. Laboratory investigation
      (1) Urine should be tested for toxic substances.
      (2) Liver function tests should be performed, and serum levels of ceruloplasmin should be measured for evidence of Wilson disease.
      (3) Psychometric testing also might be helpful.

4. Therapy. The course of childhood schizophrenia is usually chronic. A number of treatments should be considered, including:
   a. Antipsychotic medication
   b. Psychotherapy and support for the child and family (hospitalization during acute episodes may be necessary)
   c. Education (a specific educational program for the psychotic child is often necessary)

C. **Oppositional–defiant disorder**

   1. Definition. This diagnosis is given to children who demonstrate a persistent pattern (longer than 6 months) of angry, negative, and often defiant behavior. These children easily lose their temper and frequently refuse to comply with adult rules or requests.

   2. Etiology. Although this behavior pattern is more common in families with other mental health disorders, its origins are probably multifactorial and stem from interaction of biologic vulnerabilities and psychosocial stressors.

   3. Assessment. Other syndromes that should be ruled out include:
      a. ADHD
      b. Impaired language
      c. Normative stage behavior

   4. Treatment and course. Psychological intervention, working with the child and family, is the standard treatment. For many children, oppositional–defiant disorder is the developmental precursor of conduct disorder.

D. **Conduct disorder**

1. **Definition.** This disorder constitutes a pattern of behavior in which an individual violates the basic rights of others in a manner exceeding age-appropriate expectations. It may occur before age 10 years (childhood-onset) or after age 10 (adolescent-onset). Clinical presentations include:
   a. Aggression (i.e., causing or threatening physical harm)
   b. Destruction of property
   c. Deceitfulness or theft
   d. Serious violations of rules, usually truancy or running away

2. **Etiology.** The etiology is multifactorial, with genetic, neurologic, cognitive, and environmental contributions that vary from child to child. The disorder may be exacerbated by underlying ADHD, learning disabilities, and poor self-esteem; it occurs far more frequently in boys.

3. **Assessment.** The differential diagnosis includes:
   a. Oppositional–defiant disorder
   b. Manic episodes
   c. ADHD

4. **Treatment and course.** No single approach ameliorates all antisocial behavior. Individual, family, and community-based psychotherapy, education, and medication all are part of a comprehensive approach. Despite interventions, children with conduct disorders frequently have continued problems with substance abuse and antisocial behavior.

BIBLIOGRAPHY

American Psychiatric Association: *Diagnostic and Statistical Manual of Mental Disorders*, 4th ed. Washington, DC, American Psychiatric Association, 1994.

Levine MD, Carey WB, Crocker AC: *Developmental–Behavioral Pediatrics*, 2nd ed. Philadelphia, WB Saunders, 1992.

STUDY QUESTIONS

DIRECTIONS: Each of the numbered items or incomplete statements in this section is followed by answers or by completions of the statement. Select the ONE lettered answer or completion that is BEST in each case.

1. Which of the following symptoms would suggest a diagnosis of recurrent abdominal pain?

(A) Pain awakening a child from sleep
(B) Pain associated with vomiting
(C) Pain located periumbilically
(D) Pain radiating to the back

2. A 16-year-old girl presents with signs of depression, including social withdrawal, anorexia, sadness, and inability to concentrate. Initial evaluation of this teenager should include

(A) measurement of serum ceruloplasmin levels to rule out Wilson disease
(B) a toxic screen for evidence of drug abuse
(C) a computed tomography (CT) scan
(D) an electroencephalogram

DIRECTIONS: Each of the numbered items or incomplete statements in this section is negatively phrased, as indicated by a capitalized word such as NOT, LEAST, or EXCEPT. Select the ONE lettered answer or completion that is BEST in each case.

Questions 3 and 4

A 9-year-old boy presents with a 1-year history of vague nighttime leg pains that awaken him from sleep but are responsive to acetaminophen. He has no limp or pain in the morning on arising, and is otherwise well.

3. Which of the following is NOT necessary at the initial phase of evaluation?

(A) Measuring the circumference of legs
(B) Examining legs for strength
(C) Magnetic resonance imaging scan of legs
(D) Erythrocyte sedimentation rate

4. Which of the following therapeutic strategies is NOT appropriate initially?

(A) Pain diary
(B) Use of analgesics
(C) Referral to a mental health professional
(D) Scheduled follow-up visits

5. All of the following conditions may cause sensorineural hearing loss EXCEPT

(A) rubella
(B) meningitis
(C) perinatal asphyxia
(D) otitis media
(E) aminoglycoside administration

6. All of the following statements regarding the use of stimulant medication in attention-deficit hyperactivity disorder (ADHD) are correct EXCEPT

(A) Tourette syndrome is a possible complication of stimulant use
(B) stimulant drugs are the initial treatment for ADHD
(C) stimulants increase attention span
(D) methylphenidate, dextroamphetamine, and pemoline are the major stimulants in use at this time

DIRECTIONS: Each set of matching questions in this section consists of a list of four to twenty-six lettered options (some of which may be in figures) followed by several items. For each numbered item, select the ONE lettered option that is most closely associated with it. To avoid spending too much time on matching sets with large numbers of options, it is generally advisable to begin each set by reading the list of options. Then, for each item in the set, try to generate the correct answer and locate it in the option list, rather than evaluating each option individually. Each lettered option may be selected once, more than once, or not at all.

Questions 7–10

Match each description below with the disorder that it best characterizes.

(A) Depression
(B) Oppositional–defiant disorder
(C) Schizophrenia
(D) Conduct disorder

7. Physically aggressive or threatening

8. Socially withdrawn

9. Disturbances of thought

10. Angry and negative

Questions 11–13

For each case scenario described below, select the most appropriate diagnosis.

(A) Asperger syndrome
(B) Autistic disorder
(C) Pervasive developmental disorder

11. A 7-year-old child with a lifelong history of profound language delays and social skill deficits who has stereotypic movements and tests in the retarded range intellectually

12. An 11-year-old boy with no friends, poor social skills, and an intense interest in locomotive engines who flaps his hands when excited and whose intellectual testing is in the average range

13. A 6-year-old girl whose intellectual functioning is in the retarded range, who has a number of stereotypic movements and poor social skills, but whose language and play are commensurate with her developmental level

1. The answer is C *[VI D 2 a]*. Recurrent abdominal pain typically is periumbilical and diffuse. Well-localized pain, radiating pain, pain associated with other symptoms, and pain so severe as to awaken a child from sleep are less likely to be recurrent abdominal pain and more likely to be organic.

2. The answer is B *[VII A 3 c, B 3 b]*. Symptoms of drug abuse can mimic those of depression. Wilson disease is more likely to mimic schizophrenia, and, for diagnosis, an associated family history should exist. A computed tomography (CT) scan should be ordered only if there is evidence of increased intracranial pressure, and an electroencephalogram only if seizures are suspected.

3. The answer is C *[VI D 1–3]*. The case description implies that this child most likely has growing pains, a benign, self-limited, recurrent pain syndrome. The 1-year history without progression and the lack of focality make an organic explanation unlikely. Nonetheless, the physical examination should certify that there is no swelling, erythema, joint involvement, or atrophy. A magnetic resonance imaging scan is unnecessary if there are no focal findings.

4. The answer is C *[VI E 2, 3 b, c]*. Recurrent pain syndromes usually are not associated with underlying psychopathology. The typical treatment is supportive and involves analgesics and other comfort measures. It is important that the child believes he is being listened to; pain diaries and scheduled follow-up visits allow for the careful monitoring of the pain and the further development of a trusting physician–child relationship. Referral to a mental health professional is indicated only when psychological factors are strongly implicated as being responsible for the symptoms.

5. The answer is D *[Table 4-3]*. Otitis media is associated with conductive hearing loss, not sensorineural hearing loss. Rubella and other prenatal infections can cause sensorineural hearing loss, as can meningitis and other postnatal infections. Perinatal asphyxia has also been implicated. Aminoglycosides are ototoxic in high doses, and should be carefully monitored.

6. The answer is B *[III B 4 c]*. Treatment of attention-deficit hyperactivity disorder (ADHD) with stimulant drugs should be initiated only after academic and behavioral approaches to the disorder have been attempted. As part of an overall approach to ADHD, stimulants can improve attention span and decrease distractibility. A number of side effects, such as sleep and eating problems, headaches, growth retardation, and, rarely, Tourette syndrome, have been associated with stimulant use.

7–10. The answers are: 7-D *[VII D 1 a]*, **8-A** *[VII A 1]*, **9-C** *[VII B 1 a (1)]*, **10-B** *[VII C 1]*. Children with conduct disorder violate basic societal norms and may frequently initiate physical fights, brandish or use a weapon, or bully and intimidate others. Although children with oppositional–defiant disorder may be negative and angry, they are not physically threatening or aggressive. None of the other disorders is associated with this type of behavior.

Depression is categorized by sadness and unhappiness, social withdrawal, and a generalized loss of interest or pleasure in most activities. Although social withdrawal may occur in childhood schizophrenia, it is not necessarily a hallmark of that condition.

One of the main characteristics of schizophrenia is a disturbance in the content of thought. Types of thought disturbances include delusions of persecution, in which a patient feels spied on, and delusions of reference, in which a patient might feel her thoughts are being broadcast over the television or discussed by television commentators.

11–13. The answers are: 11-B *[IV A 1 b (1)]*, **12-A** *[IV A 1 b (2)]*, **13-C** *[IV A 1 b (3)]*. This child fulfills all of the criteria for a diagnosis of autism. These include profound deficits of language and social skills, stereotypic patterns of movement, and onset of symptoms before 3 years of age.

Children with Asperger syndrome function in the normal range intellectually but have deficits in social skills, often resulting in limited friendships, and have intense interests. They also often have stereotypic movements.

Children with pervasive developmental disorder have many but not all of the characteristics of autism. Although this child has stereotypies, her language delays and social skill deficits are commensurate with her level of retardation.

Chapter 5

Adolescent Medicine
Aric Schichor

I. SCOPE AND GENERAL CONCEPTS OF ADOLESCENT MEDICINE

A. **Objectives.** Adolescence begins at puberty, a time of physical growth and personality development. The transition from childhood to adulthood is a confusing and ambiguous period for adolescents, parents, and health care providers. The time of onset of puberty and the manner of coping with the many physical, social, and emotional changes associated with adolescence vary widely from one adolescent to another. Adolescent medicine should focus on more than strictly medical issues—it also should consider the issues that affect a teenager's day-to-day well-being. Pediatric health care providers are required to:

1. Deal with acute health needs

2. Provide comprehensive health care, including:
   a. General medical care
   b. Care in high-risk health areas (e.g., sexual activity, substance abuse, depression, suicide, injuries, violence)
   c. Guidance in general issues (e.g., peer relationships, school progress, home environment, relationship with parents)

3. Produce educated consumers of health services by providing health education

4. Encourage independence in health-seeking behavior

5. Support and counsel parents in providing supervision and guidance to their adolescents

6. Educate, assist, and work with other adults in the community who deal with adolescents

B. **General concepts**

1. **Common terms** are used to define the rights of adolescents.
   a. **Mature minors** are individuals 14 years of age or older who understand the risks and benefits of the services being provided and hence can give informed consent.
   b. **Emancipated minors** are individuals 16 years of age or older who are married, have joined the armed forces, or have proven in a court of law that they are living on their own and managing their own financial affairs. Emancipated minors are allowed to receive any form of health care services without parental consent. Women who are pregnant or are parents are often given the rights associated with being emancipated.

2. **State laws** vary regarding the right of adolescents to receive care without parental consent. In many states, mature minors may be treated for drug abuse and sexually transmitted diseases (STDs), and may be given mental health counseling as well as family planning, pregnancy, and abortion counseling without parental consent. More recently, several states have required parental consent or permission from a local court for a mature minor to have an abortion.

3. **Confidentiality** is a central concept for adolescent health care. It permits the patient to form a relationship with the health care provider in which the patient can share

information that is not given to anyone else without the formal consent of the patient. The adolescent needs to be informed that confidentiality may be breached when life is at risk.

4. **The physician's office** should reflect the needs of adolescents and enhance the adolescent's attitude toward seeking health care. The decor of the waiting area and examination room should attract the adolescent. If possible, infants and children should not be seen in the same space at the same time.

5. **Family involvement** can result in additional information about and support for adolescents and can increase adolescents' health care compliance.

II. HEALTH SUPERVISION ISSUES

A. History

1. **Goals** of the patient history include:
   a. Obtaining information about high-risk areas in the adolescent's life from both the patient and the parents
   b. Determining specific concerns of the adolescent
   c. Establishing the uniqueness of each adolescent

2. **Methods**
   a. Information can be obtained through **interviews, discussion,** and **written questionnaires**. Although questionnaires cannot replace verbal questioning, they can provide a focus for discussion, help for adolescents who are less verbal, and a way to use waiting time effectively.
   b. A **variety of approaches** to asking questions should be used, so that the patient has several opportunities to speak openly on the topics discussed. Three approaches to asking questions are:
      (1) **Direct approach** (e.g., Have you ever been in a hospital overnight?)
      (2) **Indirect approach** (e.g., Some people who get down or depressed sometimes think of ending it all or killing themselves. . . . Have you ever had such thoughts?)
      (3) **Open-ended approach** (e.g., What do you do for fun? What three things would you change to make your life better? On a scale of 1 to 5, with 1 being poor, 3 being average, and 5 being great, how would you rate your general health?). Follow-up to such questions should focus on what changes could be made to improve the situation and which changes the adolescent would like to pursue.

3. Discussing **key topics** can help address complex issues in the adolescent's life.
   a. **Sexual activity** (e.g., What are your plans for starting your own family? What would you use for protection against pregnancy?)
   b. **Substance abuse** (e.g., Do you ever get high? Do you have friends who use drugs and alcohol? What do you do when they ask you to try drugs and alcohol with them?)
   c. **Mental health** (e.g., Do you ever get down or depressed? What gets you down and depressed? Who do you talk to when you get down and depressed?)
   d. **Home situation** (e.g., What are your responsibilities at home? What would you change about your parents to make them better?)
   e. **Self-image** (e.g., How do you feel when you look at yourself in the mirror in the morning? What would you change to make yourself feel better when you look in the mirror?)

B. Anticipatory guidance (Table 5-1) provides an opportunity to deal with the developmental issues of adolescence with both the adolescent and the parents (see Chapter 1).

TABLE 5-1. Issues of Anticipatory Guidance in Adolescence

Early Adolescence (Age: < 15 years)	Midadolescence (Age: 15–16 years)	Late Adolescence (Age: ≥ 17 years)
Puberty	Peer network	Separation
Privacy	Cognitive development	Decision making
Independence	Control over life	Continue to develop adult identity
Peers as confidants	Bundles of energy	
Adult role models	Developing adult identity	
Mood swings		
School transition		

 C. **Physical examination** provides the physician with an opportunity to teach health maintenance, especially about routine breast and testicular examination. The adolescent's
increasing need for privacy should be addressed by the use of appropriate drapes and
gowns during the examination.

1. **Areas requiring special focus**
   a. **Skin.** The degree of acne and the patient's level of concern about acne should be
   evaluated. Facial and axillary hair development are markers used for the assessment
   of pubertal development.
   b. **Eyes.** Myopia may occur during pubertal development. The adolescent may ignore
   eye problems because of reluctance to wear glasses. Contact lenses are often a good
   solution.
   c. **Dentition.** Evaluation of the level of hygiene, discussion of the frequency of dental care,
   and a review of the development of the third set of molar teeth should be undertaken.
   d. **Neck.** The size of the thyroid gland should be noted.
   e. **Breast** examination should include determination of the stage of development, as
   described in Table 5-2. Tenderness, erythema, dimpling, asymmetric masses or size,
   discharge, and axillary adenopathy should be noted. Routine breast self-examination
   should be encouraged.
   f. **Heart sounds** may be accentuated because of a thin chest wall, and functional murmurs may become more apparent.
   g. **Male genitourinary tract** examination includes determination of the stage of development (Tables 5-3 and 5-4) and evaluation for urethral discharge, scrotal masses,
   testicular size, inguinal adenopathy, and evidence of inguinal hernia. In a boy with
   an uncircumcised penis, hygienic practices should be reviewed and particular attention given to possible lesions below the foreskin. Routine testicular self-examination
   should be encouraged.

TABLE 5-2. Stages of Female Breast Development

Stage 1	Preadolescent—The juvenile breast has an elevated papilla (nipple-shaped projection) and small, flat areola.
Stage 2	The breast bud forms under the influence of hormonal stimulation. The papilla and areola elevate as a small mound, and the areolar diameter increases.
Stage 3	Continued enlargement of the breast bud further elevates the papilla. The areola contin-ues to enlarge; no separation of breast contours is noted.
Stage 4	The areola and papilla separate from the contour of the breast to form a secondary mound.
Stage 5	Mature—The areolar mound recedes into the general contour of the breast. The papilla continues to project.

Reprinted from Hoffmann A: *Adolescent Medicine*. Reading, MA, Addison-Wesley, 1983, p 18. Adapted from Tanner JM: *Growth at Adolescence*. Oxford, Blackwell, 1962.

TABLE 5-3. Stages of Pubic Hair Development

	Male	**Female**
Stage 1	Preadolescent—No pubic hair is present; a fine vellus hair covers the genital area.	Preadolescent—No pubic hair is present; a fine vellus hair covers the genital area.
Stage 2	A sparse distribution of long, slightly pigmented hair appears at the base of the penis.	A sparse distribution of long, slightly pigmented straight hair appears bilaterally along the medial border of the labia majora.
Stage 3	The pubic hair pigmentation increases; it begins to curl and spread laterally in a scanty distribution.	The pubic hair pigmentation increases; it begins to curl and spread sparsely over the mons pubis.
Stage 4	The pubic hair continues to curl and becomes coarse in texture. An adult type of distribution is attained, but the number of hairs remains fewer.	The pubic hair continues to curl and becomes coarse in texture. The number of hairs continues to increase.
Stage 5	Mature—The pubic hair attains an adult distribution, with spread to the surface of the medial thigh. Pubic hair grows along the linea alba in 80% of men.	Mature—The pubic hair attains an adult feminine triangular pattern, with spread to the surface of the medial thigh.

Reprinted from Hoffman A: *Adolescent Medicine.* Reading, MA, Addison-Wesley, 1983, p 16. Adapted from Tanner JM: *Growth at Adolescence.* Oxford, Blackwell, 1962.

    h. Female genitourinary tract examination includes determination of the stage of development (see Table 5-3) as well as an assessment of delayed puberty or abnormal pubertal development. A pelvic examination is indicated in evaluating vulvar lesions, vaginal symptoms (e.g., itching, unusual discharge, burning), lower abdominal pain, dysmenorrhea of greater than a 3-day duration, menstrual dysfunction, and exposure to an STD (see IV A). Examination is also warranted in cases of desire for contraception, premarital assessment, and history of sexual intercourse.

    i. Musculoskeletal examination should include inspection of individual large joints as well as the back. (For screening for scoliosis, refer to section IX A 2.)

  2. Pubertal development (for disorders of pubertal development, see Chapter 17)

    a. The pubertal growth spurt (Figure 5-1) is the third and last rapid growth stage during childhood. (The first and second rapid growth stages occur in utero and shortly after birth.)

      (1) Adolescents gain up to 25% of adult height and 50% of adult weight during this period.

      (2) Individuals vary widely in the onset and rate of pubertal development. It is important to talk about this variability with adolescents and, where appropriate, reassure them about the normal nature of their pubertal development.

TABLE 5-4. Stages of Male Genital Development

Stage 1	Preadolescent—The testes, scrotum, and penis are the same as in childhood.
Stage 2	As a result of canalization of seminiferous tubules, the testes enlarge. The scrotum enlarges, developing a reddish hue and altering in skin texture. The penis enlarges slightly.
Stage 3	The testes and scrotum continue to grow. The length of the penis increases.
Stage 4	The testes and scrotum continue to grow; the scrotal skin darkens. The penis grows in width, and the glans penis develops.
Stage 5	Mature—The testes, scrotum, and penis are adult in size and shape.

Reprinted from Hoffman A: *Adolescent Medicine.* Reading, MA, Addison-Wesley, 1983, p 17. Adapted from Tanner JM: *Growth at Adolescence.* Oxford, Blackwell, 1962.

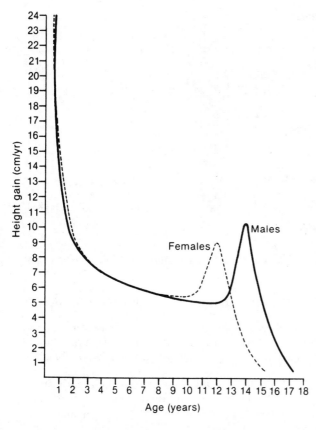

FIGURE 5-1. Graph showing the height gain (postnatal and pubertal growth spurts) in males and females between birth and age 18 years. (Reprinted from Tanner JM, et al: Standards from birth to maturity for height, weight, height velocity, and weight velocity in British children, 1965. *Arch Dis Child* 41:454, 1965.)

   (3) This growth spurt is associated with muscle development in boys and fat deposition in girls.
   b. Female pubertal changes (Figure 5-2) start between 8 and 13 years of age, and changes take place for 3–4 years. Breast development commonly precedes pubic hair development. Most girls reach adult height midway through puberty.
   c. Male pubertal changes (Figure 5-3) start between 9 and 13 years of age, and changes take place for about 3 years. Testicular enlargement is usually the first sign of male pubertal development. Most boys reach adult height during the latter half of puberty.

D. **Procedures**

   1. Routine evaluations
      a. Height, weight, and blood pressure should be measured and the data plotted in the appropriate charts. An adult blood pressure cuff should be used.
      b. Vision, hearing, and immunizations should be checked. A tetanus booster should have been given within the past 10 years. Measles reimmunization should be performed if not administered by age 11–12 years (see Chapter 1). Hepatitis B immunization is recommended for all adolescents who have not been previously infected or immunized.

   2. Laboratory studies
      a. Routine screening
         (1) A complete blood count is helpful, especially to monitor changes in hematocrit levels due to increased erythropoietin activity subsequent to changes in the level of circulating androgens.
         (2) Sickle cell testing should be done in all black and Hispanic patients if it has not been done previously.
         (3) Other screening studies include urinalysis, and tuberculin skin test (Mantoux) for high-risk adolescents (see Chapter 1).

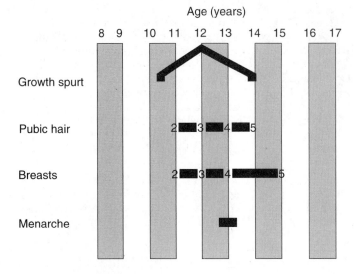

FIGURE 5-2. The average age in years of onset and duration of the stages of female pubertal development. (Adapted from Grumbach MM, Grave GD, Mayer FE: *Control of the Onset of Puberty.* New York, John Wiley, 1974, p 460.)

b. Special tests
   (1) A Papanicolaou (Pap) test should be done annually on all sexually active adolescent girls.
   (2) Pregnancy testing with a rapid urine immunoenzymatic assay for human chorionic gonadotropin (hCG) should be performed in sexually active girls who are not using any form of contraception or who experience a delayed or abnormal menstrual period.
   (3) Cholesterol (nonfasting) level should be done on initial visit and as indicated by dietary/family histories. If elevated (above 200 mg/dl), fasting cholesterol and triglyceride levels should be measured (see Chapter 1).

III. GENITOURINARY AND GYNECOLOGIC DISORDERS

A. **Disorders of menarche.** Normal menarche occurs at an average age of 12 years, with bleeding lasting an average of 4–5 days. Menses may be irregular in the first 2 years. Twenty percent of young women are anovulatory into their late teens.

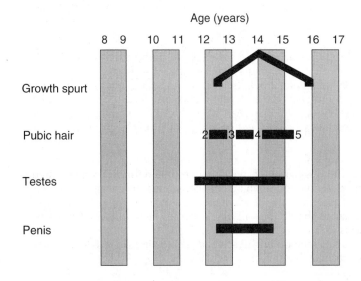

FIGURE 5-3. The average age in years of onset and duration of the stages of male pubertal development. (Adapted from Grumbach MM, Grave GD, Mayer FE: *Control of the Onset of Puberty.* New York, John Wiley, 1974, p 460.)

1. **Amenorrhea**
   a. **Etiology.** Causes for amenorrhea include delayed pubertal development, significant weight gain or loss, stress or depression, pregnancy, medications, structural obstruction or agenesis, gonadal dysgenesis, polycystic ovary syndrome, and tumors.
   b. **Primary amenorrhea** is the failure of menstruation and any other signs of pubertal development by 14 years of age, or the failure of menstruation in spite of pubertal development by age 16 years.
   c. **Secondary amenorrhea** is the cessation of menstruation after it has been established at puberty (i.e., 6 months since the last menstrual period or a period of time equal to three or four previous cycles).
   d. **Oligomenorrhea** is marked by diminished menstruation, with each cycle occurring 2–3 months apart.

2. **Dysfunctional uterine bleeding** is characterized by regular menstrual cycles with heavy bleeding lasting more than 10 days, menstrual periods occurring more frequently than every 21 days, and irregular menstrual periods aside from those that commonly occur in the first 2 years after menarche.
   a. **Etiology**
      (1) Causes associated with the vagina and cervix include foreign bodies (tampons) and trauma or irritation (rape, rupture of the hymen, intercourse).
      (2) Causes associated with the uterus, ovaries, and adnexa include intrauterine devices (IUDs), oral and injectable contraceptives, endometriosis, and polycystic ovary syndrome.
      (3) Other factors to consider include infections, masses (polyps, tumors), ectopic pregnancy, miscarriage, pregnancy termination, systemic disease, and bleeding disorders.
   b. **Evaluation**
      (1) **History.** The patient history should focus on the possible etiologies. The level of dysfunctional uterine bleeding should be determined.
         (a) **Mild dysfunctional bleeding** is characterized by an increase in duration of menses, a decrease in length of menstrual cycle, and a moderate increase in bleeding during menses.
         (b) **Moderate dysfunctional bleeding** is characterized by repeated episodes of prolonged menses, decreased length of menstrual cycle to the extent that menses occur every 2–3 weeks, and moderate to severe bleeding during menses.
         (c) **Severe dysfunctional bleeding** is characterized by menses that are so prolonged that the timing of the menstrual cycle is no longer clear, and by very heavy bleeding during the menstrual cycle.
      (2) **Physical examination** should review the skin for signs of bleeding disorders and the organs (e.g., thyroid gland, liver) for indications of systemic disease. A pelvic examination should include a rectovaginal examination.
      (3) **Laboratory studies** should initially include a complete blood count, a pregnancy test, and wet preparations and cultures for vaginitis or cervicitis. Thyroid and liver function tests as well as clotting studies should be done if indicated, or as a secondary consideration. Gonadotropin and prolactin levels should also be evaluated.
   c. **Therapy**
      (1) For **mild dysfunction** and normal hematocrit, the nature of the menstrual cycle should be reviewed and the adolescent reassured. The case is monitored for changes over time.
      (2) For **moderate dysfunction** and mild anemia, therapy may include a trial of oral contraceptives or medroxyprogesterone acetate. Iron and folic acid supplements are useful with repeated blood loss or associated anemia.
      (3) **Severe dysfunction** and moderate anemia may initially require hospitalization for stabilization and blood transfusion. Regulation of menses is achieved with administration of estrogen or an oral contraceptive with a higher estrogen dose on a more frequent basis until bleeding stops or slows down. Once this occurs, the medication is tapered over a number of days.

(4) Gynecologic consultation is recommended in cases in which the preceding guidelines do not result in menstrual regulation.

3. **Dysmenorrhea** is menstrual pain (usually in the lower abdomen).
   a. **Primary dysmenorrhea,** which accounts for 75% of all cases of dysmenorrhea, is not associated with any other pelvic abnormality, and lasts from a few hours to 2–3 days.
      (1) Symptoms include nausea, vomiting, headaches, back pain, and dizziness.
      (2) The exact etiology of the pain is unclear, but it may be related to increased myometrial activity (contractions of the smooth muscle coat) of the uterus associated with increased production of prostaglandin.
   b. **Secondary dysmenorrhea** is caused by a definable pelvic abnormality such as inflammation, structural abnormalities, adhesions, endometriosis, tumors, polyps, ovarian cysts, and IUDs.
   c. **Evaluation**
      (1) **History.** The patient history should focus on the relation of pain to the menstrual cycle, the duration of pain, associated symptoms and degree of dysfunction, and familial history of similar pain. Knowledge about the level of sexual activity and exposure to an STD (see IV A) is helpful. Systemic disease (e.g., gastroenteritis, urinary tract infection) should be ruled out.
      (2) **Pelvic examination** is indicated when the patient is in severe pain that lasts longer than 3 days and does not respond to treatment for primary dysmenorrhea.
      (3) **Laboratory evaluation** should be considered for cases that do not fit the definition of primary dysmenorrhea. Such studies should include a complete blood count and sedimentation rate for pelvic infection, vaginal wet smear, cultures for an STD, ultrasound of the pelvis for ovarian cysts, and laparoscopy for severe unresolved cases.
   d. **Therapy**
      (1) **Mild pain** with no limitation of activity may not need any treatment or may respond well to aspirin or a prostaglandin inhibitor (e.g., ibuprofen).
      (2) **Moderate pain,** with some limitation of activity but a situation in which the adolescent does not miss school, may be eased by regular use of an over-the-counter prostaglandin inhibitor.
      (3) **Severe pain** that causes the adolescent to miss school may be relieved by a prescription-strength prostaglandin inhibitor or a trial of oral contraceptives.

B. **Maternal exposure to diethylstilbestrol (DES).** DES was used from the 1940s to the early 1970s to prevent miscarriage and was subsequently associated with disorders such as vaginal adenosis and adenocarcinoma of the cervix in women and microphallus and hypospadias in men. It is useful to obtain a history of possible exposure to DES; however, most children exposed in utero to this drug will now be in their third decade or older.

C. **Pelvic masses**

1. **Sites**
   a. The **vagina** may contain foreign bodies or hematocolpos from an imperforate hymen.
   b. The **uterus** may contain a fetus or a fibrous lesion.
   c. **Adnexal sites** may hide an ectopic pregnancy, endometriosis, ovarian cysts, teratomas (tumors), or hydrosalpinx subsequent to inflammation.
   d. Masses also may be located in the bowel, kidneys, or liver.

2. **Evaluation**
   a. **History.** A history regarding menses, nature and frequency of symptoms, and level of sexual activity should be taken.
   b. **Examination** can be augmented by pelvic ultrasound or laparoscopy if indicated.
   c. **Laboratory studies** include complete blood count and sedimentation rate, analysis of any vaginal discharge, culture for an STD (see IV A), a pregnancy test, and appropriate cytologic studies of any unidentified mass.

3. **Therapy** includes the following:
   a. Perforation of the hymen to drain hematocolpos
   b. Referral of cases involving ectopic pregnancy or tumors to a gynecologist
   c. Hormonal or surgical therapeutic approach to endometriosis
   d. Treatment of the cause of pelvic inflammation to resolve hydrosalpinx
   e. Drainage of follicular cysts with laparoscopic guidance if they do not resolve spontaneously

D. **Disorders of the breast and breast development**

1. **Abnormal development.** Initial breast development may be asymmetric. Congenital lack of glandular tissue and hypertrophy of the breasts both can be surgically corrected.

2. **Gynecomastia** is excessive development of the male mammary glands. Such development is often asymptomatic and unilateral. Gynecomastia occurs in up to 60% of all boys and usually lasts 6 months to 2 years.

3. **Galactorrhea** is a discharge from the female breasts when lactation is not occurring. Evaluation for a pituitary tumor and hypothyroidism should be considered.

4. **Masses.** It is important to reassure the patient that most masses found during adolescence are benign.
   a. **Fibroadenoma** is the most common mass found in breasts of adolescents. These masses are rubbery, well defined, movable, and usually unilateral. Fibroadenomas are benign and can be surgically removed if desired.
   b. **Fibrocystic disease** is characterized by typically bilateral changes in breast tissue (thickening, small cyst formation). The cysts usually require routine follow-up. Occasionally, surgical removal of large or malignant cysts is needed.
   c. **Malignancy** occurs very rarely in adolescents; however, a biopsy specimen should be taken of any persistent breast lesion of unclear etiology.

E. **Testicular and scrotal disorders** (see also Chapters 14 and 16)

1. **Varicocele** is dilatation of the veins of the spermatic cord. This disorder occurs in 15% of adolescents, more commonly on the left side of the scrotum, and, if extensive, may result in decreased fertility in adulthood.

2. **Priapism** is a sustained, painful erection. This disorder may be associated with sickle cell anemia, leukemia, or urethral inflammation.

3. **Inguinal hernias** occur up to five times more often in boys than in girls; they occur more often on the right, but frequently are bilateral.
   a. **Common terms** used to describe hernias include:
      (1) **Reducible.** The physician can displace hernia contents back into the abdomen.
      (2) **Incarcerated.** The hernia is not reducible.
      (3) **Strangulated.** An incarcerated hernia is likely to become gangrenous (i.e., the blood supply is cut off from the contents of the hernia).
      (4) **Sliding.** The wall of the hernia sac is composed of another organ (e.g., the colon).
   b. **Types.** Inguinal hernias are direct or indirect.
      (1) **Indirect** inguinal hernias are most common, and protrude through the internal inguinal ring.
      (2) **Direct** inguinal hernias result from a weakness in the medial inguinal canal floor.

4. **Hydrocele** is a fluid-filled structure in the tunica vaginalis or the processus vaginalis located in the scrotum.

5. **Spermatocele** is cystic swelling of the epididymis or the rete testis containing spermatozoa.

IV. GENITOURINARY AND GYNECOLOGIC INFECTIONS

A. **STDs** are acquired by sexual contact and intercourse (including genital, rectal, and oral penetration). These diseases are most common in the adolescent and young adult population (15–24 years of age).

1. **Agents of specific STDs** (Table 5-5)
   a. *Chlamydia trachomatis* is the cause of the most common nonviral STD in the United States. It is an intracellular organism found in columnar lining cells of the cervix, uterus, fallopian tubes, liver capsule, urethra, rectum, pharynx, and skin. *C. trachomatis* is the most common cause of **nongonococcal urethritis** in men. It also causes **lymphogranuloma venereum** and **inclusion conjunctivitis**. It is one of the leading causes of infertility in women. It can also cause epididymitis in men.
   b. *Neisseria gonorrhoeae* is an intracellular, gram-negative diplococcus found in a distribution similar to that of *C. trachomatis*; in addition, joint involvement can cause arthritis.
   c. **Human immunodeficiency virus (HIV)** is acquired through sexual transmission or intravenous spread from blood products or illicit drug use (see Chapter 9).
   d. *Ureaplasma urealyticum* is the second most common cause of nongonococcal urethritis in men. It is a T-strain mycoplasma with genital and pelvic distribution similar to that of *C. trachomatis*.
   e. *Treponema pallidum*, the cause of **syphilis**, is a less common cause of infection in adolescents compared to adults. It is seen more regularly in association with other STDs and in adolescents involved with illicit drug use. *T. pallidum* is a motile spiral microorganism 5–20 mm long. The infection usually starts in the genital area but can affect other parts of the body.
   f. *Haemophilus ducreyi* causes chancroid. It should be considered in the differential diagnosis of a painful genital ulcer often accompanied by tender inguinal lymphadenopathy.
   g. **Herpes simplex virus (HSV)** infection has increased in incidence to more than 1 million cases per year in the United States. HSV is a DNA virus. The most common form causing genital involvement is HSV type 2.
   h. **Condylomata acuminata** (venereal warts) are a form of DNA papillomavirus infection and the most common STD in adolescents.
   i. **Molluscum contagiosum** is a poxvirus infection found in any part of the body, but it is usually present in greater concentration in the genital area when it is sexually transmitted.
   j. *Trichomonas vaginalis* is a flagellate protozoon present most commonly in the vagina, but also found near the urethra of both sexes.
   k. *Phthirus pubis* (pediculosis pubis, crab lice) is a parasite that is less than 4 mm long.

2. **Therapy** for STDs should include all exposed individuals, whenever possible. The specific treatment depends on accurate identification of the causative organism; the choice of antibiotic must take into consideration the organism's sensitivity and the patient's age and history of allergies. Two general treatment recommendations should be taken into consideration:
   a. Whenever possible, treat the STD with a single dose of medication right on the spot to ensure compliance. This is possible for gonorrhea, chlamydial and trichomonal infections, and bacterial vaginosis (see IV B 2). The latest treatment guidelines for STDs are published by the Centers for Disease Control and Prevention (refer to the Bibliography).
   b. If either gonorrhea or chlamydial infection is suspected, treatment should be given for both diseases.

3. **Prevention.** Proper use of condoms can reduce the risk of transmitting most STDs.

TABLE 5-5. Sexually Transmitted Diseases

Agent	Clinical Features	Diagnosis
Chlamydia trachomatis	Cervical ectopy and friability Mucoid cervical discharge with ↑ leukocyte count Dysuria (in men may not be accompanied by discharge) Pelvic tenderness in women Pharyngitis Rectal irritation/tenderness	Chlamydia inclusion bodies identified through cell culture or rapid test such as fluorescent antibody staining or spectrometric evaluation
Neisseria gonorrhoeae	Similar clinical features as with chlamydial infection Infection in men more likely to include purulent urethral discharge	Positive culture for gonorrhea Gram-negative diplococci in male urethral discharge
Human immunodeficiency virus (HIV)	Different from adult presentation: Lower male-to-female ratio More prevalent in black/Hispanic urban youth Higher percentage of heterosexual transmission	Specific blood assay for HIV virus (see Chapter 9)
Ureaplasma urealyticum	Similar characteristics to chlamydial infection	Culture
Treponema pallidum (syphilis)	Stage of disease: Primary (10–40 days): chancres, regional lymphadenopathy Secondary (2–6 months): generalized malaise, lymphadenopathy, skin changes/alopecia Late (2–10 years): central nervous system changes, cardiovascular changes, musculoskeletal involvement	Darkfield examination or direct fluorescent antibody tests of lesion Serologic tests: Nontreponemal Treponemal
Haemophilus ducreyi (chancroid)	Painful genital ulcer Tender inguinal lymphadenopathy	Culture Clinical picture
Herpes simplex virus	Vesicles/ulcers on external genitalia, in vagina, on cervix, and around rectal area Tender inguinal lymphadenopathy Dysuria Dyspareunia	Viral culture Tzanck test
Condylomata acuminata	Single or group of painless warts	Clinical appearance Biopsy
Molluscum contagiosum	Small papule with umbilical centers	Clinical appearance Potassium hydroxide smear of contents Biopsy
Trichomonas vaginalis	Presence of flagellated protozoan Malodorous yellow–green vaginal discharge Vaginal irritation	Microscopic identification of organism
Phthirus pubis (pediculosis pubis, crab lice)	Pruritus in pubic hair Tan egg cases in pubic hair	Crab lice or egg cases in pubic hair

B. | **Vaginitis**

1. ***Candida albicans,*** the most common cause of vaginitis, is a form of fungus (yeast) that normally inhabits the vagina. Vaginitis occurs when the growth of *C. albicans* is not limited by the vaginal environment (i.e., when vaginal flora becomes more alkaline than normal).

   a. **Clinical features.** Patients present with a cheesy white discharge associated with vulvar pruritus. The infection occurs after systemic antibiotic therapy, with diabetes, and during pregnancy, and is also associated with the use of birth control pills.

   b. **Diagnosis** is based on the presence of budding yeast and hyphae in a sample of vaginal discharge mixed with potassium hydroxide. The diagnosis is confirmed by culture.

   c. **Therapy.** Candidiasis is treated by the topical application of an antifungal preparation (e.g., miconazole nitrate) in the vagina at bedtime for 3–7 days.

2. **Bacterial vaginosis** is a syndrome in which normal vaginal *Lactobacillus* is replaced by anaerobic bacteria (e.g., *Bacteroides* and *Mobiluncus* species), *Gardnerella vaginalis,* and *Mycoplasma hominis.*

   a. **Clinical features** include a white, noninflammatory discharge with a "fishy" odor.

   b. **Diagnosis** is made by identifying clue cells (vaginal epithelial cells covered with fragments of gram-negative rods) in the vaginal discharge.

   c. **Therapy** includes metronidazole orally, or clindamycin cream or metronidazole gel applied vaginally.

3. **Other causes** of vaginitis are *T. vaginalis* infection and foreign bodies. Vaginal discharge can also be attributed to leukorrhea.

C. | **Toxic shock syndrome (TSS)** was initially associated with menstruating women who used tampons. It has also been seen in women who use a diaphragm or contraceptive sponge for an extended period of time. TSS is caused by the release of endotoxin from a *Staphylococcus aureus* infection, and is potentially fatal.

1. **Clinical features.** The patient presents with a fever higher than 102°F; a macular rash followed by desquamation, especially on the palms and soles; hypotension; and three or more of the following symptoms and systemic changes:

   a. Vomiting and diarrhea

   b. Muscle cramps accompanied by elevation of creatine phosphokinase levels

   c. Disorientation

   d. Hyperemia of the mucous membranes

   e. Hepatic changes (elevation of serum aspartate aminotransferase, serum alanine aminotransferase, and bilirubin levels)

   f. Renal changes [elevation of blood urea nitrogen (BUN), creatinine levels, or both]

   g. Hematologic changes (decreased platelet count)

2. **Therapy** includes controlling the symptoms of shock, removing any device from the vagina, and administering intravenous antibiotics. It may be useful to irrigate the vagina with normal saline or povidone–iodine. Counseling against the use of tampons and for the appropriate use of barrier contraceptives is important, because there is a potential 30% recurrence of the problem.

D. | **Pelvic inflammatory disease (PID)** is the spread of an infection from the vagina to the cervix, uterus, fallopian tubes, and peritoneum, potentially resulting in endometritis, salpingitis, parametritis, perihepatitis, and peritonitis. Such infections are most commonly seen in women 15–24 years of age and may cause subsequent infertility, especially where significant fallopian tube damage occurs. PID is strongly associated with the use of an IUD.

1. **Clinical features.** The patient presents with significant abdominal pain, and adnexal and cervical motion tenderness. The infection commonly starts during the menstrual period, and may be associated with fever. The patient may have a history of recent or past exposure to an STD. The erythrocyte sedimentation rate is elevated. An ultrasound of the pelvic area may show increased fluid outside these organs or formation of an abscess.

2. **Etiology.** The most common causes of PID are *N. gonorrhoeae* and *C. trachomatis.* Other causative organisms include *M. hominis, S. aureus, Streptococcus* species, *Escherichia coli,* and anaerobic bacteria such as *Bacteroides* species. PID often is caused by multiple organisms.

3. **Therapy** for PID needs to be tailored to each individual case. Many experts recommend initial hospitalization of adolescents with PID for stabilization of the disease, followed by outpatient therapy and repeat cultures for the diagnosed STD after the course of treatment. Refer to the 1993 Centers for Disease Control and Prevention guidelines for the latest recommendations (see Bibliography).

E. **Perihepatitis** is perihepatic inflammation caused by such organisms as gonococci (Fitz-Hugh Curtis syndrome) or by *C. trachomatis* subsequent to pelvic infection.

1. **Clinical features.** The patient may present with right upper quadrant pain, pleuritic irritation, and pain radiating to the right shoulder.

2. **Therapy** involves inpatient intravenous antibiotic treatment for the pelvic infection followed by outpatient oral antibiotic therapy depending on the causative organism.

F. **Epididymoorchitis** occurs subsequent to an STD (usually gonorrhea or chlamydial infection) or after a urinary tract infection.

1. **Clinical features.** The patient presents with dysuria and urethral discharge. The involved area may be swollen and tender.

2. **Therapy** involves the administration of an appropriate antibiotic agent for the STD or the urinary tract infection.

V. **REPRODUCTIVE HEALTH ISSUES** have become increasingly more important to adolescents. Half of all adolescents are sexually active by 17 years of age. Fewer than one-third of sexually active adolescents use any effective form of birth control. The most common reasons adolescents give for not using birth control are a denial of the ability to get pregnant, and the unexpected nature of the intercourse. Helping the adolescent choose the right birth control method is a very important step. Men are encouraged to use condoms at all times. With women, it is important to review such issues as past methods used, how often they are having sexual intercourse, what their friends use for birth control, and how comfortable they are in putting a tampon or a spermicidal suppository into their vagina. Parental support for birth control use improves compliance, especially with birth control pills. Such support can prove to be the most important factor leading to successful use of contraception.

A. **Contraception** (Table 5-6 and Figure 5-4)

1. **Oral contraceptive pill.** The "pill" is the form of contraception most commonly used by adolescent females. The failure rate of this method is 2%–4%.
   a. **Mechanism of action.** The pill suppresses ovulation, decreases the likelihood of implantation of the fertilized egg, and makes the cervical mucus more hostile to sperm.
   b. **Contraindications**
      (1) Absolute contraindications include pregnancy or a history of breast cancer, estrogen-stimulated reproductive tract neoplasm, thromboembolic disease, cerebrovascular accident, sustained hypertension, systemic disease involving the liver or coronary arteries, hyperlipidemia, or undiagnosed abnormal genital bleeding.
      (2) Relative contraindications include a history of labile or borderline hypertension, migraine headaches, diabetes, seizure disorder, oligomenorrhea, amenorrhea, sickle cell disease, or heavy cigarette smoking (especially in women older than 35 years of age).

TABLE 5-6. Advantages and Disadvantages of Birth Control Methods

Type	Advantages	Disadvantages
Oral contraceptive pills	Decreased menstrual bleeding Decreased dysmenorrhea No interference with intercourse Improvement of acne	Weight gain Bleeding between periods Nausea Headaches Having to take a pill each day Mood changes Period of anovulatory cycles after the pill is stopped
Barrier methods Diaphragm Cervical cap Female condom Spermicides Condom	No systemic effects No contraindications for use Easily available without prescription Helps prevent passage of STDs, including HIV Used only at the time of intercourse	Interferes with spontaneity Has to be inserted into vagina May decrease sensation Irritation or allergic reactions Are considered messy Interrupt lovemaking
Injectable progesterone	Lasts for 3 months Works independently	Need for shot every 3 months Irregular or absent menses Weight gain
Subdermal implant	Lasts up to 5 years Works independently	Placement into skin Need for eventual removal Irregular or absent menses Weight gain

STD = sexually transmitted disease; *HIV* = human immunodeficiency virus.

   c. Types of pills
     (1) The **combination pill** contains both estrogen and progesterone and may have fixed doses of each (monophasic pills) or may vary the dose of these hormones through the cycle (triphasic pills).
     (2) The **progesterone-only pill** works in a manner similar to the combination pill except that it may not regularly prevent ovulation. The failure rate is higher partly because the pill causes irregular menstrual periods, resulting in users stopping these pills from fear that they may be pregnant. The progesterone-only pill is reserved for women who cannot tolerate estrogen.
     (3) The **"morning after" pill** is an intermediate- or high-dose estrogen preparation used 24–72 hours after intercourse to prevent pregnancy.
   d. Common side effects of the pill are listed in Table 5-6.
   e. Advantages of the pill are listed in Table 5-6. Other advantages include the potential help in decreasing or preventing problems with ovarian cysts, fibrocystic and fibroadenoma breast changes, and ovarian and endometrial cancer.
   f. Evaluation before starting the pill should include a patient history for risk factors, a complete physical examination including a pelvic examination, and documentation of weight and blood pressure. **Clinical studies** should include a Pap smear; screening for gonorrhea, chlamydia, and syphilis; a blood count and urinalysis; and pregnancy test if indicated.
   g. Choosing the right pill for an adolescent is important for consistent compliance. Most adolescents can be started on a low-dose combination pill. An obese adolescent needs a combination pill with the lowest dose of estrogen that can be tolerated. An adolescent with severe acne may be helped by a combination pill with a slightly higher dose of estrogen for a few months, and then a switch to a lower-dose pill. A 28-pill package can increase compliance because of the necessity of taking a pill every day.

  2. Barrier methods of contraception are used regularly by less than one-fifth of the adolescent population who use any form of contraception. These methods tend to be more popular with older adolescents and young adults. The **failure rate** varies from

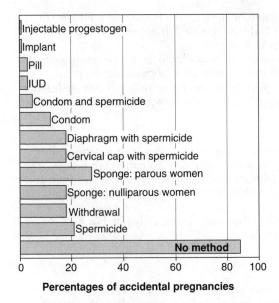

Injectable progestogen
Implant
Pill
IUD
Condom and spermicide
Condom
Diaphragm with spermicide
Cervical cap with spermicide
Sponge: parous women
Sponge: nulliparous women
Withdrawal
Spermicide
No method

0   20   40   60   80   100

Percentages of accidental pregnancies

FIGURE 5-4. Percentages of accidental pregnancies during first year of use of various contraceptive methods. *IUD* = intrauterine device. (Adapted from Trusell, et al. *Obstet Gynecol* 76:565, 1990.)

10%–20%, depending on the form of barrier contraceptive being used. Condom use has increased dramatically over the past decade, with more than 50% of adolescents indicating condom use; however, many of these adolescents do not use condoms all the time.

a. **Mechanisms of action.** Barrier contraceptives prevent sperm from entering the uterus, kill sperm while they are in the vagina, and absorb sperm.

b. **No contraindications** exist for the use of a barrier method of contraception.

c. **Types of barrier contraceptives** include:
   (1) The **diaphragm**—a circular rubber dome that, when properly placed, is an effective barrier between the vagina and cervix
   (2) The **cervical cap**—a firm plastic cap held in place by suction at the cervical opening
   (3) The **female condom**
   (4) **Spermicides**—foams, jellies, or suppositories
   (5) The **condom,** which seems to be the most effective single barrier method of contraception. The combination of a condom and a spermicide approximates the effectiveness of the pill as a contraceptive method, but with significantly fewer side effects. This method also serves as the most effective known deterrent to the spread of acquired immune deficiency syndrome (AIDS), barring celibacy.

d. **Side effects** from barrier contraceptives are listed in Table 5-6. TSS can occur when the diaphragm or sponge is left in the vagina for extended periods of time (see IV C).

e. **Evaluation** for the use of these methods may not always occur because all of the methods except the diaphragm are available without a prescription. Sexually active adolescents should have a complete health evaluation (see V A 1 f). Women wishing to use a diaphragm must be measured for the appropriate size.

f. **Advantages and disadvantages** of barrier contraceptives are listed in Table 5-6.

3. **IUD.** This method should not be prescribed for use in sexually active teens.
   a. **Mechanism of action.** The IUD blocks the implantation of a fertilized egg in the lining of the uterus, either by causing a mild endometritis or by affecting endometrial enzymes.
   b. **Side effects** include pelvic infection, uterine perforation, ectopic pregnancy, and subsequent infertility.

4. **Injectable progesterone** (medroxyprogesterone acetate) is a frequently used form of contraceptive outside the United States and has increased in popularity in the United States since it recently was approved for general use.
   a. **Mechanism of action.** Injectable progesterone is similar to the progesterone-only pill [see V A 1 c (2)] but is more effective in the suppression of ovulation.
   b. **Side effects** are similar to those seen with the progesterone-only pill and are listed in Table 5-6. There may also be a delay of 6–24 months between stopping this method and achieving pregnancy.

5. **Subdermal implants**
   a. **Subdermal implants** consist of polymeric silicone rods that release levonorgestrel once placed in the skin. Preparations now available can last either 3 or 5 years. The need for intradermal placement with this method often deters adolescents from giving it serious consideration. This method has proven more acceptable to adolescents who already have had children.
   b. **Mechanism of action** is similar to that of the progesterone-only pill, but with decreased likelihood of ectopic pregnancy.

B. | **Pregnancy**

1. **General considerations.** Pregnancy occurs in more than 1 million teenagers in the United States each year, a frequency that is two to six times greater than that seen in other developed countries. More than half the women who become pregnant while in high school drop out of school. Nearly half the women who depend on state or federal support for their families had children before the age of 20 years. Teenage mothers have a 20%–40% chance of becoming pregnant again 1–2 years after the initial delivery.

2. **Medical complications** of teenage pregnancy include toxemia and anemia. Infants born to mothers who are younger than 15 years of age have a high mortality rate and a high incidence of low birth weight. All of the developmental consequences for teenage mothers and their infants have not yet been clearly identified. Greater consequences for the younger adolescent are partially explained by the incomplete development of the pelvis.

3. **Causes of teenage pregnancy**
   a. **During the concrete operational stage** (see Chapter 1), many teenagers deny their ability to get pregnant, are unable to think of events 9 months in the future, and exhibit poor compliance with contraception.
   b. **Family influence.** Often the mother or a sibling became a parent as a teenager. Lack of an extended family decreases family support. In single-parent families or in families where both parents work, teenagers are not supervised much of the time.
   c. **Gradually decreasing age of menarche** has made pregnancy possible at an early age.
   d. **Situational stress** (e.g., school performance, family relations, pressure from a sexual partner or peer group) can also contribute to the problem.
   e. **Societal influences** may also play a role through lack of positive role models, lack of opportunities in the job market, increased emphasis on sex in the media, and relaxation of moral codes.
   f. **Desire to become pregnant** also has to be considered, because teenagers often feel that becoming a parent will give them someone to take care of, provide them with unconditional love, and offer them a way to become independent.
   g. **Often the men involved are older** (in their late teens or early twenties). In these men, physical feelings and self-image interfere with their understanding of the consequences and responsibilities of their actions.

4. **Evaluation for possible pregnancy**
   a. **History.** A patient history should correlate the frequency of sexual activity and the menstrual cycle with the understanding that often some menstrual bleeding can occur even in the presence of a pregnancy. Associated symptoms of pregnancy should be noted, including swelling of the breasts, nausea and vomiting, fatigue, and urinary frequency.

   b. Physical examination should check the size and color of the cervix as well as the size and consistency of the uterus.

   c. Clinical studies, including a urine evaluation for hCG, can determine the presence of a pregnancy within 10 days of conception. A subsequent blood analysis for hCG can quantitate the duration of the pregnancy.

5. **Decision-making for a pregnant teenager.** Allowing a teenager time to consider her options and having her talk to other teens who have been through the experience may be helpful. Involvement of the parents and the sexual partner in discussions should be encouraged when possible.

   a. Options. Alternatives include keeping the baby, putting the baby up for adoption, placing the baby in foster care (thus allowing for a later decision), and abortion.

   b. Factors influencing the decision. Issues that may influence a pregnant adolescent's decision include decreased freedom when the child is born, financial and physical responsibility for the infant, need to develop a support system, and the effects of a pregnancy on her lifestyle and career goals.

6. **Care and support for a pregnant teenager.** When the pregnancy is to be carried to term, it is important to assist the teenager with early prenatal care, to facilitate continuation of school, and to help develop a support system, especially for future parenting.

C. **Abortion.** Teenagers undergo 500,000 abortions each year, nearly one-third of the total number of abortions performed. Nearly half (47%) of the pregnant teenagers from middle- and upper-income families choose abortion, compared to one-fourth (26%) of the pregnant teenagers from low-income families.

1. **Types of abortions**

   a. First trimester abortions, which account for most abortions, are performed by vacuum curettage and are done as an outpatient procedure.

   b. Second trimester abortions are high-risk procedures, are more expensive than those performed in the first trimester, and often require overnight hospitalization. Few centers perform abortions in the second trimester. Methods include intraamniotic cavity administration of hypertonic saline, urea, or dilation and curettage; and placement of prostaglandin as a suppository in the vagina.

2. **Mortality.** The mortality rate ranges from 1 in 400,000 when the abortion is done before 9 weeks' gestation to 1 in 10,000 when it is done after 16 weeks' gestation.

3. **Evaluation** should include a discussion of the meaning of abortion and related fears. The likely procedure should be reviewed, and the adolescent should be encouraged to have a support person with her. Examination and laboratory studies should confirm pregnancy, approximate gestational size, and rule out any STDs. An ultrasound can be used to confirm gestational size.

4. **Follow-up.** A contraceptive method should be encouraged and made available immediately after the abortion. Follow-up pelvic examination is done 2 weeks after the abortion. This is a good time to assess the psychological consequences of the abortion, to plan future counseling visits to deal with unresolved feelings about the abortion, and to help prevent another pregnancy.

VI. MENTAL HEALTH ISSUES

A. **Depression** (see also Chapter 4). More than half (60%) of teenagers surveyed while receiving routine health care indicated that they feel down or depressed as frequently as once a month to daily. Women experience depression more commonly than men.

1. **Etiology.** A number of factors may lead to depression, including:

   a. Changes in peer relationships (e.g., loss of a boyfriend or girlfriend, exclusion from the peer group, lack of peer group support, inability to be with peers)

    b. Family influences (e.g., lack of independence, poor communication, decreased availability of parents, problems between the parents)

    c. School experiences (e.g., poor performance, conflict with teachers, peer conflict or pressure, unrealistically high expectations from parents)

    d. Poor self-image (e.g., dissatisfaction with one's physical appearance, lack of self-confidence, a hopeless vision of the future)

2. Clinical features. Associated signs and symptoms include:

    a. Recurrent somatic complaints (e.g., headaches; chest, abdominal, or back pains; changes in eating habits, sleep patterns, and levels of activity)

    b. Mood swings (manifested as restlessness; withdrawal from peers and family; decreased ability to function on a day-to-day basis; and "acting out" behavior such as violence, substance abuse, risk-taking, and little or no recognition of authority)

    c. A decline in the level of school performance

    d. Apathy (a loss of interest in sports, hobbies, and community-related activities)

3. Therapy. Attempts to prevent or treat depression include counseling programs associated with health services, school-based support services, and intervention in parent–adolescent conflict. The 24-hour phone availability of a health network can provide reassurance.

B. **Suicide** is the third most common cause of death in adolescents and young adults; suicide attempts outnumber successful suicides by as much as 200 to 1. Women make more attempts than men, but successful suicide is four times more common in men. More than half (60%) of teenagers who commit suicide have attempted suicide previously.

1. Methods. The most frequent methods by which adolescent suicide is committed in the United States are (in order) firearms, hanging, and drug overdose. (Women most commonly commit suicide by drug overdose.)

2. Attempts to prevent suicide should include the following steps.

    a. Questioning. All adolescent patients should be asked about suicidal thoughts, not just those who seem depressed. No clearly documented correlation exists between asking about suicidal thoughts and an increased incidence of suicide.

    b. Assessment of risk. If the adolescent has suicidal thoughts, the level of risk should be evaluated by identifying any history of suicide attempts and level of familial support.

        (1) The **degree of depression** should be assessed. A severely depressed teenager may be unable to mobilize to commit suicide, but a teenager who is recovering from depression is more likely to commit suicide.

        (2) **Danger signs** should always be ascertained in depressed teenagers (e.g., getting affairs in order, giving away favorite possessions, withdrawing from friends and from social and school activities, a history of suicide or alcohol abuse in the family).

        (3) A **precipitating event** should be noted (e.g., a breakup with a girlfriend or boyfriend, a conflict with peers, pregnancy, and, most frequently, a conflict with parents).

    c. Therapy for a suicidal adolescent works well in a team approach, including the services of a physician, a social worker, and a consulting psychiatrist. Appropriate information should be obtained to determine whether the patient can be treated on an ambulatory basis or requires inpatient evaluation (Table 5-7).

C. **Delinquency.** More than 50% of all arrests for major crimes in the United States involve individuals younger than 21 years of age, and more than one-third of these arrests involve individuals younger than 18 years of age. Men account for more than 75% of these arrests and for more than 90% of the arrests for violent crimes. A high level of delinquency is reported in the poorer population.

TABLE 5-7. Factors to Be Considered in Deciding Between an Ambulatory and an Inpatient Treatment Plan for a Suicide Attempt

Ambulatory	Inpatient
No significant history of depression or suicide attempt	Past suicide attempt
Method used less lethal and not requiring medical treatment	More lethal method used or further medical treatment needed
Suicide attempt occurred when help was available or note left in accessible place before attempt	Suicide attempt occurred without warning
Family supportive and recognizes problem	Family not supportive and does not feel that a problem exists
Adolescent and family willing to follow up on an ambulatory basis	Ambulatory care arrangement cannot be found *and* safe environment is needed

1. **Definitions**
   a. A **juvenile delinquent** is a minor 7–17 years of age who commits a criminal act. Such a case usually is processed through juvenile or family court, with emphasis on rehabilitation rather than punishment. Some cities have juvenile advisory teams who try to resolve such cases before they come to court. The youth usually is given a chance to clear his record.
   b. A **youthful offender** is an individual 16–21 years of age who commits a criminal act. Such a case usually is processed through criminal court for punishment, but the youthful offender may be tried in family or juvenile court if the act committed is minor and if the youth will benefit from rehabilitation.
   c. A **minor in need of supervision** is an individual 7–17 years of age who commits an act that would not be illegal if he were an adult (e.g., running away or skipping school). These cases may be processed through juvenile or family court, but an attempt usually is made to resolve them outside the court system.

2. **Factors relating to delinquency** include medical, behavioral, and school problems; conflict with authority; disorder at home; and influence of peers.

3. **Prevention** may be aided by:
   a. Development of **early identification programs** that foster positive youth development, such as those run by boys' clubs
   b. Greater emphasis on **positive adult role models** (e.g., Big Brother or Big Sister programs)
   c. **A change in national social priorities**
      (1) The emphasis on material possessions, living for the moment, and sexual preoccupation should be decreased.
      (2) It would also help to increase emphasis on education, family support, and self-achievement, as well as to facilitate career development for the youth at risk.

D. **Eating disorders**

1. **Anorexia nervosa**
   a. **Definition.** Anorexia nervosa is an eating disorder characterized by the following features:
      (1) **Refusal to maintain appropriate body weight** for height, resulting in a weight that is at least 15% less than expected for the given height
      (2) Intense **fear of gaining weight** or being fat
      (3) **Disturbed body image,** such as feeling fat when actually being almost emaciated
      (4) Absence of at least three consecutive **menstrual cycles** in women

b. Occurrence. Anorexia nervosa is most commonly seen in middle to late adolescence, traditionally in about 1% of white women of higher socioeconomic groups. More recently, this disorder has been seen in younger adolescents of other socioeconomic groups. Men make up less than 10% of the patient population.

c. Etiology
   (1) Norms that promote thinness as beautiful are pervasive cultural influences.
   (2) The patient often displays obsessive, overachieving, and controlling personality traits.
   (3) Disordered family relationships may contribute to the etiology.

d. Evaluation
   (1) History
      (a) Understand the patient's body image: what is acceptable, what is too fat, what is too thin.
      (b) Attempts should be made to document the chronology of the weight loss, and an extensive dietary history should be obtained.
      (c) Queries should be made about vomiting, excessive exercise, laxative abuse, and willingness to eat with friends and family.
      (d) Identify and explore relationships with family and friends.
      (e) Review of systems should consider chronic illness or pain, menstrual history, signs of depression, and assessment of level of self-esteem.
   (2) Physical examination should include accurate vital signs, weight with only a dressing gown, and body temperature. Skin may have a dry, mottled appearance with signs of lanugo (fine hair) and lack of subcutaneous fat. There may be a weak pulse. Muscle tone may be decreased with generalized weakness.
   (3) Laboratory studies
      (a) Routine laboratory tests such as hemoglobin, erythrocyte sedimentation rate, urinalysis, electrolyte levels, calcium, phosphorus, and serum protein usually are negative. BUN may be elevated with dehydration.
      (b) Special studies. Levels of triiodothyronine, luteinizing hormone, and follicle-stimulating hormone may be low, whereas cholesterol, cortisol, and endorphin levels may be elevated. An electrocardiogram is useful to assess for bradycardia, decreased QRS amplitude, nonspecific ST segment and T-wave changes, and prolonged QT interval.
      (c) A computed tomography (CT) scan should be obtained in boys who present with weight loss because the incidence of brain tumor is higher in boys. It also may be possible to document cerebral atrophy.

e. Therapy involves making an initial decision whether to treat on an ambulatory basis or to hospitalize. Findings of greater than 20% weight loss associated with electrolyte, cardiovascular, or neurologic signs suggest need for hospitalization, along with failure to gain weight on an ambulatory program.
   (1) Medical management
      (a) Nutritional support ranging from high-caloric diet to replacement by nasogastric tube or hyperalimentation if necessary
      (b) Vitamin supplement as indicated
      (c) Estrogen supplement to reinitiate menses
   (2) Psychological management
      (a) Behavior modification. Strategies include positive reinforcement for eating and negative contingencies for refusing to eat. A system of privileges often is established, depending on the patient's intake.
      (b) Psychotherapy, both individual and family, is essential.
   (3) Psychopharmacology. Antidepressant agents may be helpful.
   (4) Goals of therapy include weight gain up to 10% of expected body weight, associated with a contract to maintain this weight gain and enrollment in a comprehensive program that deals with nutritional, medical, and psychological needs.

f. Prognosis is variable, with mortality as high as 20%. Early identification and comprehensive care can reduce the mortality rate to as low as 2%.

2. **Bulimia** is considered a disorder distinct from anorexia nervosa; however, 50% of teenagers with anorexia nervosa may exhibit binging and purging behavior.
   a. **Definition.** Bulimia is characterized by the following features:
      (1) Repetitive binge eating involving rapid consumption of a large amount of food over a short period of time
         (a) Feeling of lack of control over eating during binge episodes
         (b) Minimum of two binge episodes per month for 3 months
      (2) Weight loss by vomiting, use of laxatives or diuretics, fasting, or vigorous exercise
      (3) Overconcern with body shape and weight
   b. **Prevalence.** Bulimia is seen mainly in **older teenagers** (average age is 18 years), with a rate of 3% in a college population and a female-to-male ratio of 10 to 1.
   c. **Clinical features.** The patient commonly presents with a poor self-image associated with depression (especially after a binge episode), thoughts about suicide, substance abuse (see VII), antisocial behavior (e.g., stealing), and self-mutilation.
   d. **Medical complications** may include esophagitis, gastric dilatation and possible rupture, aspiration, cardiac arrhythmia, pancreatitis, metabolic alkalosis associated with hypochloremia and hypokalemia, swelling of the parotid and submandibular glands, and dental problems such as erosion of dental enamel and dentin and loss of teeth.
   e. **Evaluation**
      (1) **History.** A patient history should consider eating patterns and food intake history, purging behavior, past weight fluctuations, body image, level of depression, risk-taking behavior, and family dynamics.
      (2) **Physical examination** includes assessment of vital signs for possible hypovolemia, assessment of dentition, and evaluation of cardiac function. The abdomen should be palpated for tenderness or distention. The skin should be evaluated (the hands should be checked for scars from repeated induced vomiting).
      (3) **Laboratory studies** should evaluate electrolyte level, hydration, and cardiovascular status.
   f. **Therapy** should initially stabilize the patient's medical condition. The focus of treatment is to normalize the metabolic state and encourage the adolescent to become involved in counseling. Antidepressant medication may be helpful in specific cases.

E. | **Sexual abuse**

1. **Rape**
   a. **Definition.** Rape is sexual intercourse without the victim's consent. Penetration need not involve rupture of the hymen or entrance into the vagina; only contact of male genitalia with labia majora is necessary. Similarly, ejaculation need not occur for rape to be alleged. Women usually are the victims (in more than 90% of cases), with teenagers making up half of all rape victims. A significant number of rape cases go unreported.
   b. **Evaluation** should be done in a supportive setting by an experienced physician. The teenager needs to have a sense of control as well as a guarantee of confidentiality and privacy during the evaluation. All procedures should be explained before they are done.
      (1) **History.** A patient history should establish date, time, and nature of the rape as well as any acute symptoms. It is important to determine if the vaginal environment has changed since the rape (has the victim douched or bathed?). Menstrual, sexual, and contraceptive histories are helpful.
      (2) **Physical examination** aims to document the event as much as possible, with pictures when appropriate. Before the examination is begun, local legal requirements should be determined.
      (3) **Clinical studies** include checking for sperm, STDs, and pregnancy. Follow-up testing for HIV should be performed if the perpetrator is unavailable or unwilling to undergo tests or if the perpetrator tests positive.
   c. **Therapy** focuses not only on possible pregnancy and STD but on the mental health needs of the victim.

d. **Sequelae of rape** initially include fear and shock, fatigue, and systemic responses (e.g., inability to eat, keep food down, or sleep). Later findings include impaired functioning at school, work, and home; sexual fear and dysfunction; poor self-image and depression; and decreased contact with peers.

2. **Incest**
   a. **Definition.** Incest is sexual intercourse or molestation with a relative or guardian. Incest is most commonly reported between father (usually stepfather) and daughter, and may also occur between siblings.
   b. **Associated behavioral changes** include somatic complaints, low self-esteem, substance abuse, running away, prostitution, depression, and thoughts about suicide.
   c. **Family dynamics** include a father figure with poor impulse control and associated alcohol abuse, and a passive mother who has a poor relationship with the father and a tendency to neglect and eventually reject the daughter.

3. **Molestation** is sexual contact short of intercourse without the victim's consent. It is most often committed by men through either exhibitionism, genital contact, or forced oral or anal sex. The evaluation, treatment, and sequelae are similar to those of rape.

VII. SUBSTANCE ABUSE

A. Overview

1. **Definition.** Substance abuse is consumption of cigarettes, alcohol, or drugs to the point of compromising health or causing dysfunctional behavior. Chronic substance abuse causes arrest of psychosocial development (Tables 5-8 and 5-9).

2. **Prevalence** of illicit drug use as reported by graduating high school seniors has shown a marked decrease over the past two decades. Initiation of use of drugs such as alcohol and cigarettes increased for younger teens (eighth graders) by the end of the 1980s. In general, men are more likely than women to use illicit drugs, except for amphetamines, barbiturates, and tranquilizers, which women may use as much or slightly more than men.

TABLE 5-8. Stages of Substance Abuse

Stages	Description
Stage 1: Experimentation	Usually starts with peer pressure Few if any behavioral changes User struggles between the euphoria achieved and associated guilt
Stage 2: To relieve stress	Use is more than occasional and in nonsocial situations Supply of the substance is maintained and peer group develops around substance abuse Exhibits mood swings and school performance declines
Stage 3: Regular abuse	Becomes involved with drug-oriented culture Most, if not all, peers use drugs Behavioral problems are chronic, may include problems with the law Depression when not using drugs Needs to raise money to support habit
Stage 4: Dependence	Drug is used to prevent depression May drop out of school and become involved in destructive family dynamics Physical changes may include weight loss, fatigue, blackouts, and chronic cough

TABLE 5-9. Hazards Associated with Drug and Alcohol Abuse

Substance	Hazards
Tobacco	Altered lung function Chronic symptoms such as productive cough and chest pain Decrease in performance endurance Lung cancer, coronary heart disease
Snuff	Associated with development of oral squamous carcinoma
Marijuana	Lung impairment greater than with cigarettes Short-term memory and learning changes Decreased reaction time, coordination, visual perception
Alcohol	Decreased reaction time, coordination, visual perception Acute illness (hangover) Liver changes leading to cirrhosis Chronic depression Withdrawal syndrome if used long term
Hallucinogens	Self-inflicted physical harm "Bad trips," "flashbacks" Chronic CNS changes Overdose
Stimulants	Depression Cardiovascular impairment Psychosis Overdose Rapid addiction Slurred speech Ataxia Impulsive behavior Respiratory depression Severe withdrawal reaction
Narcotics	Complications from injectable drugs Addiction Overdose
Inhalants	Nasal and bronchial irritation Systemic effects such as liver and renal toxicity, cardiac arrhythmias, and CNS changes
Anabolic steroids	Impaired excretion by liver Hypertension Impaired glucose tolerance Aggressive behavior

CNS = central nervous system.

3. **History**
   a. Determine **substance use pattern** by adolescent, peers, family members, other students at school.
   b. Determine **level of dysfunction:** school absences/failure, intoxication, relationship with family, problems with the law.
   c. Determine **degree of depression,** potential suicide ideation.
4. **Physical examination.** Signs of chronic drug abuse are ascertained (e.g., weight loss, skin and mucous membrane changes, compromise in lung function, mood, and affect).
5. **Laboratory studies** can confirm drug abuse through urine or blood tests and can check for systemic changes in liver and pulmonary function.
6. **Therapy** for adolescents in the first and second stages of involvement can usually be accomplished on an ambulatory basis, whereas those in the third and fourth stages may

require hospitalization or placement in a residential rehabilitation facility. Difficulties arise because many substance abusers do not realize or do not admit that they have a problem.

B. **Tobacco** abuse by teenagers strongly correlates with use by parents and peers. It is the most commonly used illicit drug. Over a 30-day period in 1991, almost one in five adolescents smoked one or more cigarettes on a daily basis. The rate of smoking in female adolescents now has equaled or surpassed that in males. Smoking is initiated about 2 years before the habit is established. Using smokeless tobacco (snuff) is a male-oriented activity (as many as 25% of American male adolescents report some involvement).

C. **Marijuana,** the most prevalent illicit drug, is derived from leaves of the hemp plant and is smoked in cigarettes (joints) or pipes, or cooked in food. The active ingredient is tetrahydrocannabinol (THC). Hashish (hash), the resin from the hemp plant, is a purer form of THC. THC is metabolized in the liver but is also stored in body fat, resulting in a long half-life. Therapeutic effects of marijuana include reduction of nausea in patients undergoing cancer chemotherapy and reduction of intraocular pressure in patients with glaucoma.

D. **Alcohol** is the most commonly abused substance. Men more frequently use and abuse alcohol, and beer is the most common form of alcohol consumed. Adolescents are more likely to abuse alcohol if their parents and peers have a history of use.

E. **Hallucinogens.** The most common hallucinogens are **lysergic acid diethylamide (LSD),** which is derived from rye fungus; **mescaline,** which is derived from a cactus; **psilocybin,** which is derived from a mushroom, *Psilocybe mexicana*; and **phencyclidine (PCP),** a drug initially developed as a general anesthetic.

F. **Stimulants.** The most frequently used stimulants are **amphetamines** and **cocaine**. Cocaine is derived from leaves of *Erythroxylon coca* and other species of *Erythroxylon*. In the 1980s, crack cocaine, a "free-base," smokable form of the drug, became popular. It proved to be very dangerous, resulting in high drug levels in the brain.

G. **Depressants.** The most commonly abused depressants are barbiturates and tranquilizers.

H. **Narcotics**

  1. The most common narcotics are **heroin, methadone, meperidine,** and **propoxyphene**.

  2. **Naloxone** is effective in counteracting the effects of narcotics and is used in treating overdose.

I. **Inhalants** usually have depressant and sedative effects. They are more commonly used by younger adolescents.

VIII. SKIN PROBLEMS

A. **Acne** is the major skin problem in adolescents.

  1. **Pathophysiology.** Acne starts with increased sebum production stimulated by androgens during puberty. Sebum consists of a mixture of follicular keratin and secretions of the sebaceous glands. Bacteria (*Propionibacterium acnes*) in the follicles use substrate from the sebum to attract a white blood cell response. The white blood cell activity releases a variety of hydrolytic enzymes, which cause a local inflammatory reaction. Gradual resolution of the inflammation may lead to scarring.

2. **Definition of terms**
   a. A **comedo** is hyperkeratosis of follicular epithelium, and its presence is the initial observable change in acne.
      (1) **Whiteheads** are closed comedones, resulting in slightly elevated papules in the skin.
      (2) **Blackheads** are a later stage of enlarged comedones that contain melanin and eventually open, leading to inflammatory responses.
   b. **Cystic acne** is not actually composed of cysts but of **nodules** formed during the inflammatory reaction, resulting in **erythematous papules (pimples)** or **pus-filled papules (pustules)**.

3. **Therapy.** Acne is treated by reducing sebum production and decreasing bacterial activity with various agents.
   a. **Comedolytic and antikeratolytic agents** include topical retinoic acid and benzoyl peroxide (also noted to have an antibacterial effect) and systemic isotretinoin.
   b. **Antibacterial agents** usually consist of topical or systemic antibiotics.
   c. **Sebaceous gland inhibitor agents** include systemic isotretinoin and agents that decrease or counteract androgen production (e.g., birth control pills, dexamethasone).
   d. Other methods include **surgical removal** of comedones, use of **exfoliating agents** (e.g., ultraviolet light, cryotherapy), and use of **antiinflammatory agents** such as steroids.
   e. The use of water-based instead of oil-based cosmetics is helpful.
   f. Diet manipulation has not proven effective.

B. **Fungal infections** are the second most common skin infection in an adolescent population.

1. **Agents.** The most common organisms causing fungal infection are dermatophytid fungi such as *Microsporum, Trichophyton, Epidermophyton,* and *Pityrosporon* species.
   a. **Tinea corporis** (ringworm) develops on the trunk, extremities, and face and is marked by circular lesions of varying size with raised borders and flat, erythematous centers.
   b. **Tinea cruris** (jock itch) is common in the groin and thigh area of men (the scrotum is spared) and is demarcated by a raised border. This infection often follows from the prolonged use of an athletic supporter.
   c. **Tinea pedis** (athlete's foot) is marked by scaling between the toes and may result from poor foot care and infrequent change of socks.
   d. **Tinea versicolor** is marked by flat patches of hypopigmented or hyperpigmented areas with a distribution similar to that of tinea corporis. It is easily confused with **vitiligo,** an autoimmune condition.
   e. **Tinea capitis** is marked by scaly patches on the scalp and hair loss, and frequently is caused by such organisms as *Microsporum* and *Trichophyton*. This infection often is associated with the use of hair products that contain significant amounts of grease or oil that remain on the scalp for extended periods of time. Superinfection with staphylococcal species is common in severe cases.

2. **Diagnosis** is made by the examination of a scraped specimen placed in potassium hydroxide and viewed under a microscope to reveal hyphae forms. A Wood's lamp is helpful in examining tinea capitis and tinea versicolor. Diagnosis may also be made by obtaining fungal cultures.

3. **Therapy.** Fungal infections are treated with topical antifungal preparations. Tinea versicolor responds to selenium sulfide therapy. Tinea capitis usually requires the use of systemic griseofulvin as well as treatment of any bacterial superinfection with the appropriate antibiotic. Tinea pedis is helped by improved foot hygiene. Tinea infections require several weeks of therapy before results are noticeable.

IX. DISORDERS OF THE MUSCULOSKELETAL SYSTEM

A. **Scoliosis** is lateral curvature of the spine involving the thoracic and lumbar vertebrae. Incidence of scoliosis varies, but is in the range of 3%–5% of the pediatric population. Seventy-five percent or more of the cases in adolescents have no known etiology. Scoliosis occurs more frequently in women when onset is in adolescence.

1. **Causes** of scoliosis other than idiopathic include congenital failure of spinal development, musculoskeletal disease (e.g., cerebral palsy), neurofibromatosis, Marfan syndrome, juvenile rheumatoid arthritis, trauma (e.g., fracture and destruction of vertebrae, severe burns), and structural defects (e.g., different leg lengths).

2. **Evaluation** includes determining an identifiable cause for the scoliosis. Physical examination of the back with the patient in an erect and a bent-at-the-hips position ascertains vertebral, scapular, and muscular asymmetry. Leg lengths should be checked, as well as symmetry at the hips and shoulders. A radiograph of the spine can quantitate any curvature greater than 10°.

3. **Therapy** depends on the degree of back curvature.
   a. If curvature is less than 15° but greater than 10°, the adolescent should be seen by a physician every 6 months. Back exercises may be recommended.
   b. Scoliosis progresses more quickly during the pubertal growth spurt, and should be checked every 3 months if the curvature is 15°–20°.
   c. If curvature is 20° or more, the patient should be referred to an orthopedic surgeon for additional therapy, which may include bracing and exercise or surgical stabilization for more advanced curvature.
   d. Change in scoliosis is not as rapid after the pubertal growth spurt but still occurs; thus, continued follow-up into adulthood is recommended.

4. **Sequelae** of uncontrolled scoliosis include deformity of the chest, limitation of lung function leading to polycythemia and pulmonary hypertension, and compromise in cardiac function from pressure on the chest cavity.

B. **Kyphosis** is excessive roundback of the thoracic spine, most often (in 95% of cases) caused by postural problems.

1. **Evaluation** consists of obtaining a history of postural difficulties and back pain. Physical examination should check for thoracic curvature, rounded shoulders, winging of the scapulae, excessive lumbar lordosis, and forward displacement of the head and neck. A radiograph of the back differentiates between a postural and a structural cause.

2. **Therapy** for mild curvature includes a review of posture in standing and sitting positions, back exercises, and appropriate supportive furniture (e.g., firm beds and chairs). Moderate to severe cases require referral to an orthopedic specialist for additional structural support.

C. **Slipped capital femoral epiphysis** is a displacement of the femoral head, usually posteriorly and medially off the femoral metaphysis. It occurs most often in men and is associated with obesity during the pubertal growth spurt.

1. **Evaluation** initially should include a history of any pain in the hip or the knee, antalgic gait, and obesity. Physical examination may reveal few positive findings except a limitation in the range of motion of the hip. A radiograph of the hip shows femoral head changes.

2. **Therapy** consists of referral of the patient to an orthopedic specialist for surgical correction.

D. **Osgood-Schlatter disease** causes stress changes in the tibial tuberosity at the site of attachment of the patellar tendon. The disease usually occurs during the pubertal growth spurt, and is more common in men who are active in sports.

  1. **Evaluation** includes a history of tenderness around the tibial tuberosity and a review of the patient's physical activities. Physical examination may identify some swelling of the tibial tuberosity with associated point tenderness. A radiograph helps to rule out any other knee pathology.

  2. **Therapy** is mainly supportive and includes reduced physical activity when pain is severe. Bracing may become necessary if supportive care is not sufficient.

E. **Osteochondritis dissecans** is the separation of bone from cartilage in the medial or lateral femoral condyle. Most cases (90%) are unilateral. This condition occurs more often in men. In addition to the femur, it may be located in the elbow, hip, and ankle.

  1. **Evaluation** includes obtaining a history of recurrent, diffuse knee pain and a limp from holding the knee rigid. Physical examination may identify pain and swelling over the site of the lesion, which inhibits full flexion of the knee, and may reveal the absence of other physical deformities of the knee. A radiograph of the knee reveals bone separation.

  2. **Therapy** with a long-leg cast is possible in cases identified early. Patients with more advanced disease may need to undergo surgery.

F. **Chondromalacia patellae** is instability of the patella leading to gradual destruction of the patellar cartilage. This is a common cause of knee pain, especially in women. The disease develops over a period of time and becomes worse with increased activity, especially when full knee flexion is required. This problem usually is unilateral but can be bilateral.

  1. **Evaluation** includes a history of knee pain associated with the patella, episodes during which the knee gives out, trauma to the patella, and difficulty maintaining the knee in a flexed position for any length of time. Physical examination shows displacement of the patella with knee extension, and tenderness and crepitation with manipulation of the patella. The disease is limited to the patella and usually is not associated with limitation of the range of motion of the knee. A radiograph is not often diagnostic but is helpful in identifying other causes of pain.

  2. **Therapy** includes limitation of activities requiring deep flexion of the knees (e.g., bicycling), pain control with aspirin or nonsteroidal antiinflammatory agents, and improvement of muscle tone with isometric exercises. A rehabilitation program includes a gradual return to more complete physical activities under the direction of an orthopedist. Patients with severe damage and pain may require casting of the knee.

BIBLIOGRAPHY

Centers for Disease Control and Prevention. 1993 STD treatment guidelines. *MMWR* 42 (RR-14):1–102, 1993.

Choice of contraceptives. In *The Medical Letter: On Drugs and Therapeutics.* Edited by M Abramowicz. 37(941):9–12, 1995.

Emans SJH, Goldstein DP: *Pediatric and Adolescent Gynecology*, 3rd ed. Boston, Little, Brown, & Company, 1990.

Friedman SB, Fisher M, Schonberg SK: *Comprehensive Adolescent Health Care.* St. Louis, Quality Medical Publishing, 1992.

McAnarney ER, Kreipe RE, Orr DP, Comerci GD: *Textbook of Adolescent Medicine.* Philadelphia, WB Saunders, 1992.

Neinstein LS: *Adolescent Health Care: A Practical Guide*, 2nd ed. Baltimore, Urban and Schwarzenberg, 1990.

STUDY QUESTIONS

DIRECTIONS: Each of the numbered items or incomplete statements in this section is followed by answers or by completions of the statement. Select the ONE lettered answer or completion that is BEST in each case.

1. A 13-year-old boy comes to his physician's office for his sports physical. He is planning to try out for the football team at his middle school. He asks if he can start to work out, especially by lifting weights, so that he can increase his muscle mass and strength. At what stage of pubertal development will lifting weights help him to increase his muscle mass?

(A) Stage 1
(B) Stage 2
(C) Stage 3
(D) Stage 4

2. A 14-year-old girl comes in for a general physical. The physician learns that she is sexually active but she does not want to get pregnant. She is interested in using some form of birth control, but does not know which kind. The physician tries to get some additional information about her so that she can better counsel her about available birth control methods. Which of the following would be most helpful to the physician?

(A) What birth control method(s) she has used in the past
(B) What birth control methods her friends use
(C) Whether her parents know that she is sexually active and has come for birth control
(D) How often she has sexual intercourse
(E) Whether she ever uses tampons

3. An 18-year-old woman presents to her physician for evaluation of a vaginal discharge. She states that she uses condoms for protection most of the time and that her partner is asymptomatic. She last had sexual intercourse 2 weeks ago. She does have some dysuria, but no urinary frequency. On pelvic examination, the physician finds a thick, purulent vaginal discharge, some cervical motion tenderness, and a friable cervix. Which of the following is the most likely cause of the infection?

(A) Gonorrhea
(B) Genital herpes
(C) Chlamydial infection
(D) Syphilis
(E) Bacterial vaginosis

4. A 15-year-old girl is requesting to start oral contraceptive pills. She has not had sexual intercourse to date, but feels that she may become sexually active in the near future. She has insulin-dependent diabetes. What is the most likely side effect she will experience?

(A) Hair loss
(B) Decreased control of her diabetes
(C) Bleeding between periods
(D) Dysmenorrhea
(E) Longer menstrual periods

5. A 17-year-old woman comes to her physician requesting a pregnancy test. Her menstrual period is 3 days overdue. She has always used condoms for protection; however, about 2 weeks ago she had a condom failure. She prefers using a condom, but wants additional protection without significant systemic side effects. Which one of the following methods would you recommend?

(A) Subdermal implant
(B) Spermicidal vaginal suppository or foam
(C) Depomedroxyprogesterone acetate
(D) Oral contraceptive pills

DIRECTIONS: Each of the numbered items or incomplete statements in this section is negatively phrased, as indicated by a capitalized word such as NOT, LEAST, or EXCEPT. Select the ONE lettered answer or completion that is BEST in each case.

6. A physician is asked to give a talk about suicide to a high school health class. Which of the following should NOT be included in the physician's talk?

(A) Suicide is the third leading cause of death for teenagers
(B) Death by suicide is more frequently seen in male adolescents
(C) Suicide is most commonly committed by overdose
(D) A history of a previous attempt is common
(E) Attempts are more common in female adolescents

7. A 15-year-old boy comes in for a physical for a summer youth employment program. Although somewhat embarrassed, he is able to say that he is worried about his facial acne. He has tried a number of over-the-counter acne preparations without success. When talking to him about his acne care, which of the following factors should the physician tell him is LEAST important?

(A) Diet
(B) Local hygiene
(C) Sebum production
(D) Inflammatory response
(E) Bacterial activity

8. All of the following statements regarding substance abuse in adolescents are true EXCEPT

(A) substance abuse may retard psychosocial development
(B) cocaine is the most commonly abused substance
(C) tobacco use is associated with use by parents
(D) the frequency of most forms of substance abuse is decreasing in adolescents

DIRECTIONS: Each set of matching questions in this section consists of a list of four to twenty-six lettered options (some of which may be in figures) followed by several items. For each numbered item, select the ONE lettered option that is most closely associated with it. To avoid spending too much time on matching sets with large numbers of options, it is generally advisable to begin each set by reading the list of options. Then, for each item in the set, try to generate the correct answer and locate it in the option list, rather than evaluating each option individually. Each lettered option may be selected once, more than once, or not at all.

Questions 9–12

The diagnosis of genital infections is made from a smear of vaginal, cervical, or urethral discharge, or by culture from the appropriate site of infection. For each microscopic finding listed below, select the causative organism with which it is most likely associated.

(A) *Neisseria gonorrhoeae*
(B) *Trichomonas vaginalis*
(C) *Candida albicans*
(D) *Chlamydia trachomatis*
(E) *Gardnerella vaginalis*

9. Budding hyphae

10. Flagellate protozoa

11. Inclusion bodies

12. Gram-negative diplococci

ANSWERS AND EXPLANATIONS

1. The answer is D *[II C 2 a (3); Figure 5-3]*. Muscle development is a major change that occurs in boys during puberty. This change accompanies the rapid increase in height that occurs at male pubertal development stage 4. Attempts to increase muscle mass at an earlier stage of pubertal development will lead to frustration. Male adolescents can know they are entering this stage of physical development when they start to grow axillary or facial hair.

2. The answer is C *[V]*. Understanding the level of parental knowledge and involvement is the most important issue. If parents are not involved, then additional efforts are needed to keep the medical visit confidential. The adolescent has to consider how she will be able to use the chosen birth control method without her parents finding out. More time will have to be given to promoting and reensuring compliance with the birth control method because female adolescents tend to have lower compliance rates if they do not have parental knowledge or support. Past history of contraceptive use is helpful in identifying what has or has not worked. What friends use for birth control is often what is most familiar and acceptable. Friends share their experiences about what methods do not work and pass rumors about various birth control methods that may not be true. The frequency of sexual intercourse may also influence the method she would like to use. Someone who is sexually active only several times a year may not want to take a pill every day. Using a tampon implies that the adolescent is comfortable with her body, and hence may be more likely to use a vaginal spermicidal or barrier method.

3. The answer is C *[IV A 1; Table 5-5]*. Findings on the examination are consistent with a sexually transmitted disease (STD) and possible early pelvic infection. *Chlamydia trachomatis* is the most common of the organisms that cause these symptoms, but also is asymptomatic in men. Gonorrhea can also cause these symptoms, but is rarely asymptomatic in men. Herpes, syphilis, and bacterial vaginosis are less likely to result in these physical findings. Active herpes is accompanied by ulcer-like lesions. Bacterial vaginosis causes a white discharge, but rarely the cervical findings.

4. The answer is C *[Table 5-6]*. Bleeding between periods, or breakthrough bleeding, is one of the most common side effects of oral contraceptive pills. This usually resolves after the second or third cycle of pills. Hair loss can occur but is much less common. Birth control pills can result in changes in control of insulin-dependent diabetes, but these changes are usually minor and easily corrected. Birth control pills usually reduce dysmenorrhea and the length of the menstrual period.

5. The answer is B *[V A 2 c (5)]*. The combination of a condom and vaginal spermicide is an excellent birth control method, almost as effective as the oral contraceptive pills. This combination method has no systemic side effects and few, if any, signs of vaginal irritation. The remaining three methods, although very effective as birth control methods, have significant systemic effects such as weight gain, breakthrough bleeding, and irregular menses.

6. The answer is C *[VI B]*. In the United States, many suicides are committed by drug overdose and poisoning, but they are not as common as those caused by firearms and hanging. Over two-thirds of those who commit suicide have tried it before, and many of those people have a history of depression or other mental health problems. Men are three to four times more likely to commit suicide than women, although women make more attempts. The ratio of suicides between men and women is influenced by the local culture. For example, the suicide rate is equal in men and women in Israel, but more women than men commit suicide in India.

7. The answer is A *[VIII A 3]*. Successful acne therapy involves counteracting the increased sebum production stimulated by elevated androgens and counteracting bacterial activity and the resulting local inflammatory response. Keeping the skin free from excessive oils has also proved to be helpful. Dietary restrictions, such as eliminating chocolate, have not proven very effective.

8. The answer is B *[VII D]*. Alcohol is the most commonly abused substance among adolescents, although cocaine abuse is a significant problem. Most forms of substance abuse in the adolescent population have gradually decreased in frequency in the 1980s from the levels seen in the late 1970s. Chronic substance abuse results in dissociation from normal socialization activities and leads to delay of psychosocial development.

9–12. The answers are: 9-C *[IV B 1 b; Table 5-5]*, **10-B** *[IV A 1 j; Table 5-5]*, **11-D** *[IV A 1; Table 5-5]*, **12-A** *[IV A 1 b; Table 5-5]*. Candidal vaginal infections are diagnosed by the presence of hyphae. This infection often is accompanied by a cheesy white discharge and vulvar pruritus. This infection often occurs after a course of systemic antibiotics taken for an unrelated infection. The antibiotics tend to decrease the normal vaginal flora and allow the yeast to proliferate.

Trichomonas vaginalis is a flagellate protozoon that causes vaginitis usually associated with a foul-smelling, greenish discharge and vulvar tenderness. The organism tends to die quickly in a normal saline preparation. Such a preparation should be reviewed without delay.

Chlamydial infections are identified by inclusion bodies located in columnar lining cells in the endocervix of the woman and about an inch into the urethra in the man. Unless samples of these cells are taken for culture or for a rapid analysis, a diagnosis of chlamydial infection is impossible to confirm. Samples of the cervical or urethral discharge may not contain the organism.

Gram-negative intracellular diplococci present in a smear from a male urethra are diagnostic for gonorrhea. In women, a culture is needed to confirm the presence of gonorrhea, because other gram-negative diplococci may be part of the normal vaginal flora.

Chapter 6

Neonatology

Ted S. Rosenkrantz

I. **GENERAL PRINCIPLES.** Many problems that arise in the newborn are discussed in detail in other chapters. This chapter emphasizes those problems that are unique to the perinatal period. In this section, some general concepts are introduced, which are amplified in subsequent sections.

A. Definition of terms

1. The normal human **gestational period** is 280 days, or 40 weeks, calculated from the first day of the mother's last menstrual cycle.
   a. **Preterm gestation** refers to delivery at less than 38 weeks' gestation.
   b. **Term gestation** refers to delivery at 38 to less than 42 weeks' gestation.
   c. **Postterm gestation** refers to delivery at or after 42 weeks' gestation.

2. The **neonatal period** is defined as the first 28 days (4 weeks) of life for term infants, although, from a practical standpoint, it is extended in the case of a prematurely delivered infant.

B. Major concepts and concerns inherent to the neonatal period

1. **Transition from fetal to neonatal life.** Changes in body and organ function occur as the fetus adapts to extrauterine life and begins to function independently. Organs mature at different rates and times during gestation. A preterm or complicated delivery may alter the normal sequence of these events (see I C 2). Some major changes occur in the following organ systems during the transition from fetal to neonatal life.
   a. **Cardiovascular system** (see Chapter 12)
      (1) **Prenatal circulation** (Figure 6-1)
         (a) Oxygenation of the blood occurs in the **placenta**—an organ of low vascular resistance—and the oxygenated blood returns to the fetus via the **umbilical vein,** which enters the liver at the porta hepatis.
         (b) Blood passes through the **ductus venosus** to the inferior vena cava. Preferential shunting allows oxygenated blood to be shunted through the **foramen ovale** to the left atrium and left ventricle and on to the coronary, carotid, and cerebral arteries, while the desaturated blood of the inferior and superior venae cavae travels to the right atrium and right ventricle and on to the pulmonary artery.
         (c) Owing to the high vascular resistance in the lung, 90% of the pulmonary artery blood bypasses the lung and is shunted through the **ductus arteriosus,** which enters the aorta below the takeoff of the brachiocephalic artery and left common carotid artery. In this way, the most highly oxygenated blood is supplied to the heart and brain.
         (d) Blood in the descending aorta, which is intermediately deoxygenated, is returned to the placenta by way of the **umbilical arteries**.
      (2) **Postnatal circulation**
         (a) At birth, there is a rise in systemic vascular resistance as a result of the cessation of blood flow through the placenta.

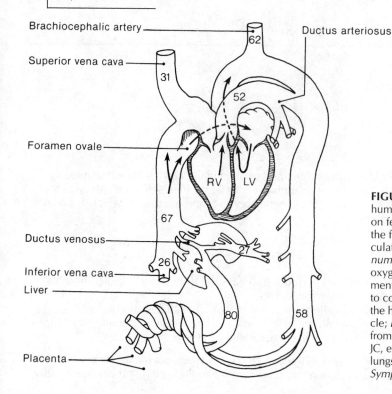

Brachiocephalic artery
Ductus arteriosus
62
Superior vena cava
31
52
Foramen ovale
RV   LV
67
Ductus venosus
27
26
Inferior vena cava
Liver
80   58
Placenta

FIGURE 6-1. Knowledge of the human fetal circulation is based on fetal animal studies, such as the fetal lamb. The fetal lamb circulation is diagramed here, with *numbers* representing the percent oxygen saturation in various segments. These values are believed to correspond closely to those in the human fetus. *RV* = right ventricle; *LV* = left ventricle. (Reprinted from Born GVR, Dawes GS, Mott JC, et al: Changes in the heart and lungs at birth. *Cold Spring Harbor Symp Quant Biol* 19:102, 1954.)

    (b) With the first few breaths, pulmonary vascular resistance falls, the foramen ovale closes, and the ductus arteriosus begins to constrict. These processes allow all deoxygenated blood returning to the right ventricle to go on to the lung and become oxygenated.

    (c) The oxygenated blood returns to the left ventricle and then is pumped throughout the body.

  b. Pulmonary system (see Chapter 13)

    (1) By the end of gestation, the major airways and alveoli are filled with fluid that contains large amounts of **surfactant**.

    (2) At birth, the negative pressure created by the first breaths draws air into the lungs, and an air–fluid interface is formed. The surfactant spreads along the epithelial lining of the alveoli and decreases surface tension at the end of expiration.

  c. Hepatobiliary system. Prenatally, bilirubin conjugation in the liver is suppressed. In the first days of life, increased **glucuronyl transferase** activity results in conjugation and elimination of bilirubin, via reduction products, in the stool.

  d. Renal system (see Chapter 14). Glomerular function, which is relatively low in fetal life as reflected by the glomerular filtration rate, increases with gestational age as well as with postnatal age. Tubular function also improves with age, which has important consequences for the elimination of many drugs from the body.

2. Growth. The growth rate of the fetus is greater than that of the infant or older child. Growth slows just before birth, limited by placental substrate transport, and a loss of body weight occurs in the first few days after birth owing to loss of extracellular water and to inadequate nutritional intake. As the newborn acclimates to the extrauterine environment and improves her behavioral organization, feeding improves and growth accelerates again. Adequate nutrition along with control of possible hyperbilirubinemia or infection are crucial to normal growth and development in the newborn. (See IV B 2, 3 for further discussion of growth and the nutritional needs of the newborn.)

3. **Initial examination of the newborn.** It is the pediatrician's responsibility to perform a thorough physical examination and a series of screening tests so that common, preventable illnesses and congenital anomalies may be identified and rapidly treated, because a poor outcome often is related to a delay in detection and therapy. (See Chapter 1 for details of the newborn examination.)

C. Somatic growth, organ maturation, and gestational age

1. **Somatic growth** refers to the process by which the body and its constituent parts increase in size. Somatic growth occurs by two processes: hyperplasia and hypertrophy.
   a. **Hyperplasia** is an increase in the size of a tissue or organ due to an **increase in cell number**. Growth during the first half of pregnancy is achieved by hyperplasia.
      (1) Problems that interfere with somatic growth early in pregnancy inhibit cell division, causing a decrease in total body cell number. As a result, the fetus may be **symmetrically growth retarded** or small for weight, length, and head circumference.
      (2) Factors that adversely affect hyperplastic growth of the fetus include:
         (a) Congenital infection
         (b) Chromosomal defects
         (c) Nonchromosomal congenital syndromes
         (d) Cell toxins (e.g., alcohol, narcotics)
   b. **Hypertrophy** is an increase in the size of a tissue or organ due to an **increase in cell size**. Growth during the last trimester of pregnancy and postnatally is achieved primarily by hypertrophy.
      (1) Aberrations in fetal nutrition in the last stage of pregnancy inhibit normal cell growth and may result in **asymmetric growth retardation**. Body weight is primarily affected, with preservation of brain growth.
      (2) Factors that adversely affect fetal nutrition include:
         (a) Maternal malnutrition
         (b) Placental abnormalities or abnormal cord insertion
         (c) Preeclampsia
         (d) Multiple gestation
         (e) Maternal use of cigarettes

2. **Organ maturation** refers to the structural and functional development of an organ system. Maturational growth is measured by comparison to the adult level of organ function.
   a. The various **organ systems mature at different rates and at different times** during gestation. Premature birth may alter the normal sequence of organ maturation.
      (1) The term infant has sufficient function of most organs to allow it to be independent at birth. Some organs (e.g., the liver, kidney) accelerate in function during the immediate perinatal period, whereas a few organs (e.g., the brain, lung) continue to mature for many years after birth.
      (2) The preterm infant has inadequate function of some vital organs (e.g., the lung) at birth, but within a short period of time many of these organs will have accelerated development and function compared with a fetus of similar conceptional age. This allows for independent function of the preterm infant at a gestationally young age.
   b. Usually, there is a **close correlation between the somatic growth and maturation of vital organs** (e.g., the lung), although various factors may accelerate or retard either or both of these processes. In the case of lung development, both fetal malnutrition and administration of betamethasone to the mother are factors that accelerate biochemical maturation, whereas maternal diabetes and the associated fetal hyperglycemia and hyperinsulinemia lead to delayed biochemical maturation of the lung.

3. **Gestational age.** Norms have been established for somatic growth at each week of gestation and are based on weight, length, and head circumference. However, size, per se, should not be used to infer gestational age or maturation.

a. If an infant's growth parameters are between the tenth and ninetieth percentiles for a specific time of gestation, the infant's growth is said to be **appropriate for gestational age**.

b. If an infant's weight is less than the tenth percentile for a specific time of gestation, the infant is said to be **small for gestational age** [see I C 1 a (2), b (2) for causative factors].

c. If an infant's weight is greater than the ninetieth percentile for a specific time of gestation, the infant is said to be **large for gestational age**. Causes include:
  (1) Maternal diabetes
  (2) Beckwith-Wiedemann syndrome
  (3) Genetic predisposition (i.e., maternal history of large infants)
  (4) Hydrops fetalis

d. If an infant's head circumference is greater than the ninetieth percentile for a specific time of gestation, regardless of other parameters, specific cerebral pathology should be investigated (see V G 4 and Chapter 18).

II. PERINATAL ASPHYXIA

A. Pathophysiology. The ability of the fetus or infant to survive episodes of asphyxia is related to the mechanisms that regulate blood flow to the organs of the body. These mechanisms are designed to maintain oxygen delivery to the vital organs (i.e., the brain, heart, adrenal gland) during periods of hypoxia.

1. **During periods of hypoxia or hypercapnia,** blood flow to the brain is increased. The result is a stable delivery of oxygen to the brain to meet metabolic demands and maintenance of a normal intracellular pH. These flow changes are operational unless the infant is extremely hypotensive.

2. **During periods of mild asphyxia,** adaptive changes in blood flow allow adequate oxygen delivery to the brain, heart, and adrenal gland. This is accomplished through an increase in and a redistribution of the cardiac output. Blood flow to the skin, muscle, kidney, and gastrointestinal tract is sacrificed to maintain perfusion of the vital organs.

3. **During periods of severe or prolonged asphyxia,** the underperfused (sacrificed) tissues and organs gradually become acidotic because of anaerobic metabolism and lactic acid production. This leads to myocardial depression and a gradual decrease in blood pressure so that blood fails to perfuse the vital organs, with resultant permanent tissue damage in such organs. The extent of the tissue damage depends on the amount of time that has elapsed between the failure of blood flow (i.e., tissue hypoxia) and the institution of resuscitation (i.e., reoxygenation of the tissues).

B. Clinical features. The ability to recognize the clinical signs and symptoms of perinatal asphyxia requires knowledge of the predisposing risk factors for asphyxia, as well as the prenatal and postnatal symptoms of asphyxia.

1. Prenatal **risk factors for asphyxia** are listed in Table 6-1.

2. **Events that occur with the onset of asphyxia**
   a. Sequence. A clear understanding of the sequence of events that occur with the onset of asphyxia is of utmost importance in determining the condition of the asphyxiated infant and in initiating therapy (Figure 6-2; see also III E).
   (1) Respiratory effort ceases abruptly, and the fetus (infant) experiences primary apnea. This is followed by a phase of gasping, and, if resuscitation is not initiated, progression to terminal apnea.
   (2) A rapid decrease in the oxygenation of blood occurs, with resultant respiratory acidosis followed by a combined respiratory and metabolic acidosis.
   (3) The onset of hypoxia results in a rapid decrease in heart rate.

TABLE 6-1. Prenatal Risk Factors for Asphyxia

Extremes in maternal age (i.e., < 20 years or > 35 years)	Fetal bradycardia
	Malpresentation
Placental abruption	Multiple gestation
Placenta previa	Prolonged rupture of the fetal
Preeclampsia	membranes
Preterm gestation	Maternal diabetes
Postterm gestation	Maternal use of illicit drugs
Meconium-stained amniotic fluid	

    (4) Blood pressure rises initially but, with progression to terminal apnea, falls to hypotensive levels.

    (5) The fall in blood pressure causes a decrease in the flow of blood to the organs and consequent tissue damage.

b. Recovery. These events can be reversed with appropriate resuscitative measures [i.e., reoxygenation of the central nervous system (CNS); see III E].

    (1) As a result of such intervention, heart rate and blood pressure improve; gasping then occurs, followed by regular breathing. Last to recover are body functions that are controlled by the higher regions of the brain.

    (2) The longer the episode of asphyxia, the longer it takes for heart rate, breathing, and other body functions to recover.

3. Postnatal symptoms of asphyxia vary with the degree of asphyxia. It is not clear why some infants exhibit multiorgan involvement, whereas others have only one or two organ systems involved. Some specific effects of asphyxia are listed by organ system.

a. Brain

    (1) Mild asphyxia. The infant who experiences mild asphyxia initially will be depressed. This is followed by a period of hyperalertness, which resolves within 1 or 2 days. There are no focal signs, and the prognosis is excellent for a normal outcome.

    (2) Moderate asphyxia. The infant who experiences moderate asphyxia will be very depressed. This is followed by a prolonged period of hyperalertness and hyperreflexia. Generalized seizures often occur 12–24 hours after the episode of asphyxia but are controlled easily, resolving in a few days regardless of therapy. The prognosis is variable; negative results on electroencephalogram (EEG) are predictive of a normal outcome.

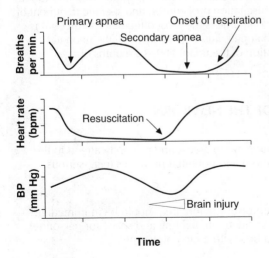

FIGURE 6-2. The sequence of events associated with perinatal asphyxia and recovery after institution of resuscitation. (Adapted from Dawes GS: *Fetal and Neonatal Physiology.* Chicago, Year Book Publishers, 1968, p 149.)

TABLE 6-2. Complications Associated With Perinatal Asphyxia

Hypotension	Adrenal hemorrhage and necrosis
Hypoxic encephalopathy and seizures	Hypoglycemia
Persistent pulmonary hypertension	Polycythemia
Hypoxic cardiomyopathy	Hypocalcemia
Ileus and necrotizing enterocolitis	Disseminated intravascular
Acute tubular necrosis	coagulation (DIC)

       (3) Severe asphyxia is associated with coma, intractable seizure activity, cerebral edema, and intracranial hemorrhage. The infant often becomes progressively more depressed over the first 1–3 days, as the cerebral edema develops, and death may occur during this period. Survival usually is associated with a poor long-term outcome.

    b. Heart. Severe or prolonged episodes of asphyxia may result in **hypoxic cardiomyopathy**. Signs and symptoms include hypotension, poor myocardial contractility, cardiomegaly, and congestive heart failure.

    c. Lung. Respiratory distress and a need for oxygen can occur owing to a delayed fall in pulmonary vascular resistance (see V A 2 h).

    d. Kidney. Decreased renal blood flow during the asphyxial event causes **acute tubular necrosis**. This usually is self-limited.

    e. Gastrointestinal tract. Asphyxia often is associated with poor gastrointestinal motility or ileus. The hypoxia also predisposes to secondary bacterial invasion and to the development of **necrotizing enterocolitis** (see V B).

    f. Blood. Hypoxia depresses bone marrow function and initiates an intravascular coagulopathy, which results in thrombocytopenia, prolonged prothrombin time (PT) and partial thromboplastin time (PTT), and clinical evidence of bleeding.

C. **Therapy**

    1. General principles. The primary objective in treating perinatal asphyxia is to restore an oxygen supply to the body tissues, especially the brain. This requires ventilation with oxygen and ensuring an adequate cardiac output. The secondary objective is to evaluate the degree of hypoxic injury and to plan treatment.

    2. Specific therapy. Specific delivery room resuscitation procedures are discussed in III E. Problems commonly associated with asphyxia are listed in Table 6-2. These conditions should be anticipated or considered and treated if present.

D. **Prognosis.** Outcome is related to the severity and duration of the asphyxial insult and to the adequacy of compensatory mechanisms, resuscitation procedures, and specific treatment of multiorgan system involvement. Neurologic outcome is the most difficult to predict but is best related to the degree of hypoxic encephalopathy and EEG activity in the neonatal period, and to findings on physical examination of the infant at 9–12 months of age.

III. **DELIVERY ROOM MANAGEMENT OF THE NEWBORN**

A. **Goals.** The goals of delivery room management are to assess and promptly attend to the immediate needs (e.g., oxygenation, ventilation) and potential problems (e.g., serious anomalies) of the newborn.

B. **Physical layout and equipment.** The newborn resuscitation area should be in immediate proximity to the delivery room. It should have adequate lighting and space for personnel and equipment for resuscitation, including a bed with a radiant warmer.

TABLE 6-3.   Essential Parts of Obstetric History

Maternal age

Medical and previous obstetric history

Length of gestation

Blood group incompatibilities

Maternal infection [e.g., syphilis, gonorrhea, rubella, herpes, human immunodeficiency virus (HIV), hepatitis]

Maternal drug use

Ultrasound evaluation of fetal growth and amniotic fluid volume, as well as for the possibility of congenital anomalies

Signs of chorioamnionitis, including prolonged rupture of the fetal membranes, maternal fever, and leukocytosis on complete blood count

Results of other fetal evaluations, including lecithin/sphingomyelin ratio [see V A 1 b (1) (b)], nonstress test, and biophysical profile

C. **Preparation for delivery**

1. **Obtaining perinatal information.** The pediatrician must have specific information concerning the mother and fetus to prepare for routine care of the mother and newborn as well as treatment of specific problems related to a particular delivery.
   a. **Obstetric history** should include all information that may be pertinent to the immediate fetal (newborn) condition. The information is best obtained from the obstetrician and the medical chart and by direct communication with the parents. Important items are listed in Table 6-3.
   b. **Labor history** should be obtained (Table 6-4).

2. **Composition of the resuscitation team.** Personnel and their tasks vary with the type of delivery that is anticipated. High-risk deliveries or pregnancies include those with such complications as listed in Table 6-5.
   a. **Low-risk delivery team** includes:
      (1) **Team leader** to assess the newborn and institute any necessary resuscitation
      (2) **One assistant** to assist in basic newborn resuscitation, including drying and warming the infant and assessing heart rate
   b. **High-risk delivery team** includes:
      (1) **Team leader** to direct resuscitation and, possibly, to direct and institute airway management
      (2) **Three assistants**
         (a) One to assess heart rate and to initiate cardiac compression if needed
         (b) One to assist with drying, suctioning, ventilating, and preparing drugs for injection
         (c) One to gain intravenous access and to administer drugs

3. **Equipment for resuscitation** (Table 6-6). The equipment needed is directly related to the basic principles of newborn resuscitation (see III E).

TABLE 6-4.   Essential Parts of Labor History

Fetal heart tracing
Duration of fetal membrane rupture
Evaluation of amniotic fluid (color and quantity)
Progress of labor
Fetal scalp blood pH

TABLE 6-5. Factors Associated With High-Risk Pregnancies or Deliveries

Maternal diabetes	Severe preeclampsia
Maternal antibody sensitization (Rh, ABO)	Intrauterine growth retardation
Preterm gestation (delivery at < 38 weeks)	Maternal narcotic addiction
Postterm gestation (delivery at > 42 weeks)	Known fetal anomalies
Multiple gestation	Breech presentation
Maternal bleeding (placental abruption, placenta previa)	Cesarean delivery
	Fetal distress

D. **Assessment of the newborn and the Apgar score.** The goal of the initial assessment is to determine the newborn's state of oxygenation and ventilation. This usually is done by performing an abbreviated Apgar evaluation (Table 6-7).

1. The Apgar score was devised as a means of assessing the oxygenation, ventilation, and degree of asphyxia in a uniform manner that quickly communicates information to all people involved in the resuscitation of the newborn. The Apgar evaluation is performed at 1 and 5 minutes after birth. Five signs—heart rate, respiratory effort, muscle tone, reflex irritability, and skin color—are examined and assigned a score of 0, 1, or 2. The Apgar score is obtained by adding all individual scores.
   a. A **score of 8–10** reflects good oxygenation and ventilation and indicates no need for vigorous resuscitation.
   b. A **score of 5–7** indicates a need for stimulation and supplemental oxygen.
   c. A **score of less than 5** indicates a need for assisted ventilation and possible cardiac support (see III E 1 c, d).

2. The Apgar score is a useful method of communicating the well-being of the newborn. However, urgently needed resuscitation should not be delayed while a full examination is performed. Bradycardia or a poor respiratory effort alone indicates a need for immediate resuscitation.

TABLE 6-6. Equipment for Resuscitation

Airway management	Wall-unit suction pump with regulator*
	DeLee suction catheter with trap
	Oral airway (various sizes)
	Endotracheal tubes of appropriate sizes
	Laryngoscope
	Suction catheters
	Endotracheal tube adapter for suctioning of meconium
Ventilation and oxygenation	Oxygen source (preferably warmed and humidified)
	Masks of appropriate sizes
	Bag with oxygen reservoir, mechanism to deliver positive end-expiratory pressure (PEEP), and manometer to measure airway pressure
Intravenous access	Umbilical catheters (3.5 F and 5.0 F)
	Instruments for umbilical cutdown
	Saline solution (0.9%)
Drugs	Epinephrine
	Plasma volume expanding agent (i.e., 5% albumin or 5% purified protein fraction solution)
	Sodium bicarbonate
	Naloxone

*A pressure of 80 cm H_2O is appropriate for most suctioning.

TABLE 6-7. Apgar Evaluation of the Newborn

Sign	Score		
	0	**1**	**2**
Heart rate	Absent	< 100 beats/min	> 100 beats/min
Respiratory effort	Absent	Weak, irregular	Strong, regular
Muscle tone	Flaccid	Some flexion	Well flexed
Reflex irritability (response to catheter in nostril)	No response	Grimace	Cough or sneeze
Skin color	Blue, pale	Body pink, extremities blue	Entire body pink

   3. The Apgar score at 5 minutes reflects the adequacy of resuscitation and the degree of perinatal asphyxia.

E. **Resuscitation.** The purpose of resuscitation is to reoxygenate the CNS of the newborn by providing oxygen, establishing ventilation, and ensuring an adequate cardiac output. Although it may be difficult to differentiate primary apnea from secondary apnea, a quick assessment of the newborn's skin color, respiratory activity, and heart rate should allow prompt institution of appropriate resuscitation (Figure 6-3).

   1. Routine procedures. The evaluations and procedures that constitute the resuscitation of the newborn are listed in the order in which they should be initiated.
      a. Maintenance of body heat. The infant should be dried and provided with radiant heat to maintain body temperature. It is important to avoid hypothermia, which will increase the newborn's oxygen consumption.
      b. Establishment of an airway. Immediately after delivery, the infant's head should be placed in a neutral or slightly extended position and an airway established by clear-

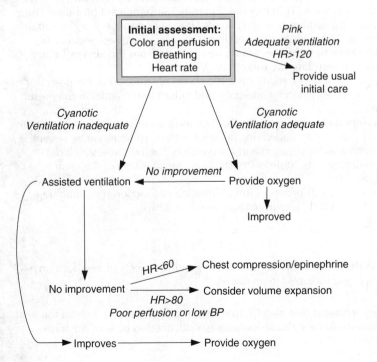

FIGURE 6-3. Scheme for assessment and resuscitation of the newborn.

ing the mouth, nose, and pharynx of thick secretions or meconium (see III E 2 a). Deep and frequent oropharyngeal suctioning should be avoided because it will increase vagal output, causing apnea and bradycardia.

c. **Ventilation.** The adequacy of air exchange in the newborn must be assessed. In most cases, drying off, suctioning, and tactile stimulation (e.g., gentle flicking of the feet or rubbing of the back) are adequate to induce effective spontaneous ventilation (see Figure 6-3).

   (1) If ventilation is adequate, **supplemental oxygen** may be given to improve heart rate or skin color.

   (2) If supplemental oxygen does not improve heart rate or skin color, or if ventilation is inadequate, **mechanical ventilation** should be initiated, using mask and bag ventilation.

      (a) If spontaneous ventilation improves, mechanical ventilation should be stopped and supplemental oxygen resumed.

      (b) If the response is poor or if airway obstruction occurs, an endotracheal tube should be inserted and mechanical ventilation continued.

d. **Circulation.** If mechanical ventilation does not improve the heart rate or skin color, one of the following steps is taken.

   (1) **If heart rate is less than 60 beats/minute,** or between 60 and 80 beats/minute and not improving, **cardiac compression** is initiated; if heart rate does not improve, **epinephrine** is administered via an umbilical venous catheter or endotracheal tube.

   (2) **If heart rate is 80 beats/minute or greater** but there is poor perfusion or weak pulse, a plasma volume-expanding agent is administered at a dose of 15 ml/kg.

e. **Drug support.** The following medications may be useful during resuscitation.

   (1) **Sodium bicarbonate** should be reserved until it is clear that a metabolic acidosis exists.

   (2) **Naloxone** may be helpful for poor spontaneous respiratory effort secondary to maternal narcotic use during labor. Naloxone is contraindicated in an infant born to a mother who is addicted to narcotics.

2. **Special problems requiring resuscitation,** which are listed below, are discussed in further detail in section V.

   a. **Meconium aspiration syndrome** (see V A 3 c). Meconium-stained amniotic fluid may be a sign of perinatal asphyxia. Thin meconium rarely is a significant problem. Thick meconium, however, is a serious concern because it may be aspirated and result in aspiration pneumonia. Although an affected infant may be depressed because of asphyxia, **it is imperative that the meconium be removed from the airway before any attempt is made to ventilate the infant** [see V A 3 c (3)].

   b. **Choanal atresia** (see V A 2 b) is a membranous or bony obstruction of the posterior nasal passages. It is a life-threatening anomaly, and failure to recognize it may result in respiratory arrest.

   c. **Progressive respiratory distress or cyanosis** that occurs in an infant despite appropriate resuscitation usually suggests an underlying disorder of the cardiopulmonary system, which requires immediate investigation and intervention. Such disorders include:

      (1) Cyanotic heart disease (i.e., pulmonary stenosis, transposition of the great vessels; see Chapter 12)

      (2) Congenital or acquired disorders of lung formation or function [i.e., diaphragmatic hernia (see V A 2 d), pneumothorax (see V A 3 b)]

      (3) Sepsis (see V F 2)

IV. CARE OF THE NEWBORN.

In this section, some specific aspects of newborn physiology, pathophysiology, and therapy are reviewed.

A. | **Fluid and electrolyte requirements** (see also Chapter 14). Water represents 94% of the fetal weight at 3 months' gestation. At term, water content has declined to 80% of the birth weight of the newborn.

1. **Fluid loss and replacement**
   a. **Fluid loss**
      (1) During the first week of life, the extracellular fluid space contracts, resulting in a large reduction in body water. This water loss is responsible for 5% of the weight loss observed in term infants. The preterm infant may lose up to 10%–15% of his birth weight.
      (2) Water loss through evaporation from the skin and from expired air is referred to as **insensible water loss**. Water loss through the urine and stool is referred to as **sensible water loss**. Stool accounts for a very small amount of sensible water loss.
   b. **Fluid replacement** is based on fluid loss and is calculated as the sum of insensible and sensible water losses. Initial parenteral fluid replacement should be accomplished with a 10% dextrose solution.
      (1) Insensible water loss varies with gestational age and factors related to the nursing environment, such as the heat source, humidity, and use of phototherapy (for treatment of hyperbilirubinemia).
      (2) In addition to water lost in the urine, other sensible losses such as gastric secretions (i.e., vomitus) should be included in the calculation of total water loss.
   c. **Fluid balance** is monitored by examining:
      (1) Urine output
      (2) Change in body weight
      (3) Serum sodium concentration
      (4) Urine specific gravity

2. **Electrolyte loss and replacement**
   a. **Sodium, potassium, and chloride** are the principal salts that are lost through the urine and should be replaced accordingly. Assuming an adequate urine output, replacement is begun 24 hours after birth at the following rates:
      (1) **Sodium:** 1–3 mEq/kg/day
      (2) **Potassium:** 1–2 mEq/kg/day
      (3) **Chloride:** 1–3 mEq/kg/day
   b. **Calcium.** A decrease in serum calcium concentration frequently occurs during the first week of life. Serum calcium concentrations below 7 mg/dl (total) or below 3–3.5 mg/dl (ionized) are considered hypocalcemic.
      (1) **Early neonatal (physiologic) hypocalcemia.** Nearly all infants experience a small decline in total serum calcium during the first few days of life owing to intrauterine parathyroid hormone suppression. Early neonatal hypocalcemia rarely requires treatment except in preterm infants, infants of diabetic mothers, and asphyxiated infants.
      (2) **Late neonatal (nonphysiologic) hypocalcemia** is seen at the end of the first week of life. Etiologies include:
         (a) Increased phosphate ingestion, as occurs in infants who are fed cow's milk or high-phosphate rice cereal
         (b) Hypomagnesemia
         (c) Hypoparathyroidism
      (3) **Therapy** usually consists of calcium replacement with calcium gluconate and treatment of any underlying cause of the hypocalcemia.
   c. **Other required minerals** include:
      (1) Phosphorus
      (2) Magnesium
      (3) Iron
      (4) Trace metals

B. **Nutritional requirements.** Adequate caloric intake with the correct balance of carbohydrate, protein, and fat is needed for homeostasis and growth. The specific nutritional requirements of the newborn are reviewed here, after a brief overview of prenatal gastrointestinal system development and fetal and neonatal growth.

1. Prenatal development of the gastrointestinal tract

   a. Anatomic development proceeds in a series of orderly steps. By 4 weeks' gestation, the primitive foregut is identified; by 6 weeks, foregut, midgut, and hindgut divisions are present. Malformations of the gastrointestinal tract occur secondary to failure in division or normal rotation or because of vascular accidents.

     (1) Esophagus

        (a) Normal development. The esophagus begins as a common tubular structure that invaginates to form the esophagus, the pharynx, and the respiratory tree.

        (b) Developmental anomalies include **esophageal atresia** and **tracheoesophageal fistula,** which result from failure in division. (The latter disorder rarely occurs in the absence of the former; see also V A 2 a.)

     (2) Stomach

        (a) Normal development. The stomach is formed by dilation of the caudal end of the foregut. Development is complete by 5 weeks' gestation.

        (b) Developmental anomalies of the stomach are rare.

     (3) Intestines

        (a) Normal development. The **duodenum** is formed as the terminal foregut and proximal midgut grow and form a loop. The remainder of the midgut forms the **jejunum** and **ileum**. Between 5 and 10 weeks' gestation, the growing midgut is forced out of the abdominal cavity and into the umbilical cord. The **mesentery** grows within the loop. By the end of this period, the intestines reenter the abdominal cavity, proceeding cranially to caudally and making a 270-degree rotation.

        (b) Developmental anomalies

           (i) Small bowel atresia is thought to result from a vascular accident, probably during rotation and reentry of the bowel into the abdominal cavity.

           (ii) Malrotation results from failure of normal rotation and fixation, which predisposes to the development of a **volvulus** (i.e., twisting of the bowel about the superior mesenteric artery with resulting obstruction).

           (iii) Omphalocele is a herniation of intraabdominal viscera into the umbilical cord. A membranous sac containing bowel, liver, or both arises from failure of reentry of the bowel from the yolk sac. The sac has a common insertion with the umbilical cord into the abdominal wall.

           (iv) Gastroschisis results from a defect in the closure of the abdominal wall, through which a variable portion of intestine protrudes.

     (4) Colon

        (a) Normal development. The colon develops from the hindgut and cloaca, which divides into the urogenital sinus and rectum by 6 weeks' gestation.

        (b) Developmental anomalies include:

           (i) Imperforate anus, which results from failure of the cloacal membrane to rupture

           (ii) Hirschsprung disease (congenital megacolon), which is failure of the normal innervation of the distal colon (see Chapter 11)

   b. Biochemical development

     (1) Gastric functional development begins during the second trimester. Gastric acid activity does not begin until after 32 weeks' gestation and increases rapidly in the first 24 hours of life.

     (2) Small intestine functional development also extends into postnatal life.

        (a) Disaccharidase activity. Sucrase, maltase, and isomaltase activity begins by 12 weeks' gestation and is at 70% by 34 weeks. Lactase activity remains low until term.

        (b) Disaccharidase deficiency. The most common congenital enzyme deficiency is a combined deficiency of sucrase and isomaltase. Congenital lactase deficiency is much less common, but a transient lactase deficiency frequently follows an episode of infectious gastroenteritis.

2. Fetal and neonatal growth

    a. Fetal growth. The fetal growth rate is 5 g/day at 14–15 weeks' gestation, 10 g/day at 20 weeks, and 30 g/day at 32–34 weeks. The growth rate slows after 36 weeks' gestation.

        (1) During the first trimester, growth parameters (i.e., weight, length, head circumference) are fairly uniform in all fetuses.

        (2) Variability in fetal growth during the last trimester is the result of several factors, including genetic endowment, fetal nutrition, and multiple gestation (fetal growth rate declines at 31 weeks' gestation in twins and at 29 weeks' gestation in triplets).

        (3) Abnormalities of fetal growth and their etiologies are discussed in I C 1.

    b. Neonatal growth

        (1) After birth, there is a loss of weight due to a loss of extracellular water and suboptimal caloric intake. Term infants lose 5% of their birth weight; preterm infants lose up to 15% of their birth weight.

        (2) Term infants regain their birth weight by the end of the first week of life, and thereafter gain 20–30 g/day.

3. Nutritional considerations. The composition of the nutritional solution and the route of delivery depend on the gestational age, general medical condition, and possible special nutritional needs of the newborn.

    a. Enteric nutrition

        (1) Route of feeding

            (a) The **term infant** can be bottle-fed or breast-fed on demand, as long as attention is paid to intake and fluid balance.

            (b) The otherwise healthy **preterm infant who is between 34 and 38 weeks' gestational age** should be fed every 3 hours by bottle, breast, or gavage, depending on the infant's strength and alertness.

            (c) The **preterm infant who is less than 34 weeks' gestational age** does not have a well-coordinated suck-and-swallow reflex, and therefore should be fed via a feeding tube. The feedings may be gastric bolus every 2–3 hours, except in infants weighing less than 1000 g.

            (d) Continuous gastric or transpyloric feeding is employed in the **infant who weighs less than 1000 g,** because this infant has a limited gastric volume and may experience intermittent hypoglycemia and hypoxia when given bolus feedings.

            (e) Continuous transpyloric feedings should be considered for the **infant who requires an endotracheal tube and mechanical ventilation** to prevent gastric reflux and aspiration.

        (2) Feeding solution. The composition of the feeding solution depends on the presence or absence of special protein, carbohydrate, or fat requirements or intolerances, which, in turn, depend on gestational age, gastrointestinal motility status, and the possibility of intestinal enzyme deficiencies or other metabolic disorders [e.g., phenylketonuria (PKU)].

            (a) Term infants who do not have complicating metabolic problems. All of the water, calorie, protein, and vitamin requirements of the normal term infant are met by human milk or 20 kcal/oz cow's milk-based formula. The specific nutritional needs of these infants for normal growth are as follows.

                (i) The normal term infant needs 100–120 kcal/kg/day to meet basal and growth requirements.

                (ii) The infant also needs 2–3 g/kg/day of protein for cellular growth, which represents approximately 10% of the total daily calorie intake.

                (iii) In addition, 40% of the daily calorie requirements should be derived from carbohydrates, with the remainder provided by dietary fats.

            (b) Preterm infants have decreased gastric motility and intestinal lactase activity as well as increased calcium and phosphorus requirements, among other nutritional problems. The initial feeding solution should be a dilute, whey-based formula or human milk. As positive nitrogen balance is achieved, the infant may be advanced to a formula that is high in calcium, phosphorus, and protein, or to supplemented human milk. A 24 kcal/oz formula is reserved for infants whose water intake must be restricted and infants who cannot tolerate adequate feeding volumes.

(c) **Infants with special metabolic needs.** Special formula solutions are available for infants with selected intestinal enzyme deficiencies (e.g., sucrase–isomaltase deficiency) or metabolic diseases (e.g., PKU).

(3) **Vitamins and minerals.** Commercially available formulas now are fortified with vitamins, minerals, and trace elements. Therefore, formula-fed term infants do not routinely require vitamin or mineral supplementation.

(a) **Special vitamin needs**

(i) Infants who are fed human milk may receive a multiple-vitamin supplement containing vitamins A, D, and C.

(ii) Owing to small body stores and inadequate feeding volumes, preterm infants should routinely receive a multiple-vitamin supplement containing the fat-soluble vitamins (A and D) and the water-soluble vitamins (B and C). In addition, the preterm infant who is less than 36 weeks' gestational age should receive vitamin E to prevent hemolytic anemia.

(b) **Special mineral and trace element needs**

(i) **Iron.** All infants require iron supplementation, which may be obtained via iron-fortified formula or through a separate supplement. Iron supplementation may be delayed in the preterm infant until enteric feedings are tolerated. Because of the increased bioavailability of iron in human milk, iron supplementation in term breast-fed infants may await the introduction of iron-fortified cereal at 4–6 months of age.

(ii) **Fluoride** supplements probably should not be given to infants younger than 6 months of age, even when otherwise indicated, because of the danger of fluorosis (see Chapter 1).

(iii) **Calcium and phosphorus.** The needs of the growing term infant are met by either commercial formula or human milk (see Chapter 1). Owing to rapid bone growth, the calcium and phosphorus requirements of the preterm infant are greater and necessitate special fortified formulas or supplementation if fed human milk.

b. **Total parenteral nutrition.** Preterm and other sick infants may require total parenteral nutrition because of gastrointestinal disorders (e.g., neonatal necrotizing enterocolitis) as well as nongastrointestinal disorders (e.g., respiratory disease, sepsis). An intravenous solution of dextrose, amino acids, fat, vitamins, and minerals can be administered by either peripheral or central venous access. Appropriately used, total parenteral nutrition can provide adequate calories and protein to support the basal needs and growth of the sick infant.

C. **Principles of drug therapy.** The administration and dosing of drugs are different in neonates. Disregarding this fact may result in toxicity or nontherapeutic use of drugs. After administration of a drug, the effect and disposition depend on a number of the factors discussed following. A neonatology or pharmacology text always should be consulted regarding dosages of drugs for preterm and term infants.

1. **Route of administration** determines the peak drug level, how quickly the peak level is reached, and how long the peak drug level is sustained.

2. **Solubility and pH** determine the compatibility of drugs, tissue penetration, and excretion rate.

3. **Protein binding.** The plasma total protein and albumin levels of the newborn are lower than the adult levels.

a. At similar total drug concentrations, there will be a larger unbound drug fraction for drugs with strong protein binding in the newborn compared to the adult.

Because the unbound fraction is the active fraction in the blood, lower total drug concentrations are needed to achieve a therapeutic effect in newborns.

   b. Drug competition for albumin-binding sites in the infant with hyperbilirubinemia (see V C) also poses a problem. If all the albumin binding sites are occupied with bilirubin, there will be a larger free fraction of drug in the blood. Conversely, if the drug displaces bilirubin or is already occupying the binding site, the increase in free bilirubin may increase the risk of kernicterus.

4. Metabolism of drugs by the liver often is suboptimal because of low levels of glucuronyl transferase. This often results in an increase in plasma drug levels and excretion of unchanged drug compared to the adult.

5. Excretion of drugs by the kidney often is impaired owing to low renal blood flow, low glomerular filtration rate, and immature tubular function.

V. **SPECIAL MANAGEMENT PROBLEMS IN THE NEWBORN.** Many of the disorders mentioned in this section are covered more extensively in other chapters of this book. However, their clinical presentation and management warrant special consideration in the newborn.

A. **Disorders of the respiratory system.** The newborn may present with a variety of respiratory disturbances, which may be developmental in origin or may occur at birth or soon after. Specific respiratory disorders of the newborn are reviewed here, after a brief overview of prenatal respiratory system development.

1. Prenatal development of the respiratory system
   a. Anatomic development begins at 3 weeks' gestation, with the division of the foregut into the esophagus and trachea. Major bronchial branching occurs by 4 weeks' gestation.
   (1) The **pseudoglandular stage of lung development** (5–16 weeks) is characterized by further branching of the conducting airways, the development of tracheal cartilage, and the appearance of bronchial arteries. At 10 weeks, goblet cells appear within the bronchioles. By 15 weeks, capillaries have developed and undifferentiated cuboidal cells have appeared. By 16 weeks, all of the major branching is complete.
   (2) The **canalicular stage of lung development** (16–25 weeks) is characterized by formation of terminal alveolar sacs, capillary approximation with the alveolar sacs, and differentiation of types I and II alveolar cells.
   (3) The **alveolar,** or **terminal sac, stage** (26–40 weeks) is characterized by a progressive increase in the number of alveolar sacs, which creates a greater surface area for gas exchange. Surfactant also appears during this stage of development.
   b. Biochemical development. The most important prenatal event is the production of surfactant by type II alveolar cells.
   (1) Function and composition of surfactant
      (a) The major function of surfactant is to decrease alveolar surface tension and increase lung compliance. Surfactant prevents alveolar collapse at the end of expiration and allows for opening of the alveoli at a low intrathoracic pressure.
      (b) The group of phospholipids comprising surfactant also is referred to as lecithin. The ratio of **lecithin (L)** to **sphingomyelin (S)** in the amniotic fluid is a reflection of the amount of intrapulmonary surfactant and lung maturity. An **L/S ratio** of 2:1 or greater usually indicates biochemical lung maturity. The presence of phosphatidylglycerol in the amniotic fluid is an additional indicator of biochemical maturity.
      (c) The most abundant component of surfactant is **phosphatidylcholine**. Less abundant but essential for optimal reduction in surface tension is **phosphatidylglycerol**.

(2) Pathways for surfactant production. There are two major pathways.
    (a) The **methylation pathway** is functional by 22–24 weeks' gestation but is easily inhibited by acidosis and hypoxia.
    (b) The **choline incorporation pathway** matures at 35 weeks' gestation and is resistant to hypoxia and acidosis.
(3) Rate of surfactant production. Factors that accelerate or retard the production are listed in Table 6-8.

2. Developmental disorders
  a. Esophageal atresia with tracheoesophageal fistula (see also Chapters 11 and 13). Esophageal atresia is a lack of continuity of the esophagus. Although it may occur alone, it most often is accompanied by a fistula between the trachea and the distal esophagus (tracheoesophageal fistula). These developmental disorders are the result of defective differentiation.
    (1) Clinical features. These infants have difficulty with copious oral and pharyngeal secretions. If the secretions obstruct the airway or if aspiration occurs, respiratory distress can result.
    (2) Diagnosis is suggested by failure to pass a nasogastric tube into the stomach and is confirmed by a chest radiograph that reveals the tube coiled up in the blind pouch of the esophagus.
    (3) Therapy. Emergency management involves constant suction of the esophagus, 30-degree elevation of the head to prevent reflux of gastric contents into the lungs, and preparation for definitive therapy (i.e., surgical repair).
  b. Choanal atresia is a unilateral or bilateral obstruction of the posterior nasal airway by a membranous or bony septum. This life-threatening anomaly results from failure of the bucconasal mucosa to rupture.
    (1) Clinical features. Because most newborns are obligate nose breathers, bilateral atresia usually presents in the delivery room as airway obstruction, apnea, and cyanosis. Unilateral obstruction may be asymptomatic.
    (2) Diagnosis is confirmed either by inability to pass a suction catheter through the nostrils into the oropharynx or by radiography using radiopaque dye to show the area of nasal obstruction.
    (3) Therapy. Emergency management consists of establishing an airway either with an oral airway or by endotracheal intubation. Definitive therapy is surgical reconstruction, performed in the neonatal period.
  c. Pulmonary hypoplasia is seen histologically as a decrease in the number of alveoli and capillary beds. The level of bronchial branching that is affected depends on the time during gestation when the insult occurs.

TABLE 6-8. Factors That Affect Fetal Lung Surfactant Production

Increase Production	Decrease or Delay Production
Maternal steroid administration in the presence of a female fetus	Combined fetal hyperglycemia and hyperinsulinemia as observed in maternal diabetes
Prolonged rupture of the fetal membranes	Acute hypoxia
Maternal narcotic addiction	
Preeclampsia	
Chronic fetal stress (i.e., placental insufficiency)	
Thyroid hormone (i.e., a long-acting thyroid stimulator-associated maternal hyperthyroidism or hypothyroidism with secondary fetal hyperthyroidism)	
Theophylline	

(1) Etiology. Major causes of pulmonary hypoplasia include:
  (a) Diminution of amniotic fluid volume due to:
    (i) Rupture of the fetal membranes
    (ii) Lack of fetal urine secondary to nonfunctioning (e.g., dysplastic, poly-cystic) kidneys or to urinary tract obstruction
  (b) Intrathoracic space-occupying lesion, such as:
    (i) Diaphragmatic hernia
    (ii) Pulmonary tumor
(2) Clinical features. The clinical presentation is one of severe respiratory distress and cyanosis.
  (a) The chest radiograph may show a small thoracic cavity and small lungs. Pneumothorax, pleural effusion, or both are frequently seen bilaterally.
  (b) When oligohydramnios is present, the characteristic facies of **Potter syndrome** are present.
  (c) On palpation, kidneys may be normal, absent, or large, if there is a renal etiology.
(3) Diagnosis. With severe hypoplasia, chest radiography is helpful for establishing the diagnosis.
(4) Therapy consists of vigorous ventilatory support and treatment of coexistent persistent pulmonary hypertension. Almost all infants with associated renal anomalies die shortly after birth, and treatment should be tailored accordingly.

d. Diaphragmatic hernia is a displacement of abdominal contents into the thoracic cavity through a defect in the diaphragm.
  (1) Types
    (a) Hernias through the foramen of Bochdalek are by far the most commonly seen diaphragmatic hernias. The defect, which almost always is on the left, occurs in the posterolateral portion of the diaphragm. It results from failure of the pleuroperitoneal canal to close, which normally occurs between 6 and 8 weeks' gestation. This is the most urgent of all neonatal thoraco-abdominal emergencies.
    (b) Hernias through the foramen of Morgagni are somewhat rare. The hernia, which usually is on the right, occurs in the anterior portion of the diaphragm through defects that are secondary to a developmental failure of the retrosternal segment of the septum transversum. Frequently, the hernia contains only omentum, and the affected newborn is asymptomatic.
  (2) Pathophysiology. Ipsilateral pulmonary hypoplasia results from compression of the affected lung by the displaced gastrointestinal organs. A shift of the mediastinal structures, resulting in compression of the contralateral lung, may cause hypoplasia of that lung to a lesser degree.
  (3) Clinical features. Severe respiratory distress, with cyanosis and dyspnea, usually is apparent shortly after birth. Breath sounds are diminished on the affected side, and heart sounds are shifted to the right. The abdomen may be scaphoid in cases of extensive displacement.
  (4) Diagnosis is confirmed by a chest radiograph demonstrating air-filled bowel in the left hemithorax.
  (5) Therapy includes intubation, vigorous oxygenation and mechanical ventilation, decompression of the intestinal tract with a nasogastric tube, correction of metabolic acidosis, and surgical removal of the abdominal contents from the thorax with repair of the hernia.
    (a) Mask and bag ventilation should be avoided or minimized because it results in distention of the bowel and further compromises the pulmonary function of the affected newborn.
    (b) Pulmonary hypertension frequently complicates the preoperative and postoperative course.
    (c) Extracorporeal membrane oxygenation may be helpful in selected infants.

      (6) Prognosis. Survival rates depend on the degree of lung hypoplasia and the presence of other anomalies. With conventional therapy, survival rates are approximately 50%; however, the use of extracorporeal membrane oxygenation may improve survival.

  e. Congenital lobar emphysema is caused by developmental abnormalities in either the conducting airways or the alveoli that result in the trapping of air in the affected lobe of the lung.

      (1) Clinical features. Infants usually present at birth or soon after with mild to severe respiratory distress, including tachypnea and cyanosis.

      (2) Diagnosis is established by chest radiography, which initially reveals a dense, opaque, overinflated area of lung. Later, with further air trapping, the area may display hyperlucency.

      (3) Therapy varies with the particular clinical presentation. The asymptomatic infant needs little immediate treatment. The severely affected infant may be helped by bronchoscopy, but in most cases eventually requires removal of the involved lobe.

  f. Hyaline membrane disease (respiratory distress syndrome of the newborn) is a respiratory disorder that primarily affects preterm infants who are born before the biochemical maturation of their lungs.

      (1) Pathophysiology. The lungs are poorly compliant owing to a deficiency of surfactant, resulting in the classic complex of progressive atelectasis, intrapulmonary shunting, hypoxemia, and cyanosis. The hyaline membrane that forms and lines the alveoli is composed of protein and sloughed epithelium—the result of oxygen exposure, alveolar capillary leakage, and the forces generated by the mechanical ventilation of these infants.

      (2) Clinical features. Affected infants characteristically present with tachypnea, grunting, nasal flaring, chest retraction, and cyanosis in the first 3 hours of life. There is decreased air entry on auscultation.

      (3) Clinical course. The natural course is a progressive worsening over the first 48–72 hours of life.

        (a) After the initial insult to the airway lining, the epithelium is repopulated with type II alveolar cells.

        (b) Subsequently, there is increased production and release of surfactant, so that there are sufficient quantities in the air spaces by 72 hours of life. This results in improvement in lung compliance and resolution of the respiratory distress.

      (4) Diagnosis is confirmed by a chest radiograph that reveals a uniform ground-glass pattern and an air bronchogram that is consistent with diffuse atelectasis.

      (5) Therapy and prognosis

        (a) Conventional therapy for the affected premature infant includes supportive care as well as the administration of **oxygen**. It also may be necessary to increase the mean airway pressure by use of continuous positive airway pressure, intermittent assisted **ventilation,** or high-frequency oscillation. Outcome with conventional therapy is good.

        (b) Exogenous surfactant replacement therapy with artificial or bovine surfactant has become an important intervention for those infants with severe surfactant deficiency. Alveolar opening and improvement in oxygenation and ventilation occur almost immediately.

      (6) Prevention. When amniotic fluid assessment reveals fetal lung immaturity and preterm delivery cannot be prevented, administration of corticosteroids to the mother 48 hours before delivery can induce or accelerate the production of fetal lung surfactant.

      (7) Complications associated with hyaline membrane disease are a result of organ immaturity associated with asphyxia, and mechanical ventilation. Common complications and associated findings include pneumothorax, patent ductus arteriosus, intraventricular hemorrhage, necrotizing enterocolitis, bronchopulmonary dysplasia, and retinopathy of prematurity (retrolental fibroplasia).

g. Transient tachypnea of the newborn is thought to result from decreased lymphatic absorption of fetal lung fluid. It most commonly occurs in infants born near term by cesarean section, without preceding labor. (The catecholamine surge associated with labor and delivery, which is thought to enhance pulmonary lymphatic drainage, does not occur in this setting.)

   (1) Clinical features. The tachypnea is quiet or mild and usually not associated with retractions. The infant appears comfortable and rarely is cyanotic.

   (2) Diagnosis is based on the delivery history and a chest radiograph, which characteristically reveals fluid in the major fissure, prominent vascular markings, increased interstitial markings, and hyperinflation. Auscultation may reveal rales.

   (3) Therapy is supportive. The tachypnea resolves in a few days. Low concentrations of supplemental oxygen may be required.

h. Persistence of the fetal circulation, or persistent pulmonary hypertension of the newborn, usually is a disease of term infants who have experienced acute or chronic in utero hypoxia. It is seen frequently in infants with meconium aspiration syndrome (see V A 3 c).

   (1) Pathophysiology. The primary abnormality is a failure of the pulmonary vascular resistance to fall with postnatal lung expansion and oxygenation.

   (a) Normally, at birth, the systemic vascular resistance rises as a result of cessation of blood flow through the placenta, and pulmonary vascular resistance falls with the first breaths.

   (b) With persistence of the fetal circulation, the pulmonary vascular resistance continues to be high, and may in fact be higher than the systemic resistance. This results in shunting of the deoxygenated blood, which is returning to the right side of the heart, away from the lungs. The right-to-left shunt can occur at both the atrial level (foramen ovale) and through the ductus arteriosus. Because the lungs are bypassed, the blood is not oxygenated and hypoxemia ensues.

   (2) Clinical features. These infants have rapidly progressive cyanosis associated with mild to severe respiratory distress. There is a varied response to oxygen administration, depending on the size of the shunt.

   (3) Diagnosis

   (a) The diagnosis is suggested by a history of perinatal hypoxia and clinical cyanosis at birth combined with a negative cardiovascular examination and negative chest radiograph, although parenchymal disease may coexist (e.g., group B streptococcal pneumonia, hyaline membrane disease, meconium aspiration syndrome).

   (b) Echocardiography should be used to establish the diagnosis, and should demonstrate:

   (i) The absence of cyanotic heart disease

   (ii) An increased pulmonary vascular resistance

   (iii) The presence of right-to-left shunt at the foramen ovale, ductus arteriosus, or both

   (4) Therapy includes supplemental oxygen, mechanical ventilation, hyperventilation, support of systemic blood pressure, and administration of sodium bicarbonate and pulmonary vasodilators.

   (5) Prognosis. The overall mortality rate associated with this disease is high. Extracorporeal membrane oxygenation may improve the outcome in certain patients.

3. Acquired disorders

a. Pneumonia

   (1) Etiology. Pneumonia often is associated with chorioamnionitis and may be caused by aspiration of infected amniotic fluid. The infectious agent also may cross the placenta, enter the fetal circulation, and spread to the lungs. Sepsis often is present (see V F 2).

   (2) Clinical features. The infant presents with signs of respiratory distress, including tachypnea, cyanosis, and retractions. Auscultation may reveal rales, rhonchi, or diminished breath sounds. Other signs of systemic infection may be noted, including poor perfusion, hypotension, acidosis, and leukopenia or leukocytosis.

(3) Diagnosis is confirmed by a chest radiograph that reveals any one of a variety of patterns, including diffuse or patchy infiltrates or consolidation. The process may be unilobar or multilobar. A tracheal aspirate also may reveal bacteria and an increased number of neutrophils.

(4) Therapy and prognosis. Treatment includes administration of appropriate antibiotics (see V F 2 f), supplemental oxygen, and mechanical ventilation (if needed). The outcome usually is good.

b. Pneumothorax is the presence of free air in the pleural space. The air often is under tension (i.e., at greater than atmospheric pressure), and in this setting is referred to as **tension pneumothorax**.

(1) Incidence and etiology. Asymptomatic, spontaneous pneumothorax occurs in 1%–2% of otherwise healthy newborns at birth. Symptomatic pneumothorax more commonly occurs in the infant who is receiving mechanical ventilation or who has underlying lung disease (e.g., hyaline membrane disease, pulmonary interstitial emphysema, meconium aspiration pneumonia).

(2) Clinical features. Symptoms and signs include cyanosis, tachypnea, and elevation of the affected hemithorax. Auscultation reveals diminished breath sounds on the affected side.

(3) Diagnosis

(a) The diagnosis is made by a chest radiograph that demonstrates a dense, partially collapsed lung surrounded by a large area of radiolucent air within the hemithorax. Depending on the degree of tension and lung compliance, the mediastinal structures are shifted toward the opposite side of the chest.

(b) Transillumination of the thorax may aid in the diagnosis of pneumothorax in emergencies; positive evidence is the transmission of light through the affected side.

(4) Therapy varies with the severity of the symptoms.

(a) If no other lung disease exists and there is minimal respiratory distress, supplemental 100% oxygen (nitrogen washout technique) for several hours usually is sufficient.

(b) If a significant degree of tension, respiratory distress, or some other lung disease exists, the air should be evacuated by aspiration with a syringe and needle or by a chest tube. Constant suction should be applied to the chest tube if a continuous air leak exists.

c. Meconium aspiration syndrome is a multiorgan disorder with perinatal asphyxia as the underlying cause. It most commonly occurs in postterm infants and infants who are small for gestational age due to intrauterine growth retardation. Both have placental insufficiency as a common pathway for fetal hypoxia.

(1) Pathophysiology. The fetal hypoxia triggers, via a vagal reflex, the passage of thick meconium into the amniotic fluid. The contaminated amniotic fluid is swallowed into the oropharynx and aspirated at birth with the initiation of breathing. With severe fetal asphyxia and acidosis, the meconium may be aspirated prenatally because of fetal gasping. Other organs affected by the perinatal hypoxia include the brain, heart, gastrointestinal tract, and kidneys.

(2) Diagnosis is established by the presence of meconium in the tracheal or amniotic fluid combined with symptoms of respiratory distress and a chest radiograph that reveals a pattern of diffuse infiltrates with hyperinflation.

(3) Therapy. Because most episodes of aspiration occur with the initiation of respiration, the most effective therapy is prevention. This consists of removal of the meconium before the initiation of ventilation. The meconium is removed from the infant's airway as follows:

(a) The oropharynx is suctioned before both delivery of the thorax and initiation of breathing, and again when the infant is on the warmer bed.

(b) The vocal cords are visualized using a laryngoscope, and a large endotracheal tube or DeLee catheter is inserted.

(c) Direct wall-unit suction (at a pressure of 80 cm H_2O) is applied to the tube or catheter as it is removed. The procedure is repeated if significant meconium is recovered. **Only after the trachea is cleared of any meconium should spontaneous or artificial ventilation be initiated.**

(d) If aspiration has occurred and the infant is in distress, therapy consists of administration of oxygen and mechanical ventilation.

(e) Persistent pulmonary hypertension also may coexist and should be vigorously treated.

   d. Bronchopulmonary dysplasia (see Chapter 13). This is a chronic pulmonary disease of infants that can result from oxygen and mechanical ventilation therapy for hyaline membrane disease in a preterm infant. It is characterized by the need for oxygen therapy beyond 28 days of life. A characteristic series of changes is seen on radiography.

4. Breathing disorders

  a. Regulation of breathing

    (1) Initiation of breathing. Although the fetus has periodic breathing movements in utero, it is not until after birth that breathing becomes regular and sustained. It is still not clear what mechanism initiates the infant's first breath.

      (a) With the first breath, the pulmonary stretch receptors do not cause complete exhalation; instead, a second inhalation follows. This is called the **Head paradoxical reflex**. It never occurs again throughout life.

      (b) Before birth, the alveoli are only minimally distended with lung fluid, and surface tension is high. The first few breaths must create a large negative intrathoracic pressure to open and distend the alveoli.

      (c) The first few breaths also allow dispersion of surfactant, which prevents alveolar collapse at the end of expiration by lowering the surface tension. Therefore, minimal negative pressure must be created by subsequent breaths to reexpand the alveoli.

    (2) Maintenance of breathing. Normal function of the respiratory center in the brain results in rhythmic inhalation and exhalation. The respiratory rate and depth of each breath are modulated by the Hering-Breuer reflex, carotid bodies, diaphragmatic strength, and cerebrospinal fluid (CSF) pH.

  b. Apnea (see also Chapter 13) is the cessation of breathing for longer than 20 seconds. Apnea often occurs in preterm infants (**apnea of prematurity**) and reflects immaturity of the respiratory control mechanisms in the brain stem.

    (1) Clinical features. Bradycardia (i.e., heart rate < 80 beats/minute) often is associated with apnea. Apnea of prematurity is characterized by periodic breathing and intermittent hypoxia, which further diminish respiratory drive.

    (2) Diagnosis of apnea of prematurity is made after excluding other reasons for the apnea (Table 6-9).

    (3) Therapy

      (a) Apnea of prematurity. Treatment measures include tactile stimulation, maintenance of the neutral thermal zone and core body temperature, supplemental oxygen, use of an oscillating water bed, and administration of respiratory stimulants (e.g., theophylline, caffeine). It also may be necessary to increase the mean airway pressure by use of continuous positive airway pressure or intermittent assisted ventilation.

      (b) Other causes of apnea. Treatment of the underlying disorder usually leads to cessation of the apneic episodes.

TABLE 6-9. Causes of Apnea

Infection	Pulmonary edema
Intracranial hemorrhage	Metabolic disturbances (e.g., hypo-
Airway obstruction	glycemia, hypocalcemia,
Gastroesophageal reflux	hyponatremia)
Seizures	Inappropriate environmental tem-
Hypoxia	perature (hot or cold)

B. **Neonatal necrotizing enterocolitis** refers to a spectrum of varying degrees of acute intestinal necrosis usually following ischemic injury of the bowel with secondary invasion and devitalization of the bowel wall.

1. **Incidence.** This is a serious and common problem, affecting 1%–5% of all newborns admitted to intensive care units. Affected infants most commonly are premature, asphyxiated, and suffering from other medical problems. Necrotizing enterocolitis rarely is observed in healthy term infants.

2. **Etiology and pathogenesis**
   a. **Bowel ischemia** secondary to preceding perinatal asphyxia generally is regarded as the cause of bowel wall injury. The introduction of formula or human milk then provides the substrate for bacterial overgrowth. Bacterial invasion of the bowel wall, often with gas production (**pneumatosis intestinalis**), leads to tissue necrosis and perforation.
   b. **Other predisposing factors** include:
      (1) Systemic hypotension
      (2) Patent ductus arteriosus
      (3) Placement of an umbilical artery catheter
      (4) Exchange transfusion
      (5) Previous treatment with systemic antibiotics
      (6) Use of hyperosmolar formula
      (7) Rapid advancement of the feeding volume

3. **Clinical features and diagnosis**
   a. **Signs and symptoms** usually are noted during the first 2 weeks of life, shortly after enteric feeding has begun (Table 6-10).
   b. **Laboratory findings**
      (1) Suggestive blood findings include:
         (a) Leukocytosis or neutropenia
         (b) Thrombocytopenia
      (2) Suggestive findings on abdominal radiography include:
         (a) Dilated, thickened bowel loops
         (b) Pneumatosis intestinalis, which usually starts in the right lower quadrant
         (c) Perforation, with free abdominal air and portal vein air

4. **Clinical course.** Two distinct clinical patterns are noted.
   a. Most infants follow a course characterized by feeding intolerance, abdominal distention, occult blood in the stool, and dilated bowel loops on radiography. These infants improve rapidly with therapy.
   b. The other group of infants has severe, progressive symptoms, including gross blood in the stool, extreme abdominal tenderness, hypotension, disseminated intravascular coagulation (DIC), and sepsis. Pneumatosis intestinalis and perforation frequently occur in this setting.

5. **Therapy**
   a. Treatment should begin with discontinuation of enteric feeding, gastric drainage, and administration of intravenous fluids.

TABLE 6-10. Signs and Symptoms of Necrotizing Enterocolitis

Gastric residuum, which often is bile stained	Poor perfusion, with hypotension or shock
Abdominal distention	Abdominal wall discoloration
Blood in stool (occult or gross)	Unstable temperature
Apnea	Hyperglycemia
Lethargy	Metabolic acidosis

b. Once cultures have been taken, systemic antibiotics (e.g, ampicillin, genta-micin) should be given. Also, any accompanying disorders (e.g., DIC) should be treated.

c. Surgical resection of the necrotic bowel segment is indicated for infants who have had a progressive downhill course and for those in whom intestinal perforation has occurred.

6. Prognosis. The mortality rate associated with necrotizing enterocolitis, which is highest in the most premature infants, is approximately 30%.

C. **Neonatal hyperbilirubinemia** is a condition characterized by an excessive concentration of bilirubin in the blood. There are two types of hyperbilirubinemia: **unconjugated,** which can be physiologic or pathologic in origin, and **conjugated,** which always stems from pathologic causes. Both types may lead to **jaundice.** Neurotoxic concentrations of unconjugated bilirubin can cause **kernicterus.**

1. Normal bilirubin metabolism (Figure 6-4). Bilirubin is a bile pigment formed from the degradation of heme that is mainly derived from red blood cell destruction (75%), but also from ineffective red blood cell production (25%).

a. The intermediary product of hemoglobin degradation—**biliverdin**—is converted to bilirubin through a reduction reaction.

b. Fat-soluble bilirubin normally circulates in plasma bound to albumin, from which it is transported into hepatocytes.

c. Conjugation with glucuronide converts bilirubin to a water-soluble product, which is excreted into the bile.

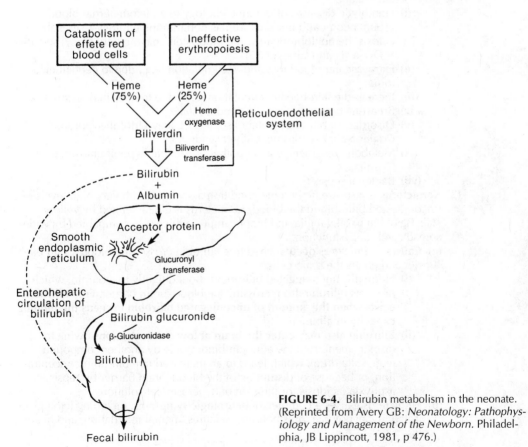

FIGURE 6-4. Bilirubin metabolism in the neonate. (Reprinted from Avery GB: *Neonatology: Pathophysiology and Management of the Newborn.* Philadelphia, JB Lippincott, 1981, p 476.)

2. **Unconjugated or indirect hyperbilirubinemia** may occur because of excessive bilirubin production (hemolysis), defective bilirubin clearance from the blood, or defective bilirubin conjugation by the liver. The most common cause in the neonatal period is a physiologic delay in the ability of the liver to clear, metabolize, and excrete the relatively large bilirubin burden at birth. At extremely high levels, fat-soluble unconjugated bilirubin enters the brain and causes neuronal dysfunction and death.

   a. **Clinical manifestations**

      (1) **Jaundice** occurs in 50% of all newborns and reflects an accumulation of unconjugated bilirubin in the blood and other tissues. Jaundice can be clinically observed at blood concentrations of 5 mg/dl or greater. Unconjugated hyperbilirubinemia or jaundice may be the result of physiologic or nonphysiologic causes.

         (a) **Physiologic jaundice** refers to the increased serum concentration of unconjugated bilirubin that is observed during the first few days of life (see Chapter 1).

            (i) **Causative factors** include delayed activity of glucuronyl transferase, increased bilirubin load on hepatocytes, and decreased bilirubin clearance from the plasma.

            (ii) **Clinical features.** Physiologic jaundice is associated with an umbilical cord serum bilirubin concentration of less than 2 mg/dl, a peak serum bilirubin level of less than 12–15 mg/dl on the third day of life, and a return to normal levels by the end of the first week of life. In preterm infants, bilirubin levels usually are higher and the physiologic jaundice lasts longer. Breast-fed infants also may have higher bilirubin levels.

         (b) **Nonphysiologic jaundice** refers to hyperbilirubinemia that is secondary to a pathologic process. Specific causes of nonphysiologic indirect hyperbilirubinemia include:

            (i) Hemolytic diseases of immune etiology (e.g., fetomaternal blood group incompatibilities) as well as nonimmune etiology [e.g., spherocytosis, hemoglobinopathy, red blood cell enzyme deficiency; see also V D 1 a (1) and Chapter 15].

            (ii) Extravascular blood loss and accumulation (e.g., due to cephalhematoma)

            (iii) Increased enterohepatic circulation (e.g., due to intestinal obstruction)

            (iv) Breast-feeding associated with poor intake

            (v) Disorders of bilirubin metabolism (e.g., Lucey-Driscoll syndrome, Crigler-Najjar syndrome, Gilbert syndrome)

            (vi) Metabolic disorders (e.g., hypothyroidism, panhypopituitarism, galactosemia)

            (vii) Bacterial sepsis

      (2) **Kernicterus** is a severe neurologic condition associated with very high levels of unconjugated bilirubin in the blood. Kernicterus is characterized by yellow staining of the basal ganglia and hippocampus, which is accompanied by widespread cerebral dysfunction.

         (a) **Causes.** Kernicterus occurs when free bilirubin crosses the blood–brain barrier and enters the brain cells.

            (i) Normally, unconjugated bilirubin is bound tightly to albumin, which prevents bilirubin from crossing the blood–brain barrier. **Free bilirubin exists when the amount of unconjugated bilirubin exceeds the binding capacity of albumin.**

            (ii) **Bilirubin also may enter the brain at low concentrations** owing to displacement from the albumin-binding site by another compound (e.g., sulfa drug), which leads to an increased free bilirubin concentration, or because of disruption of the blood–brain barrier by sepsis, asphyxia, acidosis, or infusion of hyperosmolar solutions.

         (b) Kernicterus causes a complex of **neurologic symptoms,** including lethargy or irritability, hypotonia, opisthotonos, seizures, mental retardation, and hearing loss.

b. Diagnosis

(1) Physiologic jaundice should be suspected if underlying pathologic causes of the hyperbilirubinemia can be excluded. Because the most common causes of unconjugated hyperbilirubinemia are physiologic and hemolytic, the initial evaluation should include:

(a) Complete blood count with peripheral smear and reticulocyte count

(b) Determination of maternal and infant blood types

(c) Coombs' test (indirect and direct)

(d) Determination of direct and indirect concentrations of bilirubin

(2) Nonphysiologic jaundice should always be suspected when the umbilical cord serum bilirubin concentration is elevated, when the clinical appearance of jaundice is within the first 24 hours of life, or when the conjugated fraction of the serum bilirubin concentration exceeds 2 mg/dl.

c. Therapy consists of treatment of any underlying causes of hyperbilirubinemia and the prevention of kernicterus.

(1) Treatment modalities

(a) Phototherapy converts unconjugated bilirubin into several water-soluble photoisomers that can be excreted without conjugation. **Lumirubin,** a structural isomer, is the major excretory product; **4Z, 15E-bilirubin,** a geometric isomer, is a minor photoconversion product.

(b) Exchange transfusion is used principally in hemolytic disease or when the bilirubin concentration is very high. This procedure directly removes the bilirubin from the intravascular space. Unbound antibodies that initiate the hemolytic process also are removed.

(2) Specific indications for the use of phototherapy and exchange transfusion are discussed in detail in most neonatology texts. In the term infant, phototherapy may be initiated when the serum bilirubin concentration reaches 12–15 mg/dl before the third day of life. Exchange transfusion usually is performed when the serum bilirubin concentration is 20 mg/dl or more. The specific bilirubin concentration that requires treatment varies with gestational age, the cause of the jaundice, and the presence of medical complications (e.g., sepsis, acidosis).

3. Conjugated or direct hyperbilirubinemia

a. Clinical manifestations. Jaundice associated with conjugated hyperbilirubinemia always is pathologic in origin.

b. Causes

(1) TORCH infections (toxoplasmosis, rubella, cytomegalovirus, herpes simplex) [see Chapter 8]

(2) Metabolic disorders (e.g., galactosemia)

(3) Bacterial sepsis

(4) Obstructive jaundice (e.g., due to biliary atresia; see Chapter 11)

(5) Prolonged administration of intravenous protein solutions

(6) Neonatal hepatitis

c. Diagnosis is based on a conjugated fraction of the serum bilirubin concentration that exceeds 2 mg/dl. Further evaluation should be directed to possible underlying causes of the direct hyperbilirubinemia.

d. Therapy is directed to the underlying causes of the hyperbilirubinemia.

D. Hematologic disorders

1. Anemia (see also Chapter 15). In the newborn, anemia is defined as a hematocrit less than 40%. Normally, the hematocrit at term gestation is 50%–55%.

a. Etiology. The principal causes of anemia in the newborn can be divided into those associated with acute blood loss, those associated with chronic blood loss, and those associated with impaired red blood cell production (Table 6-11). The most frequent cause—**hemolytic disease of the newborn**—is discussed first in somewhat more detail than the other causes.

TABLE 6-11. Causes and Clinical Features of Anemia

Anemia Associated With:	Causes	Clinical Features
Acute blood loss	Placenta previa Placental abruption Fetomaternal transfusion Fetoplacental transfusion Cord rupture Internal hemorrhage	Acute distress Shallow, rapid respirations Tachycardia Weak to absent pulse Hypotension Absence of hepatosplenomegaly Low blood volume

Chronic blood loss	Hemolytic disease
	Twin-to-twin transfusion
	  (monochorionic)
	Fetomaternal transfusion
	Chronic phlebotomy
		Pallow disproportionate to the
		  degree of distress
		Weak to normal pulse
		Normal blood pressure
		Signs of congestive heart failure
		Hepatosplenomegaly
		Normal blood volume

Impaired red blood
  cell production
	Diamond-Blackfan syndrome
	  (congenital hypoplastic
	  anemia)
		Pallor
		(See also Chapter 15)

(1) **Hemolytic disease of the newborn** (erythroblastosis fetalis) usually results from blood group incompatibility between the mother and the fetus. Hemolysis occurs when maternal antibodies to a particular blood group antigen cross the placenta and bind to fetal red blood cells, which are then destroyed in the spleen.

    (a) The most commonly involved antigen is **Rh$_O$(D)**—from the Rh blood group system. Rh incompatibility is associated with **extravascular hemolysis**.

    (b) ABO blood group antigens are less commonly involved.

    (c) Rarely, hemolytic disease of the newborn is caused by other blood group incompatibilities (e.g., c, E, Kell), a congenital defect or deficiency in red blood cell enzymes [e.g., glucose-6-phosphate dehydrogenase (G6PD)], a red blood cell membrane defect, infection, or vitamin deficiency (e.g., vitamin E).

    (d) In utero, if the anemia is severe (usually involving Rh incompatibility), the fetus (infant) will exhibit the signs and symptoms of **hydrops fetalis** (see V E 3).

(2) Anemia can be caused by a number of problems. Table 6-11 lists the symptoms and related etiologies.

b. **Diagnosis.** The specific cause of the anemia is established on the basis of information collected from the following sources:

    (1) History

    (2) Complete blood count with peripheral smear and reticulocyte count

    (3) Evaluation of maternal and infant blood for Rh or ABO incompatibility

    (4) Coombs' test

    (5) Other tests [e.g., Kleihauer test (to identify and quantify fetal red blood cells), hemoglobin electrophoresis, G6PD evaluation]

c. **Therapy**

    (1) **Hemolytic disease of the newborn.** Therapy is indicated when the hemoglobin and hematocrit are low enough to compromise the oxygen-carrying capacity of the blood, which can cause congestive heart failure, respiratory distress, acidosis, poor perfusion, and hypotension. The blood volume usually is normal. Therefore, the anemia is corrected by performing a partial exchange transfusion with packed red blood cells.

    (2) **Acute blood loss** should be treated rapidly. Therapy includes restoration of blood volume and red blood cell mass and elimination of the cause of blood loss, if it is still present.

(3) Chronic blood loss. Therapy varies depending on the clinical condition and cause of blood loss and may consist of transfusion of packed red blood cells, partial exchange transfusion with packed red blood cells, iron therapy, or no intervention.

2. **Polycythemia** occurs in 2%–5% of all newborns and is defined as a hematocrit of 65% or greater when a freely flowing blood sample is taken from a large vein. **Hyperviscosity** of the blood almost always exists in association with polycythemia.
   a. **Etiology.** Polycythemia has been associated with the following conditions:
      (1) Fetoplacental transfusion associated with birth asphyxia or delayed cord clamping
      (2) Twin-to-twin transfusion
      (3) Chronic intrauterine hypoxia secondary to placental insufficiency (e.g., pregnancy-induced hypertension with fetal growth retardation) or increased fetal metabolism (e.g., with maternal diabetes)
      (4) Endocrine disorders (e.g., hyperthyroidism)
      (5) Genetic disorders (e.g., Down syndrome, Beckwith-Wiedemann syndrome)
   b. **Pathophysiology**
      (1) Many of the problems associated with polycythemia were originally thought to be caused by organ ischemia and hypoxia secondary to an increase in blood viscosity. It is now known that most of the blood flow reduction is the result of an increased oxygen content in the arterial blood. This reciprocal relationship of decreased blood flow and increased arterial oxygen content results in a normal or increased delivery of oxygen to most organs.
      (2) Therefore, most of the problems associated with polycythemia are more likely the result of the perinatal events (i.e., acute or chronic hypoxia) that also are responsible for the development of the polycythemia, rather than any flow disturbances attributable to the polycythemia itself.
   c. **Clinical features**
      (1) Symptoms and signs associated with polycythemia include:
         (a) Tachypnea and cyanosis
         (b) Jitteriness and seizures
         (c) Hypoglycemia
         (d) Renal dysfunction
         (e) Necrotizing enterocolitis
      (2) Complications. Polycythemia is associated with an abnormal long-term neurologic outcome.
   d. **Therapy** generally is supportive. Reduction of the hematocrit by partial exchange transfusion may be helpful in alleviating respiratory distress, renal dysfunction and hypoglycemia, but may increase the risk of necrotizing enterocolitis. No study has shown a beneficial effect of partial exchange transfusion on long-term neurologic outcome.

E. **Hydrops fetalis** is a condition that develops in utero, usually as a result of chronic anemia due to hemolytic disease, although many etiologies exist. Its chief features include anemia, edema or anasarca, and hypoproteinemia.

1. **Etiology.** The causes of hydrops fetalis are varied and include:
   a. Severe chronic anemia due to:
      (1) Isoimmunization (i.e., Rh incompatibility)
      (2) Homozygous α thalassemia
      (3) Twin-to-twin or fetomaternal transfusion
   b. Cardiac disease, such as:
      (1) Structural defects
      (2) In utero closure of the foramen ovale
      (3) Paroxysmal atrial tachycardia
   c. Hypoproteinemia
   d. Intrauterine infection, including syphilis, toxoplasmosis, and cytomegalovirus
   e. Chromosomal disorders (e.g., Turner syndrome, 45,XO)
   f. Idiopathic causes

2. **Pathophysiology.** The exact pathophysiology is unknown, but the central factor in the development of hydrops fetalis appears to be severe chronic anemia with loss of oxygen-carrying capacity, leading to hypoxia and acidosis. A contributing factor is hypoproteinemia, which together with anemia causes the development of congestive heart failure, edema, pleural effusions, and ascites. All of these problems contribute to the respiratory distress seen at birth.

3. **Clinical features**
   a. **Signs and symptoms** include:
      (1) Congestive heart failure
      (2) Pallor
      (3) Ascites
      (4) Pleural effusions
      (5) Peripheral edema
      (6) Hepatosplenomegaly
   b. **Laboratory findings** include:
      (1) Anemia
      (2) Hypoproteinemia
      (3) Hypoxia
      (4) Acidosis

4. **Diagnosis** is based on the maternal medical and obstetric history (e.g., Rh sensitization of the mother) and the clinical and laboratory findings.

5. **Therapy** is aimed at correcting the anemia and treating the congestive heart failure and respiratory distress. In addition, appropriate treatment should be provided for associated etiologies and conditions (e.g., infections).

6. **Clinical course and prognosis** vary depending on the etiology, how severely affected the infant is at birth, the presence of perinatal asphyxia or congenital anomalies, and the response to therapy. Idiopathic causes of hydrops fetalis are associated with a high mortality rate.

F. **Infection** continues to be a major cause of neonatal morbidity and mortality despite advances in therapy. Although perinatally acquired bacterial infections are the most common, infections that are acquired in utero remain an important source of long-term disability.

1. **General considerations**
   a. **Predisposing factors.** The newborn is particularly susceptible to infection owing to immaturity of immune system mechanisms, including:
      (1) Neutrophil chemotaxis
      (2) Neutrophil phagocytosis
      (3) Bactericidal activity
      (4) Humoral components
   b. **Timing and route of infection.** The causative organism and abnormalities associated with neonatal infections vary with the time and route of infection.
      (1) **Organisms responsible for transplacental infections before birth** are listed in Table 6-12 (see also Table 8-6). Abnormalities associated with infection acquired in utero are listed in Tables 6-13 and 6-14.

TABLE 6-12. Organisms Responsible for Transplacental Infections Before Birth

Cytomegalovirus	Rubella virus
Treponema pallidum (the agent of syphilis)	*Toxoplasma gondii*
Human immunodeficiency virus, the agent of acquired immune deficiency syndrome	Echovirus
	Listeria monocytogenes

TABLE 6-13. Abnormalities Associated With Infection Acquired in the First Trimester

Congenital malformation	Hydrocephalus
Intrauterine growth retardation	Stillbirth
Microcephaly	

    (2) Perinatal infections include infections acquired through the fetal membranes, ascending infections acquired after rupture of the fetal membranes, and infections acquired via the birth canal. Common **causative organisms** are listed in Table 6-15, and **associated abnormalities** are listed in Table 6-16.

    (3) Postnatal infections most often are acquired as a result of nosocomial or community exposures. Hospitalized newborns who are premature or require instrumentation are particularly susceptible. Common **causative organisms** are listed in Table 6-17, and **associated abnormalities** are listed in Table 6-18.

2. Bacterial infection and neonatal sepsis. Bacterial infections most frequently are acquired via the birth canal or nosocomially. The infection almost always is bacteremic (often with seeding of the meninges by way of the blood) and associated with systemic symptoms—a condition referred to as **neonatal sepsis**.

    a. Incidence. Neonatal sepsis is common in premature infants. About 1%–4% of these infants have at least one episode of sepsis during their hospitalization. Sepsis in term infants is rare, occurring in less than 1%.

    b. Risk factors for early neonatal sepsis include:
      (1) Premature labor
      (2) Prolonged rupture of the fetal membranes
      (3) Low birth weight
      (4) Chorioamnionitis
      (5) Maternal fever

    c. Etiology. The most common causative organisms include:
      (1) Gram-positive cocci, especially group B β-hemolytic streptococci, but also *Staphylococcus aureus* and *Staphylococcus epidermidis*
      (2) Gram-negative rods, especially *Escherichia coli* and *Klebsiella pneumoniae*
      (3) Gram-positive rods (e.g., *Listeria monocytogenes*)

    d. Clinical features
      (1) Signs and symptoms of bacterial infection include:
        (a) Unexplained respiratory distress
        (b) Unexplained feeding intolerance
        (c) Temperature instability
        (d) Hypoglycemia or hyperglycemia
        (e) Apnea
        (f) Lethargy
        (g) Irritability
      (2) Laboratory findings include:
        (a) Abnormal white blood cell count, including neutropenia or neutrophilia
        (b) Prolonged PT and PTT
        (c) Tracheal aspirate containing bacteria and neutrophils

TABLE 6-14. Abnormalities Associated With Infection Acquired Later in Pregnancy

Microcephaly	Intracranial hemorrhage
Hydrops fetalis	Hepatosplenomegaly
Disseminated intravascular coagulation (DIC)	Jaundice
	Skin and eye lesions
Anemia	Stillbirth

TABLE 6-15. Organisms Responsible for Perinatal Infections

Group B β-hemolytic streptococcus	Herpes simplex virus
Escherichia coli	*Chlamydia trachomatis*
Klebsiella species	*Neisseria gonorrhoeae*
Streptococcus pneumoniae	*Neisseria meningitidis*

- e. **Diagnosis.** In addition to the physical examination, the laboratory evaluation for neonatal sepsis should include:
    - **(1)** Complete blood count [neutropenia (< 1800/mm³) or an elevated ratio of immature to total neutrophils suggests sepsis]
    - **(2)** Blood cultures
    - **(3)** A lumbar puncture
    - **(4)** Culture and counterimmunoelectrophoresis or latex agglutination testing of the urine
    - **(5)** Gram stain and culture of a tracheal aspirate, if the infant is intubated
    - **(6)** Chest radiograph
    - **(7)** Gastric aspirate (at the time of delivery) for neutrophil count, Gram stain, and culture
- f. **Therapy**
    - **(1)** Empiric antibiotic therapy should begin after the diagnostic workup and consist of a broad-spectrum penicillin (usually ampicillin) and an aminoglycoside (usually gentamicin). Once culture data are available, therapy should be tailored to the specific organism.
    - **(2)** The initial choice of antibiotics for nosocomial infection depends on nursery, community, and individual patient exposure information.
    - **(3)** The duration of therapy usually is 7–10 days except for invasive infections (e.g., meningitis, osteomyelitis), which require longer courses of antibiotic therapy.
    - **(4)** Other complications (e.g., DIC) always should be investigated and treated.
- 3. **Viral infection** is uncommon in the newborn but can be devastating. Viral infections can be divided into those acquired prenatally and those acquired perinatally or postnatally.
    - a. **Prenatal viral infections**
        - **(1)** **Common agents** include rubella virus, cytomegalovirus, echovirus, herpes zoster virus, and human immunodeficiency virus (see Chapter 9).
        - **(2)** **Clinical features** are listed in Table 6-19 (see also Chapter 8).
    - b. **Perinatal and postnatal viral infections**
        - **(1)** **Common agents** are listed in Table 6-20.
        - **(2)** **Clinical features**
            - **(a)** **Herpes virus infections.** Symptoms do not appear until at least 3–7 days and up to 4 weeks after birth. These infections manifest as vesicular skin eruptions, DIC, shock, pneumonia, and encephalitis.
            - **(b)** **Respiratory syncytial virus** infections manifest as temperature instability, respiratory distress, apnea, clear nasal discharge, and poor feeding.
    - c. **Diagnosis** begins with a high index of suspicion and is based primarily on infant culture data, cord immunoglobulin M level, changing infant serum antibody titers,

TABLE 6-16. Abnormalities Associated With Perinatal Infections

Respiratory distress	Thrombocytopenia
Temperature instability	Meningitis
Septic shock	Death
Neutropenia	

TABLE 6-17. Common Organisms Involved in Postnatal Infections

Staphylococcus aureus	*Klebsiella pneumoniae*
Staphylococcus epidermidis	*Clostridia* species
Pseudomonas aeruginosa	*Bacteroides* species
Candida albicans	Enterococcus
Escherichia coli	

results of rapid antigen or antibody tests, maternal medical history and culture data, and time of the year.

   d. Therapy is available for herpes virus and respiratory syncytial virus infections.
   (1) Herpes virus infections are treated systemically with vidarabine or acyclovir and ophthalmologically with vidarabine ointment.
   (2) Respiratory syncytial virus infections are treated with aerosolized ribavirin.

G. | **Neurologic disorders** generally result in abnormalities of tone, strength, and state of consciousness. The most common neurologic problems occurring in newborns are reviewed here.

1. Asphyxial brain injury (see also Section II) is the most common neurologic abnormality in the neonatal period.
   a. Risk factors for perinatal asphyxia (see II B 1)
   b. Pathophysiology (see also II A, B 2)
      (1) During mild to moderate perinatal asphyxia, blood flow to the brain is preserved owing to redistribution of the cardiac output.
      (2) During severe perinatal asphyxia, cerebral hypoxia and ischemia occur, initially in the cerebral cortex and eventually in the cerebellum and brain stem.
   c. Clinical features (see II B 3 a)
   d. Therapy (see also II C)
      (1) Treatment primarily is supportive (i.e., ventilation with oxygen and maintenance of cardiac output) while awaiting spontaneous recovery, especially with a mild insult.
      (2) Severely asphyxiated infants may require more extensive support of neurologic function as well as respiratory, cardiac, and renal function.
      (3) Anticonvulsants are helpful in controlling seizures, although the seizure activity usually is self-limited.
      (4) Therapy to reduce cerebral edema or to lower the cerebral metabolic rate has not been shown to improve outcome.
   e. Prognosis is variable and sometimes difficult to predict. Mild asphyxia almost always is associated with a good outcome, whereas severe asphyxia frequently is associated with significant morbidity and mortality. The EEG in the neonatal period is somewhat predictive of long-term outcome.

2. Seizures (see also Chapter 18) are not uncommon in the neonatal period. Subtle seizures—which manifest as rhythmic eye deviation or blinking, lip smacking, "bicycling," or apnea—are the most common form, followed by generalized tonic, multifocal clonic, focal clonic, and myoclonic seizures.

TABLE 6-18. Abnormalities Associated With Postnatal Infection in the Newborn

Respiratory distress	Disseminated intravascular coagulation (DIC)
Feeding intolerance	
Apnea	Hypoglycemia or hyper-glycemia
Anemia	Temperature instability
Shock	

TABLE 6-19. Clinical Features Associated With Prenatal Viral Infection

Intrauterine growth retardation	Hepatosplenomegaly
Congenital anomalies	Ocular lesions
Skin lesions	Coagulopathy
Central nervous system (CNS) defects	Hearing loss

a. **Etiology.** Underlying causes of seizure activity include:
(1) Asphyxia
(2) Brain anomalies (e.g., holoprosencephaly)
(3) Intracranial hemorrhage, particularly within the brain parenchyma
(4) Systemic metabolic disorders (e.g., hypoglycemia, hyponatremia, hypocalcemia, hypernatremia, hyperammonemia) and inborn errors of amino acid and organic acid metabolism
(5) Meningitis and encephalitis
(6) Pyridoxine dependency
b. **Diagnosis.** The following evaluations should be made in an effort to pinpoint the cause of the seizure activity:
(1) Neurologic examination
(2) EEG
(3) Ultrasound and computed tomography scanning, especially in the presence of lateralization of the seizure or EEG
(4) Screening for metabolic disorders (e.g., involving glucose, calcium, or sodium), for inborn errors of metabolism (e.g., involving amino acids or organic acids), and for pyridoxine dependency
(5) Lumbar puncture (in the absence of increased intracranial pressure) and evaluation of the CSF for sepsis
c. **Therapy** should be initiated with phenobarbital. Alternative or additional therapeutic agents include lorazepam, diphenylhydantoin, paraldehyde, and valproate. Pyridoxine dependency should be considered in term infants who show no clear cause for the seizure activity and who do not respond to routine therapy. Resolution of the seizure activity after pyridoxine administration is diagnostic of dependency.
d. **Prognosis** varies with the underlying etiology.

3. **Pericranial and intracranial hemorrhage** (see also Chapter 18) can be classified according to the location of the bleeding within the brain.
a. **Subaponeurotic, or subgaleal, hemorrhage** is a collection of blood beneath the thin, tendinous sheet covering the skull and above the periosteum of the bones of the skull; this is a large potential space that crosses cranial suture lines. Subaponeurotic hemorrhage generally follows head trauma at birth. On examination, the scalp and head feel firm and boggy over a large area, and there may be scalp discoloration and a large amount of blood loss. Failure to recognize subaponeurotic hemorrhage may yield disastrous results because of shock.
b. **Cephalhematoma** is a subperiosteal collection of blood; hence, it does not cross cranial suture lines. It is seen after birth trauma and is self-limited, almost always disappearing without residual effects. Therapy to evacuate the collection of blood is contraindicated because it is associated with a significant risk of infection.

TABLE 6-20. Common Viruses Responsible for Perinatal and Postnatal Infection

Herpes simplex virus	Echovirus
Herpes zoster virus	Coxsackievirus
Hepatitis A and B viruses	Cytomegalovirus (vertical transmission from mother or via blood transfusion)
Respiratory syncytial virus	

c. **Subarachnoid hemorrhage** may occur after a normal or traumatic delivery. Bleeding is self-limited, and symptoms (e.g., irritability, seizure activity) resolve in a few days. The infant may be asymptomatic in some cases.

d. **Subdural hemorrhage** also is seen with birth trauma. A significant amount of blood can accumulate and cause focal neurologic deficits owing to pressure exerted on the brain. However, drainage is necessary only if symptoms are severe or do not resolve.

e. **Intraventricular hemorrhage** is seen almost exclusively in preterm infants and is the result of bleeding of the germinal matrix, frequently after an asphyxial insult.
   (1) Small intraventricular hemorrhages that are confined to a germinal matrix (grade I) or that are associated with a small amount of blood in the ventricle (grade II) often resolve without sequelae.
   (2) Large intraventricular hemorrhages that are associated with ventricular dilatation (grade III) or with extension into the brain parenchyma (grade IV) are associated with permanent functional impairment and hydrocephalus.

4. **Hydrocephalus** (see also Chapter 18) refers to an excessive collection of CSF within the ventricular system due to imbalanced production and absorption of CSF.
   a. **High-pressure, or obstructive, hydrocephalus** results when normal drainage and reabsorption of CSF do not occur. It is seen in congenital aqueductal stenosis, Dandy-Walker malformation, and myelomeningocele with Arnold-Chiari malformation, and after intraventricular hemorrhage and meningitis.
   b. **Low-pressure, or communicating, hydrocephalus** (also called **hydrocephalus ex vacuo**) is seen after intracranial hemorrhage and in some malformations. This is to be distinguished from the fluid seen in the large intracerebral space in some malformations, such as holoprosencephaly. Communicating hydrocephalus does not require therapeutic intervention.

5. **Hypotonia,** a condition characterized by diminished tone of the skeletal muscles, is the most common neurologic motor disorder of the neonatal period. An evaluation must be performed to determine at which level in the progression of nerve impulse to muscular contraction the defect exists. Table 6-21 lists common etiologies.

6. **Myelomeningocele** (see also Chapter 18) is the most common congenital anomaly of the nervous system. It results from failure of the neural tube to close.
   a. **Clinical features** depend on the location of the myelomeningocele. Not uncommonly, there is an associated Arnold-Chiari malformation, hydrocephalus, or both.
   b. **Diagnosis.** Prenatal screening (see Chapter 8) of maternal serum and amniotic fluid for α-fetoprotein and fetal ultrasonography allow for early diagnosis of myelomeningocele and potential intervention.
   c. **Therapy.** Primary surgical closure of the sac is the treatment of choice to prevent infection. Hydrocephalus often develops after closure of the sac. A shunting procedure may be necessary to relieve the hydrocephalus and prevent intracranial hypertension.
   d. **Prognosis** depends on the location of the myelomeningocele, the presence or absence of associated brain lesions, the occurrence of shunt infections, and the effectiveness of physical therapy and other supportive care.

TABLE 6-21. Common Causes of Hypotonia

Asphyxia (brain defect)
Werdnig-Hoffmann disease (spinal cord defect)
Congenital myasthenia gravis (neuromuscular junction defect)
Muscular dystrophy (muscle defect)
Myotonic dystrophy (muscle defect)
Hypothyroidism (metabolic defect)

H. **Ophthalmologic disorders** are unusual in the newborn, which is fortunate, because the pediatrician's ability to detect specific abnormalities is limited. However, a careful examination of the newborn's eyes usually allows for gross detection of all ophthalmologic problems, which can then be delineated further by a pediatric ophthalmologist.

1. **Ophthalmia neonatorum** is an acute conjunctivitis of the newborn that has a limited number of common etiologies. Because the routine eye examination does not allow for a specific diagnosis, a Gram stain and culture should be obtained. (See Chapter 1 for further discussion of ophthalmia neonatorum.)

2. **Cataract** refers to any clouding of the lens. Early intervention is important if future blindness and amblyopia are to be prevented.
   a. **Etiology.** Cataracts result from numerous causes, including hereditary disorders, intrauterine infections (e.g., rubella), and metabolic diseases (e.g., galactosemia). The cause in some cases is unknown.
   b. **Therapy** includes removal of the lens combined with either corrective glasses or intraocular artificial lens implantation.

3. **Glaucoma** is characterized by increased intraocular pressure resulting in ocular damage and vision impairment. Glaucoma may be inherited or may be acquired as a component of some other disorder (e.g., retinopathy of prematurity, chorioretinitis, rubella).
   a. **Clinical features** include conjunctival injection, excessive lacrimation, light sensitivity, blepharospasm, and corneal clouding.
   b. **Therapy** is surgical and should be instituted as soon as possible.
   c. **Prognosis** is related to the duration of the glaucoma. Early intervention most frequently is associated with good vision.

4. **Retinopathy of prematurity** (retrolental fibroplasia) was first seen during the 1940s and 1950s, after oxygen therapy became commonly used in the nursery to sustain life in very small premature infants. Incidences of 10%–70% have been reported in infants with a birth weight less than 1500 g.
   a. **Etiology and pathogenesis.** The development of retinopathy of prematurity appears to be related to **immaturity of the retinal vessels** of preterm infants. Contributing factors include **hyperoxia,** hypercarbia, and intermittent hypoxia.
      (1) The hyperoxia induces vasospasm and endothelial damage in the retinal vessels, with resultant tissue edema and injury.
      (2) Over the following weeks, reactive proliferative neovascularization occurs, causing traction (i.e., pulling up) of the retina, which may result in retinal detachment. This sequence occurs without further insult, but may regress at any time before detachment.
   b. **Therapy.** The retinopathy usually resolves spontaneously. In infants with active, rapidly progressive disease, cryotherapy or laser therapy is indicated to prevent traction and retinal detachment.
   c. **Prognosis** is related to the severity of the vascularity and subsequent spontaneous regression. Myopia is common. Blindness follows retinal detachment.

5. **Neuroblastoma** should be suspected when an abnormal red reflex (leukokoria) is observed in a newborn.

6. **Intrauterine infection associated with ophthalmologic abnormalities**
   a. **Toxoplasmosis** is associated with a chorioretinitis. Focal or multifocal lesions are seen. Prognosis is poor.
   b. **Cytomegalovirus** infection is associated with chorioretinitis. No therapy is available.
   c. **Rubella** is associated with glaucoma, cataract, microphthalmos, and uveitis. Therapy is symptomatic.

7. **Aniridia** is a rare developmental disorder characterized by a lack of development of the iris. It is associated with other congenital abnormalities, especially Wilms' tumor (see Chapter 16), which always must be suspected when aniridia is detected.

I. **Multiple gestation** always should be seen as a high-risk event owing to its increased association with intrauterine accidents, growth abnormalities, prematurity, and problems at the time of delivery (e.g., abnormal fetal position, asphyxia).

1. **Incidence.** Approximately 1%–1.3% of all live births are the result of twin gestation. The true incidence of twin gestation probably is slightly higher. The monozygotic twinning rate is 3.5–4.0 in 1000 live births, or 35%–40% of all twins who are born.

2. **Etiology**
   a. **Monozygotic twinning** may be viewed as a teratogenic event because it occurs more frequently with increasing maternal age, is associated with more congenital malformations, and can be caused by teratogens. A problem of symmetry in the developing embryo may result in conjoined twins.
   b. **Dizygotic twinning** is caused by double ovulation, which may be related to elevated gonadotropin levels.

3. **Placentation**
   a. **Monochorionic placentation** always is associated with monozygotic twins; 1% of monozygotic twins are monoamniotic.
   b. **Dichorionic placentation** almost always is associated with dizygotic, diamniotic twins.
   c. **Twin placentas** are associated with a sixfold to ninefold increase in the incidence of velamentous cord insertion, and with a high incidence of vasa previa.

4. **Prenatal problems**
   a. **Death.** Monoamniotic twins have only a 40% chance of both surviving. Death may occur because of cord accidents and twin-to-twin transfusions, which may lead to the death of one fetus, with thromboplastin release and subsequent DIC in the second twin.
   b. **Growth disturbances** are the rule.
      (1) **Intrauterine growth retardation.** There is decreased potential for growth in twin fetuses compared to a single fetus, probably owing to the limitations of placental surface area for nutrient transfer.
      (2) **Twin-to-twin transfusion,** resulting in a large, polycythemic twin and a small, anemic twin, is a significant risk in monochorionic placentation.
   c. The incidence of **congenital malformations** is doubled in twin pregnancy.
   d. The incidence of **spontaneous abortion** also is increased.
   e. **Preterm delivery** is the most common complication of multiple gestation. It occurs in up to 50% of twin pregnancies; the incidence is even higher in triplet and quadruplet pregnancy.
      (1) Preterm delivery is a significant factor in the increased morbidity and mortality associated with multiple gestation.
      (2) The incidence of preterm delivery and growth retardation can be decreased by early identification of multiple gestation and by placing the mother on strict bed rest. Maternal compliance is higher in the hospital setting.
   f. **Maternal complications include:**
      (1) Pregnancy-induced hypertension
      (2) Polyhydramnios
      (3) Hyperemesis and nausea
      (4) Anemia

5. **Postnatal problems**
   a. **Prematurity,** with all of its sequelae, is the most common management problem. Complications of prematurity include:
      (1) Low birth weight
      (2) Hyaline membrane disease, which occurs more often and is more severe in the second-born twin
      (3) Intracranial hemorrhage
      (4) Infection

    b. Growth retardation, both symmetric and asymmetric, occurs more frequently in multiple gestation. This may be associated with developmental abnormalities as well as long-term growth disturbances.

    c. Perinatal asphyxia, especially of the second-born twin and in instances of malpresentation or vasa previa, may result in long-term morbidity or mortality.

  6. Management is aimed at:

    a. Identifying multiple gestation as early as possible

    b. Managing other medical problems

    c. Controlling preterm labor

    d. Identifying the ideal route of delivery

    e. Avoiding asphyxia in the second twin (in twin pregnancy) or in subsequent infants (in other multiple pregnancies)

J. **Hypoglycemia** is defined as a plasma glucose concentration less than 30 mg/dl during the first 24 hours of life and less than 45 mg/dl thereafter. Hypoglycemia is very common in infants of diabetic mothers as well as in infants who are born after various perinatal complications, including prematurity, intrauterine growth retardation, and asphyxia.

  1. Pathogenesis. The pathogenesis varies depending on the clinical setting and the associated conditions affecting the infant.

    a. Maternal diabetes. The hypoglycemia in infants of diabetic mothers is the result of a hyperinsulinemic state that persists after the umbilical cord is cut and the maternal supply of glucose is interrupted.

    b. Prematurity. Preterm infants become hypoglycemic owing to diminished glycogen stores and to immaturity of gluconeogenic enzymes.

    c. Growth retardation. Growth-retarded infants frequently are depleted of hepatic glycogen and quickly become hypoglycemic.

    d. Perinatal asphyxia forces the fetus (infant) to use anaerobic metabolism, which quickly depletes stored glycogen and results in hypoglycemia.

    e. Cold stress increases oxygen consumption as well as glucose consumption. It also may increase free acids and result in hypoglycemia.

    f. Sepsis may cause hypoglycemia, although hyperglycemia also is observed, which presumably is caused by insulin insensitivity.

    g. Beckwith-Wiedemann syndrome is characterized by hypoglycemia, visceromegaly, macroglossia, and omphalocele. Hyperinsulinism secondary to pancreatic islet cell hyperplasia is responsible for the hypoglycemia.

    h. Nesidioblastosis and **pancreatic islet cell adenoma** are associated with hyperinsulinemia and hypoglycemia.

    i. Metabolic disorders, such as galactosemia and panhypopituitarism, also are associated with hypoglycemia.

  2. Clinical features. Infants with hypoglycemia are not always symptomatic. However, the following symptoms may occur:

    a. Hypotonia or jitteriness

    b. Apnea or tachypnea

    c. Seizures

  3. Diagnosis. Screening for hypoglycemia may be done using any of a number of bedside reagent strips. The diagnosis is confirmed by the actual measurement of the plasma glucose concentration by the clinical laboratory.

  4. Therapy

    a. Primary therapy is intravenous glucose. The glucose infusion may be required for several days until the basal insulin secretion rate decreases, glycogen stores are replenished, or gluconeogenesis improves. Bolus infusions of hypertonic glucose should be avoided because they may result in a rebound hypoglycemia.

(1) Intravenous glucose should be administered as a constant infusion begun at a rate of 6–8 mg/kg/minute. This may be increased to a rate of up to 20 mg/kg/minute. (A central venous access should be used for infusions given at a rate above 12–15 mg/kg/minute.)

(2) A small (0.5–1.0 g/kg) bolus of glucose may be used for extreme hypoglycemia or if severe symptoms related to hypoglycemia occur. This should always be followed by a constant infusion.

b. Hypoglycemia that is secondary to hyperinsulinemia and resistant to intravenous glucose should be treated with corticosteroids or diazoxide. If drug treatment fails, pancreatectomy should be performed. These more aggressive forms of therapy rarely are necessary except for hypoglycemia that is associated with Beckwith-Wiedemann syndrome, nesidioblastosis, or islet cell adenoma.

K. **Disorders associated with maternal diabetes.** The pregnancy of a diabetic woman is one that is associated with multiple complications affecting both mother and fetus. The key to an optimal outcome is consistent euglycemia in the mother.

1. **Diabetic embryopathy**
   a. **Caudal regression** is a congenital anomaly that is specifically associated with infants of diabetic mothers. It clearly is related to maternal hyperglycemia during organogenesis.
   b. **Other anomalies** also occur at an increased rate. The specific genetically related anomalies vary depending on geographic location and race. In the United States, congenital anomalies of the heart and CNS are the most common.

2. **Prenatal growth abnormalities.** Glucose easily crosses the placenta, whereas insulin does not; therefore, maternal hyperglycemia causes fetal hyperglycemia and a reactive fetal hyperinsulinemia. This combination results in increased somatic growth of the fetus due to cellular hyperplasia and hypertrophy. The large size of the fetus often results in dystocia. The brain is the only organ whose growth is not affected by the fetal hyperglycemia and hyperinsulinemia.

3. **Late fetal death** occurs more frequently in the poorly controlled diabetic pregnancy than in the normal pregnancy or euglycemic diabetic pregnancy. Animal studies show that fetal hyperglycemia and hyperinsulinemia are associated with an increase in fetal metabolism and respiration. As the fetus approaches term, oxygen transport becomes limited, and the hypermetabolic state may lead to fetal hypoxia and death.

4. **Preterm delivery** is common and the result of fetal distress or a planned early delivery. Complications largely depend on the gestational age and lung maturity of the infant at the time of delivery. Effective production of surfactant is delayed in these infants; therefore, an L/S ratio always should be determined before an elective delivery to indicate the level of lung maturity.
   a. An L/S ratio of 3:1 or greater indicates lung maturity in an infant of a diabetic mother.
   b. A lower ratio reflects lung maturity only if significant amounts of phosphatidylglycerol are present.

5. **Hypoglycemia** is very common in infants of diabetic mothers and is related to the mother's overall glycemic control as well as the intrapartum glucose levels (see V J).

6. **Other metabolic disturbances** seen in infants of diabetic mothers include hypocalcemia and hyperbilirubinemia (see V C).

7. **Polycythemia** associated with elevated erythropoietin levels is observed and probably reflects chronic fetal hypoxia.

8. **Alterations in normal neonatal behavior** commonly are observed in infants of diabetic mothers. Abnormalities include lethargy, hypotonia, and poor feeding. An etiology is not clear.

9. **Large body size.** Those infants who are large for gestational age are more likely to continue to be large for age beyond infancy.

L. **Intrauterine drug exposure.** Studies have documented fetal exposure to numerous drugs, including antibiotics, caffeine, nicotine, alcohol, aspirin, and antihistamines. Over the past decade, the use of illicit drugs (e.g., heroin, cocaine, marijuana) by pregnant women also has grown. The intravenous use of illicit drugs is associated with a high risk for preterm birth as well as a significant risk of hepatitis and acquired immune deficiency syndrome (AIDS) in both the mother and infant. The drug-seeking behavior of these mothers often makes it difficult for them to care for their infants. The following are some commonly used drugs that may have major effects on the developing fetus and newborn.

1. **Nicotine** is absorbed through the lungs from cigarette smoke and is accompanied by the diffusion of carbon monoxide across the alveoli into the mother's blood. Nicotine is a vasoconstrictor that may limit uterine blood flow, and carbon monoxide decreases the arterial oxygen content. Together the two substances reduce the transfer of oxygen and nutrients from mother to fetus. The result is decreased intrauterine growth and chronic hypoxia.

2. **Alcohol** is a well-established teratogen. Fetal exposure may result in a spectrum of effects ranging from mild reduction in cerebral function to classic **fetal alcohol syndrome** (see also Chapter 8). Features of this syndrome include microcephaly with cerebral dysfunction, characteristic facies (short palpebral fissures, diminished philtrum, small upper lip), and intrauterine and extrauterine growth failure. The amount of alcohol consumed by the mother appears to correlate with the degree to which the fetus is affected.

3. **Heroin and methadone**
   a. Narcotic use by the mother is associated with intrauterine growth retardation, infant narcotic withdrawal syndrome, and increased risk of sudden infant death. There is accelerated maturation of several fetal organs, including the liver and lung (surfactant production).
   b. It is not clear whether the abnormalities of fetal growth and maturation are caused directly by the effects of the drugs or by other environmental factors (e.g., poor maternal nutrition) often associated with maternal narcotic use.
   c. Many of these infants will experience **narcotic withdrawal syndrome,** which is characterized by irritability, poor sleeping, high-pitched cry, diarrhea, sweating, sneezing, seizures, poor feeding, and poor weight gain. Naloxone should never be given to such infants in the delivery room because it precipitates acute withdrawal.
   d. The long-term neurologic consequences of fetal narcotic exposure have not been investigated completely.

4. **Cocaine** use by pregnant women has increased dramatically over the past decade. Such use is associated with congenital anomalies, intrauterine growth retardation, intracranial hemorrhage, placental abruption, and preterm birth. Infants may undergo withdrawal (irritability, poor feeding). Studies have demonstrated abnormalities in control of respiration and an increased risk for sudden infant death.

VI. **CARE OF THE PARENTS AND ETHICAL DECISION MAKING.** Whether the parents have the happy experience of bonding to a healthy newborn or the tragic experience of mourning a dying infant, it is the pediatrician's role to provide the parents with support and information and to answer their questions.

A. **Parent–infant bonding**

1. **Bonding between the healthy term infant and her parents**
   a. Bonding, or the process of psychological attachment of the parents to the newborn, appears to begin during pregnancy and to intensify as the fetus begins to move inside the uterus and react to external stimuli. During this period, the parents often form a mental image of what the infant will look like at birth.

b. At the time of delivery, it is thought that the mother experiences a unique psychological state or "window." This close contact with the infant in the delivery room fosters ideal bonding and promotes optimal future mother–infant interactions.

  (1) The **maternal behavior pattern** typically begins with touching of the infant's fingers and palms followed by central caressing. Eye contact is also made.

  (2) **Paternal behavior** is quite similar.

  (3) Although every effort should be made to ensure parent–infant bonding in the delivery area, medical problems (e.g., hypothermia, respiratory distress) must take precedence.

c. The process of bonding continues for hours and days after birth. Even if the delivery room bonding experience does not occur, it has been shown that strong mother–infant ties will be established if the mother and infant are given long periods of contact together over the next few days.

2. Problems in bonding between the sick infant and his parents

  a. The establishment of neonatal intensive care units, the advancement of technology, and the honing of clinical skills have allowed the survival of an increasing number of small and sick infants. The size and fragility of the newborn, the equipment used to care for the infant, and the long periods of hospitalization may make the normal bonding process more difficult for parents.

  b. At the turn of the century, it was recognized that institutional care improved the outcome of the feeble infant, yet the separation of the infant from the mother often led to abandonment. The ideal solution to this problem has not been found, as evidenced by the high rate of child abuse among infants who have been cared for in neonatal intensive care units. The following procedures are recommended to minimize the physical separation of the infant from the parents and to encourage the formation of a strong bond.

  (1) Whenever possible, the mother should be transported to a tertiary care center before delivery.

  (2) When the infant is transported to another hospital, the father should travel immediately to the referral center so that he may keep close contact with the infant and bring photographs and information back to the mother.

  (3) Visitation should be available 24 hours a day.

  (4) A strong line of communication should be established between the medical staff (i.e., physicians, nurses, social workers) and the parents.

  (5) The parents should be encouraged to keep in contact by telephone when visitation is difficult.

  (6) The parents should be prepared regarding what to expect during their first visit to the nursery, and they should be made aware of any sudden change in the infant's condition.

  (7) Information should be conveyed in a positive and truthful manner.

  (8) Psychological evaluation and support should be made available to parents who are having a particularly difficult time coping with their sick infant or the intensive care unit setting. Parents' groups often are helpful.

  (9) Plans for discharge should be made in advance and should include the parents. Having the parents stay overnight in the hospital before discharge can significantly help them adapt to new roles that they will perform after they leave the hospital. Any current or future medical problems and follow-up plans should be explained to the parents.

B. | **Support of the parents of a malformed infant.** The birth of a malformed infant is a tragedy that creates a complex challenge for the pediatrician, who must care for the child and help the parents through the disappointment and period of adjustment.

1. Stages of parental reaction. Parents go through four stages in reacting to their malformed infant, starting with mourning the loss of the expected healthy infant and ending with acceptance of the actual infant. These stages are:

  a. Shock

      b. Denial

      c. Sadness and anger

      d. Reorganization and acceptance

  2. Supportive actions that help the parents through this tragic period include the following:

      a. The parents should be encouraged to spend as much time as possible with the infant.

      b. The infant should be shown to the parents as soon as possible, because a mental image of the anomaly is often worse than the actual malformation.

      c. Good lines of communication should be maintained, and information should be conveyed in a truthful manner.

      d. The parents need support through each stage of adjustment and should not be rushed through the various stages.

      e. Plans for adequate support of the infant and parents should be made before discharge.

C. **Support of the parents of a dying infant during the illness and after the death**

  1. Parental reactions

      a. Grief experienced after the loss of a newborn is unique in that the attachment one has for a parent, sibling, spouse, or older child has not been formed. Rather, the newborn is perceived as a part of the parent, especially the mother. As such, the grieving behavior of the parents includes both the classic grieving behaviors plus behaviors reflecting detachment, similar to the feelings experienced when a limb has been amputated. The feelings include anger, guilt, fury, helplessness, and horror. As opposed to the feelings when a spouse or sibling dies, the feelings after the loss of an infant are not relieved by identification.

      b. Loss of a newborn often results in a **breakdown in communication** between the parents owing to their difficulty in expressing emotions and their feelings of guilt, blame, or both.

  2. Supportive actions. The parents can best be supported through the following actions.

      a. The parents should be prepared if death is anticipated.

      b. The parents should be together when they are told of the death.

      c. Every effort should be made to allow the parents to hold the infant before and after death if they desire to.

      d. Time for the immediate grieving should be allowed to pass before discussion of autopsy and burial arrangements.

      e. Support should be offered to the parents 3–4 months after the death. This may be in the form of an office visit or contact with a parents' group.

      f. Autopsy reports should be made available and discussed with the parents in a timely fashion.

D. **Ethical decision making.** Over the past 25 years, advances in knowledge of fetal and neonatal physiology and improvements in clinical skills and technology have allowed the survival of many immature and congenitally malformed infants. Ethical problems arise when this "high-tech" care is given to potentially nonviable infants. Some guidelines for ethical decision making are as follows (see also Chapter 7 VIII):

  1. The parents always should be involved, with the physician, in the decision-making process. It is the role of the physician to provide knowledge so that the parents can participate in life-or-death decisions regarding their infant.

  2. When viability is in doubt because of inadequate knowledge concerning the nature and severity of the infant's condition or prognosis, life support always should be provided until adequate data can be gathered.

3. All hospitals should have an ethics committee to assist the pediatrician when issues of life support or proper treatment are not clear, when the parents' wishes conflict with the physician's, or when the parents are not competent and cannot participate in the decision-making process.

4. The decision to terminate life support should be made only when it is clear that therapy is prolonging the dying process or when the burden of therapy outweighs any potential benefit to the infant.

BIBLIOGRAPHY

Avery GB, Fletcher MA, MacDonald MG: *Neonatology: Pathophysiology and Management of the Newborn,* 4th ed. Philadelphia, JB Lippincott, 1994.

Avery ME, Ballard RA, Taeusch HW: *Schaffer and Avery's Diseases of the Newborn,* 6th ed. Philadelphia, WB Saunders, 1991.

Creasy RK, Resnik R: *Maternal–Fetal Medicine,* 2nd ed. Philadelphia, WB Saunders, 1989.

Klaus MH, Fanaroff AA: *Care of the High-Risk Neonate,* 4th ed. Philadelphia, WB Saunders, 1993.

Polin RA, Fox WW: *Fetal and Neonatal Physiology.* Philadelphia, WB Saunders, 1992.

Volpe JJ: *Neurology of the Newborn,* 2nd ed. Philadelphia, WB Saunders, 1987.

DIRECTIONS: Each of the numbered items or incomplete statements in this section is followed by answers or by completions of the statement. Select the ONE lettered answer or completion that is BEST in each case.

1. An infant is born at term to a woman who has had an uncomplicated pregnancy. Immediately after delivery, the infant has severe respiratory failure. Breath sounds are diminished bilaterally. The abdomen is flat. The chest radiograph shows a multicystic mass in the left chest with a shift of the mediastinum to the right. The most likely diagnosis is

(A) respiratory distress syndrome
(B) diaphragmatic hernia
(C) tracheoesophageal fistula
(D) congenital lobar emphysema
(E) persistence of the fetal circulation

2. A newborn is brought to the delivery room. After assessing the infant's heart rate, color, and respiratory effort, a decision is made that the infant should receive ventilatory assistance. After 30 seconds of this therapy, cardiac compressions are initiated. The most likely Apgar score at this point in time is

(A) 9
(B) 7
(C) 6
(D) less than 5
(E) 8

DIRECTIONS: Each of the numbered items or incomplete statements in this section is negatively phrased, as indicated by a capitalized word such as NOT, LEAST, or EXCEPT. Select the ONE lettered answer or completion that is BEST in each case.

3. Newborns often require lower doses of drugs compared to adults (adjusted for body mass and weight) for all of the following reasons EXCEPT

(A) newborns have lower blood protein and albumin concentrations
(B) newborns have a lower glomerular filtration rate
(C) glucuronyl transferase activity is reduced in newborns
(D) renal tubular secretion is lower in newborns
(E) newborns have a lower normal blood pH

4. An infant is admitted to the nursery for evaluation of persistent hypoglycemia. As part of the workup for the hypoglycemia, a serum insulin level is obtained. The level comes back elevated. The differential diagnosis includes all of the following EXCEPT

(A) Beckwith-Wiedemann syndrome
(B) nesidioblastosis
(C) maternal diabetes
(D) asymmetric growth retardation
(E) pancreatic islet cell adenoma

5. An infant is born prematurely at 28 weeks' gestation and weighs 1028 g. The infant is started on enteric feedings at 3 days of age. Three days later, he is not tolerating his feedings. The signs and symptoms exhibited by the infant that make you suspect he has neonatal necrotizing enterocolitis include all of the following EXCEPT

(A) bile-stained gastric fluid
(B) pneumatosis intestinalis
(C) guaiac-positive stools
(D) apnea
(E) jaundice

6. A pregnant woman is admitted with vaginal bleeding. The fetal heart tracing is indicative of fetal distress, and a decision is made to perform an immediate cesarean delivery. Immediate preparation for a high-risk delivery involves all of the following steps and procedures EXCEPT

(A) obtaining the obstetric history
(B) gathering the appropriate personnel
(C) requesting a neonatology consultation
(D) obtaining the labor history
(E) readying the resuscitation equipment

7. You are called on to evaluate a newborn infant whose neurologic examination results are abnormal. It is suspected that the infant may have suffered perinatal asphyxia. All of the following complications of pregnancy are risk factors for perinatal asphyxia EXCEPT

(A) placental abruption
(B) hyperemesis gravidarum
(C) prematurity
(D) preeclampsia
(E) meconium-stained amniotic fluid

8. An infant was born at 26 weeks' gestation. The infant is now 8 weeks old and has bronchopulmonary dysplasia and retinopathy of prematurity. Which of the following statements regarding the pathogenesis and treatment of retinopathy of prematurity is FALSE?

(A) Its development is related to retinal vessel immaturity and hyperoxia
(B) The retinopathy resolves spontaneously in most infants
(C) Cryotherapy is the treatment of choice for all stages of disease
(D) Myopia is a common sequela

9. In both term and preterm infants, there are major shifts of water from various compartments, as well as diuresis. True statements concerning fluid balance in the newborn include all of the following EXCEPT

(A) sensible water loss includes urine, stool, and pulmonary and gastric fluid losses
(B) insensible water loss is increased by the use of radiant warmers, phototherapy, and an elevated environmental temperature
(C) replacement of sodium, potassium, and chloride in physiologic amounts is begun at 24 hours of age in the presence of normal urine output
(D) water loss in the first week of life is greater in the preterm infant

10. An infant born at 30 weeks' gestation begins to experience apnea on the second day of life. Included in the initial management of this infant should be all of the following EXCEPT

(A) therapy with theophylline
(B) evaluation for evidence of hypoxia, infection, or intracranial hemorrhage
(C) evaluation of the upper and lower airway
(D) complete blood count, arterial blood gas studies, and plasma glucose and electrolyte measurement

ANSWERS AND EXPLANATIONS

1. The answer is B *[V A 2 d]*. All of these problems cause respiratory disease in the newborn. Respiratory distress syndrome is the result of surfactant deficiency in preterm infants. The respiratory failure associated with diaphragmatic hernia usually is severe and presents at birth. The abdomen is scaphoid because the abdominal contents are in the chest. The air-filled bowel gives the appearance of a cystic mass in the left hemithorax and pushes the normal thoracic structures into the right hemithorax. The respiratory distress is caused by a combination of lung hypoplasia and persistently elevated pulmonary vascular resistance. Tracheoesophageal fistula does not present with severe respiratory failure, and the lung fields should be normal. Congenital lobar emphysema may present with mild to severe respiratory failure, but the chest radiograph reveals a dense, opaque, overinflated area of lung. Persistence of the fetal circulation as the sole etiology of respiratory failure is associated with a negative radiograph. Usually there is a history of meconium aspiration or perinatal asphyxia.

2. The answer is D *[III D 1; Table 6-7]*. The Apgar score determines the state of oxygenation and ventilation as reflected by heart rate, respiratory effort, muscle tone, reflex irritability, and skin color. An infant who requires ventilatory support and cardiac compression must have a score of less than 5 because the scores for heart rate, color, and respiratory effort would be less than 1, 0, and 0, respectively.

3. The answer is E *[IV C]*. Several factors must be considered when administering drugs to newborn infants, but blood pH is not one of them; normal pH is similar in infants and adults. The lower blood protein concentration in newborns compared to adults results in higher unbound fractions of drugs at given total drug concentrations. Lower drug metabolism in the newborn liver and lower renal clearance result in longer drug half-lives in newborns compared to adults. These factors require appropriate adjustments in drug dosing and monitoring of drug concentrations in neonates.

4. The answer is D *[V J 1]*. Infants with asymmetric growth retardation usually are the result of a pregnancy complicated by placental insufficiency; these infants have been "starved" in utero. They have virtually no glycogen

stores and become hypoglycemic soon after birth. Conditions that cause hypoglycemia due to hyperinsulinemia include Beckwith-Wiedemann syndrome (a condition associated with pancreatic islet cell hyperplasia), nesidioblastosis, and pancreatic islet cell adenoma. Infants of diabetic mothers are both hyperglycemic and hyperinsulinemic in utero. The hyperinsulinism continues after birth and results in hypoglycemia if proper therapy is not provided.

5. The answer is E *[V B 3, 4, C 2 a (1) (b)]*. Jaundice is not a feature of necrotizing enterocolitis, although it may occur if sepsis develops. Neonatal necrotizing enterocolitis is accompanied by an ileus as evidenced by abdominal distention, loss of bowel sounds, and bile-stained gastric fluid. The bacterial invasion of the intestinal wall leads to inflammation and tissue breakdown, which result in blood in the stool. Gas formation by the bacteria in the intestinal wall can be seen on radiography, and is referred to as pneumatosis intestinalis. Apnea, a nonspecific sign of infection, often is seen in association with necrotizing enterocolitis and other infections in the newborn.

6. The answer is C *[III C]*. To prepare for a high-risk delivery, the pediatrician must gather information about problems in the present and past pregnancies, such as Rh sensitization, herpetic infections, and malformations. The length of gestation and the results of fetal evaluation must also be ascertained. In addition, the labor history yields information concerning the risk for asphyxia. An optimal resuscitation requires an appropriate number of trained personnel and properly functioning equipment. Although a neonatology consultation may be needed for some high-risk deliveries, it is not part of the immediate preparation.

7. The answer is B *[Table 6-1]*. Hyperemesis gravidarum is not a risk factor for perinatal asphyxia. Placental abruption, prematurity, preeclampsia, and meconium-stained amniotic fluid do predispose to perinatal asphyxia. Placental abruption is the separation of the placenta from the uterine wall. With progressive separation, there is decreasing surface area for oxygen transfer from mother to fetus, and an increasing degree of fetal hypoxia results. Premature infants frequently suffer perinatal asphyxia owing to their inability to tolerate labor and to respiratory problems at birth. The incidence of perinatal asphyxia increases with decreasing gestational age at birth. Preeclampsia predisposes newborns to hypoxia and perinatal asphyxia due to chronic placental insufficiency and superimposed intermittent uteroplacental hypoperfusion during labor. Meconium-stained amniotic fluid is the result of fetal passage of meconium, which is triggered by hypoxia-stimulated vagal reflexes.

8. The answer is C *[V H 4]*. Retinopathy of prematurity usually resolves spontaneously. In the few infants with active, rapidly progressive disease, cryotherapy has been shown to be effective in many, but not all, cases. Retinopathy of prematurity appears to be related to immaturity of retinal vessels in preterm infants and to hyperoxia. The degree of insult to the retina varies with the severity of the vascularity and subsequent spontaneous regression. Myopia is a common outcome.

9. The answer is A *[IV A 1]*. Total body water and extracellular water and fluid loss are greater in the preterm infant than in the term infant; these parameters increase in an exponential manner with decreasing gestational age. Electrolyte replacement begins at 24 hours of age, after the establishment of an adequate urine output. An overload of total body sodium, potassium, and chloride may result if electrolytes are replaced before 24 hours of age or before an adequate urine output is established. Insensible water loss is increased by the use of radiant warmers, phototherapy, and an elevated environmental temperature, because these factors all increase evaporative water loss through the relatively thin and poorly keratinized skin of the infant. Pulmonary water losses are not directly measured and are not sensible water losses.

10. The answer is A *[V A 4 b (2)]*. Although apnea of prematurity is the most common cause of apnea in a 2-day-old preterm infant, other etiologies must be evaluated before initiating therapy. Failure to perform the appropriate evaluations may result in a delay in the diagnosis and thus in the appropriate treatment of correctable and potentially life-threatening causes of the apnea (e.g., infection, hypoxia, airway obstruction, metabolic disturbances).

Chapter 7

Critical Care
Betty S. Spivack

I. **GOAL AND SCOPE OF CRITICAL CARE MEDICINE.** Critical care is a specialty concerned with the management of patients whose homeostatic mechanisms have failed. The goals of the specialty are to maintain physiologic balance, while treating the underlying derangement. Intensive care physicians have special expertise in ventilatory support, promotion of cardiac output, treatment of acute electrolyte disorders and acute coma, and the nutritional support of the critically ill patient. They also frequently deal with families in the context of end-of-life decision making. The boundaries of critical care medicine intersect with those of many other specialties, most notably pulmonology, cardiology, neurology, and surgery.

II. **RESUSCITATION**

A. **Primary concerns**

1. **Basic life support** must precede any advanced life support techniques.

2. **Prompt intervention** with **advanced techniques** is provided after basic life support has been established.

3. **Reassessment** is required after any intervention.

4. The material in this portion of the chapter is a summary, and is not meant to replace the need for adequate training in basic and advanced life support techniques.

B. **Basic life support**

1. **Airway and breathing.** Ventilation is the most important intervention in the apneic child. The correct amount of ventilation will provide a moderate, but not excessive chest rise.
   a. The **airway** is assessed for patency. If breathing is not apparent, help is summoned, and the head is repositioned in the sniffing position.
   b. **Breathing** is reassessed. If breathing is not apparent, two slow breaths are given.
   c. If **air entry** is impeded, reposition the head and repeat the sequence. If it is still obstructed, use maneuvers recommended for the obstructed airway (see II B 3).

2. **Circulation**
   a. Palpate the **femoral or brachial pulse** in infants younger than 1 year of age. In children older than 1 year, the **carotid pulse** should be palpated.
   b. If no pulse is present, begin **chest compressions,** coordinated with ventilation. Rate and ratio are summarized in Table 7-1.

3. **Airway obstruction.** Foreign body aspiration should be suspected in children with sudden onset of respiratory distress associated with gagging, coughing, or stridor.
   a. **Infant.** Alternating sequences of four back blows and four chest thrusts are administered until spontaneous breathing is reestablished or until a manual breath can be given.

TABLE 7-1. Basic Life Support Maneuvers in Infants and Children

Component	Infants	Children
Maintenance breathing	20 breaths/min	15 breaths/min
Pulse check	Brachial/femoral	Carotid
Compression site	Lower third of sternum	Lower third of sternum
Compression depth	0.5–1.0 inch	1.0–1.5 inches
Compression rate	≥ 100/min	80–100/min
Compression:breath ratio	5:1, with pause for ventilation	5:1, with pause for ventilation

      (1) Back blows. Straddle the infant over the rescuer's arm, with the head below the trunk, while supporting the head. Deliver the blows with the heel of the hand between the infant's shoulder blades.

      (2) Chest thrusts. Turn the infant over onto the thigh, with the head and neck still supported. The thrusts are performed as for chest compressions, but at a slower rate.

    b. Child. Subdiaphragmatic thrusts (the **Heimlich maneuver**) are performed until the object is clearly expelled or 10 thrusts have been given, at which time the victim is reassessed.

      (1) Unconscious child. The maneuver is performed with the child on the ground, and the rescuer straddling the child. The heel of a fisted hand is placed in the subxiphoid region of the abdomen, and the fist is covered by the other hand. The thrust is given upward, taking care to stay in the midline.

      (2) Conscious child. The rescuer stands or sits behind the victim, holding the thumb side of his fist against the subxiphoid region of the abdomen. The thrust is given as a quick upward movement, avoiding the xiphoid and the internal organs.

    c. Contraindications

      (1) Airway clearing maneuvers should not be attempted if there is **gradual onset of respiratory symptoms** over hours or days, especially if these are associated with fever or other signs of infection.

      (2) The Heimlich maneuver should not be performed on children younger than 1 year of age.

C.   **Advanced life support** involves quick cardiopulmonary assessment and reevaluation after every intervention.

    1. Quick cardiopulmonary assessment. This initial evaluation takes 30–60 seconds and determines treatment priorities.

      a. Assessment areas

        (1) Airway. The airway is assessed for patency. It is described as patent, maintainable with positioning, or unmaintainable (i.e., requiring assisted ventilation, intubation, or other intervention).

        (2) Breathing is assessed with regard to rate, air entry, work of breathing, and skin color.

        (3) Circulation is assessed on the basis of heart rate, blood pressure, peripheral and central arterial pulses, and skin and central nervous system perfusion.

      b. Sequence of assessment

        (1) Inspection of the patient's rate and work of breathing, skin color, and alertness

        (2) Palpation of peripheral and central pulses, skin temperature, capillary refill, response to painful stimulation, and localization of the liver edge

        (3) Auscultation of the quality of air entry and the cardiac sounds

        (4) Blood pressure measurement

      c. Physiologic classifications

        (1) Stable: airway, breathing, and circulation are adequate

        (2) Respiratory distress: work of breathing is increased, but ventilation and oxygenation (with supplemental oxygen) are adequate, and alertness is maintained

(3) **Respiratory failure:** ventilation or oxygenation is impaired, but circulation is adequate

(4) **Early shock:** perfusion is decreased, but blood pressure is maintained

(5) **Late shock:** there is marked hypoperfusion with frank hypotension

(6) **Cardiopulmonary failure:** an agonal state with bradycardia, agonal respirations, and absence of pulses (it is impossible to know whether cardiopulmonary failure is the result of respiratory or circulatory embarrassment)

(7) **Cardiopulmonary arrest:** no breathing or effective cardiac output is present

2. **Therapeutic interventions**

a. **Stable condition.** Pursue evaluation suggested by more detailed history and physical examination. **Reassess** physiologic status periodically.

b. **Respiratory distress.** Keep the child in a position of comfort with parent, with professional staff nearby. Cardiac monitor and oximetry are appropriate. Apply oxygen as tolerated. Continue diagnostic and therapeutic course as indicated by more complete history and physical examination.

c. **Respiratory failure.** Separate the child from the parent and monitor with cardiac monitor and oximetry. Administer high-concentration oxygen and ventilate via bag and mask or intubation.

d. **Shock.** Separate child and parents, monitor with cardiac monitor, and reassess frequently. Vascular access should be quickly established, using peripheral venous, central venous, or intraosseous routes. Shock due to arrhythmia or congestive heart failure should be distinguished from shock arising from other causes.

(1) If there are no signs of dysrhythmia or congestive heart failure, give a 20-ml/kg fluid bolus using crystalloid or colloid and reassess. Repeat boluses may be required.

(2) If congestive heart failure is present, inotropic support with continuous infusion may be necessary. This is relatively uncommon in childhood.

(3) If a dysrhythmia is present on the cardiac monitor, treat appropriately as described later (see II C 2 g).

(4) **Reassess** status frequently.

e. **Cardiopulmonary failure.** Assist ventilation with 100% oxygen by bag and mask or endotracheal intubation, then reassess. Initiate cardiac monitoring.

(1) If circulatory status improves, the event was most likely respiratory in origin. Treat appropriately as in II C 2 c.

(2) If the patient appears to be in shock, circulatory embarrassment is the apparent triggering event. Treat as described in II C 2 d.

f. **Cardiopulmonary arrest.** Ventricular tachycardia and fibrillation are rare causes of cardiac arrest in childhood, and should be treated as described in II C 2 g.

(1) Initiate basic life support, begin cardiac monitoring, and ventilate with bag and mask or intubate.

(2) Establish vascular access if possible, but do not delay therapy.

(3) If there is no restoration of circulation with assisted ventilation and cardiac compressions, administer epinephrine 1:10,000 intravenously or via endotracheal tube.

(4) **Reassess.** If there is persistent asystole or bradycardia, atropine may be given intravenously or endotracheally in a dose of 0.02 mg/kg, and a minimum dose of 0.1 mg.

(5) Reassess, including blood gas analysis.

(6) If there is a marked metabolic acidosis, and assisted ventilation is adequate, $NaHCO_3$ may be given, but only via a vascular route. **Do not give bicarbonate through an endotracheal tube.**

g. **Dysrhythmia.** Only unstable dysrhythmias require emergent treatment. Dysrhythmias without cardiac or circulatory instability may await definitive consultation with a pediatric cardiologist before treatment.

(1) **Bradydysrhythmias (unstable).** Most childhood bradycardia is caused by hypoxemia. Cardiac output is decreased owing to the low rate.

(a) **Oxygenate and ventilate,** then reassess.

       (b) If bradycardia persists despite adequate oxygenation and ventilation, **drug therapy** with atropine or isoproterenol should be initiated.

       (c) If these modalities are ineffective, and bradycardia persists, **pacing** should be considered.

    (2) Tachydysrhythmias (unstable). Instability results from small stroke volume.

       (a) Determine whether the rhythm is **narrow complex** or **wide complex.** If the rhythm shows a narrow-complex tachycardia, distinguish **sinus tachycardia** from **supraventricular tachycardia (SVT;** Table 7-2).

       (b) Sinus tachycardia

          (i) Sinus tachycardia in an unstable patient suggests a primary problem with respiration or perfusion, which should be appropriately treated.

          (ii) Sinus tachycardia in a stable patient may be the result of fever, anxiety, dehydration, or pain. Treat the source of the tachycardia, not the symptom.

       (c) Unstable SVT is treated by prompt use of adenosine (intravenous bolus of 0.1 mg/kg) or synchronized cardioversion, starting at 1 watt-second/kg of discharge. If the patient is conscious, use sedation before cardioversion. Be prepared to assist ventilation. If the patient is in shock and venous access is not present, treat immediately with synchronized cardioversion.

       (d) Unstable, wide-complex tachycardia is treated by synchronized cardioversion, as described in (c).

       (e) A pediatric cardiologist should be contacted as soon as possible to coordinate further therapy. **Do not delay treatment of unstable patients to get a consultation.**

    (3) Absent pulse rhythms are most commonly caused by asystole, but may be the result of ventricular tachycardia, ventricular fibrillation, or electromechanical dissociation.

       (a) Ventilate with 100% oxygen and initiate basic life support.

       (b) If there is **asystole,** proceed as for cardiac arrest (see II C 2 f).

       (c) If there is **ventricular fibrillation** or **pulseless ventricular tachycardia, defibrillation** should be performed using an unsynchronized discharge of 2 watt-seconds/kg. This may be doubled or increased to a maximum of 300 watt-seconds. If three consecutive shocks are ineffective, epinephrine, lidocaine, bretylium, or procainamide may assist defibrillation. **Note: Ingestion of sympathomimetic or anticholinergic drugs is the most common cause of ventricular tachycardia in childhood.**

       (d) Electromechanical dissociation may be caused by reversible mechanical problems such as tension pneumothorax or cardiac tamponade, or by reversible metabolic problems such as extreme hypovolemia, hypoglycemia, hyperkalemia, or hypocalcemia. Consider therapy for these entities, guided by the context of presentation.

TABLE 7-2. Distinguishing Sinus Tachycardia and Supraventricular Tachycardia

Measurement	Sinus Tachycardia	Supraventricular Tachycardia
Heart rate	Usually < 200, but may exceed 200	Usually > 230
Electrocardiogram	Usually P waves Variability	No P wave Very regular
History	Cause for increased rate found (e.g., fever, dehydration, respiratory distress)	Nonspecific symptoms
Physical examination	Consistent with history	Instability greater than suggested by history Congestive heart failure usually present in infants

III. **RESPIRATORY INTENSIVE CARE.** The goal of respiratory support is to maintain oxygenation and ventilation at levels that can support physiologic needs, while minimizing oxygen toxicity and barotrauma.

A. Derangements of oxygenation and ventilation

1. Oxygenation defects
   a. **Tissue oxygenation** may be impaired with or without associated impairment of **alveolar** or **arterial** P_{O_2} (Table 7-3). Other causes include decreases in **oxygen content, oxygen delivery,** or **oxygen utilization.**
   b. **Alveolar** P_{O_2} depends on **barometric pressure** (PB) or altitude, **water vapor pressure** (PH$_2$O), the **fraction of inspired oxygen** (FIO$_2$), P_{CO_2}, and **respiratory quotient** (R):

   $$\text{Alveolar } P_{O_2} = F_{IO_2} (PB - PH_2O) - P_{CO_2}/R$$

   c. **Arterial** P_{O_2} depends on **distribution** of inspired gas in the alveoli ("$\dot{V}/\dot{Q}$ matching"), **diffusion** of oxygen across the alveolar–capillary membrane, which depends on time available for diffusion, the nature of the membrane, and **alveolar** P_{O_2}.

   $$\text{Alveolar-arterial (A-a) oxygen gradient} =$$
   $$\text{alveolar } P_{O_2} \text{ (calculated)} - \text{arterial } P_{O_2} \text{ (measured)}$$

   Note: Arterial hypoxemia may occur with or without an increase in A-a gradient (see Table 7-3). Conditions that do not increase the gradient lower arterial P_{O_2} by lowering alveolar P_{O_2}. Conditions that result in an increased A-a gradient impair distribution or diffusion.
   d. **Arterial oxygen content** depends on hemoglobin concentration, hemoglobin saturation, arterial P_{O_2}, and type of hemoglobin.

   $$O_2 \text{ Content} = 1.34 \times HGB \times SAT + (0.003 \times P_{O_2})$$

   e. **Oxygen delivery** to the tissues depends on the oxyhemoglobin dissociation curve, cardiac output, perfusion of the tissue bed involved, and arterial oxygen content.

   $$\text{Delivery} = O_2 \text{ Content} \times Q \times 10$$

   f. **Oxygen utilization** by the tissues depends on the availability of other substrates (e.g., glucose) and enzymes, the coupling of oxidative phosphorylation and the electron transport chain, and on oxygen delivery.

2. Ventilation defects
   a. P_{CO_2} may be elevated because of a decrease in **alveolar minute volume** or an increase in CO_2 **production.**

TABLE 7-3. The A-a Gradient and Arterial Hypoxemia

Cause of Hypoxemia	Gradient	Mechanism
Shunt	Increased	Unsaturated hemoglobin does not come into contact with alveolar O_2
Low $\dot{V}/\dot{Q}$ ratio	Increased	Insufficient alveolar O_2 to completely saturate hemoglobin present in pulmonary capillary
Hypoventilation	Normal	P_{CO_2} rises, decreasing alveolar P_{O_2}
"Diffusion defect"	Increased	Oxygen diffusion is mechanically obstructed (e.g., fibrosis) or is limited by time available before exhalation
Altitude	Normal	Lower atmospheric pressure causes decreased alveolar P_{O_2}

b. Alveolar minute ventilation depends on **dead space volume** (VD, the volume of gas inspired in each breath that does not end up in a functional alveolus), **tidal volume** (VT, the volume of gas inspired in each breath), and **respiratory rate**.

$$\text{Alveolar minute ventilation} = (VT - VD) \, RR$$

B. **Respiratory support techniques.** Oxygenation and ventilation may be assisted by providing supplemental oxygen; by mechanical or pharmacologic techniques that alter patient mechanics, thereby improving the patient's ability to oxygenate and ventilate spontaneously; or by mechanical ventilation.

1. **Supplemental oxygen** may be provided by nasal cannula, face mask, or tent, or in association with other techniques of assisted ventilation.
   a. Purpose. Supplemental oxygen is used to provide sufficiently high P_{O_2} to maintain the body's physiologic activities. It has no major role in treatment of hypoventilation or hypercarbia.
   b. Limitations
   (1) Toxicity. In high concentrations (80%–100%), oxygen is damaging to biologic membranes (including the alveolar–capillary membrane) in as little as 24 hours. With more prolonged exposure, even 40%–50% O_2 may cause permanent injury.
   (2) Effectiveness. Supplemental oxygen is moderately useful for treating low V/Q processes, but of little or no use in treating processes characterized by significant shunt or diffusion defect. In general, if adequate oxygenation ($P_{O_2} > 60$ mm Hg) is not obtained using 60% O_2, and the expected need for therapy extends beyond 24 hours, another modality of therapy is needed.

2. **Aids to spontaneous ventilation and oxygenation**
   a. Continuous positive airway pressure (CPAP), or the related use of **positive end-expiratory pressure (PEEP),** improves end-expiratory lung volumes in poor compliance–low volume states. CPAP or PEEP may be used in combination with supplemental oxygen, pressure-supported ventilation, or mechanical ventilation.
   (1) CPAP/PEEP provides an end-expiratory pressure that exceeds barometric pressure (Figure 7-1). This causes an increase in end-expiratory volumes (functional residual capacity), which yields improved V/Q ratios, decreased shunting, and improved oxygenation.
   (2) Higher lung volumes generate improved lung compliance, reducing the work of breathing. This encourages the patient to breathe in a slower, deeper pattern, which is more consistent with good gas distribution and diffusion. This improves both oxygenation and ventilation.

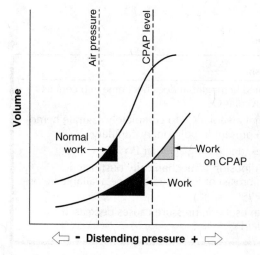

FIGURE 7-1. Effect of the use of continuous positive airway pressure (*CPAP*) on end-expiratory lung volumes in respiratory failure. *FRC* = functional residual capacity.

b. Pressure-supported ventilation is an advanced technique that decreases the work of breathing and increases spontaneous ventilation in patients with respiratory failure. It may be used in association with supplemental oxygen, PEEP, or mechanical ventilation.

   (1) At the initiation of a spontaneous breath, the machine increases airflow through the tubing. This substantially reduces the resistance, resulting in a larger tidal volume for a given amount of work performed by the patient.

   (2) Although the machine senses the initiation of the breath and increases airflow, the patient is in full control of tidal volume, respiratory rate, and inspiratory time. Therefore, this mode of assisted ventilation requires a respiratory drive and some ability to do mechanical work on the part of the patient.

c. Helium–oxygen (He-O$_2$) mixtures also reduce airway resistance, because helium is a lighter and therefore less viscous gas than nitrogen. He-O$_2$ mixtures may be used in conjunction with supplemental oxygen, and in some, but not all, mechanical ventilators.

   (1) Mixtures containing more than 50% helium may improve spontaneous ventilation, breathing pattern, gas distribution, and oxygenation.

   (2) This modality is of little or no benefit in patients requiring a high FIO_2.

d. Bronchodilating agents reduce airway resistance by increasing the diameter of the smaller airways (see Chapter 13). These agents may be used in conjunction with supplemental oxygen, CPAP/PEEP, and pressure-supported or mechanical ventilation.

   (1) Bronchodilating agents may be administered orally, intravenously, or as aerosols (see Chapter 13).

   (2) Continuous nebulization of aerosols may provide additional relief in severe asthmatic episodes; however, this method precludes the use of pressure support to assist in spontaneous ventilation.

e. Artificial airways, such as nasopharyngeal tubes, endotracheal tubes, and tracheostomy tubes, can improve airway mechanics by bypassing obstructions. All of these can be used in conjunction with supplemental oxygen, but only endotracheal tubes and tracheostomy tubes can be used with mechanical ventilation. Tracheostomy tubes can also improve alveolar ventilation in the patient with neuromuscular weakness or chronic respiratory failure by decreasing dead space and airway resistance.

3. Mechanical ventilation

   a. Positive-pressure ventilation supplies gas directly to the trachea via endotracheal tube or tracheostomy. The delivery of gas may be controlled by direct setting of flow rate and inspiratory time, volume, or pressure. All modes may be used with supplementary oxygen and PEEP.

   (1) Time-cycled, pressure-limited ventilation delivers gas by setting flow rate, inspiratory time, and a pressure limit. Pressure is determined by the patient's lung compliance and tidal volume.

   (a) Flow rate is constant unless the pressure limit is reached. If the pressure limit is reached, flow ceases.

   (b) If the pressure limit is not reached, volumes increase linearly during inspiration. This will tend to worsen gas distribution.

   (2) Volume-cycled, pressure-limited ventilation delivers gas by directly setting tidal volume, gas flow pattern, and a pressure limit. Pressure is determined by the patient's lung compliance and the tidal volume.

   (a) Flow pattern may be constant or decelerating. A constant flow generates a breath indistinguishable from a time-cycled ventilator. A decelerating flow pattern provides most of the gas early in inspiration, improving gas distribution, diffusion, and oxygenation.

   (b) If the pressure limit is reached, the remaining volume is dumped. Thus, in a patient with worsening compliance, preset volumes may not be reached, causing unrecognized hypoventilation.

(3) Pressure-cycled ventilation delivers gas by setting inspiratory pressure and inspiratory time. Volume depends on the patient's lung compliance and the preset inspiratory pressure.

    (a) Inspiratory pressure levels are reached almost instantly, and continue throughout inspiration.

    (b) This pattern yields extremely high flows initially, decreasing over the remainder of the inspiratory period. This is the most effective way to distribute gas in a patient with poor compliance and impaired diffusion secondary to restriction of time of gas in the alveoli. It is most effective combined with a relatively long inspiratory time.

    (c) In a patient with worsening compliance, tidal volumes may decrease at a constant inspiratory pressure level. This mode of ventilation requires continuous monitoring of expired tidal or minute volumes.

(4) Oscillating ventilators deliver gas by setting mean airway pressure, frequency of oscillation (cycles/second or Hz), and amplitude of oscillation.

    (a) The oscillations provide a wave of alveolar ventilation, and the normal rules of lung mechanics (e.g., dead space ventilation) do not apply.

    (b) Oscillating ventilators are useful in ventilating patients with poor compliance as a means of limiting barotrauma.

(5) Jet ventilators deliver gas by setting frequency and volume of jet through a special endotracheal tube inserted to deliver the jet of gas.

    (a) The jet delivery entrains additional gas, increasing laminar flow at low pressures. Conventional mechanics do not apply.

    (b) Jet ventilation is limited by the size availability of the required, special endotracheal tubes. It is an experimental technique.

b. Negative pressure ventilators establish a vacuum around the patient's chest, and the preset negative pressure yields a tidal volume that depends on the patient's lung–thorax compliance.

(1) This mode of ventilation is appropriate only for patients with neuromuscular problems.

(2) Limitations on the negative pressure will unduly limit the tidal volumes and minute ventilation of the patient with poor chest or lung compliance.

IV. CARDIOVASCULAR INTENSIVE CARE

A. **Invasive monitoring techniques.** In a critically ill patient, any parameter that may indicate a life-threatening change before severe deterioration should be monitored frequently or continuously. Such parameters include cardiac rate and rhythm, arterial pressure, central venous pressure, pulmonary arterial pressure, and cardiac output.

1. Arterial pressure. A vascular catheter is placed percutaneously or by cutdown in a peripheral or central artery.

    a. Indications include shock, hypertensive crisis, and intravenous therapy with sympathomimetic medications.

    b. Complications primarily relate to thrombosis within the arterial vessel.

2. Central venous pressure. A vascular catheter is placed percutaneously or by cutdown, with the tip in the central venous vessels of the chest, or in the right atrium. The latter is more dangerous.

    a. Indications include all states in which volume status is a key to critical management, such as severe congestive heart failure or renal failure.

    b. Complications include hemorrhage, air embolus, pneumothorax, and arrhythmias.

3. Pulmonary artery pressure. A vascular catheter is introduced, either percutaneously or by cutdown, into one of the central venous vessels. The catheter is advanced through the right atrium, right ventricle, and into one of the pulmonary arteries, aided by balloon flotation.

    a. Data supplied
      (1) With the balloon deflated, a **pulmonary arterial pressure wave** is displayed. With the balloon inflated, and properly positioned, a **pulmonary capillary wedge** tracing is displayed, reflecting left atrial filling pressures.
      (2) The catheter may be used to determine **cardiac output** by thermodilution technique.
      (3) After the pressure and output data have been obtained, other variables may be calculated including systemic vascular resistance, pulmonary vascular resistance, and right and left myocardial work.
    b. Indications include any situation in which central venous pressure may not accurately reflect left atrial filling pressure, or in which accurate measurement of cardiac output may be repeatedly required. This includes septic shock, cardiogenic shock, adult respiratory distress syndrome, and postoperative management of patients with impaired cardiovascular function.
    c. Complications include all those caused by central venous catheterization, plus pulmonary infarction, ventricular arrhythmias, perforation of the pulmonary artery or cardiac chambers, or rupture of cardiac valves.

B. | **Shock** is a complex metabolic state characterized by impaired delivery of oxygen and other substrates to the tissues.

  1. General principles
    a. Causes
      (1) Noncardiovascular causes include hypoxemia, hypoglycemia, and toxins (e.g., cyanide) that impair delivery and utilization of oxygen by the tissues.
      (2) Cardiovascular causes include derangements of preload, contractility, and afterload.
    b. Phases. All forms of untreated shock go through three phases, which vary in duration depending on the cause. These are:
      (1) Compensated shock (normal blood pressure)
      (2) Uncompensated shock (low blood pressure)
      (3) Irreversible shock (multiple organ system damage)

  2. Types of cardiovascular shock
    a. Hypovolemic shock is caused by decreased circulating volume (preload; see also Chapter 14).
      (1) Compensatory mechanisms
        (a) Secretion of antidiuretic hormone (ADH)
        (b) Secretion of aldosterone–renin–angiotensin
        (c) Secretion of endogenous catecholamines
      (2) Physiologic response
        (a) Decreased urine output
        (b) Vasoconstriction
        (c) Tachycardia
        (d) Increased contractility
      (3) Clinical features
        (a) Tachycardia
        (b) Cool, pale extremities
        (c) Prolonged capillary refill time (> 2 seconds)
        (d) Decreased level of consciousness (late)
        (e) Hypotension (**very late**—this implies a greater than 40% decrease in circulating volume in infants)
      (4) Therapeutic approach
        (a) Reestablish circulating volume with crystalloid or colloid solutions.
        (b) Inotropic support is used only in very late hypovolemic shock, when myocardial damage has been done by prolonged hypoperfusion. It should be started only after **adequate volume has been provided**.

        (c) Reassess fluid balance and physical examination frequently. If there is a poor response to fluid therapy, central venous or pulmonary artery pressure monitoring may be necessary.

  b. Cardiogenic shock is caused by decreased contractility.

    (1) Compensatory mechanisms

      (a) ADH secretion

      (b) Aldosterone–renin–angiotensin secretion

      (c) Endogenous catecholamine secretion

    (2) Physiologic response

      (a) Decreased urine output leading to hypervolemia

      (b) Vasoconstriction leading to increased afterload

      (c) Tachycardia

      (d) Further decrease in contractility and cardiac output due to increased demands resulting from (a), (b), and (c)

    (3) Clinical features

      (a) Tachycardia

      (b) Cool, pale extremities

      (c) Delayed capillary refill

      (d) Impaired mental status

      (e) Hypotension (early)

    (4) Therapeutic approach

      (a) Inotropic support with dopamine, dobutamine, epinephrine, or amrinone

      (b) Vasodilation with nitroprusside, phentolamine (acute), or captopril (chronic). Dobutamine and amrinone have vasodilator properties in addition to their inotropic effect.

      (c) Diuresis

      (d) Continuous monitoring of cardiac rhythm, arterial blood pressure, and urine output is indicated. Central venous pressure monitoring is likely to be beneficial. In very unstable patients, therapy can be controlled best with pulmonary artery catheter guidance.

  c. Distributive shock is caused by poor perfusion of tissue beds (afterload).

    (1) Compensatory mechanisms are limited to catecholamine secretion.

    (2) Physiologic response

      (a) Tachycardia

      (b) Increased contractility

    (3) Clinical features

      (a) Early signs include fever, extreme tachycardia, low diastolic pressure, normal or slightly increased systolic pressure, bounding pulses, prolonged capillary refill, and impaired level of consciousness.

      (b) Late signs are those features seen in cardiogenic shock.

    (4) Therapeutic approach

      (a) Maintain circulating volume.

      (b) Prolong the hyperdynamic phase by using inotropic support.

      (c) Promote vasoconstriction if needed, using alpha-agonist agents.

      (d) Attempt to correct triggering derangement.

      (e) Monitor cardiac rhythm, arterial and central venous pressure, and urinary output; pulmonary arterial catheterization may be helpful.

C.   **Postoperative cardiovascular management**

  1. Acute management. Patients who have been placed on cardiopulmonary bypass for open heart procedures frequently exhibit decreased myocardial contractility for the first 24–48 postoperative hours. This is exaggerated in those patients who have undergone ventriculotomy.

    a. In such patients, there is continuous monitoring of arterial pressure, central venous pressure, and left atrial or pulmonary artery pressure, as well as electrocardiograph (ECG) tracing.

b. Cardiac output may be supported by infusion of **inotropic agents** such as dopamine, dobutamine, or epinephrine.

c. Perfusion may be enhanced by use of **vasodilators** such as nitroprusside and phentolamine.

d. Monitoring devices and drainage tubes are removed as the patient continues to stabilize.

2. **Complications**

a. Pleural or **pericardial effusions** may appear in the first postoperative week, or even later, as part of the **postpericardiotomy syndrome**. These usually disappear untreated, but should be monitored until they do so, and may require intervention if cardiac output or ventilation is impaired.

b. Patients with intracardiac repairs may have **conduction defects** that predispose them to dysrhythmias. Such patients may require medication to suppress the arrhythmias, or may need implantable pacemakers or defibrillators (rare).

c. Patients with indwelling grafts or valve devices are at increased risk for **thrombogenesis** and **bacterial colonization**. Such complications may lead to **stroke** or **endocarditis**.

V. NEUROLOGIC INTENSIVE CARE

A. Increased intracranial pressure

1. **Normal physiology**

a. Intracranial pressure (ICP) is generated as a function of the **compliance of the cranial vault** and the **volume of the intracranial contents,** which include brain parenchyma, cerebrospinal fluid (CSF), intravascular blood, and interstitial fluid. Compliance of the system may vary depending on the degree of ossification of the skull, splitting of the sutures, or the presence or absence of fontanelles. Significant increased intracranial pressure may occur with an open fontanelle.

b. In the normal situation, cerebral blood flow remains stable over a wide range of states of hydration and blood pressures owing to **autoregulation**.

2. **Causes of increased ICP** include:

a. Increased intracerebral mass (e.g., brain tumor)

b. Increased CSF volume (hydrocephalus)

c. Increased intravascular blood volume (e.g., arteriovenous malformations)

d. Increased interstitial fluid (cerebral edema)

e. Presence of extravascular fluid collections (epidural, subdural, subarachnoid, or intracerebral hemorrhages)

3. **Pathophysiology**

a. ICP may remain constant for a variable length of time after intracranial volume begins to increase by:

(1) Shunting of blood out of the venous sinuses to the central veins of the chest

(2) Shunting of CSF out of the ventricles into the spinal cord

b. Whenever intracranial volume exceeds the capacity of the cranial vault to expand, and when shunting of CSF and venous blood have been maximally accomplished, intracranial pressure begins to rise dramatically.

(1) The capacity for autoregulation may be lost (i.e., cerebral blood flow may become directly proportional to mean arterial blood pressure).

(2) Pressure exerted on the brain stem may cause the **Cushing reflex** (bradycardia and hypertension).

(3) Continued increase in intracranial pressure may cause **herniation** and death by compression of brain stem structures. This is more likely with a mass lesion than with a more uniform increase in pressure, but may occur with any source of increased ICP.

4. Therapy
  a. Monitoring
  (1) ICP may be measured directly by a number of devices.
  (2) Arterial pressure should be continuously assessed in any patient requiring ICP monitoring.
  (3) Central venous pressure monitoring may be required.
  (4) Cardiac rate and rhythm should be monitored continuously.
  b. Reduction of intracranial volume
  (1) **Brain mass** may be normalized by partial or total resection of a tumor. Other interventions may be required first in a quickly progressive, unstable situation.
  (2) **CSF** may be removed directly from the ventricles via ventriculostomy. This is useful only when the increased ICP is associated with hydrocephalus.
  (3) **Intravascular blood volume** may be reduced.
  (a) **Hyperventilation** (Pco_2 25–30 mm Hg) reduces ICP because cerebral blood flow is directly proportional to Pco_2 within the physiologic range (20–60 mm Hg).
  (b) **Infusion of short-acting barbiturates** (e.g., pentobarbital) also causes cerebral vasoconstriction, as well as decreasing cerebral metabolic demand.
  (c) **Elevation of the head** may promote drainage of venous blood into the internal jugular veins.
  (4) **Interstitial fluid** may be reduced by:
  (a) **Osmotic diuresis** with agents such as mannitol
  (b) **Restriction of fluids**
  (c) **Infusion of short-acting barbiturates,** which act by decreasing the metabolic rate, therefore decreasing the water generated during the catabolism of glucose.
  (d) **Glucocorticoids** (limited utility)
  (5) **Extravascular fluid collections** should be removed if they demonstrate a significant mass effect. Other, quicker techniques such as hyperventilation should be used initially in the emergent situation.

B. **Brain death** is a state characterized by **complete and irreversible brain and brain stem failure**. Physical examination or other testing reveals no brain or brain stem function at any level.

  1. General principles
  a. Somatic death. Brain death is invariably followed by somatic death even if the body is maintained by mechanical ventilation and inotropic support.
  (1) The usual mechanism of somatic death is progressive hypotension that becomes increasingly unresponsive to catecholamines.
  (2) This process may take anywhere from several days to several weeks.
  b. Legality of brain death. All states now accept brain death as actual death.
  (1) Some states have legislation declaring that brain death is actual death.
  (2) Other states have appellate court rulings declaring that brain death is equivalent to somatic death, obviating any need for treatment.
  c. Pediatric brain death
  (1) Brain death is difficult to assess in young children owing to developmental issues. States of apparent brain death have been followed by prolonged survival and some degree of recovery in very young infants, and, more frequently, in premature babies. Therefore, standards in these age-groups differ from those in older children or in adults.
  (2) Standards for diagnosis of brain death in various age-groups are summarized in Table 7-4.

  2. Physical examination must be performed when the body temperature is greater than 35°C, blood pressure is normal for age, and when no medications or toxins are present in concentrations that may cause coma. Because brain-dead patients commonly have difficulty or inability in maintaining body temperature or vasomotor tone, this may

TABLE 7-4. Standards for Pediatric Brain Death Determination

Age Range*	Observation Period	EEG Testing
7 days to 2 months	Two examinations separated by 48 hours	Two examinations separated by 48 hours
2 months to 1 year	Two examinations separated by 24 hours	Two examinations separated by 24 hours
Older than 1 year	Two examinations separated by 12–24 hours	None required; observation period may be reduced if isoelectric EEG is obtained

EEG = electroencephalogram.
*No standards exist for premature infants or for full-term infants during the first week of life.

require artificial warming or use of pressor drugs to guarantee the validity of the examination. An examination revealing any level of brain function in the following areas is incompatible with the diagnosis of brain death.
  a. **Cortical functions**
    (1) Any pain response other than simple withdrawal, which may be a spinal cord–mediated response
    (2) Preservation of muscle tone (nonflaccid limbs)
    (3) Voluntary movement, localization, decorticate or decerebrate posturing
  b. **Midbrain functions**
    (1) Oculocephalic reflexes ("doll's eyes")
    (2) Oculovestibular reflexes ("caloric" responses)
  c. **Cranial nerve functions**
    (1) Pupillary reflex
    (2) Corneal reflex
    (3) Gag reflex
    (4) Sucking movements
  d. **Respiratory drive** is assessed with the **apnea test**.
    (1) The patient is preoxygenated with 100% O_2 for 5 minutes, but must not be hypocapnic (i.e., Pco_2 must be ≥ 35 mm Hg) at the beginning of the test.
    (2) Mechanical ventilation is stopped, and heart rate and respiration are observed continuously for 10 minutes or until heart rate begins to fall.
    (3) An arterial blood gas sample is drawn at the end of the testing period, before reinstituting mechanical ventilation. The Pco_2 must rise by 20 mm Hg without spontaneous ventilation for the test to be confirmatory.

 3. **Neurophysiologic testing** may be used to rule out continued activity or perfusion of the brain. Absence of expected findings is compatible with brain death. Any test that reveals function of the brain at any level is incompatible with brain death.
  a. **Electroencephalography (EEG)** is the oldest technique available for this assessment, but it is prone to produce artifacts. It is required in the determination of brain death in children younger than 1 year of age (see Table 7-4). To be reliable, the EEG requires:
    (1) Body temperature > 35°C
    (2) Absence of significant levels of drugs, such as barbiturates, which may reversibly suppress cortical function
    (3) Careful attention to eliminate electrical artifact caused by life support equipment
    (4) Recording of response to painful stimulation
    (5) ECG and muscle tracings as well as the standard cephalic leads
    (6) High-sensitivity (3 mV) recording
  b. **Evoked brain stem potentials** assess brain stem transmission of external stimuli and may be helpful in assessing absence of brain stem function at certain levels. Both auditory and somatosensory evoked responses have been studied in this setting.
  c. **Four-vessel cerebral angiography** studies cerebral blood flow after injection of dye into the internal carotid and vertebral arteries. Brain death is associated with absence

of cerebral blood flow, without anatomic obstruction, for reasons that are not well understood. This test is very invasive and difficult to perform in a child who is on multiple forms of life support.

   d. Isotope brain scanning may be used in the pediatric intensive care setting, if a portable gamma counter is available. Otherwise, it too may be difficult to perform in a critically ill child, although less so than angiography. Isotope brain scanning is somewhat less reliable than four-vessel angiography.

VI. TRAUMA

A. General principles

1. **Mortality**
   a. **Injuries** are the leading cause of death in children older than 1 year of age (see Chapter 2).
   b. **Inflicted trauma** (child abuse) may be the leading cause of death in children between 1 month and 1 year of age. Child abuse death estimates range from 1300 to 4000 deaths a year (see Chapter 3).

2. **Management.** Children with severe trauma are best treated in a hospital with pediatric surgeons and a pediatric intensive care unit. They should be rapidly transferred to such a facility after initial stabilization, and not delayed in an inappropriate facility for time-consuming diagnostic tests. Studies have corroborated excessive mortality resulting from young adolescents receiving care in adult intensive care settings.

3. **Prevention.** Although appropriate management of the injured child improves survival and morbidity statistics, the largest improvement in these areas comes from injury prevention programs and early identification of abusive families.

B. Initial assessment

1. Quick assessment of **airway stability, respirations, circulation,** and **organ function** is required. Large-bore intravenous access is established at this time.

2. A rapid **physical examination** is done, assessing external evidence of trauma and neurologic status after the neck has been stabilized.

3. Initial **emergent interventions** (see VI C) are performed.

4. Appropriate **radiographs,** including cervical spine films, are done rapidly, preferably in an appropriately equipped trauma room rather than in a radiology suite.

5. **Blood tests** are performed, including arterial blood gas, hematocrit, coagulation studies, electrolytes, hepatic enzymes, amylase, and lipase.

6. The **bladder is cannulated** and urine is evaluated for flow and presence of blood.

7. **Further radiologic tests,** such as cystogram and head or abdominal computed tomography (CT) scans, are done if indicated.

8. **Diagnostic peritoneal lavage** is done if emergent treatment of another site requires immediate surgery and precludes abdominal CT studies.

C. Therapy. The patient should be observed and treated in a pediatric intensive care unit.

1. **Airway instability** is treated by endotracheal intubation, tracheotomy, or cricoidotomy.

2. **Respiratory distress** is treated by manual or mechanical ventilation, and, depending on the examination or setting, by placement of thoracostomy tubes both to diagnose and treat potential pneumothorax and hemothorax.

3. **Hypoperfusion** is treated by volume therapy with isotonic crystalloid, colloid, or blood. In the appropriate setting, a pericardial tap may be indicated to rule out and treat potential cardiac tamponade from hemopericardium. Inotropic support is rarely indicated.

4. **Surgical intervention** is guided by the patient's status and the results of the diagnostic evaluation.

D. | **Specific injuries**

1. **Head injuries** may require neurosurgical procedures for relief of **intracranial hematomas**. Fewer than 20% of children with severe head injury have such lesions. Most have severe **cerebral edema** associated with increased ICP not susceptible to surgical intervention.
   a. **Patients with cerebral edema and evidence of increased ICP** on physical or radiologic examination should have an intracranial pressure monitoring device placed, and be treated as described in V A 4. Appropriate rehabilitation should begin as early as possible, with passive range-of-motion exercises (to prevent joint contractures) performed as soon as such stimulation does not cause a dangerous rise in ICP.
   b. **Infants with intracranial injuries suggestive of child abuse** must be completely evaluated for other occult injuries, especially **occult fractures** (see Chapter 2).
      (1) Intracranial injuries highly suggestive of abusive etiology include interhemispheric subarachnoid/subdural bleeds, acute and chronic subdural hematomas, retinal hemorrhages, and cerebral edema.
      (2) The likelihood of abuse increases dramatically if these injuries are found in a child with no history of severe impact or deceleration trauma. Falls from less than 3 feet are insufficient to explain such injuries. Falls of less than 3 stories are unlikely to cause such injuries, and the reliability of the history should be examined carefully.

2. **Hepatic and splenic lacerations** are best diagnosed by abdominal CT examination. Surgical repair or resection is rarely required; usually such lesions tamponade, followed by hemostasis and healing.
   a. **Nonoperative management,** best accomplished in a pediatric intensive care unit, is predicated on close observation for evidence of hypoperfusion, hypotension, falling hematocrit, or any change in physical examination.
   b. **Operative management** is indicated when continued bleeding necessitates large-volume transfusions, shock is present, or associated trauma or medical conditions make appropriate observation impossible.

3. **Seat belt injuries**
   a. **Types.** Inappropriate use of lap belts in small children may lead to a triad of **abdominal injuries,** including hepatic or splenic laceration, dislocation of the lumbosacral spine, and visceral contusion. The small bowel and pancreas are frequent sites of injury; vascular trauma may occur as well.
   b. **Signs.** Seat belt injury may be indicated by external bruising of the abdomen where the lap belt applied pressure.
   c. **Therapy** is specific as indicated for the discovered lesions.

4. **Spinal cord trauma**
   a. **Evaluation**
      (1) Evaluation of the spinal column should be done immediately in all cases of multiple or severe trauma. Cervical support should be continued until the entire cervical spine including the odontoid has been adequately evaluated and cleared.
      (2) The comatose "drowning" victim must also be evaluated for cervical trauma secondary to vertex compression from a diving accident.
   b. **Complications.** Unrecognized fractures or dislocations of the spinal column may lead to paraplegia, quadriplegia, or death because of inappropriate handling.
   c. **Therapy**
      (1) Stabilization of the vertebral column by halo traction or operative spinal fusion is mandatory.

    (2) Glucocorticoid or GM_1 ganglioside administration in the initial posttrauma period may limit ultimate severity of sequelae.

    (3) Supportive care may include mechanical ventilation, bladder catheterization, and adaptive equipment.

    (4) Associated injuries must be treated appropriately.

5. Orthopedic Injuries. Any fracture occurring in a child younger than 6 to 12 months of age is highly suggestive of abuse and should be followed by a complete plain film and isotope skeletal survey to rule out other occult fractures. Metabolic bone diseases should be ruled out by appropriate radiography and blood testing.

  a. Fractures especially indicative of abusive trauma include:

    (1) Metaphyseal corner fractures

    (2) Posterior rib fractures

    (3) Spiral or oblique fractures in a premobile child

    (4) Stellate or widely diastatic skull fractures

  b. Abusive fractures in infancy are frequently associated with intracranial injury, and head CT scanning should be done in all such cases.

  c. Damage to growth plates in young children may be difficult to assess radiographically, and may result in disparity of growth in those regions.

VII. NUTRITIONAL SUPPORT DURING CRITICAL ILLNESS

A. High-stress states (sepsis and multiple trauma)

1. Metabolic pathophysiology

  a. Secretion of counterregulatory hormones (endogenous catecholamines, glucocorticoids, glucagon, and the like) leads to **relative insulin resistance** and **hyperglycemia**.

  b. Hyperpyrexia, increased cardiac demands, and healing of wounds lead to a **marked increase in metabolic activity, oxygen** and **energy consumption,** and **carbon dioxide generation**.

  c. These increased metabolic demands lead to a requirement for **increased alveolar ventilation** and may predispose to early **respiratory failure**.

  d. In the absence of adequate caloric and protein sources, muscle proteins are broken down for gluconeogenesis and amino acids for protein synthesis.

  e. These processes may lead to severe **malnutrition** in a short period. This state is associated with anergy, infectious complications, and high mortality.

2. Nutritional support

  a. General guidelines

    (1) Multiple organ failure or abdominal trauma may prevent early enteral feeding. In this case, parenteral alimentation should be established within the first 48 hours of treatment.

    (2) Enteral feeding during the hypermetabolic phase should also conform to the need for increased protein sources. This may be accomplished by using parenteral or enteral formulas designed for the severely stressed patient, or by adding protein supplements to standard enteral formulas.

  b. Specific guidelines

    (1) A **positive nitrogen balance** should be provided as soon as possible. This requires higher protein–calorie ratios than a normal diet because carbohydrates are being handled inefficiently.

    (2) Provision of **fat** in the early period prevents essential fatty acid deficiency and may decrease carbon dioxide production by lowering the metabolic rate. This may help prevent or ameliorate respiratory failure.

    (3) The increased metabolic requirements in such patients imply that calories must be provided in substantially greater than normal amounts to prevent muscle breakdown for energy generation.

B. **Renal failure** (see Chapter 14)

    1. Metabolic pathophysiology

        a. Impaired excretion of nitrogen as urea leads to **uremia,** which potentially contributes to platelet dysfunction and hyperosmolar states. Limited caloric intake causing muscle breakdown for gluconeogenesis may increase urea production and worsen uremia.

        b. Impaired ability to excrete water leads to **hypervolemia,** exacerbated by excess sodium ingestion.

        c. Impaired ability to synthesize vitamin D_3 leads to **hypocalcemia, hyperphosphatemia,** and **secondary hyperparathyroidism**.

    2. Nutritional support may be provided parenterally using relatively low amounts of well-balanced essential amino acid preparations in conjunction with carbohydrate and lipid sources. Enteral nutrition should be provided with a diet or enteral formula that conforms to the following guidelines.

        a. The nutritional source must be low in protein, sodium, and phosphate.

        b. The nutritional source must provide adequate calories to meet metabolic needs.

C. **Hepatic failure** (see Chapter 11)

    1. Metabolic pathophysiology

        a. Extreme hepatic insufficiency causes an inability to detoxify NH_3 to urea, and thus may result in **hyperammonemia,** a state that is highly toxic to the brain.

        b. A relative inability to metabolize aromatic amino acids may lead to high concentrations of these substances. In association with hyperammonemia and the other derangements caused by fulminant hepatic failure, this may lead to **hepatic encephalopathy**.

        c. An inability to store glucose as glycogen and impaired hepatic gluconeogenesis create an intolerance of fasting and result in **hypoglycemia**.

        d. Impaired production and secretion of bile acids may cause **impaired absorption of long-chain fatty acids**.

    2. Nutritional support

        a. Protein sources must be limited to help prevent hyperammonemia. Some authorities recommend also limiting sources containing aromatic amino acids.

        b. High-density carbohydrate sources should be used as continuous infusions (parenteral or enteral) to prevent hypoglycemia.

VIII. ETHICAL ISSUES IN PEDIATRIC INTENSIVE CARE (see also Chapter 6)

A. **Brain death.** Although the legal validity of brain death determination has been established (see V B), a single physician caring for the possibly brain dead patient, as well as for a potential transplant recipient, may face an ethical dilemma.

    1. Areas of potential conflict

        a. Potentially transplantable organs may be made nonviable by delays in establishing cerebral death.

        b. Evaluation to determine whether one or more organs may be suitable for transplantation, or treatments designed to enhance the viability of donated organs, may be of no benefit to the prospective donor. Indeed, if such a protocol requires invasive procedures or trips away from the intensive care unit, it may limit the patient's small chances of improvement and survival (procedures done before final determination that brain death is present).

    2. Ethical resolution

        a. The attending physician has an ethical responsibility to establish brain death promptly, and to participate in decisions as to what benefit or risk a procedure that may benefit a potential recipient may present to that physician's patient.

        b. Questions of risk and benefit that are not easily resolved should be presented to the hospital ethics committee.

B. **Do not resuscitate (DNR) orders**

1. **Areas of potential conflict.** By definition, minors have never been legally competent, and therefore would have been unable to create a **"living will"** or **durable power of attorney** before catastrophic, life-threatening illness or injury. Therefore, decisions relating to resuscitation in the event of further deterioration or cardiopulmonary arrest must be based on the **substituted judgment** of others, such as relatives, physicians, judges, or other interested parties. Such parties may not be in agreement over the proper course of action, necessitating mediation by courts or other third parties.

2. **Ethical resolution.** In general, in the absence of mental incompetency or evidence of child abuse or neglect, the parents are considered the guardians of the child's best interests.
   a. Conflicts between the parents as to the aggressiveness of future therapy should be discussed with the attending physician and other significant support figures, such as clergy. In the absence of uniform agreement, intervention will continue to be provided.
   b. Conflicts between parents and medical staff as to indications for emergent intervention may necessitate consultation with the hospital ethics committee. However, if the medical staff insists that DNR status is unwarranted and tantamount to medical neglect, legal resolution may be required.

C. **Removal of supportive therapy** may be requested by families or recommended by physicians in situations in which a child is unlikely to survive or to regain a significant level of function. The substituted judgment of the family is required in this case (see VIII B).

1. **Areas of potential conflict**
   a. Many people believe that a decision not to initiate a therapy is fundamentally different from a decision to discontinue an administered therapy. This perception is by no means universal.
   b. The legal status of the decision to remove a patient who is not brain dead from life support currently varies from state to state, but the **right to die** has been upheld by the Supreme Court in very narrowly defined circumstances. Some states have enacted legislation further defining and expanding this right. Some of these state acts apply to minors.

2. **Ethical resolution**
   a. Discontinuation of life-supporting therapy in a patient who is not brain dead is predicated on consensus of parents and physicians (where legally permissible).
   b. Conflict between parents and physicians should be referred to the hospital ethics committee. However, resolution in the absence of final consensus may require adjudication.

D. **Religious objections to therapy**

1. **Areas of potential conflict**
   a. Free exercise of religion by a family may be in conflict with the state's interest in the welfare of a child, and with the child's right to adequate care.
   b. Examples of such conflicts may be seen in children of Jehovah's Witnesses who require blood transfusion, or children of faith healers who require antibiotics for life-threatening infection or treatment for some other severe illness or injury.

2. **Ethical resolution**
   a. The legal and ethical consensus is that an adult may refuse treatment for himself, but that the child's right to treatment is safeguarded by the state when lack of treatment will make death likely or probable.
   b. Because such an act does represent infringement of the parents' right to free exercise of religion, court orders for such treatment are given only when evidence of clear danger of imminent death without therapy is provided.

BIBLIOGRAPHY

Chameides L, Hazinski M (eds.): *Textbook of Pediatric Advanced Life Support*. Dallas, American Heart Association, 1994.

STUDY QUESTIONS

DIRECTIONS: Each of the numbered items or incomplete statements in this section is followed by answers or by completions of the statement. Select the ONE lettered answer or completion that is BEST in each case.

1. A 3-year-old child is a passenger during a two-car collision. The child had been restrained with a lap belt. On presentation, the child is alert and normotensive, but has a tender right upper quadrant, and the possible diagnosis of hepatic laceration is entertained. Which of the following is true concerning this lesion?

(A) The lesion is best demonstrated by radionuclide liver–spleen scan.
(B) The laceration typically requires surgical exploration and repair.
(C) This child is not at risk for hepatic laceration because a lap belt was used.
(D) Hepatic lacerations are not associated with any other significant injuries.
(E) None of the above statements is true.

Questions 2 and 3

A young infant is rushed to the emergency department by a hysterical parent who speaks no English. The infant is cyanotic, breathing with gasping respirations, and has a heart rate of 40.

2. Which of the following best describes the physiologic status of this patient?

(A) cardiopulmonary failure
(B) shock
(C) respiratory failure
(D) respiratory distress
(E) cardiopulmonary arrest

3. The first intervention that should be performed in this child is

(A) intraosseous cannulation
(B) synchronized cardioversion
(C) chest compressions
(D) 100% oxygen by face mask or hood
(E) bag-and-mask ventilation with 100% oxygen

Questions 4 and 5

A 16-year-old boy with Duchenne muscular dystrophy presents to the emergency department with increasing respiratory distress and cyanosis in room air. Physical examination reveals a diaphoretic adolescent, in marked respiratory distress, with gasping respirations, poor air entry, a heart rate of 160, and diminished responsiveness. The parents assert that no one has ever discussed end-of-life decisions with them, and they insist that they want everything possible done for their son.

4. Which of the following is the most appropriate immediate sequence of interventions?

(A) Tell family that support is futile, because of the fatal nature of Duchenne muscular dystrophy, and hence you will not institute mechanical ventilation.
(B) Bag-and-mask ventilate with 100% oxygen, followed by rapid-sequence intubation and mechanical ventilation.
(C) Provide high-flow oxygen by mask or nasal cannula, and get a chest radiograph and arterial blood gas reading before making a decision about intubation.
(D) Make a request for emergency medical ethics committee consultation to clarify the need to intervene.
(E) Send patient to pulmonary laboratory for pulmonary function tests.

5. The child is intubated and treated for pneumonia. Over the next week, his radiographic status consistently improves, with resolution of consolidation and atelectasis. However, it becomes difficult to wean him from the ventilator. Which of the following therapeutic modalities might improve his ability to breathe while off the ventilator?

(A) pressure-controlled ventilation
(B) pressure-supported ventilation
(C) supplemental oxygen
(D) tracheostomy
(E) nasopharyngeal tube

6. A 3-month-old child presents with a history of several days of nonspecific upper respiratory symptoms, and one day of poor feeding and decreased activity. On physical examination, the child has a respiratory rate of 50, with mild retractions, a heart rate of 260, and a capillary refill time of 4 seconds. Crackles are heard on auscultation of the chest. Blood pressure is 80/55, and oxygen saturation is 95% in room air. Cardiac monitor confirms heart rate of 260 with narrow complexes. Intravenous access is easily obtained. The initial therapy plan for this child should include which of the following?

(A) fluid bolus with isotonic crystalloid
(B) dopamine infusion
(C) bolus injection of adenosine
(D) bag-and-mask ventilation followed by intubation
(E) echocardiogram

Questions 7–9

A 12-year-old child presents to the emergency department with a 6-hour history of high fever, an ecchymotic rash, and decreasing mental status. On initial physical examination, the respiratory rate is 25, with deep but unlabored respirations, the heart rate is 180, the child is poorly responsive, even to noxious stimulation, and central pulses are bounding, but distal pulses are thready or absent. Capillary refill time is 7 seconds. Purpura is present at many sites, and is confluent over the distal extremities. Temperature is 40.5°C (105°F) and blood pressure is 90/32.

7. What is this child's physiologic status?

(A) respiratory distress
(B) respiratory failure
(C) cardiopulmonary failure
(D) shock
(E) cardiac arrest

8. All of the following would be appropriate as part of the early management of this child EXCEPT

(A) fluid bolus to restore circulating blood volume
(B) beta-blocking agent to decrease heart rate and thereby decrease oxygen consumption
(C) inotropic support with alpha-agonistic agents to increase contractility while increasing vasoconstriction
(D) antibiotic administration to treat the presumed infection
(E) invasive monitoring of arterial and central venous pressure

9. All of the following would be expected to occur as a result of the metabolic derangements occurring in this patient EXCEPT

(A) hypoglycemia
(B) increased carbon dioxide production
(C) anergy
(D) catabolism of muscle proteins
(E) gluconeogenesis

DIRECTIONS: Each set of matching questions in this section consists of a list of four to twenty-six lettered options (some of which may be in figures) followed by several numbered items. For each numbered item, select the ONE lettered option that is most closely associated with it. To avoid spending too much time on matching sets with large numbers of options, it is generally advisable to begin each set by reading the list of options. Then, for each item in the set, try to generate the correct answer and locate it in the option list, rather than evaluating each option individually. Each lettered option may be selected once, more than once, or not at all.

Questions 10–13

For each case listed below, match the associated principal cause of tissue hypoxia.

(A) Decreased alveolar P_{O_2}
(B) Decreased arterial P_{O_2}
(C) Decreased arterial oxygen content
(D) Decreased oxygen delivery

10. A child with new-onset leukemia presents to the hospital with a hemoglobin concentration of 3 g/dl.

11. A child experiences respiratory distress and decreased activity tolerance while vacationing in the Grand Teton Mountains.

12. A child presents to the emergency room in severe hypovolemic shock from diarrhea and dehydration.

13. A newborn is extremely cyanotic in room air. Evaluation reveals pulmonary atresia and a large ventricular septal defect.

1. The answer is E *[VI D 2]*. Hepatic lacerations are best demonstrated by abdominal computed tomography (CT) scan. Most typically, the lesion tamponades itself and does not require surgical repair. These injuries may occur in conjunction with other abdominal or extraabdominal injuries, and often occur as a result of seat belt use by inappropriately young children. In this setting, the laceration is often accompanied by surface bruising, intestinal injury, and lumbar vertebral dislocation.

2. The answer is A *[II C 1 c]*. Cardiopulmonary failure is a state characterized by agonal respirations and bradycardia. It may arise from respiratory failure or from shock, and is quickly followed by cardiac arrest if intervention is not appropriate.

3. The answer is E *[II C 2 e]*. The first intervention in the patient with cardiopulmonary failure is provision of adequate ventilation. If vital signs improve with bag-and-mask ventilation or subsequent intubation, respiratory failure was the source of the condition. Transition to a shock state after ventilation implies circulatory compromise as the etiology, and further interventions are guided by the remainder of the assessment.

4. The answer is B *[II C 2 c; VIII B]*. This child is in severe respiratory failure by physical examination, and is at high risk for imminent death if no action is taken. The parents, who are presumed to be speaking for the best interests of the child, wish aggressive treatment to be provided, and the child is not in a condition to express his own wishes. Referral to the medical ethics committee or legal resolution is impractical because of the need for immediate intervention. Therefore, the parents' wishes should be respected, and appropriate intervention performed. Definitive therapy (i.e., intubation and mechanical ventilation) should not be deferred to perform diagnostic tests.

5. The answer is D *[III B 2]*. This child's primary problem is that he is too weak to generate an adequate tidal volume, and thus his alveolar ventilation is impaired. Tracheostomy reduces both airway resistance and dead space, thus increasing his tidal volume, and wasting less of it in dead space ventilation. In addition, it provides access for direct suctioning of secretions, which may help prevent atelectasis. This may be enough to allow him to wean from mechanical ventilation.

Although pressure-supported ventilation improves his ability to breathe spontaneously, it presumes that he is attached to a mechanical device. A nasopharyngeal tube helps only when there is an obstruction between the nose and the posterior pharynx. In the absence of such an obstruction, it actually raises airway resistance by providing a smaller diameter airway. Pressure-controlled ventilation is a means of mechanical ventilation, not an aid to spontaneous ventilation. Supplemental oxygen increases Po_2, but will not assist alveolar ventilation.

6. The answer is C *[II C 2 g]*. This is a typical presentation for supraventricular tachycardia in an infant. Although this child is probably in the early phases of shock (increased capillary refill time), the source is cardiogenic because of prolonged, severe tachycardia, rather than relative or absolute hypovolemia. Administration of a fluid bolus would be likely to worsen the respiratory status and would not alleviate the shock. Dopamine infusion would be likely to exacerbate the primary problem of tachycardia. Although the child does have some mild respiratory distress (mild tachypnea and retractions), there are no indications of respiratory failure, and thus intubation is not indicated. Intravenous adenosine is likely rapidly to abort the supraventricular tachycardia. Most commonly, normal sinus rhythm is resumed immediately afterward. Appropriate treatment of this compromised child should not be delayed for diagnostic procedures that can be done more appropriately after resolution of the initial problem.

7. The answer is D *[II C 1 c]*. This child exhibits many of the features of shock. There are poor distal pulses, markedly prolonged capillary refill time, and evidence of impaired vital organ function (decreased mental status). This presentation is very typical of septic shock, one of the causes of distributive shock.

8. The answer is B *[IV B 2 c]*. The goal in treatment of distributive shock is to maintain the patient in the hyperdynamic (early) phase of shock, which helps to prevent irreversible, multiple–organ-system failure, with a high likelihood of death. This is best accomplished by addressing all components of hemodynamic support: preload, contractility, and afterload. In this setting, the patient usually exhibits significant vasodilation, which lowers mean arterial pressure, although systolic pressure may be normal. Accordingly, alpha-agonist agents are preferred because they restore some measure of vasoconstriction, which raises diastolic, mean, and systolic pressures, enhancing perfusion. It is also important to reverse the initial derangement that led to the shock. In this case, the marked elevation in temperature and the extensive purpura are suggestive of infection with *Neisseria meningitidis*, although *Streptococcus pneumoniae* and other bacterial pathogens may be the source of infection. Antibiotic therapy should be started promptly, and not delayed significantly by other procedures. Invasive monitoring may help guide inotropic support and fluid management. In addition, central access may be helpful for administration of multiple drugs, as well as nutritional support.

9. The answer is A *[VII A 1]*. Sepsis syndrome creates a metabolic pattern characterized by insulin resistance, hyperglycemia, increased metabolic rate with increased oxygen consumption and carbon dioxide production, decreased immune status, and rapid muscle catabolism for gluconeogenesis and generation of amino acids for protein synthesis. Hypoglycemia is not characteristic of this syndrome.

10–13. The answers are: 10-C, 11-A *[III A 1 b, Table 7-3]*, **12-D, 13-B** *[Table 7-3]*. Severe anemia causes marked decrease in arterial oxygen content by decreasing the amount of oxygen bound to hemoglobin. This is independent of arterial P_{O_2}, which remains normal. High elevations are associated with lower barometric pressure, which lower alveolar P_{O_2}. A child in shock has diminished oxygen delivery because of decreased cardiac output, independent of arterial P_{O_2} and oxygen content. A child with cyanotic congenital heart disease has right-to-left shunting. Arterial P_{O_2} is diminished despite normal alveolar P_{O_2} and lung structures because the blood does not contact alveolar gas.

Chapter 8
Birth Defects and Genetic Disorders
Suzanne B. Cassidy
David A. H. Whiteman

I. OVERVIEW

A. **Definition.** Medically significant birth defects are congenital anomalies that require some form of medical intervention. Birth defects range in severity from relatively minor anomalies (e.g., polydactyly) to severe or systemic conditions (e.g., hydrocephalus, Down syndrome).

B. **Incidence.** The population risk for medically significant birth defects is approximately 3% of all live-born infants. However, not all birth defects are detected at birth; for example, some forms of kidney disorders, congenital heart disease, and mental retardation are diagnosed later in life. Congenital anomalies cause 10% of all neonatal deaths.

C. **Etiologic classification.** The entire spectrum of human development is guided by the interaction of genetic makeup and the environment. Most birth defects are caused by environmental factors, genetic alterations, or a combination of both. In some cases, birth defects are caused by unknown factors and are called sporadic disorders.

1. **Environmental factors** are known to cause at least 10% of all birth defects. **Teratogens** are environmental agents that cause congenital anomalies by interfering with embryonic or fetal organogenesis, growth, or cellular physiology, or by disrupting previously normal tissue (see II).

2. **Genetic disorders.** Genetic factors are responsible for many **single birth defects** as well as many **syndromes** (see I D 2). **Contiguous gene deletion syndromes** are a newly recognized class of human genetic disorders due to the absence of several neighboring genes. These defects cause recognizable but variable conditions, often with several diverse manifestations. In some cases, microdeletions are visible by high-resolution chromosome analysis; in others, they are not. The recognition of such syndromes can be aided by review of the rapidly accumulating information on the human genome.

3. **Sporadic disorders** present no risk to future offspring. These disorders often are the result of accidents of embryonic development or gestation (e.g., blood vessel occlusion). Some birth defects probably are caused by new autosomal dominant mutations that are lethal before reproductive age or that interfere with the reproductive potential of affected individuals. These defects are difficult to distinguish from sporadic disorders.

D. **Dysmorphism and syndromes**

1. **Dysmorphism** is an abnormality in form or structural development. The presence of abnormal physical features often suggests an underlying (often genetic) disorder and sometimes portends the presence of other (internal) abnormalities of form or function.
   a. **Dysmorphic features** are those that fall outside the range of normal.
      (1) **Causes of dysmorphic features** fall into three major categories (Table 8-1).
      (2) **Objectively measurable features.** For many features (e.g., height, weight, head circumference), there are objectively measurable norms.

TABLE 8-1. Categories of Birth Defects and Dysmorphism

Category	Pathogenesis	Causes
Malformations	Poor tissue formation	Genetic Teratogenic
Deformations	Abnormal mechanical forces	Crowding Oligohydramnios Abnormal position
Disruptions	Destruction of normal tissue	Amniotic bands Thrombosis

(a) An example is interpupillary distance: Patients whose distance is measurably smaller than normal have **hypotelorism,** and patients whose distance is greater than normal have **hypertelorism**.

(b) Other measurable features include inner canthal and outer canthal distances, ear length, hand and foot length, penis and clitoral length, and upper-to-lower segment ratios.

(3) **Subjectively observable features.** Some features must be judged subjectively by contrast with the normal population.

(a) Examples of subjectively observable dysmorphic features include a flat facial profile, a small chin, a down-turned mouth, an abnormally curled ear, and abnormal palmar creases.

(b) Subjectively observable dysmorphic features require careful observation. The features of a dysmorphic-appearing child should be compared with those of the parents in an attempt to distinguish between subjectively dysmorphic features and familial characteristics. One or more dysmorphic features may be present in otherwise completely normal individuals.

b. **Minor anomalies** are unusual morphologic features that are of no serious medical or cosmetic consequence to the patient.

(1) Examples include ear pits, toe syndactyly, curved fifth fingers, and unusual ear shape.

(2) The significance of minor anomalies is that they serve as valuable clues to a possible underlying pattern of malformation or to isolated major internal malformations.

(3) The presence of **two or more minor anomalies** should lead to a more extensive evaluation of the patient.

2. **Syndromes** are recognizable patterns of internal and/or external structural and functional abnormalities or malformations that are known or presumed to be the result of a single cause. Recognizable patterns of dysmorphic features, with or without other abnormalities, often constitute syndromes; Down syndrome is a classic example of dysmorphic features in a recognizable pattern [see IV B 1 b (1)]. Some syndromes, however, have no associated dysmorphic features.

a. Every feature that is part of a syndrome need not necessarily be present in a given individual with the syndrome. People with the same syndrome share a number of features, but not necessarily any one feature or any specific combination of them. In most cases, no one feature is pathognomonic for a syndrome.

b. It is not uncommon for the features characteristic of syndromes to develop over time, so that it may not always be possible to make a diagnosis in a very young child.

c. Syndromes can be sporadic and of unknown etiology, or caused by single gene abnormalities, chromosomal anomalies, teratogens, or deformations.

3. **Patient evaluation.** The presence of dysmorphic features in a patient should lead to the search for other abnormalities and for an underlying disorder. A careful evaluation of the dysmorphic child is important so that a diagnosis can be reached (Table 8-2). Diagnosis currently is achieved in about 50% of dysmorphic children.

TABLE 8-2. Evaluation Patterns of Malformation

Evaluation	Examples of Areas of Focus
Family history	Consanguinity Similar problems Other birth defects Abnormal mental development Pregnancy loss
Prenatal history	Mechanical forces Teratogen exposure
Physical examination	Dysmorphic features Growth Development
Neurologic examination	Asymmetry Eye problems Altered tone
Laboratory studies	Chromosomes Prenatal infection titers Metabolic studies
Imaging studies	Computed tomography or magnetic resonance imaging scan of the brain Ultrasound of heart or kidneys Skeletal radiographs

    a. Prenatal history should pay particular attention to potential causes of abnormal features such as oligohydramnios, abnormal uterine structure, abnormal fetal position, abnormal fetal activity, twinning, fibroids, medications, and illicit drugs.

    b. Physical examination should focus on seeking a pattern of features that has been previously described.

E. **Genetic counseling** is made available to individuals who have a positive history of genetic disorders or other birth defects and to those who are at increased risk for having a child with a birth defect.

  1. Establishing a specific diagnosis. The ability to make a specific diagnosis allows better medical management of affected individuals, because the natural history of etiologically separate disorders with similar manifestations may be very different.

  2. Evaluating recurrence risk. Once a diagnosis has been made, and thus the pattern of inheritance, if any, is known, it becomes possible to discuss recurrence risks for birth defects and **prenatal diagnosis** for future pregnancies.

    a. If a couple has a child with a specific genetic condition, that couple's risk for having another child with a birth defect equals their risk for having a child with this specific condition plus the background risk of 3% with each pregnancy.

    b. If a birth defect is caused by a known environmental agent (e.g., radiation, alcohol), the risk for recurrence of the specific birth defect in future pregnancies can sometimes be eliminated.

  3. Pedigree analysis is the first step in most genetic counseling. A four-generation pedigree is constructed for each family, including all medical information.

    a. Ethnic background is ascertained for all family members because some conditions (especially autosomal recessive disorders) occur with increased frequency in specific populations. Certain ethnic subgroups are at increased risk for having children with specific autosomal recessive disorders owing to inbreeding (Table 8-3).

    b. Family history of birth defects and pregnancy loss is noted because they may give clues to genetic disorders.

TABLE 8-3. Populations at Increased Risk for Specific Genetic Disorders

Population	Disease
Northern European Caucasian	Cystic fibrosis
African descent	Sickle cell disease
Ashkenazi Jews, French Canadians	Tay-Sachs disease
Mediterranean descent	α-Thalassemia
Southeast Asians	β-Thalassemia

    c. Husband–wife consanguinity is noted because this leads to an increased risk for having a child with a birth defect, particularly an autosomal recessive disorder or multifactorial disorder, because people who are related are more likely to carry the same rare genes than are those who are not related.

F. **Prenatal diagnostic procedures** allow detection of birth defects and genetic disorders before delivery and usually before the third trimester. Detection of birth defects in pregnancy allows parents the option of pregnancy termination or additional time for emotional adjustment. Early detection also affects how the physician manages the remainder of the pregnancy, delivery, and neonatal period. Available prenatal diagnostic procedures include the following. Indications for prenatal testing are listed in Table 8-4.

    1. Maternal serum α-fetoprotein (AFP) level reflects a fetal protein in maternal blood.
        a. It can be offered to every pregnant woman at 15–17 weeks' gestation because there are no risks involved.
        b. Elevated AFP level indicates increased risk for neural tube defects, other open defects, and fetal bleeding. Low AFP level indicates increased risk for trisomies.
        c. Combining maternal serum testing for AFP with testing levels of unconjugated estriol and human chorionic gonadotropin, which is sometimes called the **triple test** or triple screen, allows improved ascertainment of fetuses at risk for Down syndrome. It also provides improved indication of risk for trisomies 18 and 13, as well as for Turner syndrome (45,XO) with hydrops.

    2. Fetal ultrasound is a safe test that can be offered in pregnancies in which there is a risk for structural fetal anomalies or growth abnormalities. Currently there are no known associated risks for the fetus or mother from ultrasound testing.
        a. Level I ultrasound is performed in most obstetric office settings to evaluate fetal size, growth, number of fetuses, and viability. If abnormalities are suspected, most patients are referred for level II ultrasound.
        b. Level II ultrasound is offered at centers that specialize in the care of high-risk pregnancies and management of fetal abnormalities. Major structural abnormalities of most organ systems can be diagnosed and evaluated. Level II ultrasound is often performed in conjunction with amniocentesis and chorionic villus sampling (see I F 4).

TABLE 8-4. Some Indications for Prenatal Testing

	Risk
Women $\geq$ 35 years of age	Down syndrome
Elevated maternal serum AFP or triple test	Open defect (e.g., neural tube defect)
Low maternal serum AFP	Down syndrome
Prior history of autosomal trisomy	Trisomy
Parent with balanced chromosome translocation	Unbalanced karyotype
Family history of genetic disorder or carrier parent	Specific disorder in family
Family history of isolated structural defect	Same structural defect

AFP = α-fetoprotein.

3. **Amniocentesis**
   a. **Technique**
      (1) **Timing.** Amniocentesis usually is performed at about 16 weeks' gestation. **Early amniocentesis,** performed at 12–14 weeks, is being used increasingly.
      (2) **Procedure.** In routine amniocentesis, a needle is inserted into the amniotic cavity and approximately 30 ml of amniotic fluid are removed. The fluid or living fetal cell material it contains is evaluated for fetal chromosome anomalies, specific biochemical or molecular genetic abnormalities, or for AFP level. In early amniocentesis, 1 ml/week gestation is withdrawn.
      (3) **Complications** occur in 1/200 to 1/400 tests and include:
         (a) **Spontaneous labor,** leading to spontaneous abortion
         (b) **Amniotic fluid leakage,** leading to spontaneous labor or oligohydramnios
         (c) **Needle puncture of the fetus** (rare)
         (d) **Infection** (rare, because the procedure is done aseptically)
   b. **Indications.** Amniocentesis is offered primarily to women whose risk for having an affected fetus is greater than the underlying risk for complications from the procedure. This high-risk group includes those listed in Table 8-4.

4. **Chorionic villus sampling (CVS)**
   a. **Technique.** A polyethylene catheter is placed through the cervix via the transvaginal route under ultrasound guidance, or a needle is inserted transabdominally into the developing placenta. Chorionic villus cells of the placenta are aspirated through the tube and can be used for chromosomal, DNA, or biochemical studies.
   b. **Complications.** Compared to amniocentesis, CVS poses a greater risk (1%–1.5%) for fetal loss and for maternal infection (chorioamnionitis).
   c. **Advantages.** A major advantage of CVS is the early gestational age at which the test is offered. This allows lower anxiety for the family, compared to amniocentesis, because fetal movements have not been felt yet and the fetus is not yet completely formed. If an abnormality is detected and the parents opt to terminate the pregnancy, the procedure is less psychologically traumatic and of lower risk at or before 12 weeks (when CVS results are available) than at 18–20 weeks (when amniocentesis results are available).
   d. **Disadvantages**
      (1) It is not possible to perform amniotic fluid AFP testing with CVS because this test is done so early in pregnancy and only fetal cells are obtained.
      (2) Owing to the possibility of chromosomally differing cell lines in the chorionic villi (**mosaicism;** see IV A 1 c), CVS results occasionally are ambiguous, necessitating further evaluation with amniocentesis.

5. **Percutaneous umbilical blood sampling (PUBS)** is a procedure in which fetal blood is obtained from the umbilical cord with ultrasound guidance but without direct visualization. The test is used for chromosome analysis and biochemical study of fetal blood for conditions such as hemophilia. The complication risk of the procedure is 2%–3%.

6. **Fetoscopy**
   a. **Technique.** Fetoscopy is an infrequently used procedure whereby a small fiberoptic instrument is inserted, under ultrasound guidance, transabdominally into the uterine cavity where the fetus is visualized and can be examined. The technique can also be used to obtain **fetal skin biopsy specimens** for prenatal diagnosis of genetic skin disorders such as ichthyosis.
   b. **Complications.** The risk of this procedure is approximately 3%–5%, with complications involving bleeding, pregnancy loss, infection, and amniotic fluid leakage.

7. **DNA analysis** has increased the ability to make diagnoses in single-gene disorders, even in some conditions in which the mutant gene product has not yet been identified. Through the use of restriction endonucleases from bacteria and recombinant DNA technology, it has been possible to find **restriction fragment length polymorphisms (RFLPs),** which permit detection of abnormal genes through linked gene markers.

a. Linkage analysis. Many RFLPs are not located within the gene being sought but are located sufficiently close on the same chromosome that linkage analysis can be used, because the RFLP segregates with the gene.

    (1) For many disorders, the use of this technique requires that several family members—including one affected individual—undergo DNA analysis of their leukocytes or skin fibroblasts. In informative families, this allows the possibility of prenatal diagnosis from amniocytes or CVS.

        (a) Informative families are those in which the RFLPs on the chromosome carrying the mutation are different than the RFLPs on the chromosome with the normal gene, or those in which the RFLPs in the parent with the gene are different than those of the parent not carrying the gene.

        (b) When both chromosomes or both parents have the same RFLPs, they cannot be distinguished by linkage analysis, and so are **uninformative**.

    (2) Examples of disorders in which this methodology can be used include polycystic kidney disease, neurofibromatosis, and tuberous sclerosis.

b. Direct detection. In an increasing number of disorders, genetic analysis allows direct detection of the abnormal gene itself (e.g., cystic fibrosis, sickle cell disease, fragile X syndrome) through the use of DNA probes complementary to the gene that detect alterations in the gene itself. In these cases, other family members do not need to be tested because linkage analysis is not needed.

II. ENVIRONMENTAL FACTORS

A. **General principles.** Proving the relationship between a substance to which a fetus is exposed and a birth defect involves the consideration of several important factors. Usually, not every exposed fetus shows the effect of a teratogen.

    1. Teratogen specificity. A teratogen increases the risk for a specific malformation or a specific pattern of malformations. A general increase in all malformations usually is the result of a bias of ascertainment.

    2. Timing of exposure is vital, because morphogenesis occurs for only the first 8–12 weeks, so that any structural abnormality in tissue development must occur before 12 weeks' gestation. Growth and central nervous system (CNS) development are primarily affected thereafter. Exposure before implantation (days 7–10 postconception) results in loss of the embryo or produces no effect.

    3. Dosage is important. In many cases, there is a threshold below which no effect is demonstrable.

    4. Genetic constitution of the mother and, especially, the fetus determines whether a specific fetus will be affected. For example, only 11% of fetuses whose mothers take hydantoin during pregnancy will exhibit fetal hydantoin syndrome.

    5. Interaction between a potential teratogen and other exposures also must be considered.

B. **Infectious agents,** especially the **"TORCH" organisms,** are known to be responsible for a significant proportion of birth defects (Table 8-5; see Chapter 6 V 3 b).

C. **Medication, drugs, and chemicals** can interfere with embryonic and fetal development.

    1. Hydantoin exposure during pregnancy can cause fetal growth disturbance and skeletal and CNS abnormalities. A specific pattern of anomalies, the **fetal hydantoin syndrome,** is seen in some exposed infants.

    2. Thalidomide exposure during pregnancy has been associated with limb malformations and cleft palate.

TABLE 8-5. Prenatal Infections Causing Fetal Abnormalities

Infectious Agent	Potential Effects
Toxoplasma gondii (agent of toxoplasmosis)	Poor growth, abnormal CNS development
Rubella virus	Cataracts, deafness, mental retardation, congenital heart defects
Cytomegalovirus	Poor growth, hearing loss, CNS anomalies
Herpes virus	Neonatal encephalitis (with perinatal exposure)
Treponema pallidum (agent of syphilis)	Poor growth, abnormal brain and skeletal development

CNS = central nervous system.

3. **Retinoic acid** exposure during pregnancy, especially exposure to isotretinoin, results in brain, ear, and heart malformations.

4. **Tetracycline** exposure causes dark staining of teeth.

5. **Other teratogenic chemicals** have been described, including anticonvulsants, anticoagulants, antithyroid medications, cancer chemotherapeutic agents, iodine-containing agents, lead, lithium, and mercury.

D. High-dose (usually therapeutic) **radiation** is a teratogenic agent that causes fetal malformations by interfering with cell division and organogenesis. Usually, the dose received by the fetus from diagnostic x-ray studies falls below the threshold for teratogenic effect.

E. **Maternal metabolic disorders** also can adversely influence fetal development.

1. **Diabetes.** Infants of diabetic mothers have a 10%–15% risk for birth defects, particularly those involving the heart, skeleton, brain, and spinal cord. The causative factor is believed to be hyperglycemia. Careful control of diabetes before conception and throughout pregnancy decreases the risk for birth defects.

2. **Phenylketonuria (PKU).** Infants of mothers who have PKU are exposed during pregnancy to excess metabolites of the amino acid phenylalanine. Brain and congenital heart defects occur in nearly every fetus exposed to uncontrolled maternal PKU. Dietary control in the mother, particularly if begun before conception, may significantly decrease this risk [see III B 3 b (2)].

F. **Mechanical forces**

1. **Intrauterine mechanical forces** result in **deformations**.
   a. Intrauterine tumors or fibroids or abnormal uterine anatomy may result in a fetus that is constrained, thereby causing breech presentation, facial distortions, dislocations of the hips, or club feet.
   b. Inadequate amniotic fluid (oligohydramnios) results in severe fetal constraint and may also be associated with hypoplasia of the lungs.

2. **External mechanical forces** can result in **disruptions of fetal blood supply**. These forces can include the formation of bands of tissue from the amniotic sac that can cause hypoplasia of limbs or transverse amputations.

G. **Maternal alcoholism.** Alcohol is the most common major teratogen to which the fetus may be exposed. The amount of alcohol consumed appears to correlate with the degree of adverse effect to the fetus. A genetic predisposition may play a significant role in determining which fetus will be severely or mildly affected by maternal alcohol use and which will be unaffected, although specific genetic factors have not been identified.

1. **Fetal alcohol syndrome** represents a frequent and striking example of a teratogenic disorder.
   a. **Incidence**
      (1) In most populations, fetal alcohol syndrome occurs in 1–2 in 1000 newborns. The syndrome affects 30%–45% of the offspring of women who drink more than four to six drinks per day while pregnant.
      (2) An estimated 10%–20% of cases of mild to moderate mental retardation are the result of the effects of alcohol in utero.
   b. **Clinical features** of fetal alcohol syndrome include CNS dysfunction (mean IQ of 63, infantile tremulousness, childhood hyperactivity), growth deficiencies in all parameters, facial dysmorphism (small eyes, small midface, long smooth philtrum), and other anomalies, including joint contracture and kidney malformations (Figure 8-1).

2. **Possible fetal alcohol effects.** In those offspring of alcoholic women who do not manifest the complete fetal alcohol syndrome, one or more of the anomalies seen in that syndrome can sometimes be found. This has been called possible fetal alcohol effects. It is important to rule out some other etiology for the abnormalities found in offspring of alcoholic women without the complete fetal alcohol syndrome before ascribing the effects to alcohol exposure. This is particularly important as it relates to possible associated findings and recurrence risk.

3. **Miscarriage.** There is an increase in the risk for miscarriage, which is proportional to the amount of alcohol consumed.

4. **Other effects.** Lesser amounts of alcohol have been shown to produce milder symptoms in a proportion of exposed offspring, particularly with regard to size and behavior. Although there is no demonstrated medically significant adverse effect from ingestion of small amounts of alcohol during pregnancy or from an occasional episode of greater intake (binge drinking), there are no data to support a "safe" amount of alcohol use during pregnancy. Thus, the most cautious approach is to avoid alcohol entirely during pregnancy.

H. **Environmental pollutants** of various types have been suggested as possible teratogens, although it has been very difficult to study such agents. Birth defects registries, which exist in many states, may be helpful in implicating or absolving specific environmental pollutants as causes of birth defects.

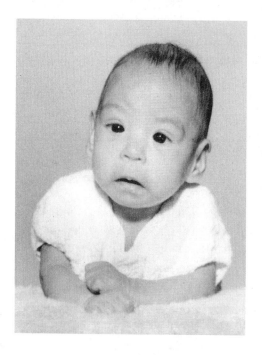

FIGURE 8-1. Characteristic dysmorphic facial features in an infant with fetal alcohol syndrome. Note mild ptosis, epicanthal folds, flat nasal bridge, short nose, long, smooth philtrum, and thin upper vermillion border. (Photograph courtesy of T. Kellerman.)

III. **SINGLE-GENE DISORDERS.** Each human normally has between 50,000 and 100,000 **genes** that are packaged in the 46 chromosomes (22 pairs of **autosomes** and 1 pair of **sex chromosomes**). All genes come in pairs except for the genes on the sex chromosomes of men. Over 5000 different single-gene disorders have been described, which are classified by their mode of inheritance (i.e., autosomal dominant, autosomal recessive, or X-linked).

A. **Autosomal dominant disorders** occur when one gene of a gene pair is altered, or mutated.

1. **General characteristics**
   a. **Defect.** Autosomal dominant disorders often are caused by a **mutation in a gene coding for a structural protein**.
   b. **Recurrence risk.** Any individual with an autosomal dominant disorder has a 50% chance of passing on the mutant gene to offspring. Thus, each child of an affected individual has a 50% chance of being affected.
   c. **Inheritance.** A mutant gene usually is inherited from one parent who is affected with the same condition. Sometimes, an individual will be the first person in a family to display an autosomal dominant trait. This is caused by a **fresh mutation** of that gene in the ovum or spermatocyte that produces the affected individual. The recurrence risk for the parents of a child with a fresh mutation is very low (i.e., equivalent to the chance that another spontaneous mutation will occur). However, the risk for the offspring of the affected individual is 50%.
   d. **Clinical features**
      (1) It is common for autosomal dominant genes to cause conditions that manifest differently and vary in degree of severity among affected individuals. This is called **variable expressivity**. For example, in polycystic kidney disease, some people present with early renal failure, whereas others have only hypertension and normal renal function at the same age. The severity or type of expression of an autosomal dominant disorder in an offspring is usually independent of the way the parent is affected.
      (2) A mutant dominant gene often has an effect on more than one tissue or organ system, which is called **pleiotropy**.

2. **Marfan syndrome** is an autosomal dominant disorder that affects at least 1 in 10,000 newborns. Marfan syndrome demonstrates variable expressivity, pleiotropy, and a high rate of new mutation.
   a. **Defect**
      (1) Marfan syndrome is caused by abnormal fibrillin (the major protein of myofibrils), which results in connective tissue abnormalities.
      (2) The gene for fibrillin (and, therefore, for Marfan syndrome) has been identified and mapped to the long arm of chromosome 15.
         (a) A large number of different mutations in this gene have been identified in people who have the condition.
         (b) Linkage analysis can be accomplished in families with more than one affected family member, allowing diagnosis of symptomatic and presymptomatic individuals and prenatal detection.
         (c) Direct diagnosis in an isolated case is not yet available.
   b. **Clinical features** are listed in Table 8-6 and illustrated in Figure 8-2.
      (1) **Diagnostic criteria**
         (a) To make the diagnosis, at least two of the following major manifestations must be present:
            (i) Typical skeletal findings
            (ii) Typical ocular findings
            (iii) Typical cardiovascular findings
            (iv) Positive family history
         (b) Once a diagnosis is made, the other manifestations should be sought by skeletal measurements, ophthalmologic evaluation, and echocardiography.

TABLE 8-6. Clinical Features of Marfan Syndrome

Skeletal	Long, thin face, limbs, and digits
	Disproportionate tall stature
	High arched palate
	Sternum deformity (asymmetric pectus excavatum/ carinatum)
	Hypermobile joints
	Scoliosis
Cardiac	Aortic root dilatation
	Mitral valve prolapse
	Risk for aortic aneurysm rupture
Ophthalmologic	Lens subluxation
	Flat corneas
	Severe myopia
Pulmonary	Spontaneous pneumothorax
	Emphysema

      (2) Diagnostic challenges. Only 70%–85% of affected people have an affected parent, owing to the high incidence of new dominant mutations in Marfan syndrome. Variability in severity and in manifestations also can make it difficult to prove a positive family history. Usually it is necessary to examine the parents and siblings of a possibly affected individual and to obtain and review medical records of family members who died suddenly or of unknown causes.

   c. Follow-up. Individuals with or suspected of having Marfan syndrome should be followed with annual physical examinations, ophthalmologic evaluations, and echocardiography. Treatment with β-blockers has been effective in reducing the progression of aortic root dilatation, and some cardiologists suggest starting them as soon as the diagnosis is made.

B. **Autosomal recessive disorders** occur when both genes of a gene pair have mutations.

  1. General characteristics
   a. Defect. Many autosomal recessive disorders are caused by mutations in genes coding for **enzymes**. Because half of the normal enzyme activity is adequate under most circumstances, a person with only one mutant gene will not be affected.
   b. Inheritance. An individual in whom both members of a gene pair have mutations is called **homozygous** for that gene. In autosomal recessive disorders, an individual with one mutant and one normal gene for a gene pair is called **heterozygous** for that gene pair and displays no clinical effects from the single mutant gene.
   c. Recurrence risk. Both parents of a child with an autosomal recessive disorder are usually heterozygous for that gene; each child of such a couple has a 25% risk of having the disorder.

  2. Cystic fibrosis is the most common autosomal recessive disorder in whites of European descent. It affects 1 in 2000 newborns in this population (see Chapters 11 and 13).
   a. Defect. A defect in membrane transport of chloride results in an inability to clear mucous secretions in the lungs and causes decreased pancreatic exocrine function.
    (1) Molecular genetic analysis has located the mutant gene on the long arm of chromosome 7.
    (2) More than 300 different mutations of this gene have been identified, and some correlations between the specific mutation and the clinical severity have been made. There is significant ethnic variation in the frequency of different mutations.
    (3) One mutation, called delta-F508, is the mutation on 70% of the chromosomes in patients with cystic fibrosis in the United States.
    (4) The protein product of this gene is a membrane-bound ion transporter called cystic fibrosis transmembrane receptor (CFTR).

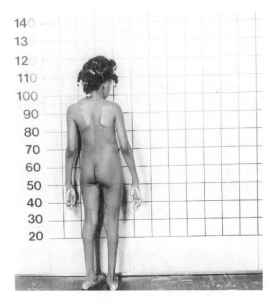

140
130
120
110
100
90
80
70
60
50
40
30
20

FIGURE 8-2. Characteristic body habitus in a 3-year-old child with Marfan syndrome. Note tall stature; thin body habitus with long limbs, long hands, and long flat feet; and scoliosis. (Photograph courtesy of R. Pyeritz, M.D.)

b. Clinical features and course
    (1) Affected children have recurrent pneumonias and intestinal malabsorption. Men are infertile. Growth is secondarily poor.
    (2) Cystic fibrosis usually causes death in early adulthood from pulmonary destruction.
    (3) Some individuals identified as having two genes for cystic fibrosis have few or no manifestations. Others have only congenital absence of the vas deferens.

c. Diagnosis
    (1) Direct DNA analysis using DNA probes can identify 85%–90% of chromosomes carrying a specific cystic fibrosis mutation. In many of the remaining cases, the mutant gene can be detected through genetic linkage of DNA markers, starting from an affected family member.
    (2) Prenatal diagnosis can be accomplished if mutations have been identified in the parents.
    (3) It is appropriate to screen unaffected relatives of individuals with cystic fibrosis who have an identified mutation.

3. Inborn errors of metabolism usually are autosomal recessive, although a few are X-linked [e.g., ornithine transcarbamylase deficiency (OTCD), discussed in III C 3], or autosomal dominant (e.g., porphyria).
  a. General features
    (1) Incidence and epidemiology
      (a) Although individual metabolic disorders are rare, the hundreds of such disorders together are responsible for a significant amount of mental retardation and mental illness.
      (b) Certain ethnic groups are at increased risk for specific metabolic errors (e.g., Tay-Sachs disease is seen most frequently in Ashkenazi Jews and French Canadians).
    (2) Defect
      (a) Metabolic disorders usually are caused by specific **defects in enzyme structure or function** or by **abnormalities of proteins that transport metabolites** to cells or across cell membranes. The consequent metabolic alterations manifest as physiologic disturbances, mental deficiencies, or both.
      (b) Inborn metabolic errors may be associated with accumulation of excess precursor, toxic metabolites of excess precursor, or deficiency of products needed for normal metabolism.

(3) Categories of common metabolic disorders are listed in Table 8-7.

(4) Clinical features that are helpful in detecting inborn errors of metabolism are listed following.

    (a) Vomiting and acidosis after initiation of feeding with breast milk or formula may herald a disorder of **amino acid** metabolism or **carbohydrate** metabolism.

    (b) Unusual odor of urine or sweat may be seen in several conditions. For example, **maple syrup urine disease** is named for the odor given off by urine of affected children.

    (c) Hepatosplenomegaly can be caused by metabolic disorders in which there is an accumulation (storage) of metabolites within the cells of the liver and spleen.

    (d) Mental retardation, especially if progressive, may be caused by inborn metabolic errors. **Brain atrophy** or other toxic effects can be caused by harmful effects of circulating metabolites, such as occurs in PKU. **Megalencephaly** (enlarged brain) with mental retardation can result from the inability to metabolize intracellular substances, such as occurs in **mucopolysaccharide** disorders.

    (e) Severe **acidosis** with a high anion gap can be caused by the presence of abnormal metabolites, most commonly in **aminoacidurias**.

    (f) Hyperammonemia usually is associated with **urea cycle** disorders and **organic acid** disorders.

    (g) A family history of **early infant death** should suggest the possibility of an inborn error in metabolism.

    (h) Growth retardation is frequently seen in infants with inborn errors of metabolism.

    (i) Seizures commonly occur when a metabolic disturbance is present.

(5) Diagnosis. In most metabolic disorders, an enzyme activity can be measured as abnormal or a metabolite can be measured as abnormally high or low. Thus, in many such disorders, it is possible to detect heterozygous gene carriers and to make a prenatal diagnosis from amniocytes or chorionic villus tissue. An increasing number of inborn errors may be diagnosed using RFLPs or DNA probes.

b. Disorders of amino acid and organic acid metabolism

    (1) General features

        (a) Defect. These disorders usually involve a block in a synthetic pathway, causing buildup of either the precursor or catabolites of the precursor.

        (b) Clinical features

            (i) Symptoms, which usually begin in early infancy, are the result of inadequate synthesis of necessary metabolic compounds. Excess precursors or their metabolites may interfere with normal metabolic function and regulation (e.g., by causing severe acidosis or alkalosis).

            (ii) Symptoms may become evident after the initiation of protein-containing feedings, which increase the substrate for the deficient enzyme.

        (c) Diagnosis. Specific diagnosis requires evaluation of urine or plasma for the concentration of amino acids, organic acids, and their metabolites.

        (d) Therapy. Some of these disorders are untreatable and associated with early death or mental retardation. Others are treatable with dietary manipulation

TABLE 8-7. Categories of Common Metabolic Disorders

Category	Common Examples
Disorders of amino acid and organic acid metabolism	Phenylketonuria, homocystinuria, isovaleric acidemia
Disorders of ammonia metabolism	Ornithine transcarbamylase deficiency
Disorders of carbohydrate metabolism	Galactosemia, glycogen storage diseases
Mucopolysaccharidoses	Hurler syndrome

or replacement of deficient cofactors. Most organic acid disorders lead to decreased level of consciousness, mental and neurologic deficiency, and death in infancy or childhood.

(2) PKU, the best studied and most common of the amino acid disorders, occurs in 1 in 12,000 live births.

    (a) Defect. A deficiency in the enzyme phenylalanine hydroxylase prevents conversion of phenylalanine to tyrosine, with subsequent buildup of the toxic metabolites phenylacetic acid and phenyllactic acid.

    (b) Clinical features. Unlike most amino acid disorders, PKU is not symptomatic early in infancy. Symptoms are seen later in infancy and during childhood, if the disorder is untreated.

        (i) The most significant manifestation is moderate to severe **mental retardation**.

        (ii) Neurologic manifestations, including hypertonicity and tremors, and behavior disorders are common.

        (iii) Because there is a block in the conversion of phenylalanine to tyrosine, **hypopigmentation** is a common sign (tyrosine is a necessary intermediate in production of the pigment melanin).

    (c) Prevention of mental retardation in PKU can be achieved by early identification of the defect and restriction of dietary intake of phenylalanine.

        (i) Most states have mandatory **newborn screening programs** to identify infants with PKU, so that the diet can be initiated sufficiently early to prevent mental retardation.

        (ii) Dietary restriction should start very early in infancy (by age 1 month) to be optimally effective, and life-long restriction is recommended to prevent loss of intellectual capability.

        (iii) Individuals with PKU who **maintain careful dietary management** are able to live normal lives. However, women with PKU who have discontinued dietary restriction are at substantially increased risk for having children with birth defects, especially microcephaly, congenital heart disease, and mental retardation.

(3) Homocystinuria occurs in several distinct biochemical forms. The incidence has been estimated from newborn screening for one biochemical form as 1 in 100,000 live births. If it were possible to screen for all biochemical forms, which can have very nonspecific symptoms, the incidence would be higher.

    (a) Defect. Homocystinuria is caused by deficiency of the enzyme **cystathionine synthetase,** leading to accumulation of homocystine, which is excreted in the urine and can be measured there. There is **genetic heterogeneity** in the cause of homocystinuria, and the disorder may also occur as a result of a **cofactor deficiency**. The cofactor involved is **5-methyl-tetrahydrofolate**.

    (b) Clinical features. There are no symptoms in infancy. The major manifestations during childhood are skeletal, ocular, and intellectual.

        (i) There is a typical **body habitus** similar to that seen in Marfan syndrome, with long, thin limbs and digits. Scoliosis, sternal deformity, and osteoporosis are common.

        (ii) Dislocated lenses are a frequent feature.

        (iii) Mental retardation, generally mild to moderate, is seen in some affected individuals.

        (iv) Vascular thrombosis occurs commonly, and childhood strokes and myocardial infarctions are reported.

    (c) Management

        (i) When the cofactor deficiency is the cause, the disorder can be treated with pharmacologic doses of vitamin B_6.

        (ii) In non–B_6-responsive homocystinuria, dietary management is extremely difficult because the necessary restriction of sulfhydryl groups leads to a very low-protein, foul-tasting diet.

(4) Isovaleric acidemia
  (a) Defect
      (i) Isovaleric acidemia is a prototypic organic acid disorder resulting from deficiency of **isovaleryl CoA dehydrogenase,** the enzyme responsible for the oxidative decarboxylation of leucine.
      (ii) A secondary deficiency of L-carnitine may develop due to consumption of dietary and body stores of carnitine by conjugation to the water-soluble isovaleryl glycine and elimination in the urine.
  (b) Clinical features
      (i) The presentation varies from severe neonatal ketoacidosis with encephalopathy (which, untreated, will progress to death) to a more indolent form with failure to thrive, developmental delay, and episodic metabolic acidosis.
      (ii) During ketoacidotic episodes, patients may demonstrate neutropenia and pancytopenia and have the odor of "sweaty feet."
      (iii) Myopathy, cardiomyopathy, or both may occur with L-carnitine deficiency.
  (c) Diagnosis is by demonstration of isovaleric acid, isovaleryl glycine, and isovaleryl carnitine in the urine.
  (d) Therapy includes moderate protein restriction and dietary supplementation with glycine and L-carnitine. If begun at an early age, treatment leads to resolution of the ketoacidotic episodes and normal development.
c. Disorders of ammonia metabolism occur in at least 1 in 50,000 newborns.
  (1) General features
    (a) Defect. Disorders of the urea cycle are associated with hyperammonemia, because they are involved with the metabolism of ammonia for excretion from the body.
    (b) Clinical features
      (i) Ammonia levels usually rise after initiation of protein-containing feedings or breast-feeding.
      (ii) Affected children are well at birth but become progressively more lethargic, and seizures or decreased level of consciousness may develop.
  (2) OTCD is a prototypic disorder of ammonia metabolism, but—unlike most metabolic disorders—it is inherited as an X-linked recessive trait (see III C 3).
  (3) Other urea cycle disorders (e.g., citrullinemia, argininosuccinic aciduria, carbamyl phosphate synthetase deficiency) have similar clinical courses to OTCD. A fifth disorder, arginase deficiency, tends to present with less severe hyperammonemia and with progressive spastic quadriplegia and mental retardation.
d. Disorders of carbohydrate metabolism
  (1) Galactosemia is a severe example of an inborn error of carbohydrate metabolism.
    (a) Defect. It is an autosomal recessive disorder caused by deficiency of the enzyme **galactose 1-phosphate uridyltransferase,** resulting in impaired conversion of galactose-1-phosphate to glucose 1-phosphate.
    (b) Clinical features are noted within a few days to weeks after initiation of formula or breast milk feedings. Initial symptoms include hepatomegaly, vomiting, anorexia, aminoaciduria, and growth failure.
    (c) Diagnosis is initially made by detection of non–glucose-reducing substances in the urine (galactose and galactose 1-phosphate) and is confirmed by demonstrating absence of galactose 1-uridyltransferase in erythrocytes. Many states have mandatory newborn screening for galactosemia because it is largely treatable when diagnosed early.
    (d) Therapy for galactosemia is the elimination of all formulas and foods containing galactose.

       (i) **Treated individuals** often have normal intelligence if the diagnosis is made and treatment is initiated early. However, there is an increase in the incidence of learning disorders even in treated individuals. Affected women have a high incidence of **ovarian hypofunction** and premature ovarian failure.

       (ii) **Untreated infants** often die, either from inanition or *Escherichia coli sepsis*. Untreated survivors suffer from growth retardation, mental retardation, and cataracts.

   (2) **Glycogen storage diseases** are a group of conditions caused by a lack of enzymes involved in glycogen synthesis or breakdown, with a resultant buildup of glycogen in tissues (see also Chapter 18). Representative autosomal recessive types listed in Table 8-8 illustrate the variable clinical picture of glycogen storage diseases.

e. **Mucopolysaccharidoses (MPSs)** are a group of disorders characterized by deficiency of lysosomal enzymes responsible for intracellular catabolism of mucopolysaccharides. All are autosomal recessive conditions except for **Hunter syndrome** (MPS type II; iduronate sulfatase deficiency), which is an X-linked recessive disorder (see III C). The incidence of this group of disorders is 1 in 25,000 newborns.

   (1) **Clinical features** are caused by intracellular accumulation (storage) of mucopolysaccharides and are not apparent at birth.

      (a) All tissues can be affected, but effects are most commonly seen in the liver and spleen (hepatosplenomegaly), skeleton (skeletal dysplasia, dwarfism, joint contracture), brain (megalencephaly, mental retardation), heart (aortic and mitral valve incompetence), and respiratory system (tracheal stenosis).

      (b) Mucopolysaccharidoses usually are associated with deterioration of neurologic function and progressive mental retardation. In some MPSs, the brain is unaffected and intelligence is normal.

   (2) **Diagnosis** of the mucopolysaccharidoses is suggested by the presence of specific mucopolysaccharides in the urine. The diagnosis is confirmed by performing specific enzyme assays on leukocytes or fibroblasts.

C. **X-linked disorders** occur when a male inherits a mutant gene on the X chromosome, which always is maternal in origin. Common X-linked disorders include hemophilia A, color blindness, Duchenne muscular dystrophy, and fragile X syndrome.

   1. **General characteristics**
     a. **Inheritance**
       (1) The affected male is termed **hemizygous** for the gene because he has only a single X chromosome and a single set of X-linked genes.

TABLE 8-8. Representative Glycogen Storage Disorders

Type	Eponym	Deficient Enzyme	Onset	Symptoms	Treatment
I	von Gierke disease	Glycogen-6-phosphatase	Infancy	Hepatomegaly, renomegaly, hypoglycemia, acidosis	Prevention of hypoglycemia, complex carbohydrate (corn starch), continuous feeds
II	Pompe disease	Acid maltase	Infancy	Cardiomegaly, hepatomegaly, hypotonia	None available. Lethal by 1 year of age
V	McArdle syndrome	Skeletal phosphorylase	Late childhood, adolescence, adulthood	Fatigue, cramps, myoglobinuria	Avoidance of exercise stress

(2) The mother of the affected individual is **heterozygous** for the gene because she has two X chromosomes, one normal and one with a mutant gene. She may demonstrate partial manifestations of the disorder because only one of the two X's in any cell is transcriptionally active (**Lyon hypothesis**).

  b. Recurrence risks for X-linked disorders differ depending on whether the mother or the father has the abnormal gene.

    (1) If the mother has the gene on one of her two X chromosomes and, thus, is a **carrier,** there is a 50% chance that the gene will pass to each offspring. If the offspring inheriting the mutant gene is a daughter, she, too, will be a carrier. If the offspring inheriting the mutant gene is a son, he will be affected because he will not have a second X chromosome to compensate for the effects of the abnormal gene. Thus, each daughter has a 50% chance of being a carrier, and each son has a 50% chance of being affected.

    (2) If the father has the gene and, thus, is **affected,** he can pass that abnormal gene only to his daughters; all his daughters, therefore, will be carriers. Because the Y chromosome is normal, all his sons will be unaffected. **There is no male-to-male transmission.**

2. Fragile X syndrome is a common cause of mental retardation, which is associated with a chromosomal marker.

  a. Incidence. An X-linked form of mental retardation is found in 1 in 1000 men, and 40% of men with X-linked mental retardation have the fragile X syndrome. Some women with mental retardation also may display the fragile X chromosome (approximately 1/2000).

  b. Diagnosis can be made in two ways.

    (1) A chromosomal marker called a **fragile site** can be detected on the distal end of the long arm of the X chromosome in a proportion of cells when lymphocytes are cultured in a **folate-deficient medium**.

    (2) Molecular genetic testing is also available and is based on the number of repeats of the nucleotide sequence CGG that are found within a specific region of the gene.

      (a) Normal (noncarrier, unaffected) people have a series of 6–52 repeated triplet nucleotides.

      (b) Carriers, who have a "pre-mutation," have 50–200 triplet repeats.

      (c) Affected men or women have more than 200 repeats, and the gene becomes inactivated, and therefore not expressed. This results in mental retardation.

      (d) The number of repeats becomes increased (amplified) when the gene is inherited from a mother, but not usually when inherited from a father.

    (3) The frequency of this syndrome calls for all children (male and female) with mental retardation of unspecified etiology to undergo a fragile X study.

  c. Recurrence risk. Because the fragile X syndrome is an X-linked disorder, recurrence risks (for the mutation) are the same as for other X-linked disorders. However, the number of triplet repeats in part determines whether the offspring will be affected. This complicates genetic counseling and prediction of risk for an affected child.

  d. Clinical features may be quite variable, and may include all or some of those listed in Table 8-9.

  e. Therapy. There is no specific therapeutic modality for the fragile X syndrome. Serotonin uptake inhibitors, such as fluoxetine, may be of value in improving behavior.

3. OTCD

  a. Defect. OTCD is a prototypic disorder of ammonia metabolism, which is inherited as an X-linked recessive trait.

    (1) Although males primarily are severely affected, up to one-third of female carriers may manifest symptoms because of lyonization [see III C 1 a (2)].

    (2) Genetic heterogeneity exists, so that some affected males have a less severe mutation and clinical course.

TABLE 8-9. Phenotypic Features of Fragile X Syndrome

Growth	Large birth size
	Macrocephaly
Facial	Long face
	Prominent forehead
	Large, prominent ears
	Long chin
Other features	Macroorchidism
	Joint laxity
	Mitral valve prolapse
	Obesity (occasional)
Neurologic findings	Mental retardation
	Autistic-like features
	Hyperactivity

b. Clinical features
   (1) Typically, overwhelming illness develops in affected males within 24–48 hours of birth (i.e., after initiation of protein-containing feedings). The newborn becomes progressively more lethargic and may manifest seizures and a decreased level of consciousness as serum ammonia levels rise to more than 500 μg/dl and, ultimately, to about 1000 μg/dl.
   (2) Female carriers may present with headache and vomiting after high-protein meals and, later, with learning disabilities or an altered response to protein loading.
c. Therapy and prognosis
   (1) Treatment may be attempted with intravenous fluids, glucose, and agents that exploit alternative pathways for nitrogen excretion (e.g., benzoic acid, phenyl-acetate).
   (2) Early aggressive treatment can improve the prognosis for survival and function, but the outlook often remains poor unless the infant is managed prospectively from birth (based on a positive family history). Even then, the management is complex and demanding of the parents.

IV. **CHROMOSOME DISORDERS.** Each human normally has 22 pairs of autosomes and 1 pair of sex chromosomes, with females having two X chromosomes and males having one X and one Y chromosome. One member of each pair of chromosomes comes from each parent, with a carefully regulated amount of genetic material. An alteration in the amount or nature of chromosome material usually is associated with birth defects or other abnormalities. Chromosome disorders are seen in 5 in 1000 live births (0.6%).

A. **General characteristics**

1. **Defect.** Most chromosome defects arise **de novo** (i.e., no other family member has a defect). The defects usually are classified as abnormalities of **number** or of **structure and content**. They may involve either the **autosomes** or the **sex chromosomes;** birth defects due to autosomal abnormalities usually are more severe than those due to sex chromosome abnormalities.
   a. Numerical defects may be **aneuploid** (chromosome number is not an exact multiple of the diploid number) or **euploid** (chromosome number is an exact multiple of the diploid number). Examples of numerical chromosome abnormalities include trisomy 21 (Down syndrome), trisomy 18, trisomy 13, Klinefelter syndrome (47,XXY), and Turner syndrome (usually 45,XO).

b. Structural defects result from chromosome breakage and include unbalanced translocation, deletion, duplication, inversion, isochromosome, and centric fragment. Examples of disorders due to structural chromosome abnormalities include Prader-Willi syndrome (15q deletion), cri du chat syndrome (5p deletion), and Wilms tumor with aniridia (11p deletion).

c. Mosaicism is another type of chromosome defect characterized by two or more cell lines with different chromosome compositions. Mosaicism occurs as a result of mitotic nondisjunction after fertilization. Therefore, recurrence risk for parents of a child with mosaicism is negligible.

2. Indications for chromosome analysis

a. Children who have **recognizable phenotypes** (clinical features) consistent with known chromosomal disorders should have confirmatory chromosome studies.

b. Children with **multiple congenital abnormalities or dysmorphic features** and no clinically identifiable etiology require chromosome studies.

c. Children with **mental retardation** and no identifiable etiology require chromosome studies, including a fragile X study.

d. Parents who have had **recurrent (two or more) pregnancy losses** should have chromosome studies.

  (1) Of couples with two or more miscarriages, 5% will have one member with a balanced reciprocal chromosome translocation.

    (a) Miscarriage can result when an embryo or fetus has an inherited unbalanced chromosome translocation that is incompatible with life.

    (b) Such couples are at risk for having a live-born child with multiple congenital anomalies due to an unbalanced translocation, and should be offered prenatal diagnosis.

  (2) Some women with recurrent pregnancy loss have been found to have mosaicisms involving the sex chromosomes; however, the etiologic significance of this, if any, is not clear.

e. Because 40% of all **spontaneous abortions** are caused by chromosome abnormalities (usually extra or missing chromosomes), all spontaneously aborted and stillborn fetuses should have chromosome studies.

f. Chromosome studies are valuable for aiding in the diagnosis and management of patients with **ambiguous genitalia**.

g. Sex chromosome abnormalities are often found in men and women with **infertility**.

h. Chromosome studies should be obtained on bone marrow samples from all patients with **leukemia** because leukemic cells often have chromosome abnormalities.

i. Solid tumors often contain cytogenetic alterations, which may give clues to their gene origin.

3. Methods of chromosome analysis. Chromosome studies can be performed on any tissue in which cells are actively undergoing mitosis. A **karyotype** is an arrangement of the chromosomes that is made from micrographs; it allows the analysis of chromosome number and structure.

a. Peripheral blood studies are the most common because blood is the easiest tissue to obtain.

  (1) The T cells are stimulated with phytohemagglutinin, which causes the cells to undergo mitosis.

  (2) Results from peripheral blood chromosome studies usually take a minimum of 3 days to obtain, because that is the time required for the cells to enter metaphase.

b. Bone marrow studies. Bone marrow cells are constantly undergoing mitosis, making it possible to obtain results within 6 hours of obtaining a sample.

  (1) Bone marrow chromosomes may be studied when management decisions regarding newborn infants who have multiple birth defects may be altered by knowing whether there is a chromosome abnormality associated with a very poor prognosis [e.g., trisomy 18 (see IV B 3)].

    (2) The most common use of bone marrow chromosome studies is for evaluation of leukemias. The exact type of chromosomal anomaly in leukemic cells aids in diagnosis, management, and determination of prognosis (see Chapter 16).

  c. Organ tissue studies. Chromosome studies also can be performed on solid tissues and organs.

    (1) Occasionally it is not possible to obtain peripheral blood, as in the case of a stillborn fetus, and another tissue is evaluated.

    (2) In the case of chromosome mosaicism, tissue biopsy specimens (usually taken from the skin) are grown in culture to diagnose or confirm the defect. Usually, it takes at least 3–4 weeks for solid tissue cells to grow in culture before chromosome analysis can be performed.

B. **Numerical autosomal abnormalities.** Characteristic phenotypes are associated with specific autosomal trisomies. **Trisomy** refers to the fact that three—rather than the normal two—copies of a specific chromosome are present in the cells of an individual. Such trisomies occur because of a meiotic division error called **nondisjunction** in either the oocyte of the mother or the spermatocyte of the father. Only a few trisomies are found in live-born infants; others are seen only in aborted fetuses.

  1. Down syndrome is the most common autosomal trisomy compatible with life.

    a. Types of defects. The characteristic finding and etiology of Down syndrome is trisomy 21, although some cases result from translocation or, more rarely, mosaicism.

      (1) Trisomy. Ninety-five percent of children with Down syndrome have 47 chromosomes, with 3 number 21 chromosomes. Trisomy 21 occurs in 1 in 700 live births.

        (a) The risk for having a child with an extra chromosome 21 increases with **advancing maternal age**. This risk rises dramatically after 35 years of age. Most children with trisomy 21 are born to women younger than 35 years of age, however, because most women give birth before 35 years of age. The mechanism for the increased incidence of trisomy 21 in fetuses of older mothers is not understood. The extra chromosome comes from the father in only a small percentage of cases.

        (b) The **recurrence risk** for parents of children with trisomy 21 increases to 1%–2% (unless age-related risk is greater).

      (2) Translocation. Four percent of children with Down syndrome have 46 chromosomes, with a translocation of the third number 21 chromosome to another chromosome—usually a **D-group** (number 13, 14, or 15) or a **G-group** (number 21 or 22) chromosome.

        (a) Of all cases of translocation Down syndrome, three fourths are **de novo** (i.e., not familial).

        (b) One fourth of translocation cases are **familial,** meaning that one of the parents has a balanced translocation involving one number 21 chromosome and another chromosome. In these cases, the **recurrence risk** may be as high as 15% in future pregnancies (depending on which other chromosome is involved and on the sex of the partner carrying the balanced translocation).

      (3) Mosaicism. One percent of children with Down syndrome has chromosome mosaicism, with some cells having 46 chromosomes and 2 number 21 chromosomes, and some cells having 47 chromosomes and 3 number 21 chromosomes. The mosaicism results from a mitotic division error that occurred during early embryonic development.

    b. Clinical features. Children with Down syndrome have a characteristic appearance that can be defined in terms of their dysmorphic features. They also have a number of other characteristic functional and structural abnormalities that are part of the syndrome. Children with mosaic Down syndrome may have a milder clinical presentation than those with trisomy 21 in all of their cells.

(1) Dysmorphic features (Figure 8-3)

    (a) Common dysmorphic facial features are a flat facial profile; short, upslanting palpebral fissures; Brushfield spots; a flat nasal bridge with epicanthal folds; a small mouth with protruding tongue; a small, retroplaced chin; and short ears with abnormal ear lobes that usually are downfolded.

    (b) Other dysmorphic features include microcephaly, flat occiput (brachycephaly), excess posterior neck skin, short stature, short sternum, small genitalia, short hands and fingers marked by incurved fifth fingers with hypoplastic middle phalanx, single palmar creases (simian creases), and a gap between the first and second toes.

(2) Functional and structural abnormalities

    (a) Hypotonia is a frequent accompaniment to the dysmorphic features of Down syndrome and is most noticeable in the newborn.

    (b) Cardiac defects, especially endocardial cushion defects and septal defects, are seen in 50% of people with Down syndrome; about half of these may be fatal.

    (c) Gastrointestinal abnormalities (especially duodenal atresia and Hirschsprung disease) are the next most common internal organ abnormalities in Down syndrome.

    (d) Developmental delay is seen in young children, and **mental retardation** is diagnosed once the age of IQ testing is reached. The mean IQ is 50, with most individuals performing in the moderately retarded range.

    (e) Hypothyroidism and **leukemia** occur at higher frequency than in the general population.

    (f) With improved medical, educational, and vocational management, life expectancy for Down syndrome patients can be well into adulthood. A newly recognized problem of the third and fourth decade is a pattern of **dementia** much like Alzheimer disease.

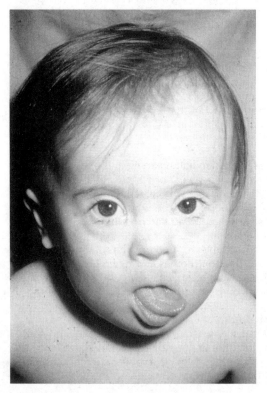

FIGURE 8-3. Characteristic dysmorphic features in an infant with Down syndrome. Note small palpebral fissures with epicanthal folds, flat nasal bridge, small nose and mouth, protruding tongue, and small chin. Brushfield spots can be seen on the iris. (Photograph courtesy of K. Jones, M.D.)

     c. Prognosis. With increased life expectancy in Down syndrome, issues relating to employment, financial security, health care, and living situation must be addressed by families and social service agencies. Supervised group home living has become a successful alternative for these and other mentally retarded adults.

2. Trisomy 13. From 1 in 4000 to 1 in 10,000 newborns are affected by trisomy 13.
    a. Types of defects
       (1) Trisomy. Seventy-five percent of cases of trisomy 13 are caused by a free extra chromosome 13—a result of a parental meiotic nondisjunction. There is a relation between the occurrence of trisomy 13 and advanced maternal age, although it is not as strong as that for trisomy 21.
       (2) Translocation. Twenty percent of cases of trisomy 13 are the result of translocation involving chromosome 13.
          (a) Three fourths of these cases are **de novo**.
          (b) One fourth are caused by a familial translocation involving the number 13 chromosome, and in these cases the **recurrence risk** can be as high as 14% in future pregnancies.
       (3) Mosaicism. Five percent of the cases of trisomy 13 are mosaics for normal 46-chromosome cell lines and cell lines with 47 chromosomes with an extra number 13 chromosome.
    b. Clinical features. Trisomy 13 is associated with severe birth defects, including:
       (1) Microcephaly with open skin lesions of the scalp (**aplasia cutis congenita**)
       (2) Cleft lip with or without cleft palate (often severe and bilateral)
       (3) Severe CNS malformations, including **holoprosencephaly** (absence of midline structures, often with a single ventricle)
       (4) Eye malformations, including **microphthalmos** and **colobomata**
       (5) Polydactyly of the hands and feet
       (6) Omphalocele
       (7) Genital malformations, including ambiguous genitalia in males
       (8) Congenital heart disease
       (9) Severe mental retardation
    c. Prognosis for patients with trisomy 13 is extremely poor: 50% of patients die before 1 month of age, 70% die before age 6 months, and 90% die before age 1 year.

3. Trisomy 18 occurs in 1 in 8000 live births. There is a relationship between advanced maternal age and the occurrence of trisomy 18, but this is less marked than that seen in trisomy 21 and trisomy 13.
    a. Types of defects. Trisomy 18 rarely is caused by a chromosome translocation.
       (1) Ninety percent of the cases of trisomy 18 are a result of **meiotic nondisjunction**.
       (2) Ten percent of the cases of trisomy 18 are **mosaics**—caused by a postzygotic (postfertilization) mitotic nondisjunction.
    b. Clinical features
       (1) Trisomy 18 is associated with **multiple congenital anomalies,** including intrauterine growth retardation, microcephaly with prominent occiput, CNS malformations and severe mental retardation, hypertonia (spasticity) after initial hypotonia, and micrognathia (small mandible).
       (2) Other congenital anomalies include characteristic overlapping of the second and fifth fingers over the third and fourth fingers, with fixed finger contractures and absence of interphalangeal flexion creases, dislocated hips, rocker-bottom feet, congenital heart disease, and occasional neural tube defects. The variability and subtlety of the dysmorphic features can sometimes make this condition difficult to recognize.
    c. Prognosis for patients with trisomy 18 is extremely poor: 30% of patients die within 1 month of birth and 90% die before 1 year of age.

C. **Sex chromosome disorders** involve abnormalities in the number or structure of the X or Y chromosome.

1. Turner syndrome affects 1 in 2500 newborn girls.

a. **Types of defects.** In Turner syndrome, only one X chromosome exists or is normal. Several different chromosomal anomalies can result in the Turner phenotype.
   (1) In 55% of girls with Turner syndrome, there is a 45,X karyotype.
   (2) In 25% of cases, the structure of one of the X chromosomes is altered. The structural anomaly usually is a **deletion** of a segment of the chromosome or a duplication of the long or short arm of the chromosome with a subsequent loss of the other arm (called an **isochromosome**).
   (3) In 15% of cases, there is a **mosaic** for two or more cell lines, one of which usually is 45,X and the other is 46,XX or 46,XY. A third cell line may be present, most commonly leading to a karyotype of 45,X/46,XX/47,XXX. Mosaicism is caused by postzygotic mitotic nondisjunction.
b. **Recurrence risk** for Turner syndrome is the same as the general population risk (i.e., 1 in 5000 live births).
c. **Clinical features** of Turner syndrome may be noted at birth, although many girls are not diagnosed until puberty.
   (1) **Dysmorphic features** include **lymphedema** of hands and feet at birth, a shield-shaped chest, **webbing of the neck,** cubitus valgus (increased carrying angle), short stature (average adult height is 135 cm), and multiple pigmented nevi.
   (2) **Functional and structural abnormalities**
      (a) **Gonadal dysgenesis** is present in 100% of patients and is associated with primary amenorrhea and lack of pubertal development due to absence of ovarian hormones. It is important to replace ovarian hormones at puberty as part of the management of patients with Turner syndrome. With rare exceptions, women are unable to become pregnant.
      (b) **Gonadoblastoma** (a tumor of abdominally located gonads with Y-containing cells) may develop in patients who have a cell line with a Y chromosome. It is essential to perform bilateral gonadectomy in girls with such a cell line.
      (c) **Renal anomalies** occur in 40% of patients and include duplication of the collecting system and horseshoe kidney.
      (d) **Congenital heart disease** occurs in 20% of patients. Defects include aortic stenosis, bicuspid aortic valve, and coarctation of the aorta.
      (e) **Autoimmune thyroiditis** is common.
      (f) **Learning disabilities** are common.
d. **Diagnosis.** Some girls suspected of having Turner syndrome have a 46,XX karyotype in peripheral blood.
   (1) Most of these girls have mosaic Turner syndrome, and a skin biopsy is necessary to find the mosaicism in fibroblasts.
   (2) Some of these patients have a phenotypically similar but genetically unrelated condition called **Noonan syndrome,** which, unlike Turner syndrome, can also affect males and has a number of additional clinical findings, including mental retardation in many cases.
e. **Prognosis** depends on the type and severity of malformations. Life span probably is normal in most cases.

2. **Klinefelter syndrome** affects 1 in 1000 newborn boys and is caused by an extra X chromosome.
   a. **Types of defects**
      (1) In 80% of boys with Klinefelter syndrome, there is a **47,XXY karyotype**.
      (2) In 20% of cases, there is a mosaic, with one cell line having a **47,XXY karyotype**.
   b. **Recurrence risk** for Klinefelter syndrome is the same as the general population risk (i.e., 1 in 2000 live births).
   c. **Clinical features** are variable and nonspecific.
      (1) Boys usually are **taller than average** in relation to their families, with an arm span generally greater than their height.
      (2) At puberty, boys are **incompletely masculinized** and usually have a female body habitus and female escutcheon with decreased body hair.
         (a) **Gynecomastia** is a common feature.

(b) The **testes remain small,** and there is hyperplasia of Leydig cells and greatly diminished spermatozoa production, with infertility. This represents **seminiferous tubule dysgenesis**.

(3) The mean IQ is 90, and there is a slight increase in the incidence of mild mental retardation.

(4) Behavioral problems and immaturity are common.

3. Other sex chromosome abnormalities

a. Men with **46,XX karyotype** have a phenotype similar to Klinefelter syndrome. The incidence of 46,XX men is 1 in 25,000 live births. This condition is caused by a translocation of genetic material from the short arm of the Y chromosome to another chromosome.

b. A **47,XXX karyotype** is seen in 1 in 1000 live-born girls. Most cases have a normal phenotype, although tall stature for the family is a frequent finding. The average IQ is 90, but there is no apparent increased incidence of mental retardation. There may be an increased tendency for schizophrenia.

c. A **47,XYY karyotype** is seen in 1 in 1000 live-born boys. The phenotype usually is normal, although most patients are taller than average for their families (the average height is 180 cm). Previous concerns about behavioral disorders in these individuals have been challenged by subsequent research.

D. **Structural chromosome abnormalities**

1. Partial deletions

a. Types of defects

(1) Some syndromes can be caused by the loss of chromosome material from the ends of a chromosome (**terminal chromosome deletion**) or loss of material from the middle or inner portion of a chromosome (**interstitial deletion**).

(2) Although most chromosome deletions arise de novo, terminal deletions may result from the child inheriting an **unbalanced chromosome translocation** (unequal exchange of chromosome material between two chromosomes) from a parent who has a balanced reciprocal translocation (equal exchange of chromosome material between two chromosomes).

b. Clinical features. Children with terminal deletions usually have growth deficiency, mental retardation, dysmorphic features, and multiple malformations.

c. Detection

(1) It often is necessary to perform special chromosome studies to detect small or subtle deletions. These **high-resolution, or prometaphase, studies** capture cells in an early stage of the mitotic cycle, so the chromosomes are longer and have more regions (bands) visible for analysis.

(2) A new and powerful technique of genetic analysis called **fluorescence in situ hybridization (FISH)** is particularly useful for detecting very small deletions.

(a) This technique uses fluorescence-labeled probes of short (submicroscopic) segments of DNA containing only a few genes to detect the presence, absence, or rearrangement of the complementary DNA segment by hybridization to it.

(i) When the DNA of interest is present on the chromosome, it is identified by a fluorescent spot (Figure 8-4).

(ii) When the DNA is deleted, no fluorescent spot is visible.

(b) The loss or rearrangement of material in a contiguous gene syndrome (see I C 2), such as Prader-Willi syndrome, can be confirmed with more accuracy than with high-resolution chromosome analysis.

(c) FISH is becoming available as a rapid and sensitive diagnostic test for a number of syndromes that previously could be diagnosed only clinically.

(3) In cases of terminal deletion, it is necessary to perform karyotypes of both parents.

(4) A family history of recurrent pregnancy loss may be found when parents have balanced chromosome translocations because other family members also may carry the translocation.

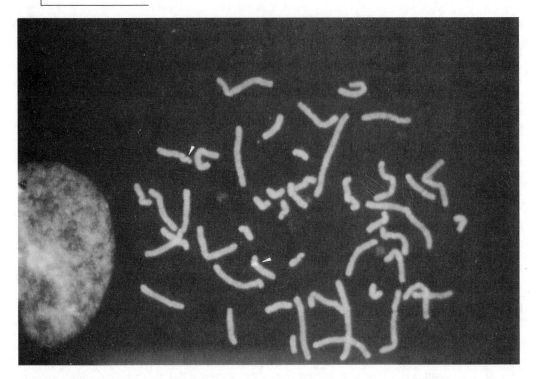

FIGURE 8-4. Fluorescence in situ hybridization (FISH) demonstrating a deletion (*arrow* pointing to absent bright spot) in chromosome 15 in a patient with Prader-Willi syndrome. (Photograph courtesy of Stuart Schwartz, Ph.D.)

d. Disorders caused by partial deletions
  (1) Cri du chat syndrome occurs in 1 in 50,000 newborns.
    (a) Defect. The syndrome is caused by a deletion of material from the terminal end of the short arm of chromosome 5 (**5p-**).
    (b) Clinical features
      (i) Affected children have a characteristic cat-like cry.
      (ii) Profound mental retardation and CNS abnormalities are consistent findings.
      (iii) Congenital heart disease is common, as are ocular malformations (e.g., cataracts, optic atrophy).
    (c) Prognosis. Many patients can survive into adulthood.
  (2) Retinoblastoma (see also Chapter 16)
    (a) Defect. Some children with retinoblastoma have an interstitial deletion of the long arm of chromosome 13 (**deletion of 13q14**), detected by prometaphase analysis.
    (b) Clinical features
      (i) The onset of retinoblastoma in these cases usually is in the first 2 years of life. The disease usually is bilateral.
      (ii) Mental retardation usually is seen.
      (iii) Patients often have some degree of facial dysmorphism.
  (3) Wilms tumor with aniridia (see also Chapter 16)
    (a) Defect. Children with Wilms tumor and aniridia (absent irises) may have an interstitial deletion of the short arm of chromosome 11 (**deletion of 11p13**), detected by prometaphase analysis.
    (b) Clinical features
      (i) Mental retardation is a consistent feature.
      (ii) Males often have ambiguous genitalia.

        (iii) Children with 11p13 deletion, as well as those with similar features in whom a deletion has not been detected, are at high risk for development of abdominal tumors, especially Wilms tumor and gonadoblastoma; therefore, they should be monitored frequently with abdominal ultrasound.

  2. Partial trisomy

    a. Defect. Partial trisomy results when extra chromosome material is found in the karyotype, but there is less than an entire extra chromosome present.

      (1) The extra chromosome material can occur at the end of the long or short arm of the chromosome, or it may be inserted into the normal chromosome at any point.

      (2) It also may occur as a separate piece of chromosome material (a chromosome **marker** or **minute**), with or without its own centromere.

    b. Clinical features. The origin of the extra chromosome material determines the phenotypic effects. When the extra material is autosomal, dysmorphic features, growth insufficiency, malformations, and developmental abnormalities are commonly seen.

    c. Diagnosis

      (1) High-resolution banding or special staining techniques sometimes can identify the origin of the extra chromosome material, especially if it is large. **DNA probe analysis** also may be helpful in identifying the origin of markers.

      (2) Parental karyotypes should be obtained because the partial trisomy sometimes results from a balanced parental translocation. Such a translocation gives a parent an increased risk for future chromosomally unbalanced offspring, with clinical consequences of increased risk for miscarriage, stillbirth, malformations, or mental retardation. It may also aid in the identification of the chromosome of origin of the extra material in the child.

      (3) In the past, in many cases of **de novo partial trisomy,** the extra material could not be identified. In such cases, it was impossible to predict specifically the prognosis for the child because the origin of the extra genetic material remained unknown. A new technique called **chromosome painting,** which colors each individual chromosome with a fluorescent color, now permits specific identification of individual chromosomes and even small pieces of individual chromosomes that have been translocated (Figure 8-5). This technique is based on unique fluorescence-tagged DNA probes along the whole length of each chromosome.

V.   **MULTIFACTORIAL DISORDERS** are conditions that are believed to be caused by a combination of genetic liability and environmental (nongenetic) factors. Many common birth defects and many common disorders of midlife are ascribed to multifactorial inheritance.

A.   **General characteristics**

  1. Incidence. The general population incidence of most multifactorial disorders is 1.0–1.5 per 1000 for each condition.

  2. Recurrence risk. Individuals who have a multifactorial disorder or who have a child with a multifactorial disorder have approximately a 2%–5% empiric risk for recurrence of the disorder with each subsequent pregnancy.

    a. The increased risk for recurrence implies that there must be some genetic factors, probably several genes, that play a role in the occurrence of these disorders.

    b. The fact that these conditions do not recur in 25% or 50% of offspring, as do autosomal recessive, autosomal dominant, and X-linked disorders, implies that environmental factors also must play a role in their occurrence.

    c. Unlike single-gene disorders, the recurrence risk for multifactorial disorders increases with an increasing number of affected relatives and increasing severity of the disorder.

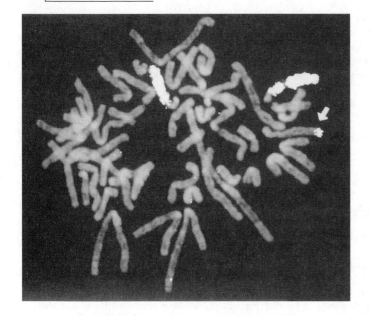

FIGURE 8-5. Chromosome painting using fluorescence-tagged DNA library for chromosome 14. There is a translocation involving the long arms of chromosomes 13 and 14. The proband has two normal chromosomes 14 and a derivative 13 with a small piece of 14 translocated to it. (Photograph courtesy of Stuart Schwartz, Ph.D.)

 d. There is a difference in male (M) to female (F) ratio of several multifactorial disorders [e.g., congenital hip dislocation (F > M) and pyloric stenosis (M > F)]. When this is the case, the recurrence risk for first-degree relatives is greater when the affected individual is of the less often affected sex.

 e. The recurrence risk is greater when the affected individual is more severely affected. For example, the recurrence risk is greater when a child has bilateral cleft lip and palate compared to isolated cleft lip.

 f. The recurrence risk for multifactorial disorders decreases rapidly with decreasing degree of relatedness.

 3. Examples. Common multifactorial disorders include:

  a. Common birth defects [e.g., clubfoot, cleft lip with or without cleft palate, neural tube defects (meningomyelocele, anencephaly), congenital heart defects, congenital hip dislocation, pyloric stenosis]

  b. Mental retardation (when a specific cause is not identified)

  c. Affective disorders (e.g., schizophrenia)

  d. Common disorders of midlife (e.g., hypertension, peptic ulcer disease, hyperlipidemia, diabetes mellitus, coronary artery disease, cancer)

B. **Neural tube defects** (see also Chapter 18) occur in 1–2 in 1000 newborns in the United States.

 1. Types of defects. The two major types of neural tube defect, anencephaly and meningomyelocele, are caused by failure of the neural groove to fuse completely into a tube by the twenty-eighth day of pregnancy.

  a. Anencephaly represents failure of closure of the cranial neural tube.

   (1) Children with anencephaly have no cranium and have only the most basal portions of the brain.

   (2) They are profoundly neurologically abnormal and usually die within the first few hours to days of life, surviving to that time on brain stem functions.

  b. Meningomyelocele represents failure of closure of the neural tube distal to the brain, leading to hernial protrusion through the vertebral column, as in **spina bifida**.

   (1) Lesions may be anywhere along the spine but most commonly occur in the lumbar area.

(2) Failure of development of normal vertebral architecture allows the cord to bulge out of the protective confines of the spine, with resultant loss of neurologic function below the level of the lesion.

(3) The dura and skin must be surgically closed over the lesion to prevent meningitis. Very often, the consequence is **hydrocephalus** due to the associated presence of an **Arnold-Chiari malformation** of the ventricular system (downward displacement of the hindbrain through the foramen magnum).

(4) Additional neurologic and other associated findings in children with meningomyelocele depend on the level of the lesion.

  (a) **Bladder control** may be absent, with consequent recurrent urinary tract infections, reflux, and the need for urinary diversion.

  (b) **Bowel function** may be lost, with consequent severe chronic constipation.

  (c) **Clubfoot** and other orthopedic problems below the level of the lesion are common.

  (d) **Mental retardation** and **seizures** are frequent when hydrocephalus is or has been present.

2. Risk factors. Anencephaly and meningomyelocele are two expressions of the same disorder, and a person at risk for this disorder may have a child with either manifestation. Neural tube defects show classic multifactorial inheritance, but the incidence varies with a number of factors.

a. Geographic location is important, with the incidence being highest in Ireland and Wales.

b. Economic class is an important variable, with a higher incidence in poorer groups.

c. Maternal age is a factor, and both teenage mothers and older mothers are at increased risk.

d. Prenatal exposure to known contributory environmental factors, such as valproic acid and maternal diabetes, results in an increased risk.

3. Recurrence risk increases with each additional first-degree relative who is affected.

a. If a couple has one child with a neural tube defect, the risk for each subsequent child to be affected is 3%–5%. It is 7%–10% after a second affected child.

b. A person with a meningomyelocele has a 2%–4% risk of having an affected child with each pregnancy.

4. Prenatal diagnosis of neural tube defects almost always can be accomplished in the second trimester.

a. Most neural tube defects, being open defects, are reflected by **elevated AFP levels** in amniotic fluid and in maternal serum (see I F 1).

b. Elevated maternal serum AFP levels can be followed by a **level II ultrasound** (to examine the fetus for anencephaly or a spinal defect) and **amniocentesis** (to determine whether amniotic fluid AFP and acetylcholine esterase levels are elevated, because the presence of both of these is more specific for neural tube defects). The parents of an affected fetus then have options of terminating the pregnancy or continuing the pregnancy with knowledge of the condition, which allows improved perinatal management and permits the parents to prepare emotionally for having a child with a serious birth defect.

5. Preventive therapy

a. Current studies suggest that the recurrence risk for neural tube defects may be lowered significantly by taking 4 mg of **folic acid** daily from the time of conception through the time of formation of the neural tube (end of first trimester). As a result, many physicians recommend starting prenatal vitamin preparations that contain adequate folate from the time conception is attempted.

b. Studies also suggest that taking 0.4 mg of folic acid daily beginning before conception and continuing through the second month of gestation (after neural tube closure is complete) may significantly lower the incidence of neural tube defects in the general population. Food grains may shortly be supplemented to provide this level of folic acid.

C. **Orofacial clefts** are common birth defects with multifactorial inheritance.

1. **Cleft lip with or without cleft palate** is seen in 1–2 per 1000 live births.
   a. **Risk factors**
      (1) Twice as many boys are born with cleft lip with or without cleft palate as girls.
      (2) The incidence of cleft lip is highest in Asian and American Indian populations and lowest in blacks.
   b. **Differential diagnosis.** There are over 50 syndromes that include cleft lip with or without cleft palate, and these must be excluded before making the diagnosis of isolated cleft lip with or without cleft palate. These syndromes may be autosomal dominant, autosomal recessive, X-linked, or sporadic.
      (1) An example is **van der Woude syndrome,** an autosomal dominant condition in which lip pits are seen in all gene carriers but only some individuals have cleft lip with or without cleft palate owing to variable expressivity. The recurrence risk for gene carriers is 50% versus 3%–5% in the multifactorial isolated cleft lip.
      (2) Cleft lip may be associated with exposure to **teratogenic agents,** particularly alcohol.
   c. **Recurrence risk**
      (1) Recurrence risk if one child or one parent is affected is 3%–5%.
      (2) Recurrence risk if two children or one child and one parent are affected is 10%.
      (3) Recurrence risk is higher if affected individuals have bilateral cleft lip and palate or if females are affected.

2. **Isolated cleft palate** is a multifactorial condition distinct from cleft lip with or without cleft palate that is seen in 1 in 2000 live births.
   a. **Risk factors**
      (1) Girls are affected more frequently than boys.
      (2) The recurrence risks for cleft palate without cleft lip are similar to those for cleft lip with or without cleft palate; however, there is no increased risk for having a child with cleft lip.
   b. **Differential diagnosis.** There are over 150 syndromes that involve cleft palate; therefore, other abnormalities must be excluded before making a diagnosis of isolated cleft palate.
   c. **Subtypes**
      (1) Microforms of cleft palate are **bifid uvula** and **submucous cleft** of the palate. These conditions usually are not of functional significance. However, the recurrence risk is 3%–5%, which includes a risk for having a child with a complete cleft of the palate.
      (2) Another form of cleft palate is caused by **micrognathia (hypoplastic mandible)** and projection of the tongue posteriorly during development, preventing closure of the palate. This phenomenon is called **Pierre Robin sequence**.
         (a) The cleft usually is U-shaped.
         (b) The **recurrence risk** generally is low because the Pierre Robin sequence usually is sporadic; however, the Pierre Robin sequence can be associated with syndromes such as **Stickler syndrome** and **Treacher Collins syndrome**. When a syndrome is present, the recurrence risk depends on the inheritance of the syndrome. There are more than 50 syndromes in which the Pierre Robin sequence may be seen.

VI. MITOCHONDRIAL DISORDERS

A. The **mitochondrion** is a structure exclusively inherited from the mother through ovum cytoplasm and is the center of cellular energy metabolism.

1. It carries some of its own genetic information in the form of a small **circular chromosome,** although several important mitochondrial enzyme functions are also coded on the nuclear chromosomes and transported into the mitochondria by a targeted active process.

2. **Mutations** causing disease are known in both the mitochondrial and the nuclear-encoded enzymes.

    a. The resulting phenotypes are considered to be **energy-deficient states**.

    b. Organs and physiologic processes that are highly energy dependent are preferentially affected, causing:

        (1) Myopathies, both peripheral and cardiac

        (2) Intestinal dysfunctions, such as transport dysfunction and chronic diarrhea

        (3) CNS dysfunction, such as developmental delay or seizures

3. In many mitochondrial disorders, intermittent elevations of blood **lactate** levels, and sometimes secondary elevation or depression of **pyruvate** levels, occur. Measuring these substances, as well as ammonia, **carnitine,** and organic acids, is a useful laboratory tool for diagnosing these disorders.

B. **Heteroplasmy** refers to the observation that the relative population of mutant mitochondria can vary both within and between individuals in the same family.

1. There can be variation in the affected organ.

2. There can be variation over time, usually increased severity.

3. Heteroplasmy produces tremendous variability in severity of expression for the same mutation, ranging from lethal disorders affecting growth and brain function, to minimally affected individuals in the same family.

C. Because mitochondria are inherited only through the mother, this **maternal transmission** can produce a unique pedigree pattern.

1. All affected individuals are related to each other through the maternal line.

2. Transmission from affected men to their offspring is not seen.

3. Differentiation from dominant and X-linked nuclear inheritance on the basis of pedigree analysis alone can be difficult, and requires **enzyme and DNA analysis,** which are available.

VII. DISORDERS DUE TO GENETIC IMPRINTING.

It has recently been recognized that some genes are expressed differently depending on the parent from whom the gene was inherited. This differential modification or marking of genes, which is a normal phenomenon, is known as **genetic imprinting**.

A. Some genes are inactivated when inherited from the father, and others are inactivated when inherited from the mother. These **inactivated genes** are not transcribed into gene products to the same extent as the gene from the other-sex parent.

1. In genetic imprinting, the gene is intact and normal, but has somehow been modified so that its expression is modulated depending on which parent it was inherited from.

2. Imprinting is a reversible process when the gene is passed to succeeding generations, again influenced by the sex of the transmitting parent.

3. Only a relatively small proportion—less than 5%—of the genes in the human genome are known to be affected by imprinting.

B. **Prader-Willi syndrome** was the first disorder recognized as resulting from genetic imprinting. Prader-Willi syndrome occurs in 1 in 15,000 newborns.

1. **Defect.** This syndrome is associated with an interstitial deletion of the long arm of chromosome 15 [**deletion of 15(q11-q13)**], detected by high-resolution chromosome analysis, FISH, or molecular genetic analysis.

    a. About 70% of patients with Prader-Willi syndrome have a chromosome deletion, always in the paternally derived chromosome 15.

    b. A small proportion of patients (about 5%) have a chromosome translocation or other structural rearrangement involving 15q.

    c. The remaining patients with Prader-Willi syndrome, who have a normal-appearing chromosome complement, recently have been found to be missing the paternal contribution to 15q on the basis of absence of the entire paternal chromosome 15 and presence of two number 15 chromosomes of maternal origin. This is called **maternal disomy,** or maternal **uniparental disomy**.

        (1) Two copies of chromosome 15 are required for survival. For most of the genes on this chromosome, it does not matter whether the genes are maternal or paternal in origin, because most of the genes on chromosome 15 are not imprinted.

        (2) Uniparental disomy probably occurs because of nondisjunction, which leads to a trisomy followed by loss of the chromosome from the parent who contributes only one copy to the trisomy. In Prader-Willi syndrome, the trisomy would contain one paternal 15 and two maternal 15s, and would be followed by loss of the paternal 15.

    d. In the normal individual, the maternal contribution to the relevant region of chromosome 15 is not expressed; only the paternal copy is normally expressed. In Prader-Willi syndrome, the paternal copy of these genes has either been deleted or is missing owing to maternal disomy, so that no active copies of these genes are present.

2. Recurrence risk. The empiric recurrence risk is less than 1 in 100, unless the chromosome 15 deletion is the result of parental translocation or some other rearrangement (very rare).

3. Clinical features

    a. Children with Prader-Willi syndrome have severe **infantile hypotonia** associated with feeding difficulties and **failure to thrive** in infancy. Later (between 1 and 4 years of age), **central obesity** develops in these children owing to an appetite disorder. They eat large amounts of food unless strict dietary control is enforced.

    b. Developmental delay is a major feature. Most patients are mildly mentally retarded, although some have a normal IQ or are more severely retarded. Behavior problems are common, and a characteristic personality type is seen.

    c. Dysmorphic features include narrow bifrontal diameter, almond-shaped palpebral fissures, a down-turned mouth, and small hands and feet.

    d. There is **hypogonadotrophic hypogonadism,** which manifests as small genitalia and incomplete puberty.

    e. Mild **short stature** in adulthood is the rule.

4. Prognosis. Life span is shortened only by the complications of obesity (e.g., diabetes mellitus, hypoventilation).

C. When **uniparental disomy** for a chromosome occurs, it can have three different consequences.

1. If there are no imprinted genes and no abnormal genes on the chromosome, there will be no consequences that have been recognized. This is the case for several of the chromosomes, including 3, 4, 6, 13, 21, and 22.

2. If there are one or more imprinted genes, abnormality may ensue, as is the case in Prader-Willi syndrome and in several other recognized conditions, including **Angelman syndrome** and **Beckwith-Wiedemann syndrome**.

3. In uniparental disomy, the two chromosomes from the same parent can be the two different chromosomes in that parent (called **heterodisomy**) or can be only one of the parent's chromosomes that has been duplicated (called **isodisomy**). If it is the latter, and a recessive single-gene mutation is present on that duplicated chromosome, an autosomal recessive disorder could result. This has been identified in a number of instances, and was first recognized in a case of **cystic fibrosis**.

D. Much is yet to be learned about the impact of genetic imprinting in causing human genetic disorders. It is known that many imprinted genes are growth related, and abnormalities relating to the dose of imprinted genes often cause undergrowth or overgrowth.

VIII. WHEN TO CONSIDER A GENETIC OR MULTIFACTORIAL DISORDER

A. Prenatally

1. **Fetal wastage** may be an indication of a balanced chromosome translocation, a lethal autosomal recessive disorder, or a new dominant disorder.

2. **Fetal growth deficiency** is seen in many chromosomally abnormal pregnancies, in some syndromes, and in many fetuses with malformations.

3. **Oligohydramnios** may reflect genetic urinary tract disorders, in which there is decreased fetal urine production.

4. **Polyhydramnios** can be seen in neurologically impaired fetuses, including those with genetic neurologic disorders, and in fetuses with malformations of the gastrointestinal tract, in which swallowing is impaired.

B. In the newborn

1. **Congenital malformations** often are caused by a genetic disorder or condition with a genetic component. A careful evaluation should consider other anomalies, dysmorphic features, and neurologic abnormalities that suggest syndromes, chromosome disorders, and multifactorial isolated birth defects.

2. Infants who are **small for gestational age** may have a genetic disorder.
   a. Examination should seek possible dysmorphic features, malformations, neurologic abnormalities, and a significant prenatal history.
   b. Chromosome disorders, syndromes, and dwarfing conditions should be considered in addition to teratogens, placental abnormalities, and in utero constraint.
   c. Infants with just **short stature at birth** may have a dwarfing condition or may be small for gestational age.

3. **Large size at birth** also may be a reflection of an abnormality. One of the disorders of overgrowth is **Beckwith-Wiedemann syndrome,** which is associated with macrosomia, omphalocele, macroglossia, and hypoglycemia. Infants of diabetic mothers often are large (macrosomic) at birth.

4. **Dysmorphism** often is an indicator of a chromosomal abnormality, a single gene or sporadic syndrome, or deformation. An evaluation for other anomalies of function or structure should be undertaken. A careful prenatal history may indicate deformation as the cause.

5. **Hypotonia** may indicate a genetic disorder, such as a CNS malformation, neuromuscular disease, or one of a variety of syndromes associated with central hypotonia (e.g., chromosomal disorders, Prader-Willi syndrome, some dwarfing conditions).

6. **Seizures** resulting from a metabolic derangement or CNS malformation associated with a genetic disorder may present in the newborn. Chromosomal disorders and single-gene disorders frequently are the cause.

7. **Ambiguous genitalia** imply a genetic disorder unless the fetus was exposed to hormones. The differential diagnosis of ambiguous genitalia includes metabolic disorders (see Chapter 17), multifactorial abnormalities, chromosome anomalies, single-gene disorders, teratogenic exposures, and sporadic syndromes.

8. **Metabolic disturbances,** such as abnormal pH (acidosis, alkalosis), elevated ammonia, or absent or excessive ketones, occur in a number of inborn metabolic errors.

C. **In the infant and toddler**

1. **Failure to thrive,** or insufficient growth rate, has many causes, some of which are genetic (see also Chapter 3). It often is helpful diagnostically to distinguish conditions with prenatal-onset growth deficiency (such as fetal alcohol syndrome and chromosomal disorders) from those with only postnatal-onset failure to thrive (such as metabolic disorders).

   a. **Inborn errors of metabolism** commonly have associated failure to thrive, as do **neurodegenerative disorders** and other severe neurologic conditions that may be genetic in origin.

   b. Many **chromosome abnormalities and syndromes** have associated growth deficiency.

   c. **Dwarfing conditions** may initially present as failure to thrive, although growth rate may eventually normalize.

   d. Some **teratogens,** such as alcohol, may also produce postnatal as well as prenatal growth deficiency.

2. **Developmental delay** also has many causes, but it should raise suspicion of a genetic condition.

   a. **Delays in motor development** alone may reflect a neuromuscular disorder, either central or peripheral.

   b. **Delays in cognitive development** alone or cognitive plus motor delays may presage mental retardation, which should raise suspicion of a genetic cause.

   c. Many syndromes have associated **developmental delays and mental retardation,** and, thus, delays should trigger the search for associated anomalies or dysmorphism.

3. **Loss of developmental milestones,** or **regression,** suggests neurodegenerative disorders, most of which are genetic in origin (e.g., neuronal storage disorders).

4. **Microcephaly** [head circumference below the second percentile or discrepant to that expected for the child's height or family background (see also Chapter 18)]

   a. Microcephaly usually is a sign of poor brain development (**micrencephaly**), because the skull generally grows in response to brain growth. There are many causes of micrencephaly, including single gene disorders, chromosomal abnormalities, syndromes, anoxic or vascular brain damage, and teratogen exposure.

   b. Occasionally, microcephaly can be a reflection of premature closure of the sutures (**craniosynostosis**). This can occur on the basis of a genetic disorder or syndrome, or can occur sporadically.

5. **Macrocephaly** (head circumference above the ninety-eighth percentile or discrepant to that expected for the child's height or family background) can be familial and isolated or can reflect an abnormality that may be genetic in origin.

   a. Macrocephaly may be caused by increased ventricular size (as in hydrocephalus), or it may be the result of increased brain size (**macrencephaly**).

   b. Some disorders and syndromes are associated with macrocephaly without apparent consequence, such as **neurofibromatosis**. Associated signs and symptoms should be sought.

   c. **Fragile X syndrome** has associated macrocephaly, so patients with macrocephaly should be evaluated for mental retardation.

   d. Some inborn metabolic errors causing **storage of material in nerve cells** can produce macrocephaly. MPSs, for example, are associated with macrocephaly.

   e. **Intracranial malformations** may present as large head size, reflecting **hydrocephalus**. In most cases, it is appropriate to do a cranial computed tomography or magnetic resonance imaging scan if macrocephaly of unknown etiology is present.

6. An **unusual growth pattern** may be an indication of a genetic condition.

a. Some disorders associated with **limb asymmetry or hypertrophy** include neurofibromatosis, **Klippel-Trenaunay-Weber syndrome,** and **Russell-Silver syndrome**. Such asymmetry should also raise suspicion of an intraabdominal tumor, such as Wilms tumor. Abdominal ultrasound is indicated when limb hypertrophy is present.

b. Generalized overgrowth may suggest Beckwith-Wiedemann syndrome or **Sotos syndrome**.

c. Disproportionate growth often is indicative of a bony dysplasia or connective tissue abnormality.

　(1) Short limbs, often resulting in short stature, should trigger the search for radiologic abnormalities of bone growth.

　(2) Unusually long limbs for race might suggest Marfan syndrome, homocystinuria, or Stickler syndrome.

　(3) A short trunk usually indicates a bony abnormality of the spine, generally a bony dysplasia, scoliosis, or structural vertebral anomalies.

7. Abnormal pigmentation, diffusely or focally, may reflect a genetic disorder (see also Chapter 18).

a. Neurocutaneous disorders often present in this age-group with dermatologic findings. Such disorders include **neurofibromatosis** (café au lait spots), **tuberous sclerosis** (hypopigmented spots), **basal cell nevus syndrome** (multiple nevi), and **incontinentia pigmenti** (swirls of hyperpigmentation).

b. Generalized hypopigmentation may be seen with **albinism** or **ectodermal dysplasias**.

8. An **unusual odor** of an infant or the infant's urine may be a manifestation of an inborn metabolic error, such as PKU (mousy odor) or maple syrup urine disease.

D. | In childhood

1. Mental retardation is the most common indication of a genetic problem that is recognized in the school-age child. Frequently, it is preceded by developmental delay.

a. The causes of mental retardation are many. Identifying the specific etiology is important because it allows the determination of prognosis, educational planning, possible associated problems, treatment if available, and the recurrence risk. Table 8-10 lists the major categories of causes of mental retardation and some examples (see also Chapter 4).

TABLE 8-10. Causes of Mental Retardation

Category	Examples
Autosomal dominant	Tuberous sclerosis Myotonic dystrophy
Autosomal recessive	Phenylketonuria Mucopolysaccharidoses
X-linked	Fragile X syndrome Aqueductal stenosis
Multifactorial	Nonspecific mental retardation Hydrocephalus
Chromosomal	Down syndrome Prader-Willi syndrome
Teratogenic	Fetal alcohol syndrome Congenital rubella syndrome
Accidental	Perinatal anoxia Intracranial hemorrhage

b. The evaluation of the child with mental retardation is discussed in Chapter 4. When no cause for mental retardation can be found, multifactorial inheritance is the most likely etiology, with a 3%–5% recurrence risk.

2. Some **metabolic disorders, genetic neurologic conditions, and neurodegenerative disorders** may present in mid-childhood.

3. **Chronic anemia** may reflect hemoglobinopathy (e.g., thalassemia) or a disorder of red blood cell metabolism (e.g., glucose-6-phosphate dehydrogenase deficiency).

E. In adolescence and adulthood

1. Failure of expected secondary sexual development and other **pubertal disorders** may indicate a genetic condition.
  a. Some single-gene disorders, such as testicular feminization, are associated with primary amenorrhea.
  b. Sex chromosome abnormalities, such as Turner syndrome (45,X) or Klinefelter syndrome (47,XXY), lead to incomplete or inadequate sexual development.
  c. Several syndrome disorders have associated delayed, precocious, or abnormal pubertal development (e.g., Prader-Willi syndrome).

2. Several genetic **neurologic disorders** may present in adolescence, such as the hereditary and sensory motor **neuropathies** [e.g., Charcot-Marie-Tooth disease (see Chapter 18)], some **spinocerebellar degenerations,** and some **ataxias** [e.g., Friedreich ataxia (see Chapter 18)].

3. **Genetic kidney disorders** (see Chapter 14) commonly present in adulthood, including autosomal dominant polycystic kidney disease and hereditary nephritis. The initial presenting symptom may be hypertension.

4. **Cancer at an earlier age** than is commonly seen may be the result of genetic predisposition (see Chapter 16).
  a. Some single-gene disorders cause a predisposition to cancer, including those causing multiple endocrine neoplasias, breast cancer, Peutz-Jeghers syndrome (colon cancer), familial polyposis, and Gardner syndrome.
  b. Some families have an increased risk for several different types of cancer. These so-called cancer families present as though they have an autosomal dominant disorder with variable expressivity.
  c. Some chromosomal deletions can predispose to cancer (e.g., deletion of 11p13 with Wilms tumor).

5. **Early onset of common disorders of midlife,** such as coronary artery disease and hypertension, are caused in some families by genetic predisposition, which may be the result of a single-gene disorder or may be multifactorial.

6. **Infertility** or **recurrent pregnancy loss** may be caused by a parental balanced translocation, a genetic lethal disorder in the fetus, or a structural uterine abnormality in the woman. Oligospermia associated with infertility in men can be seen in Klinefelter syndrome, cystic fibrosis, and immotile cilia syndrome.

7. Several autosomal dominant **seizure disorders** present during adolescence or adulthood.

8. A **family history of birth defects or mental retardation** may be indicative of an autosomal or X-linked disorder or a balanced chromosomal translocation within the family.

BIBLIOGRAPHY

Buyse ML (ed): *The Birth Defects Encyclopedia.* Cambridge, MA, Blackwell Scientific, 1990.

Emery AEH, Rimoin DL: *Principles and Practice of Medical Genetics,* 2nd ed. New York, Churchill-Livingstone, 1990.

Gorlin RJ, Cohen MM, Levin LS: *Syndromes of the Head and Neck,* 3rd ed. New York, Oxford University Press, 1990.

Jones KL: *Smith's Recognizable Patterns of Human Malformation,* 4th ed. Philadelphia, WB Saunders, 1988.

McKusick VA: *Mendelian Inheritance in Man,* 10th ed. Baltimore, Johns Hopkins University Press, 1992.

Scriver CR, et al: *The Metabolic Basis of Inherited Disease,* 6th ed. New York, McGraw-Hill, 1989.

Stevenson RE, Hall JG, Goodman RM: *Human Malformations and Related Disorders.* New York, Oxford University Press, 1993.

Thompson MW, McInnes RR, Willard HF (eds): *Thompson & Thompson: Genetics in Medicine,* 5th ed. Philadelphia, WB Saunders, 1991.

DIRECTIONS: Each of the numbered items or incomplete statements in this section is followed by answers or by completions of the statement. Select the ONE lettered answer or completion that is BEST in each case.

1. A newborn girl has been diagnosed with phenylketonuria (PKU), the most common disorder of amino acid metabolism, through state-mandated newborn screening. Which one of the following statements can be accurately made to the parents?

(A) PKU is an autosomal dominant disorder
(B) Hyperpigmentation is a common sign of PKU
(C) Dietary management should begin within 1 month of birth to prevent mental retardation
(D) Dietary restriction can be discontinued safely in adolescence
(E) Heart defects are common in people with PKU

2. Marfan syndrome would be suspected in a 14-year-old boy because of which one of the following clinical abnormalities?

(A) Aortic dilatation and loose joints, suggestive of a connective tissue disorder
(B) Excess bone length and width, suggestive of a bone metabolism disorder
(C) Floppy tendons and ligaments, suggestive of a muscle cell developmental disorder
(D) Tall stature and excess subcutaneous tissue, suggestive of a growth factor disorder

3. Which of the following statements regarding an 18-week fetus with a neural tube defect is true?

(A) The neural tube defect was produced before implantation of the embryo
(B) The defect results in an abnormally low maternal serum α-fetoprotein (AFP) level
(C) A single autosomal recessive gene is the most common cause of the neural tube defect
(D) The parents of this fetus with a neural tube defect have an increased risk for having another child with such a defect
(E) The neural tube defect is most likely part of a syndrome with birth defects of other organs

DIRECTIONS: Each of the numbered items or incomplete statements in this section is negatively phrased, as indicated by a capitalized word such as NOT, LEAST, or EXCEPT. Select the ONE lettered answer or completion that is BEST in each case.

4. A pregnant woman is referred for predelivery counseling. She has ingested significant amounts of alcohol throughout pregnancy. You explain that alcohol exposure may cause any of the following outcomes EXCEPT

(A) a normal child
(B) a child with developmental delay who is otherwise normal
(C) a child with Down syndrome
(D) a child with dysmorphic features, small size, and developmental retardation
(E) a child who is microcephalic and small for gestational age

5. A 36-year-old pregnant woman has prenatal testing that reveals trisomy 21. During counseling, you explain all of the following regarding Down syndrome EXCEPT

(A) it is the most common chromosome abnormality
(B) there is nothing that either parent did that caused this abnormality
(C) heart defects and gastrointestinal abnormalities occur with increased frequency
(D) most individuals are severely or profoundly retarded
(E) the likelihood of trisomy 21 occurring again in subsequent pregnancies to this couple is approximately 1%–2%

6. A 4-year-old boy with mildly delayed language development is found to have macrocephaly. This could be the result of any of the following EXCEPT

(A) fragile X syndrome
(B) a benign familial characteristic
(C) mucopolysaccharidosis
(D) vascular brain damage
(E) hydrocephalus

DIRECTIONS: Each set of matching questions in this section consists of a list of four to twenty-six lettered options (some of which may be in figures) followed by several items. For each numbered item, select the ONE lettered option that is most closely associated with it. To avoid spending too much time on matching sets with large numbers of options, it is generally advisable to begin each set by reading the list of options. Then, for each item in the set, try to generate the correct answer and locate it in the option list, rather than evaluating each option individually. Each lettered option may be selected once, more than once, or not at all.

Questions 7–10

Match each genetic disorder listed below with its most likely genetic cause.

(A) Autosomal recessive disorder
(B) Autosomal dominant disorder
(C) X-linked disorder
(D) Multifactorial disorder
(E) Chromosome deletion disorder

7. Prader-Willi syndrome

8. Fragile X syndrome

9. Phenylketonuria (PKU)

10. Nonspecific isolated mental retardation

ANSWERS AND EXPLANATIONS

1. The answer is C *[III B 3 b (2)]*. Phenylketonuria (PKU) is an autosomal recessive disorder of amino acid metabolism that is characterized by lack of conversion of phenylalanine to tyrosine. Dietary restriction should start early in infancy (by 1 month of age) and be maintained throughout life, especially in women with PKU, who are at a high risk for giving birth to children with microcephaly and congenital heart disease when they are not observing dietary restrictions. Because tyrosine is essential to the production of the pigment melanin, hypopigmentation is a common sign of PKU.

2. The answer is A *[III A 2 a, b]*. Marfan syndrome is an autosomal dominant disorder of connective tissue. Major manifestations include a characteristic body habitus (i.e., long, thin digits and limbs; loose joints; scoliosis and chest deformity), aortic dilatation and mitral valve prolapse, and lens dislocation and myopia. Bone metabolism, muscle cell development, and hormone status are thought to be normal.

3. The answer is D *[V B 1–4]*. Neural tube defects result from a defect of closure of the neural groove, which normally closes by 28 days' gestation. Implantation occurs by 7–10 days postconception. Cranial failure to close results in anencephaly, and distal failure to close results in meningomyelocele (spina bifida), both occurring on the basis of a multifactorial disorder with two possible manifestations. The recurrence risk for neural tube defects increases with each additional first-degree relative who is affected. A couple with one affected child has a 3%–5% risk of having another child with a neural tube defect; the risk is 7%–10% after a second affected child. High maternal serum α-fetoprotein (AFP) levels reflect an abnormal opening between the fetus and amniotic fluid, and occur in 85% of pregnancies in which a neural tube defect is present. Neural tube defects rarely are part of a syndrome.

4. The answer is C *[II G 1 b, 2]*. Alcohol exposure during gestation can produce a child who has some or all of the features of the fetal alcohol syndrome, or it can have no recognizable effect. Clinical features of fetal alcohol syndrome include central nervous system (CNS) abnormalities (e.g., intellectual defects, microcephaly), growth deficiencies, facial dysmorphisms, and other structural anomalies. Down syndrome is not known to occur at an increased rate as a result of maternal alcohol use.

5. The answer is D *[IV B 1]*. Down syndrome results in a characteristic pattern of dysmorphic features and mental retardation, with an increased risk for internal malformations, especially congenital heart defects and duodenal atresia. Mental retardation usually is moderate, with the average IQ being 50. The chance that another child with Down syndrome will be born to this couple is increased compared with parents in the general population, and is approximately 1%–2%, compared with the population incidence of 1/700.

6. The answer is D *[VIII C 4 a, 5]*. Microcephaly, not macrocephaly, may be caused by anoxic or vascular brain damage unless hydrocephalus is present as a complication. Macrocephaly has many causes, including intracranial malformations or hydrocephalus (enlarged ventricles) and enlarged brain due to storage of abnormal substances within or between the nerve cells (e.g., mucopolysaccharidosis). Certain disorders have associated macrocephaly for unknown reasons, such as fragile X syndrome and neurofibromatosis. Macrocephaly also may run in families; by definition, 5% of the normal population have a head circumference greater than the ninety-fifth percentile. In these cases, there are no known associated abnormalities, and this boy's language delay would be unrelated.

7–10. The answers are: 7-E *[VII B 1]*, **8-C** *[III C 2]*, **9-A** *[III B 3 b (2)]*, **10-D** *[VIII D 1 b]*. Prader-Willi syndrome is a multisystem disorder characterized by dysmorphic features, obesity, short stature, and mental retardation. It is associated with a detectable deletion of the long arm of chromosome 15 in 70% of patients. Fragile X syndrome is a common form of mental retardation that is X-linked. A marker, the so-called fragile X chromosome, is demonstrable on the distal end of the long arm of the X chromosome in folate-deficient cell culture studies performed in affected individuals. This karyotypic phenomenon is believed to be a consequence of the abnormal gene, which also causes mental retardation. Phenylketonuria (PKU) is an autosomal recessive disorder of amino acid metabolism resulting from deficiency of phenylalanine hydroxylase, the enzyme that converts phenylalanine to tyrosine. If not treated with dietary restriction of phenylala-

nine, mental retardation results. When no cause for mental retardation can be found and there are no associated physical or functional abnormalities, multifactorial inheritance is the most likely etiology. In this case, there is a 3%–5% empiric recurrence risk.

Chapter 9

Immunologic, Allergic, and Rheumatic Diseases

Mark Ballow
Milton Markowitz
James Robinson

I. **HOST DEFENSE SYSTEMS.** The human immune system is a dynamic network of cellular and humoral elements working in concert to allow the host to distinguish between self and nonself in order to recognize foreign substances and to eliminate, neutralize, or metabolize those substances. Functions of the immune system fall into three main categories: resistance to microbial invasion, maintenance of homeostasis, and surveillance against transformed or malignant cells.

A. Nonspecific (innate, nonadaptive) host defenses

   1. **Barriers** act as a front line in defense. There are two types:
      a. Anatomic (physical) barriers (e.g., skin, cilia, mucus)
      b. Biochemical barriers (e.g., lysozyme, lactoferrin, gastric acid)

   2. **Cells** involved in nonspecific defense include leukocytes (neutrophils, eosinophils, basophils), mast cells, macrophages, cells of the reticuloendothelial system, platelets, and natural killer (NK) cells.

   3. **Plasma or soluble factors** serving in conjunction with the cellular elements of the nonspecific defense system include proteins of the complement and coagulation pathways, proteins of the kinin–kallikrein system, acute-phase proteins, and fibronectin.

   4. **Factors released from cells** of the nonspecific defense system include α- and β-interferons, interleukins, lysosomal enzymes, and mediators of anaphylaxis.

B. **Specific (adaptive) host defenses** involve an adaptive (**immunogenic**) response to foreign materials, followed by specific recognition and long-term memory of the molecule (**antigen**) that caused the initial **immune response**.

   1. **Humoral immunity** defends primarily against the extracellular phases of bacterial and viral infections.
      a. Cellular elements consist of **B lymphocytes (B cells)** and **plasma cells**.
      b. Serum factors include five classes of **immunoglobulins (antibodies):** immunoglobulin G (IgG), IgM, IgA, IgD, and IgE.

   2. **Cellular immunity** defends against intracellular organisms (e.g., viruses, fungi, parasites) and provides immune surveillance against malignant cells and foreign tissue.
      a. Cellular elements consist of **T lymphocytes (T cells)** and their subsets.
      b. T-cell–derived factors include lymphokines, interleukins (IL), helper and suppressor factors, and γ-interferon.

II. **IMMUNODEFICIENCY DISORDERS.** Deficiencies of host defense systems result in an immunologic imbalance that can lead to a susceptibility to infection, an autoimmune disease, or a predisposition to malignancies.

A. **Complement disorders.** Activation of the complement system, by either the classic or the alternative pathway, leads to the generation of potent complement components, which have various biologic activities. The complement system is a complex system composed of many serum proteins and cellular receptors that serve as important mediators of inflammation and host defense, particularly against microbial organisms. **Faulty complement activation or regulation** can lead to immune-mediated damage of host tissues and various disorders. Most genetically determined complement deficiencies are inherited as autosomal recessive disorders.

1. **Deficiency of early complement components** (C1, C4, C2) results in a symptom complex resembling collagen vascular disorders [e.g., systemic lupus erythematosus (SLE)] and increased susceptibility to pyogenic infections.

2. **C3 deficiency** results in severe pyogenic infections. Several patients have also had SLE and glomerulonephritis.

3. **Deficiency of late complement components** (C5, C6, C7, C8) results in systemic *Neisseria* infections such as meningococcal sepsis and meningitis, and disseminated gonococcal infections.

4. **Abnormalities of the control proteins of the alternative pathway** (factor H, factor I, properdin) may result in recurrent infections.

5. **Deficiency of complement inhibitors** (C1 esterase inhibitor, carboxypeptidase N) leads to recurrent angioedema.

B. **Phagocyte disorders** (Table 9-1)

1. **Types of defects.** Phagocyte disorders affect any one or several of the cell's functions, including:
   a. Adherence to vascular endothelium
   b. Recognition of and migration toward a chemical stimulus (chemotaxia)
   c. Phagocytosis
   d. Intracellular killing

2. **Clinical features**
   a. Affected individuals are prone to infections with low-grade bacteria such as *Staphylococcus aureus* and gram-negative enteric bacteria. Infections may range from mild skin lesions to severe systemic infections. Typical infections include furunculosis, organ abscess, lymphadenitis, and perirectal abscess.

TABLE 9-1. Phagocyte Disorders in Children

Disorder	Inheritance	Clinical Features	Therapy
Chronic granulomatous disease	X-linked (66%); autosomal recessive (33%)	Infections with catalase-positive bacteria and fungi affecting skin, lungs, liver; granuloma formation; NBT test is diagnostic	Antibiotics; γ-interferon
Myeloperoxidase deficiency	Autosomal recessive	Fungal infections (candidiasis) in deep tissues, especially in presence of diabetes	Antibiotics
Leukocyte adhesion deficiency	Autosomal recessive	Delayed separation of the umbilical cord; skin infections; otitis media; pneumonia; gingivitis; periodontitis	Antibiotics
Abnormal chemotaxis	Variable	Recurrent skin infections with staphylococci, enteric bacteria	Antibiotics

NBT = nitroblue tetrazolium dye.

b. Patients with **disorders of leukocyte movement** are unable to accumulate neutrophils at the sites of infection (Chediak-Higashi syndrome, hyper-IgE syndrome) [see Chapter 15 V A 1].

c. Patients with a **leukocyte adhesion deficiency** have defective expression of cell membrane adhesion glycoproteins (e.g., CD11, CD18) and have a history of delayed separation of the umbilical cord (> 4 weeks after birth).

3. Molecular basis of disease

a. Chronic granulomatous disease arises from a defect of cytochrome b558 components in cell membrane or cytosol.

b. Leukocyte adhesion deficiency is the result of a gene defect of the β chain (CD18) of the integrin molecule.

C. | **B-cell deficiency disorders** (Table 9-2). Defects or deficiencies of B cells lead to various antibody deficiencies, or **hypogammaglobulinemias**. Patients suffer from recurrent infections.

TABLE 9-2. B-Cell Deficiency Disorders in Children

Disorder	Inheritance	Clinical Features	Therapy
X-linked agammaglobulinemia (Bruton disease)	X-linked	Recurrent pyogenic infections; infections of lungs, sinuses, middle ear, skin, central nervous system	Immune serum globulin; antibiotics
Transient hypogammaglobulinemia of infancy	Unknown	Recurrent pyogenic infections; frequent in families with other immunodeficiencies	Antibiotics; immune serum globulin (selected patients)
Selective immunoglobulin deficiency (IgA, IgM, IgG subclasses)	Various (IgA deficiency only); autosomal recessive; unknown	Recurrent infections of lungs, sinuses; gastrointestinal disease; allergy; frequent in families with common variable immunodeficiencies	Antibiotics; immune serum globulin (IgG subclass deficiencies only)
Immunoglobulin deficiency with increased IgM (and IgD)	X-linked; autosomal recessive; unknown	Infections of lungs, sinuses, middle ear; increased frequency of autoimmune disease	Immune serum globulin; antibiotics
Common variable immunodeficiency	Autosomal recessive; autosomal dominant; unknown	Infections of lungs, sinuses, middle ear; giardiasis; malabsorption; autoimmune disease	Immune serum globulin; antibiotics
Transcobalamin II deficiency	Autosomal recessive	Recurrent infections; megaloblastic anemia; intestinal villous atrophy; defective granulocyte bactericidal activity	Immune serum globulin; high dose of vitamin B_{12}
X-linked hypogammaglobulinemia with growth hormone deficiency	X-linked	Recurrent pyogenic infections; short stature	Immune serum globulin
Functional or specific antibody deficiency with normal total immunoglobulins and normal IgG subclasses	Unknown	Recurrent sinopulmonary infections	Antibiotics; immune serum globulin

1. **Causative agents** are most commonly extracellular organisms, namely pyogenic and enteric bacteria, because patients are deficient in serum opsonins (antibodies) necessary for phagocytosis. Patients with X-linked (Bruton) agammaglobulinemia may also have problems with certain enteric viruses (e.g., polio virus, echo virus, coxsackievirus). Patients with IgA deficiency or common variable hypogammaglobulinemia are affected by *Giardia lamblia,* a gastrointestinal parasite (see Chapter 10).

2. **Sites of infection** include the skin, sinuses, meninges, and the respiratory, urinary, and gastrointestinal tracts.

3. **The molecular basis** of X-linked agammaglobulinemia is a gene deletion of cytoplasmic tryrosine kinase.

D. **T-cell deficiency disorders** (Table 9-3), also known as **cell-mediated (cellular) immuno-deficiencies,** result from abnormalities in T-cell functions. Antibody production is also likely to be affected in patients with severe T-cell abnormalities because T cells are important immunoregulators of B-cell differentiation and function.

1. **Recurrent infections** also are common in patients with cellular immunodeficiencies.
   a. **Causative agents** are **intracellular pathogens** [e.g., herpesviruses, mycobacteria, fungi (*Candida*), and protozoa (*Pneumocystis carinii, Toxoplasma*)].
   b. **Sites of infection** include a variety of sites, both local and systemic.

2. **Congenital cell-mediated immunodeficiencies** represent a complex spectrum of immunodeficiencies. At one extreme are defects in lymphoid stem cell differentiation, which result in severe combined immunodeficiency disorders. At the other extreme are isolated defects that affect only cell-mediated immunity to one particular pathogen (e.g., chronic mucocutaneous candidiasis).

3. **Molecular basis of disease**
   a. Hyper-IgM syndrome arises from a gene mutation of CD40 ligand, gp 39, on T cells.
   b. Severe combined immunodeficiency disorders result from the following defects: gene mutation affecting the CD3 complex (e.g., γ, ε chains); gene mutations of adenosine deaminase enzyme; gene mutations of purine nucleoside phosphorylase enzyme; gene defect of γ-chain of IL-2 receptor; defective signal transduction pathway in T cells; defective IL-2 production; and defects of T-cell–specific regulatory factors for the transcription of cytokine genes.

E. **Acquired immune deficiency syndrome (AIDS)** is a disorder associated with a profound deficiency in T-cell immunity, and, in children, T-cell and B-cell abnormalities. AIDS currently is the eighth leading cause of death among children 1–4 years of age and the sixth leading cause of death in youths 15–24 years old. By 1992, there were 20,000 human immunodeficiency virus (HIV)-infected infants reported in the United States; this is probably an underestimate of the actual number of cases.

1. **Causative agent and mechanisms of transmission**
   a. **HIV-1,** a retrovirus, is the cause of AIDS.
   b. **Transmission**
      (1) Approximately 85% of childhood HIV infections occur because of perinatal transmission from an HIV-infected mother to her newborn. The average risk of perinatal transmission is such that 20%–25% of babies born to infected mothers will become infected. There is evidence that a large proportion of perinatal infections occur at parturition. Breast feeding can also transmit HIV infection to an infant.
      (2) Transmission to recipients of blood, blood products, or organ transplantation has diminished in importance owing to efficient screening of blood and organ donors and pretreatment of plasma products.
      (3) Adolescents acquire infection via sexual contact and intravenous drug abuse.

TABLE 9-3. T-Cell and Combined T-Cell and B-Cell Deficiency Disorders in Children

Disorder	Inheritance	Clinical Features	Therapy

Severe combined immuno-deficiency
  Sporadic
  X-linked
  Autosomal recessive
  With B cells and a mixed lympho-cyte reaction
  Nezelof syndrome
	X-linked; autosomal recessive	Recurrent infections; wasting; chronic diarrhea; failure to thrive; graft versus host disease	Bone marrow transplantation

Defects of the purine salvage pathway
  Adenosine deaminase deficiency
  Purine nucleoside phosphorylase deficiency
	Autosomal recessive	Recurrent infections; dysostosis (some adenosine deaminase deficiency); anemia and mental retardation (purine nucleoside phosphorylase deficiency)	Bone marrow transplantation; enzyme replacement therapy

DiGeorge anomaly (third and fourth pouch/arch syndrome)	None or unknown (embryologic defect)	Hypoparathyroidism (hypocalcemia); facial abnormalities; cardiovascular abnormalities; infections; mental deficiency (some patients); gastrointestinal tract malformation (some patients)	Thymus graft or thymic humoral factors (e.g., thymosin)
Chronic mucocutaneous candidiasis	Autosomal recessive	Chronic candidal infection of the skin, nails, scalp, and mucous membranes; autoimmune endocrine disorders	Topical and systemic antifungal agents; transfer factor; thymus transplantation

Major histocompatibility complex deficiency
  Class I deficiency
  Class II deficiency
	Autosomal recessive	Intestinal malabsorption (class II deficiency); recurrent infections	Bone marrow transplantation

Ataxia–telangiectasia	Autosomal recessive	Oculocutaneous telangiectasia; progressive cerebellar ataxia; bronchiectasis; malignancy; defective chromosomal repair; raised α-fetoprotein level	Bone marrow transplantation
Wiskott-Aldrich syndrome	X-linked	Eczema; thrombocytopenia; susceptibility to infections; malignancy; small, defective platelets	Bone marrow transplantation; antibiotics; splenectomy
Immunodeficiency with short-limbed dwarfism	Autosomal recessive	Short-limbed dwarfism; lymphopenia	Immune serum globulin

2. Immunologic abnormalities associated with HIV infection
   a. Progressive depletion of CD4 T cells (helper-induced T cells)
   b. Impaired T-cell immunity (even when CD4 T cells are present in normal numbers)
   c. Impaired mononuclear macrophage function
   d. Impaired production of specific antibody despite a polyclonal increase in serum immunoglobulins that lack antibody functions

3. Centers for Disease Control classification of clinical manifestations of HIV infection
   a. Category E (perinatally exposed infant) describes HIV-exposed infants in whom infection has not been confirmed or excluded.
   b. Category N (infected infant) describes HIV-infected infants that are not symptomatic.
   c. Category A (mildly symptomatic infection). Manifestations include lymphadenopathy, hepatosplenomegaly, parotitis, recurrent upper respiratory infections, and otitis media.
   d. Category B (moderately symptomatic infection). Manifestations include chronic oral candidiasis, diarrhea, failure to thrive, anemia, thrombocytopenia, lymphocytic interstitial pneumonitis, cardiomyopathy, and a variety of infectious diseases that reflect some degree of immunodeficiency, but which are not AIDS-defining conditions.
   e. Category C (severely symptomatic infection) includes AIDS-defining conditions.
     (1) Recurrent, serious bacterial infections
     (2) Opportunistic infections include *P. carinii* pneumonia, *Mycobacterium avium-complex,* candidal esophagitis, disseminated cryptococcosis, toxoplasmosis encephalitis, cryptosporidiosis, and disseminated tuberculosis.
     (3) Wasting syndrome
     (4) Progressive neurologic disease can manifest as developmental delay, encephalopathy, paresis, dystonia, and peripheral neuropathy. Cerebral atrophy and intracranial calcifications may be seen on computed tomography scan.

4. Diagnosis of HIV infection
   a. Infants born to HIV-infected mothers (category E)
     (1) Serologic testing (ELISA and Western blot). Maternal antibodies may persist for up to 18 months in exposed infants; hence, with few exceptions, a positive HIV serology in such infants is not diagnostic until after 18 months.
     (2) HIV p24 antigen detection. Not all infected infants have positive tests; a negative test does not exclude HIV infection, but a positive test generally makes the diagnosis.
     (3) HIV culture of blood lymphocytes. When available, this is the most reliable diagnostic test; but a negative culture does not rule out HIV infection.
   b. In infants and children **without known perinatal HIV exposure,** a complex of presenting signs and symptoms may raise suspicions of HIV infection [see II E 3 c–d], or children may present with AIDS-defining infections [see II E 3 e].

5. Prognosis. The majority of children with HIV infection will eventually die of complications of AIDS.
   a. Infants with significant clinical disease in the first year of life tend to progress most rapidly (about 20% of HIV-infected children).
   b. Infants remaining asymptomatic into the second year are likely to remain relatively disease free for several years; some of these children may reach adolescence.

6. Therapy. General management includes antiretroviral therapy, treatment of secondary infections, prophylaxis against *P. carinii* pneumonia, and nutritional support.
   a. Antiretroviral therapy. Nucleoside analog drugs available for pediatric use include zidovudine (AZT, ZDV), didanosine (ddI), zalcitabine (ddC), and stavudine (d4T). These drugs may provide short-term benefits, especially if used in combination; however, these drugs invariably select for emergence of resistant virus. Thus, no treatment regimen is effective in eradicating HIV or halting disease progression entirely. A newer drug, lamuvidine (3TC), used in combination with AZT, appears to manifest

more sustained antiviral effects because 3TC selects for viral mutants that remain sensitive to AZT. The efficacy of other classes of drugs, such as inhibitors of HIV protease, is being evaluated.

  b. Prophylaxis for *P. carinii* pneumonia

   (1) Prophylaxis is recommended for all perinatally exposed infants from 6 weeks to 12 months of age, or until immune status has been clarified. For infected children 12 months to 6 years of age, prophylaxis is given if the percentage of CD4 cells is less than 15% of the total T-cell number, or if the CD4 T-cell number is less than 500/µl; for children older than 6 years, prophylaxis is given when the CD4 T-cell number is less than 200/µl.

   (2) The **drug of choice is trimethoprim–sulfamethoxazole** (TMP-SMX), which is given 3 times a week. Dapsone is used in children who do not tolerate TMP-SMX.

 7. Prevention

  a. Prevention of childhood HIV infections requires decreasing the spread of HIV and decreasing the number of births to HIV-infected women. This ultimately requires a general change in behavior through education and counseling of adults, adolescents, and children about risk behavior.

  b. A recent study demonstrates that the rate of perinatal HIV transmission can be dramatically reduced (about 66%) by treating HIV-infected mothers during pregnancy and delivery with ZDV.

  c. No effective vaccine against HIV infection is likely to be available for some time to come.

F. **Evaluation for immunodeficiency disorders.** During examination of a patient with a suspected immunodeficiency disorder, several clues should be sought.

 1. History

  a. Infections. Severe, recurrent, or persistent infections strongly suggest an immunodeficiency disorder. The following points should be investigated.

   (1) Age at onset. In general, the earlier the age at onset, the more serious the underlying immunodeficiency.

   (2) Site of infection. Serious sites of infection (as in meningitis, pneumonia, sepsis, or generalized dermatitis) suggest an underlying immunodeficiency.

   (3) Causative agent

    (a) Usually, infectious agents in **phagocytic dysfunction** are low-grade bacteria (e.g., *Staphylococcus, Klebsiella,* and *Serratia* sp).

    (b) Infectious agents in **B-cell deficiency disorders** include:

     (i) High-grade (i.e., virulent) bacteria (e.g., *Streptococcus pneumoniae* and other streptococci, *Hemophilus influenzae,* meningococci)

     (ii) *Giardia lamblia*

    (c) Infectious agents in **T-cell deficiency disorders** include:

     (i) Viruses (e.g., herpesviruses, cytomegalovirus)

     (ii) Fungi (e.g., *Candida* sp)

     (iii) Opportunistic organisms (e.g., *Pneumocystis* sp, mycobacteria)

  b. Family history. A pedigree chart is helpful because many immunodeficiency disorders are autosomal recessive or X-linked.

  c. Adverse reactions to drugs, vaccines, or blood products occur more commonly in patients with immunodeficiency disorders.

 2. Physical examination

  a. Growth and development. The physical appearance is characteristic in short-limbed dwarfism and in DiGeorge anomaly. Failure to thrive is common in patients with combined T-cell and B-cell deficiencies.

  b. Skin and oral mucosa should be inspected for signs of infection (e.g., pyoderma, abscess, candidiasis). Eczema is seen in a number of immunodeficiency disorders, especially Wiskott-Aldrich syndrome.

  c. Eyes. Conjunctival telangiectasias occur in ataxia–telangiectasia.

TABLE 9-4. Tests of Immune Competence

Screening tests
  Nonspecific tests
    Absolute granulocyte count
    Total hemolytic complement (CH_{50}; for primary complement deficiency)
    Nitroblue tetrazolium test of neutrophil function (for chronic granulomatous disease)
    Flow cytometry (for leukocyte adhesion molecules on surface of monocytes)

  Tests of humoral (B-cell) immunity
    Quantitation of serum immunoglobulins
      Isotypes—IgG, IgM, IgA, IgE
      IgG subclasses
    Tests for functional antibodies
      Serum isohemagglutinin levels
      Patient's antibody response after immunization for diphtheria and tetanus toxoids or pneumo-
        coccal polysaccharide antigens, if older than 2 years
    Antibody response after infection to respiratory viruses
    Enumeration and phenotyping of B cells in blood

  Tests of cellular (T-cell) immunity
    Absolute lymphocyte count
    Chest x-ray for thymus shadow (only in first few days of life)
    Delayed hypersensitivity skin tests to recall antigens
    Enumeration and phenotyping of T cells and T-cell subsets

Special immunologic tests
  B-cell tests
    Polyclonal B-cell–induced immunoglobulin production in vitro
    Tests of immunoregulation by T cells of immunoglobulin synthesis

  T-cell tests
    Lymphocyte blast transformation response to mitogens, antigens
    Mixed lymphocyte culture assays
    Tests of lymphocyte-mediated cytotoxicity

     d. Lymphatic system
       (1) Hepatomegaly and splenomegaly may be present in patients with phagocytic
          defects or common variable hypogammaglobulinemia.
       (2) Other lymphoid tissues (e.g., lymph nodes, tonsils) are enlarged in some defects
          but are very small in others.
     e. Cardiovascular system. Congenital heart disease occurs in DiGeorge anomaly.
     f. Neuromuscular system. Ataxia may indicate ataxia–telangiectasia.
     g. Skeletal system. Nonspecific arthritis may be seen in Bruton disease and other B-cell
       immunodeficiencies.
   3. Laboratory testing. Information about immune function can be obtained from a number
    of tests (Table 9-4).

III.   **HYPERSENSITIVITY REACTIONS.** The same immunologic mechanisms that protect
    the host can cause tissue damage if they occur in exaggerated or inappropriate form.

  A.   **Types of hypersensitivity.** The widely accepted **Gell and Coombs classification** divides
    these mechanisms into four types of hypersensitivity reactions. Many immunopathologic
    processes are mediated by more than one type of hypersensitivity reaction.

    1. Type I (immediate-type, atopic, or reaginic) hypersensitivity reactions. An antigen
      reacts with IgE antibodies, triggering the release of pharmacologic mediators (chiefly

histamine) from mast cells and basophils (see also IV A 1). Examples of type I reactions include hay fever, extrinsic asthma, and anaphylactic shock.

2. **Type II (antibody-dependent cytotoxic) hypersensitivity reactions.** Antibody (usually IgG or IgM) binds to cell-associated antigens, leading to phagocytosis, killer cell activation, or complement-mediated lysis. An example of a type II reaction is autoimmune hemolytic anemia.

3. **Type III (immune complex–mediated) hypersensitivity reactions.** Complexes composed of antigen and antibody activate complement and mediate an inflammatory reaction. An example of type III reaction is acute glomerulonephritis.

4. **Type IV (cell-mediated or delayed) hypersensitivity reactions.** These reactions are caused by antibody-independent mechanisms involving sensitized T cells and natural killer (NK) cells. Examples of type IV reactions include contact dermatitis and graft rejection.

B. **Role in autoimmune disease.** In most hypersensitivity reactions, the antigen is a foreign substance that the host defense mechanisms recognize as **nonself**. For unknown reasons, the body's self-recognition system sometimes goes awry, so that substances in the body's own tissues become **autoantigens,** and the stage is set for the development of an **autoimmune disease**. Autoimmune disorders usually are type II or type III hypersensitivity reactions, but also may include type IV processes.

IV. ALLERGIC DISORDERS

A. **Principles of IgE-mediated allergic disorders.** IgE originally was called **reaginic or atopic antibody,** because it was known to react with the antigens that cause symptoms in atopic individuals (i.e., people with a familial predisposition to allergic disorders such as hay fever, asthma, and atopic eczema).

1. **Pathogenesis of IgE-mediated allergies.** In IgE-mediated allergies, IgE binds to surface receptors on **mast cells** and **basophils,** thereby sensitizing these cells. When these sensitized cells come in contact with a **specific antigen,** they release substances that are **mediators** of inflammation to trigger the immediate allergic reaction. The mediators act rapidly on local tissues, causing the patient's symptoms. In many allergic disorders, the immediate short-lived inflammatory episode is followed 4–8 hours later by a second event that persists for 24–48 hours. These **late-phase allergic reactions,** which are mediated by CD4+ T cells, eosinophils, and specific mediators and cytokines released from these cells, contribute to the clinical manifestations and prolonged inflammation in bronchial asthma (see Chapter 13), allergic rhinitis, urticaria, and atopic dermatitis.
   a. **Mediator cells**
      (1) **Mast cells and basophils**
         (a) **Mast cells** are the major cell type that is sensitized by IgE antibodies through the Fc receptor on the cell membrane. Two different mast cell phenotypes are found: mucosal and connective tissue mast cells.
         (b) **Basophils** also bind IgE antibody by their Fc receptor. The number of IgE receptors on basophils has been estimated to be about 400,000. Basophils comprise fewer than 0.2% of the leukocytes in the circulation.
         (c) Both mast cells and basophils are characterized by their intense, **deep blue granules,** which contain many pharmacologic mediators of type I hypersensitivity reactions.
      (2) **Eosinophils** comprise 2%–5% of blood leukocytes and are characterized by heavily stained **red granules**. These cells play an important role in allergic diseases and helminthic infections. Eosinophilia is used as an indicator of atopic states.

b. Antigens are molecules that induce a specific immune response, resulting in the creation of antibodies or T cells that specifically match the antigen. Antigens react with their matching antibodies or T cells. **Allergens** are antigens that cause an allergic reaction (i.e., a clinical type I hypersensitivity reaction) by eliciting IgE antibodies. Characteristics of **allergens** include the following.

    (1) Molecules larger than 70,000 daltons are too large to be allergens because they cannot cross mucosal surfaces to reach IgE-forming plasma cells.

    (2) Substances with molecular weights below 10,000 daltons are too small to link the IgE molecules on mast cells, a prerequisite for mediator release. However, smaller molecules can bind to proteins, and this **protein–hapten combination** can be allergenic.

    (3) Most allergens are **glycoproteins**.

c. Mechanisms of mediator release

    (1) Crosslinking. When adjacent cell-bound IgE molecules become crosslinked by the specific antigen, the mast cells degranulate and release the mediators of immediate hypersensitivity.

    (2) Other mechanisms also lead to mast cell activation and degranulation, including:

        (a) Complement activation products, such as anaphylatoxins (complement components C3a and C5a)

        (b) Drugs (e.g., codeine, morphine), which activate mast cells by causing an influx of calcium ions

d. Mast cell- and basophil-derived mediators

    (1) Preformed mediators found in mast cell and basophil granules include:

        (a) Histamine, which causes vasodilation, increased capillary permeability, chemokinesis, and bronchoconstriction

        (b) Heparin

        (c) Proteolytic enzymes (e.g., chymase, tryptase)

        (d) Chemotactic peptides (i.e., eosinophil chemotactic factors, platelet activating factor, and neutrophil chemotactic factor)

    (2) Newly formed mediators in the cytoplasm of mast cells and basophils include:

        (a) Lipoxygenase pathway products [e.g., leukotriene C4 (LTC4), LTB4, LTD4, monohydroxyeicosatetranoic acid], which have various vasoactive, chemotactic, and chemokinetic actions and cause bronchoconstriction and mucus secretion

        (b) Cyclooxygenase products (e.g., prostaglandins, thromboxanes), which cause bronchial muscle contraction, platelet aggregation, and vasodilation

e. Late-phase allergic reactions are mediated by antigen interaction with IgE antibody and by the release of mediators from mast cells, with subsequent recruitment of leukocytes [i.e., neutrophils, eosinophils, lymphocytes (CD4+ T cells), and monocytes]. Corticosteroids and sodium cromolyn are important pharmacologic modifiers of the late-phase response.

2. Evaluation for allergic disorders

    a. History. Information obtained can help in identifying specific allergens as well as in identifying the child's condition as allergic.

    (1) Infections

        (a) Causative agents. In allergic diseases, respiratory viruses (e.g., respiratory syncytial virus and parainfluenza in infants, and influenza and rhinoviruses in older children) are common agents.

        (b) Site of infections. Pharyngitis, sinusitis, serous otitis, and acute otitis media suggest allergy-related infections, which often are caused by boggy mucous membranes and lymphoid tissue hypertrophy.

    (2) Variations in symptoms provide clues to the allergen. Symptoms may vary with:

        (a) Time (e.g., symptoms may be seasonal, perennial, monthly, diurnal, nocturnal)

        (b) Geography [e.g., symptoms may occur indoors, outdoors, at school or work, at home, at certain places in the home (e.g., basement, bedroom)]

(c) Environment (e.g., symptoms may be induced or made worse by pets, foods, molds, tobacco smoke, perfumes, and wood-burning stoves)

(3) Family history. Information regarding family history of atopic disorders (e.g., asthma, rhinitis, eczema) should be sought.

b. Physical examination. Signs and symptoms at the upper and lower airways and skin may suggest allergic disorder.

(1) Skin (e.g., dermatitis, eczema, urticaria, angioedema)

(2) Eyes (e.g., pruritus, tearing, swelling)

(3) Ears (e.g., fullness, popping, infection)

(4) Nose (e.g., congestion, sneezing, pruritus, discharge)

(5) Throat (e.g., pruritus, scratchiness or soreness, postnasal mucous discharge, cobblestoning due to lymphoid hypertrophy of posterior pharynx)

(6) Chest (e.g., cough, dyspnea, wheezing, sputum production)

(7) Gastrointestinal tract (e.g., diarrhea, malabsorption, food intolerance)

c. Laboratory testing

(1) Pulmonary function testing may be helpful (see Chapter 13).

(2) Skin testing is based on the antigen–IgE reaction that occurs on the surface of mast cells in the skin. Usually, several potential antigens are tested at one time. Controls used for skin testing include histamine (positive) and solvent or vehicle (negative).

(a) A small amount of presumed antigen is administered, as a solution, into the superficial layers of the skin by a superficial scratch (**scratch test**), by a needle-prick through a drop of the antigen solution (**prick test**), or by intracutaneous injection (**intracutaneous test**).

(b) If the patient is allergic to the test substance, the patient's mast cells, which are coated with specific IgE antibody via the Fc receptor, recognize the allergen by binding to the specific IgE antibody. When two IgE receptors are bridged by the allergen, the patient's mast cells release histamine. The histamine causes local vasodilation and capillary permeability, producing a **wheal-and-flare reaction** at the skin test site.

(3) Quantitation of total and specific IgE

(a) Total serum IgE levels are determined by a paper radioimmunosorbent test (PRIST).

(i) At birth, cord serum contains virtually no detectable IgE. Serum concentrations in children increase slowly, reaching adult levels at 5–7 years of age.

(ii) Basal total serum IgE level is determined by complex interaction of multiple genetic and nongenetic factors.

(iii) Not all atopic subjects have high IgE levels, and, conversely, not all nonatopic individuals have low IgE levels; the adult cutoff is 95 IU/ml.

(b) Antigen-specific IgE levels in serum can be determined by a radioallergosorbent test (RAST). This in vitro analogue of skin testing is 10-fold less sensitive than intracutaneous skin testing.

(4) Provocation (challenge) testing. A presumed allergen sometimes is administered directly to the mucosa of the target organ to identify the relationship between direct contact with the allergen and the development of symptoms.

(a) Route. The oral route is used in food allergy, the nasal route in allergic rhinitis, and the bronchial route in asthma.

(b) Elimination diets for the diagnosis of food allergy and food intolerance are a form of challenge testing. The patient first eats a basic diet consisting of standard nonallergic food (the elimination diet) and then adds possible offenders to the diet one by one.

3. Drug therapy for allergic disorders. Drugs used to treat allergies act at various stages of the IgE-mediated reaction.

a. β-Adrenergic agonists target the following tissues.

(1) Bronchial smooth muscle. β_2-adrenergic agonists relax smooth muscle.

       (2) Respiratory epithelium. β_2-adrenergic agonists increase the chloride ion and water secretion, ciliary beat frequency, and mucus flow.

       (3) Mast cells and basophils. β_2-adrenergic agonists increase the level of cyclic adenosine monophosphate (cAMP) and inhibit mediator release.

       (4) Bronchial microvasculature. β_2-adrenergic agonists decrease vascular permeability.

  b. Theophylline targets the following tissues.

       (1) Bronchial smooth muscle. Theophylline relaxes bronchial smooth muscle.

       (2) Mast cells. Theophylline decreases degranulation by increasing cAMP.

       (3) Diaphragm muscles. Theophylline increases contractility.

  c. Anticholinergic agents (e.g., ipratropium bromide) target the postganglionic effects on parasympathetic receptors, and they competitively antagonize the muscarinic action of acetylcholine.

  d. Mast cell stabilizers (e.g., cromolyn/nedocromil) target mast cells and eosinophils, where they inhibit mediator release and inhibit the release of leukotrienes.

  e. Antihistamines target the following tissues.

       (1) H$_1$ receptors. Antihistamines block the effects of histamine.

       (2) Muscarinic and serotonin cholinergic receptors (first generation only). Antihistamines stimulate these receptors, which results in dry mucous membranes.

  f. Glucocorticosteroids target the following tissues:

       (1) Inflammatory cells. Glucocorticosteroids inhibit arachidonic acid metabolism and stabilize the cell membrane. They inhibit the secretion of growth factors and cytokines, and they inhibit mediator release.

       (2) Vasculature. Glucocorticosteroids decrease permeability and inhibit the response to neuropeptides.

B. **Anaphylaxis** is an acute, life-threatening systemic reaction caused by an IgE-mediated hypersensitivity reaction and characterized by urticaria, acute airway obstruction, and circulatory collapse. **Anaphylactoid reactions** are clinically identical to anaphylaxis but are caused by the nonimmunologic release of mediators from mast cells and basophils.

  1. Pathogenesis

    a. The most common **causes** are antibiotic (penicillin) injections, Hymenoptera (bee) stings, foods (e.g., peanuts, shellfish), and, more recently, latex products, particularly in high-risk groups such as patients with spina bifida. However, almost any foreign substance can cause anaphylaxis.

    b. The **route** of allergic administration most commonly is parenteral. Ingestion also is common. Inhalation is less common.

    c. The **onset of anaphylaxis** occurs within a few minutes to hours after antigen exposure. Systemic manifestations are caused by the release of inflammatory mediators from mast cells and basophils.

  2. Clinical features include:

    a. Skin manifestations, such as urticaria and angioedema

    b. Respiratory manifestations, such as edema of the larynx and epiglottis (causing hoarseness and stridor), bronchospasm, hypoxia, nasal congestion, sneezing, and rhinorrhea

    c. Circulatory manifestations, such as vasodilation, loss of intravascular volume, hypotension, circulatory collapse, arrhythmias, palpitations, and syncope

    d. Gastrointestinal manifestations, such as vomiting, diarrhea, dysphagia, and abdominal cramps

    e. Genitourinary manifestations, such as urgency

  3. Therapy must be immediate.

    a. The administration of epinephrine and antihistamines is the first-line approach to the treatment of anaphylaxis.

    b. Fluid therapy and vasopressors are given for circulatory collapse to maintain blood pressure.

    c. Airway maintenance and bronchodilating drugs may be necessary.

d. In severe anaphylaxis, corticosteroids are administered; however, these do not take effect for 6–8 hours.

e. Oxygen should be given if the patient is cyanotic or has a low oxygen tension (PO_2).

4. Prevention involves avoidance of known antigens (e.g., drugs, latex, foods), the use of emergency epinephrine self-administration kits, and identification bracelets.

C. **Allergic rhinitis** is a disorder of the nasal mucosa characterized by nasal blockage, rhinorrhea, sneezing, and pruritus.

1. Pathophysiology. Itching, sneezing, and hypersecretion are related to the effects of histamine on nerve receptors. Mast cells in the nasal mucosa also regulate the local blood flow in the mucosa by a controlled release of vasoactive mediators. Parasympathetic nerve pathways also play a major role in hypersecretion and congestion.

2. Classification and clinical features
a. Seasonal allergic rhinitis (hay fever)
(1) Nasal symptoms include congestion, pruritus, and increased mucus secretion (rhinorrhea).
(2) Other symptoms include loss of the senses of smell and taste, chronic cough and clearing of the throat due to postnasal discharge, and chronic malaise and fatigue. Epistaxis, nasal or sinus polyps, and persistent serous otitis and sinusitis may also be significant problems.
(3) Physical findings are characteristic.
(a) Children typically show certain **facial features** such as a transverse nasal crease, dark shadows under the eyes ("allergic shiners"), and dental malocclusion.
(b) The **nasal turbinates** are edematous and pale with a bluish tinge; they are covered with a thin, clear secretion.
(4) Nasal mucosal scrapings show large numbers of eosinophils.
b. Chronic or perennial rhinitis may have an allergic or nonallergic basis. **Vasomotor rhinitis** results from local autonomic imbalance.

3. Inhalant or airborne allergens
a. Pollens constitute one of the most important groups of allergens. Ragweed, other weeds, grasses, and trees are the most common offenders.
(1) To cause clinically significant sensitization, a pollen must be produced in large quantities by a common plant and must be dispersed by wind rather than by insects.
(2) Seasonal occurrence varies with geographic location and time of pollination. For example, in the North Atlantic region of the United States, the following inhalant allergens are prevalent.
(a) Trees (e.g., oak, maple) cause allergic reactions in late winter and early spring.
(b) Grasses (e.g., June, Timothy) are prevalent in spring and early summer.
(c) Molds (e.g., *Alternaria*) are most prevalent in the spring and fall.
(d) Weeds (e.g., ragweed) cause allergic reactions more often in the late summer and early fall.
(e) Dust mites tend to be more prevalent in late fall and winter.
b. Molds or fungi. Spores are ubiquitous in the environment; molds are especially present in places of high humidity and warmth.
c. Household dust. The principal allergen is the **feces of dust mite**. Dust mite–sensitive patients have perennial symptoms but usually are worse in the late fall and winter. The dust mite feeds on human dander.
d. Animal allergens. Dander, hairs, dried saliva, and feathers are the major allergens. Cats are the most highly allergenic of the common household pets.

4. Contributing factors
a. Although **odors and fumes** (tobacco smoke, perfumes) are not allergens, they are primary irritants of the mucosal epithelium.

    b. Other contributing factors include weather conditions, temperature changes, infections, air pollution, and stress.

  5. Therapy

    a. Avoidance. The most direct and safest mode of treatment is avoidance of the offending allergen, such as removal of a pet from the home. After removal of a pet from the household, it may take 20–24 weeks before the allergen levels are significantly reduced, even with extensive cleaning.

    b. Drug therapy is directed at preventing mast cell degranulation and blocking the effects of the released mediators.

      (1) Antihistamines are useful for controlling rhinorrhea and pruritus. A variety of agents are available, which fall into two main classes.

        (a) First-generation antihistamines include several pharmacologic groups of drugs that produce varying degrees of sedation.

        (b) Second-generation antihistamines are recently developed drugs that are nonsedating (they do not cross the blood–brain barrier).

      (2) Decongestants (oral only) are useful for reducing congestion.

      (3) Cromolyn sodium (topical) blocks mediator release from mast cells and is effective in both early- and late-phase allergic reactions.

      (4) Corticosteroids (topical sprays) affect mainly late-phase allergic reactions.

      (5) Atropine-like drugs (topical sprays) are useful for vasomotor rhinitis.

    c. Desensitization (immunotherapy) can be useful in patients with clear-cut seasonal allergic rhinitis to the inhalant pollen allergens.

D. | **Allergic diseases of the eyes and ears**

  1. Allergic (hay fever) conjunctivitis usually is caused by inhalant allergens. Patients often have other allergic disorders (e.g., rhinitis, eczema, asthma).

    a. Clinical features include tearing, itching, edema (chemosis), and redness of the conjunctiva. The **cornea is not involved;** thus, no scarring occurs.

    b. Therapy is primarily drug therapy with combination ocular decongestant–antihistamine preparations, or oral antihistamines.

  2. Vernal conjunctivitis is a severe bilateral inflammatory disorder that occurs mainly in the spring and summer in preadolescent boys (the male-to-female ratio is 3:1). The disease tends to resolve after puberty.

    a. Clinical features include intense itching, tearing, photophobia, and a stringy ocular mucous discharge that contains numerous eosinophils. Physical findings include giant papillae or cobblestoning of the upper tarsal conjunctiva. Unlike allergic conjunctivitis, vernal conjunctivitis **can result in corneal damage** with ulceration and scarring.

    b. Therapy is with topical lodoxamide (a mast cell stabilizer), and, if necessary, topical or systemic corticosteroids.

  3. Involvement of the lids can occur in patients with **atopic dermatitis** or **eczema.** Symptoms can range from a scaly, edematous, crusty exudate to keratoconjunctivitis, cataracts, or keratoconus.

  4. Serous otitis media and **middle ear effusions** may be allergy related. In allergic children, adenoidal hypertrophy contributes to obstruction of the eustachian tube.

E. | **Atopic dermatitis (atopic eczema).** This common pruritic skin disorder usually begins in infancy and has a chronic fluctuating course with seasonal variations. In 80% of patients, the skin problem starts in the first year of life; in up to 90%, onset is before 5 years of age.

  1. Immunologic aspects

    a. Serum IgE levels are elevated in 80% of patients, and most patients have immediate skin reactivity (i.e., specific IgE antibodies) to a variety of environmental allergens.

    b. Atopic dermatitis often occurs in combination with other atopic diseases such as asthma or hay fever.

c. The family history influences the likelihood of atopic dermatitis. If one parent is atopic, there is a 25%–30% chance of atopy in the child; if both parents are atopic, then the incidence increases to 50%.

2. Clinical features
   a. Atopic dermatitis is characterized by a chronic or relapsing course.
   b. The pruritic dermatitis has a typical morphology and distribution.
      (1) In infants and young children, the facial and extensor surfaces are affected. Lesions tend to be erythematous, papulovesicular, and exudative.
      (2) In older children, the distribution is more on the flexural surfaces, and lesions are more dry and lichenified.
   c. Other clinical features include chelitis, infraorbital folds, anterior neck folds, white dermatographism and a delayed blanch response, and facial pallor associated with infraorbital darkening.

3. Complications include repeated cutaneous infections and, occasionally, keratoconus. Anterior or posterior subcapsular cataracts are rare before puberty.

4. Therapy. It is imperative to suppress the itch–scratch cycle by using oral antihistamines (e.g., hydroxyzine) and, if necessary, mild sedation. Skin lubricants and moisturizers are used to maintain skin hydration and prevent drying. Antibiotics may be necessary for patients with weepy lesions and pyoderma. Topical corticosteroids are used only in patients with severe atopic dermatitis.

F. **Urticaria and angioedema. Hives,** the lesions of **urticaria,** are evanescent wheals of varying size affecting the superficial layers of the epidermis and mucous membranes. **Angioedema** is similar but involves the deeper layers of the dermis and submucosal or subcutaneous tissues. In both disorders, acute evanescent lesions are more common than chronic lesions lasting 6 weeks or more.

1. Pathogenesis
   a. **IgE-mediated (type I) hypersensitivity reactions** are a common cause of urticaria and angioedema. This mechanism underlies the acute urticaria commonly seen with **viral infections** and associated with parasitic, fungal, and certain bacterial infections. **Hymenoptera stings, drugs,** and certain **foods** (e.g., nuts, shellfish, eggs, milk) are other common causes of IgE-mediated urticaria and angioedema.
   b. **Immune complex disease and cutaneous vasculitis,** which are associated with activation of the complement system and the generation of anaphylatoxins, can also be associated with urticaria, angioedema, or both.
   c. **Other mechanisms** also cause urticaria and angioedema.
      (1) A variety of factors can cause urticaria or angioedema through the **nonspecific release of histamine** from mast cells or basophils. Morphine, codeine, and curare derivatives can act by this mechanism, as can bacterial toxins, crustacean secretions, and snake venom. **Physical agents** also can induce urticaria by this mechanism in some people, as in dermatographism (from pressure), solar urticaria, and cold urticaria.
      (2) Some substances activate the **arachidonic acid pathway,** with production of leukotrienes. Examples include aspirin, food dyes [e.g., tartrazine (yellow food dye no. 5)], and preservatives (e.g., metabisulfite, methylparabens, benzoic acid).
      (3) **Complement** can also be involved in the pathogenesis of urticaria and angioedema. Radiocontrast dyes and blood transfusions can induce complement-mediated urticaria or angioedema. **Hereditary angioedema** is caused by the deficiency or dysfunction of C1 esterase inhibitor.

2. Therapy
   a. **Antihistamines.** H_1-receptor antagonists are the principal drug for the management of urticaria and angioedema. The choice of antihistamine depends on efficacy and tolerance. Hydroxyzine may show a slight advantage over other classic (first-generation) antihistamines. The newer antihistamines (i.e., terfenadine, astemizole,

loratadine) have a distinct advantage of not being able to cross the blood–brain barrier to cause sedation. Some patients with chronic urticaria unresponsive to H_1-receptor antihistamines may respond to therapy with both H_1- and H_2-receptor antihistamines.

   b. Systemic corticosteroids should be used only in patients with severe, acute urticaria and angioedema and in patients with an underlying disorder that calls for their use.

   c. Avoidance. In 70% of chronic urticaria cases, the etiology cannot be found, but if it can, its removal may be sufficient to resolve the urticaria and angioedema.

G. Food allergy

1. **Pathogenesis**
   a. The **foods that most commonly cause reactions** include milk, soy, eggs, fish, peanuts, and wheat. Preservatives (metabisulfite) and dyes (yellow food dye no. 5) are a minor cause of food reactions.
   b. Many adverse reactions to foods are not true food allergy (i.e., the development of IgE-mediated hypersensitivity to a food antigen). Among the many **other causes of adverse reactions to foods** are the toxic or pharmacologic effects of bacterial toxins, chemical additives, or certain food substances; nonimmunologically mediated histamine release; an inborn enzyme deficiency; psychological reactions; and intrinsic gastrointestinal disease.

2. **Clinical features.** Food allergy can be expressed through a variety of clinical symptoms.
   a. Some patients have abdominal symptoms, such as nausea, vomiting, abdominal pain, bloating, or diarrhea. There may be an associated swelling of the lips and tingling of the mouth or throat.
   b. Other patients may have different clinical symptoms, including anaphylaxis, asthma, rhinorrhea and congestion, urticaria, angioedema, eczema, and joint pain. Whether headaches, lethargy, and behavioral disturbances can be symptoms of food allergy remains controversial.

3. **Diagnosis.** The classic diagnostic tests used in allergy (e.g., RAST, skin testing) will not reliably identify a food allergy. The diagnosis of food allergy is best made by **oral challenge testing** in which the food is given in a disguised form (double-blind) and effects on the target organ (e.g., skin, lungs, intestine) are evaluated. An **elimination diet** with a gradual add-back of foods is an approach that may help in the management of food allergy as well as in diagnosis.

4. **Therapy.** Elimination or avoidance of the offending food substance from the diet is the major approach to the treatment of patients with food allergy.

H. Allergy to stinging insects (Hymenoptera).

Allergic reactions to stinging insects (bees, yellow jackets, hornets, wasps) are mediated by IgE antibodies directed at one or more proteins in the venom of these insects. Between 0.5% and 5% of the population experience a systemic reaction after a sting, but death from insect allergy in children is very rare.

1. **Clinical features**
   a. **IgE-mediated reactions** can range from mild symptoms, such as urticaria and pruritus, to angioedema or life-threatening anaphylactic shock.
   b. **Large local reactions** that exceed 5 cm and occur within 24–72 hours after the sting are probably delayed hypersensitivity reactions.

2. **Diagnosis.** Allergy to stinging insects is identified from the history and by skin testing (or by in vitro testing with RAST), using purified venoms.

3. **Therapy** is mainly preventive. Patients should carry an emergency treatment kit containing epinephrine and antihistamines in case anaphylaxis follows an insect sting. Desensitization or immunotherapy may be helpful. Patients should avoid using perfumes and wearing brightly colored clothes, which attract stinging insects; they also should not walk barefooted outdoors.

I. Adverse drug reactions

1. **Pathogenesis**
   a. **Cause.** Adverse drug reactions (i.e., undesirable reactions that occur at an appropriate therapeutic dose) have many causes.
      (1) Fully 70%–80% of adverse drug reactions are **predictable adverse reactions** that result from the pharmacologic actions of a drug.
      (2) **Unpredictable adverse reactions** can result from immunologic hypersensitivity, from an underlying genetic susceptibility, or from idiosyncrasy. In contrast to idiosyncratic reactions, which can occur on first exposure to a drug, immunologic reactions require prior exposure or at least 7 days of continuous therapy with the drug in question.
   b. **Mechanism.** A drug hypersensitivity reaction may occur by any of the four Gell and Coombs mechanisms (see III).
   c. **Factors that may influence the development of drug allergy**
      (1) Few drugs are large enough molecules to serve as complete antigens. **Drugs** (or their metabolites) **that can serve as haptens** are most likely to cause sensitization.
      (2) **Topical application** causes sensitization more often than other routes of drug administration, probably because the carrier proteins for the drug haptens are readily available in the skin.
      (3) **Intermittent courses of moderate doses of a drug** are more likely to predispose to sensitization than prolonged treatment courses.
      (4) **Atopy.** Although the incidence of adverse drug reactions is the same for atopic and nonatopic patients, an atopic person is more prone to the development of severe reactions.

2. **Clinical features**
   a. **Skin manifestations.** The skin is the most common site of drug hypersensitivity reactions and may be affected by any of the four hypersensitivity mechanisms. Drug eruptions can take many forms. Exanthematous eruptions, urticaria, angioedema, and photosensitivity are most common and are relatively mild; the less common bullous eruptions (epidermal necrolysis, Stevens-Johnson syndrome) can be fatal.
   b. **Anaphylaxis** occurs most commonly with parenteral administration.
   c. **Serum sickness** is a type III (immune complex) hypersensitivity reaction (a type I reaction may also occur). It can be induced by various drugs, notably the penicillins and related agents, as well as by the foreign protein in serum.
      (1) **Symptoms** usually develop in 7–12 days but may be accelerated (appearing in 1–3 days or even as anaphylaxis) in patients previously exposed to the drug. Symptoms include urticaria, angioedema, erythema multiforme, fever, and arthritis.
      (2) **Therapy.** Reactions can be controlled by antihistamines or, in severe cases, corticosteroids. There are no sequelae.
   d. **Other manifestations** of drug allergy include drug fever; a reaction resembling SLE; hematologic manifestations (hemolytic anemia, thrombocytopenia, purpura); asthma; hypersensitivity pneumonitis; hepatocellular damage; cholestasis; peripheral neuritis; and seizures (rarely).

3. **Examples of drug allergies**
   a. **Penicillin and its derivatives** cause many cases of allergic drug reactions.
      (1) **Mechanism.** Metabolites of penicillin are haptens and bind with proteins to form antigenic groups known as the **major determinant** [benzyl penicilloyl (**BPO**)] and several **minor determinants,** which are part of the β-lactam ring structure.
      (2) **Types of reactions**
         (a) **Anaphylaxis** is an IgE-mediated reaction to the minor determinants.
         (b) **Serum sickness or hematologic reactions** (type II and III reactions) may be related to IgG, IgM, or even IgE antibodies to either the major or minor determinants.

      (c) **Other reactions** to penicillin (e.g., late or recurrent urticaria, arthralgia, late maculopapular reactions) also may be caused by either the major or minor determinants.

      (3) Although the **cephalosporins** have a similar structure to penicillin, a person who is sensitive to penicillin has only an 8% cross-reactivity with the second- and third-generation cephalosporins.

    b. Aspirin can cause reactions that appear to be allergic in nature, such as urticaria, angioedema, or asthma. However, such reactions to aspirin are probably not IgE mediated, but instead may be related to perturbations of the arachidonic pathways with increased production of leukotrienes, because the structurally unrelated nonsteroidal antiinflammatory drugs (e.g., indomethacin, naproxen) can produce similar reactions.

    c. Other significant hypersensitivity reactions to drugs include those to **insulin** and **anticonvulsants**.

    d. Adverse reactions to radiocontrast media, various opioids, vancomycin, angiotensin-converting enzyme inhibitors, and local anesthetics may be mediated by nonimmunologic release of mediators from mast cells.

V. RHEUMATIC DISEASES

A. **Rheumatic fever** is a multisystem, nonsuppurative, inflammatory disease triggered by a group A β-hemolytic streptococcal (GABHS) infection of the upper respiratory tract. Patients in whom rheumatic fever develops have a marked tendency to suffer recurrent attacks after subsequent GABHS infections of the upper respiratory tract. Rheumatic fever is a potentially serious disease because it may cause permanent damage to heart muscle and valves (**rheumatic heart disease**).

    1. Incidence. The peak incidence of initial and recurrent attacks of rheumatic fever is between 5 and 15 years of age, which coincides with the high frequency of GABHS infections in this age group. Although the incidence of rheumatic fever declined markedly in the United States before 1985, several focal outbreaks occurred between 1985 and 1991. These outbreaks have subsided and there has been no significant generalized increase in incidence nationally. However, rheumatic fever continues to be a major cause of heart disease in economically underdeveloped countries.

    2. Pathogenesis. The concept of "rheumatogenicity" of selected **serotypes of GABHS** was reinforced by the reappearance of specific serotypes (notably M3 and M18) during the recent outbreaks. These serotypes are known to have caused rheumatic fever in past outbreaks. What remains unknown is exactly how rheumatogenic GABHS serotypes cause the varied manifestations of rheumatic fever. An autoimmune mechanism seems most likely, and is supported by evidence such as:

    a. Antigenic cross-reactions between streptococcal cellular components and human heart tissue have been demonstrated.

    b. Cross-reactive (anti-heart) antibodies are found in rheumatic fever patients, although it is not known whether they are the cause or an effect of injury.

    3. Pathology. Exudative and proliferative inflammatory reactions occur mainly in the connective tissue and around small blood vessels in the heart, joints, skin, subcutaneous tissues, and brain. **Aschoff bodies,** which consist of clusters of large, multinucleated cells in a mass of fragmented, swollen collagen fibers, and which are found only in the myocardium, are considered specific for rheumatic fever. The site of the Aschoff body becomes a healed scar. Healing of the inflammatory reaction involving heart valve leaflets may lead to deformity and valvular dysfunction.

    4. Clinical features

    a. Polyarthritis—usually with fever—is the presenting finding in about 75% of patients. The arthritis chiefly affects large joints, is characteristically migratory, and is painful out of proportion to objective findings of redness and swelling. There are no sequelae.

b. Carditis occurs in about 50% of the patients and may be asymptomatic, unless pericarditis or heart failure is present. A pansystolic, blowing mitral murmur is the hallmark. Less common is a diastolic aortic murmur heard along the left sternal border. Murmurs may remain but often disappear if rheumatic fever does not recur.

c. Chorea occurs in from 10%–30% of the patients. Often insidious in onset, it causes emotional lability followed by characteristic, random, jerky movements and muscle weakness. Chorea runs a self-limited course of 6–13 weeks' duration, and recovery is complete.

d. Less common findings include **subcutaneous nodules** (small, painless swellings found overlying bony prominences) and **erythema marginatum** (a pink, evanescent rash over the trunk).

5. **Diagnosis**
   a. **Jones criteria.** The widely accepted Jones criteria classify the manifestations as **major** and **minor** according to their diagnostic usefulness.
      (1) **Major manifestations** include carditis, polyarthritis, chorea, erythema marginatum, and subcutaneous nodules.
      (2) **Minor manifestations** can be clinical (e.g., fever, arthralgia) or can come from laboratory findings (e.g., erythrocyte sedimentation rate, C-reactive protein, prolonged PR interval).
   b. **Making the determination using Jones criteria.**
      (1) The presence of two major criteria, or of one major and two minor criteria, indicates a high probability of the presence of rheumatic fever if supported by evidence of a preceding streptococcal infection. This evidence includes an elevated or rising streptococcal antibody titer, a positive throat culture for group A streptococcus, and a recent history of scarlet fever.
      (2) The absence of a preceding streptococcal infection should make the diagnosis suspect, except in situations in which rheumatic fever is first discovered after a long latent period from the antecedent infection (e.g., Sydenham chorea, indolent carditis).
      (3) **Laboratory tests**
         (a) Streptococcal antibody tests (e.g., antistreptolysin O) are useful for documenting a recent streptococcal infection, and the erythrocyte sedimentation rate and C-reactive protein test can provide evidence of an inflammatory process.
         (b) Throat culture is not very helpful, because it is usually negative by the time signs of rheumatic fever appear.
         (c) Doppler echocardiography may prove useful in identifying "silent" mitral insufficiency, but there is insufficient information at present to accept echocardiography to document valvular regurgitation without accompanying ausculatory findings as the sole criterion for carditis in acute rheumatic fever.
   c. **Exceptions to Jones criteria.** There are three circumstances in which the diagnosis of rheumatic fever can be made without strictly adhering to the Jones criteria.
      (1) **Chorea** may occur as the only manifestation of rheumatic fever.
      (2) **Indolent carditis** may be the only manifestation in patients who come to medical attention months after the onset of rheumatic fever.
      (3) Although most patients with recurrences fulfill the Jones criteria, some may not. It is often difficult to establish evidence of acute carditis during a recurrence in someone who already has rheumatic heart disease unless a different valve is affected or pericarditis is detected. Therefore, a presumptive diagnosis of rheumatic recurrence may be made when only one major or several minor manifestations are present in a patient with a reliable past history of rheumatic fever or established rheumatic heart disease, provided there is supporting evidence of recent group A streptococcal infection.

6. **Differential diagnosis** includes other cardiac conditions (e.g., functional murmurs, congenital heart disease, viral carditis), other causes of arthritis, and other movement disorders.

7. **Therapy** includes the following:
   a. Bed rest and close attention to changes in cardiac findings
   b. Salicylates to control fever and joint manifestations
   c. Steroids for severe carditis
   d. Chlorpromazine or haloperidol for chorea

8. **Prevention of recurrences.** Once the diagnosis is established, the patient should be given 600,000–1.2 million units of penicillin G as one injection or therapeutic doses of oral penicillin for 10 days. Penicillin-allergic patients may be treated with erythromycin. Long-term prophylaxis with penicillin or erythromycin should be started thereafter to prevent streptococcal infections and recurring attacks of rheumatic fever.

B. **Juvenile rheumatoid arthritis (JRA)** is a chronic inflammatory disease of one or more joints in children 16 years of age or younger.

1. **Pathogenesis and pathology.** The etiology is unknown. Evidence points to a major role for an immune response, possibly initiated by an as yet unidentified infectious agent(s). This immunologic reactivity results in inflammation of synovial membranes, which is followed by synovial proliferation and destruction of cartilage.

2. **Clinical features.** JRA may begin at any age, but is seen most commonly between 1 and 4 years, more often in girls than in boys. Although all children with JRA have arthritis, the disease is classified as **systemic, pauciarticular,** and **polyarticular,** based on the mode of onset, number of involved joints, systemic complications, and prognosis.
   a. **Systemic JRA** usually presents with a high, spiking fever that returns to normal levels daily. A salmon-colored, morbilliform rash anywhere over the body is characteristic. The rash is fleeting in nature and should be sought for at the height of the fever. Many of these patients have hepatosplenomegaly and lymphadenopathy. The joint involved may not become apparent until several weeks or even months after the onset of fever. About one-third of these patients go on to have disabling chronic arthritis.
   b. **Pauciarticular JRA** is characterized by involvement of up to four usually large joints, most frequently the knee. Fever is absent and iridocyclitis is the only systemic finding. This is a serious complication and occurs in a high percentage of patients, especially in girls who are antinuclear antibody (ANA) positive. Iridocyclitis may be present without any clinical signs and should be sought for by slit-lamp examination in every patient with this type of JRA. Chronic joint disease is unusual in patients with pauciarticular onset.
   c. **Polyarticular JRA** by definition involves five or more joints, both small and large. The onset is often insidious, with low-grade fever and lethargy. There is symmetric swelling of large joints, and the small joints of the hand are frequently involved. Patients are frequently ANA positive, and rheumatoid factor is positive in minorities. This form of JRA is most likely to persist and cause the typical deformities seen in adult rheumatoid arthritis.

3. **Diagnosis** is made from the history, the physical examination, and exclusion of other causes of acute and chronic arthritis, such as infectious arthritis, acute rheumatic fever, reactive arthritis, and other collagen vascular diseases. Radiographs at the onset are of value only to exclude trauma. Rheumatoid factor is rarely positive in patients with JRA. ANA may be positive, but it is not specific for JRA. The persistence of the joint manifestations in patients with JRA distinguishes this form from other forms of arthritis.

4. **Treatment.** Aspirin is the drug of choice. If salicylates are not well tolerated, other nonsteroidal agents can be used (e.g., ibuprofen). Corticosteroids have a limited role. A short course of prednisone may be used in children with acute febrile onset when nonsteroidal agents fail to control the fever. Slower-acting drugs such as gold salts are indicated during the chronic phase when antiinflammatory drugs fail to control symptoms. Cytotoxic agents have been used when all other drugs fail to control progressive arthritis. Physical and occupational therapy are essential to prevent joint deformities.

C. **Other collagen vascular diseases**

1. **Systemic lupus erythematosus (SLE)** is an immunologically mediated inflammatory disease affecting multiple organ systems. It is rare in children younger than 5 years of age and uncommon in children younger than age 10 years. SLE is seen occasionally in adolescents, particularly girls.
    a. **Pathogenesis and pathologic features.** The manifestations are caused by immune complex deposition in various organs (a type III hypersensitivity reaction), but why this occurs is unknown. Pathologic features consist of fibrinoid deposition and lupus erythematosus (LE) bodies in certain tissues (e.g., kidneys, skin, heart, brain, lungs, peripheral blood vessels).
    b. **Clinical features.** The butterfly rash across the nose and cheeks is the most characteristic sign. Nephritis may be the major presenting problem or a concomitant finding. Arthralgia is common, although severe arthritis is uncommon and deforming arthritis is rare. Other symptoms reflect involvement of other organ systems.
    c. **Diagnosis.** The appearance of the butterfly rash and the presence of LE cells in a patient with multisystem disease simplify diagnosis. ANA is present in virtually all patients, but its detection, although of diagnostic importance, is not a specific test for SLE. Testing for LE bodies is not always positive in children, but is more specific than ANA testing.
    d. **Therapy.** Prednisone is given in a dosage and frequency suitable for the severity of the disease. Immunosuppressive agents are used for steroid-resistant patients.

2. **Dermatomyositis** is an uncommon connective tissue disease of unknown etiology characterized by inflammation of the skin and muscles. The **skin lesions** are caused by perivascular infiltration by lymphocytes and histiocytes, resulting in thinning of the epidermis and dermal edema. The **muscle lesions** consist of foci of inflammation, capillary necrosis, and ischemia, causing atrophy. **Polymyositis** is the diagnosis when the disease is limited to the muscles.
    a. **Clinical features**
        (1) Onset usually is insidious, with scaly, erythematous rash over the joints, especially the knuckles, knees, and elbows, and a characteristic purplish discoloration and edema of the upper eyelids. Later in the disease course, pain and weakness develop symmetrically in distal muscle groups.
        (2) Less frequently, the patient presents with acute high fever and profound muscle weakness.
    b. **Diagnosis.** The typical skin rash and signs of myositis usually are diagnostic. Muscle enzymes are elevated and electromyography is indicative of myositis, but neither finding is specific. Muscle biopsy shows characteristic pathologic features.
    c. **Therapy.** Long-term corticosteroid therapy results in permanent remission in 90% of the patients.

3. **Scleroderma** is an uncommon disease of unknown etiology that occurs as a localized form (**morphea**) or, even more rarely, as a multisystem disorder (**progressive systemic sclerosis**). Histologic changes consist of a small artery vasculitis in the subcutaneous fat, which becomes replaced with sclerotic collagen extending into the dermis.
    a. **Clinical features**
        (1) **Morphea,** the localized form, appears as oval sclerotic plaques or linear band-like lesions. Erythematous at first, these evolve into firm, shiny, white lesions with violaceous borders. Morphea is not associated with severe organ system involvement.
        (2) **Progressive systemic sclerosis** presents as a diffuse hardening and tightening of the skin and subcutaneous tissues. The joints, lungs, heart, kidneys, and gastrointestinal tract may be involved. Raynaud phenomenon and esophageal dysfunction are often present.
    b. **Diagnosis.** The characteristic clinical findings usually are sufficient to make a diagnosis. Laboratory findings are essentially negative but help to exclude other collagen vascular diseases.
    c. **Therapy** is limited to symptomatic treatment.

4. Mixed connective tissue disease is a connective tissue disorder that combines the clinical and laboratory features of JRA, SLE, dermatomyositis, and scleroderma. Therapy is the same as that for SLE.

D. **Henoch-Schönlein (anaphylactoid) purpura** is a generalized hypersensitivity reaction that produces a characteristic clinical syndrome (see Chapter 14).

1. Etiology and pathogenesis. Anaphylactoid purpura is a vasculitis secondary to the deposition of immune complexes. The antigen(s) provoking the hypersensitivity reaction is not usually apparent. It has been suggested that in a few patients in whom there is a history of an antecedent GABHS infection, this may be the initiating event.

2. Clinical features. A maculopapular rash that becomes hemorrhagic and abdominal pain are the most common manifestations. Typically, the rash occurs initially over the lower half of the body. Pain and swelling of one or more joints are also frequent findings, as is renal involvement, manifested by gross or microscopic hematuria.

3. Diagnosis. The hemorrhagic appearance and the distribution of the rash are characteristic of this syndrome. The normal platelet count and coagulation studies differentiate it from other hemorrhagic disorders.

4. Course and therapy. The disease has a self-limited course of from 4–6 weeks. In a minority of patients, repeated episodes may occur over a period of months or years. Treatment is symptomatic. Antibacterial therapy is indicated if a throat culture is positive for GABHS.

E. **Miscellaneous conditions with arthritic symptoms**

1. Reactive arthritis is the occurrence of an aseptic arthritis after an infection elsewhere in the body, especially after gastrointestinal infections. The bacteria most frequently involved include *Yersinia, Salmonella, Shigella,* and *Campylobacter* sp. The arthritis occurs 1–2 weeks after onset of gastrointestinal symptoms. The course is self-limited and treatment of the joint manifestations is symptomatic.

2. Reiter syndrome is a form of reactive arthritis that, in addition to joint manifestations, is characterized by urethritis and conjunctivitis or iritis. It is usually associated with *Chlamydia trachomatis* infections. The arthritis is mild and chronic arthritis rarely occurs.

3. Psoriatic arthritis. The psoriatic skin lesions may precede, accompany, or follow the joint symptoms. The arthritis is chronic and is indistinguishable from JRA. Dactylitis ("sausage finger") is a characteristic finding. Therapy is the same as that for JRA (see V B 4) and psoriasis.

4. Serum sickness (see IV I 2 c) may be associated with painful swelling around the joints without warmth or redness. Treatment is symptomatic and there are no sequelae.

5. Kawasaki disease (see Chapter 10) may be associated with arthritis or arthralgia. Treatment is symptomatic and there are no sequelae.

6. Lyme disease (see Chapter 10) may be associated with asymmetric pauciarthritis or arthralgia, involving primarily the knees.

DIRECTIONS: Each of the numbered items or incomplete statements in this section is followed by answers or by completions of the statement. Select the ONE lettered answer or completion that is BEST in each case.

Questions 1–2

A 12-month-old boy was born to a 22-year-old human immunodeficiency virus (HIV)-infected mother who died only months after delivery. At 12 months, the child appears healthy and is growing and developing well, but his blood test is positive for HIV antibodies.

1. What does this result indicate?

(A) The child is definitely infected with HIV
(B) Maternal antibodies are still present in the boy's blood
(C) The positive HIV antibody test could be the result of paternal antibodies
(D) The test is not diagnostic, and the child remains in the category E, or indeterminate, classification
(E) Maternal antibodies to HIV are more likely to cause positive HIV serologic tests than antibodies produced in children

2. Which of the following tests is considered the most reliable in diagnosing human immunodeficiency virus (HIV) infection in asymptomatic infants younger than 18 months of age?

(A) HIV serologic tests (ELISA and Western blot)
(B) HIV p24
(C) HIV culture
(D) CD4 cell count
(E) CD4/CD8 ratio

3. In a teenager who gets stung by a bee, urticaria develops within 30 minutes of the sting. This reaction is most likely mediated by

(A) complement component C3
(B) immunoglobulin E (IgE) antibodies
(C) neutrophils
(D) natural killer (NK) cells

4. Pollens are important airborne allergens. Which of the following is a characteristic of pollens causing allergic rhinitis?

(A) Molecular weight greater than 70,000 daltons
(B) Dispersal largely by insects
(C) Production by flower-bearing plants
(D) Dispersal by the wind

DIRECTIONS: Each of the numbered items or incomplete statements in this section is negatively phrased, as indicated by a capitalized word such as NOT, LEAST, or EXCEPT. Select the ONE lettered answer or completion that is BEST in each case.

5. A 3-year-old boy is taking ampicillin for otitis media. On day 4 he breaks out with an urticarial rash. Past medical history indicates that he has had multiple ear infections treated with antibiotics. He also has a history of asthma and atopic dermatitis. All of the following statements could characterize his adverse reaction to ampicillin EXCEPT

(A) the reaction requires prior exposure to ampicillin
(B) multiple short courses of antibiotics place the patient at higher risk of sensitization
(C) the incidence of adverse drug reactions is higher in atopic patients than in nonatopic patients
(D) the reaction may take the form of serum sickness
(E) the reaction may take the form of interstitial nephritis

6. A 12-year-old girl presents with all the classic clinical features of allergic rhinitis. These include all of the following EXCEPT

(A) dark shadows under the eyes
(B) erythematous nasal mucosa
(C) dental malocclusion
(D) thin, watery nasal secretions
(E) a transverse crease across the nose

DIRECTIONS: Each set of matching questions in this section consists of a list of four to twenty-six lettered options (some of which may be in figures) followed by several numbered items. For each numbered item, select the ONE lettered option that is most closely associated with it. To avoid spending too much time on matching sets with large numbers of options, it is generally advisable to begin each set by reading the list of options. Then, for each item in the set, try to generate the correct answer and locate it in the option list, rather than evaluating each option individually. Each lettered option may be selected once, more than once, or not at all.

Questions 7–10

For each patient problem, choose the type of hypersensitivity reaction it represents.

(A) Type I
(B) Type II
(C) Type III
(D) Type IV

7. Urticaria after the ingestion of peanuts

8. Dermatitis from poison ivy

9. Autoimmune hemolysis of red blood cells

10. Lupus nephritis

1. The answer is D *[II E 4 a]*. In this case, detection of human immunodeficiency virus (HIV) antibody could be the result either of maternal antibody or of antibody produced by an infected child. The test does not discriminate. Hence we can say only that the child was perinatally exposed and remains in the indeterminate classification.

2. The answer is C *[II E 4 a (3)]*. Human immunodeficiency virus (HIV) culture is the most reliable test to establish a diagnosis of HIV infection in infants in whom the persistence of maternal antibodies may cause a positive HIV serology. The HIV p24 test can be diagnostic, but it is very often negative in infected infants. A very low CD4 T-cell count might suggest HIV infection, but usually low CD4 counts are accompanied by clinical disease. It should be emphasized, however, that even HIV cultures may be negative in an HIV-infected infant, because this test is not 100% sensitive. Hence, time and repeated testing may be necessary to establish or exclude HIV infection: a healthy baby with a negative antibody test at 18 months would be considered noninfected; whereas an apparently healthy baby who remains HIV antibody positive past 18 months of age would be considered to be HIV infected.

3. The answer is B *[III A 1]*. Immediate type (type I) hypersensitivity reactions are mediated by immunoglobulin E (IgE) antibodies. Type III hypersensitivity reactions are mediated by IgG antibodies, complement, and neutrophils. Type IV hypersensitivity reactions are mediated by natural killer (NK) cells.

4. The answer is D *[IV A 1 b, C 3 a]*. The inhalant pollen allergens vary with their season of pollination (e.g., trees pollinate in the northeast United States in late winter or early spring, whereas ragweed pollinates from late summer to the first frost). In general, the pollen allergens have a molecular weight less than 70,000 daltons. Structures larger than 70,000 (e.g., the pollen from pine trees) are not thought to cause allergic diseases. Plants that bear pollen allergens are from nonflowering plants, and thus rely on wind or air currents to spread the pollen. In contrast, flowering plants (e.g., roses) depend on insects to carry pollen

to other plants for reproduction, and thus do not cause allergies.

5. The answer is C *[IV I]*. The incidence of adverse drug reactions is not correlated with the atopic state of the patient; however, atopic individuals may be prone to more severe drug reactions. Immune complex reactions (e.g., serum sickness) and interstitial nephritis are among the many varieties of drug hypersensitivity reactions that can occur. Idiosyncratic drug reactions can occur on first exposure to a drug, but hypersensitivity reactions as in this child with urticaria require prior exposure or at least 7 days of continuous therapy with the drug in question. Intermittent or multiple courses of a drug are more likely to predispose to sensitization than even prolonged treatment courses with an antibiotic.

6. The answer is B *[IV C 2 a]*. In patients with allergic rhinitis, the nasal mucosa is not erythematous (red) but, instead, is pale and quite boggy. The pale appearance is caused by edema and the presence of eosinophils in the mucosa. An erythematous nasal mucosa is seen more commonly in patients with infectious rhinitis or rhinitis medicamentosa. Other physical findings in allergic rhinitis patients include dark shadows under the eyes; thin, watery nasal secretions; dental malocclusion; and a nasal crease.

7–10. The answers are: 7-A, 8-D, 9-B, 10-C *[III A]*. A type I (immediate-type, atopic, or reaginic) hypersensitivity reaction is mediated by immunoglobulin E (IgE) antibodies. Antigen attaches to its specific IgE on the surface of mast cells and basophils. This triggers the release of pharmacologic mediators that produce the inflammation seen in type I hypersensitivity reactions.

A delayed cutaneous reaction to specific antigen is a type IV (cell-mediated or delayed) hypersensitivity reaction. Type IV hypersensitivity reactions are mediated by sensitized T cells. The T cells, after binding to antigen, release a variety of lymphokines, which results in the infiltration of tissues by mononuclear cells and lymphocytes, causing destruction of the tissue. Type IV reactions are typically seen in the dermatitis of poison ivy, organ graft rejection reactions, or in infections with *Mycobacterium* (tuberculosis).

The pathogenesis of many autoimmune hemolytic anemias is an antibody-dependent cytotoxic reaction, which is a type II hypersensitivity reaction. Antibody binds to a cell membrane antigen, and, acting in conjunction with complement, causes lysis of the red cells.

Immune complex–mediated (type III) hypersensitivity reactions begin when anti-body and antigens in the circulation combine to form soluble complexes. These complexes eventually filter out along basement membranes, such as the glomerular basement membrane. The deposition of these complexes on the basement membrane, together with the activation of complement, produces the inflammatory reaction that results in glomerulonephritis.

BIBLIOGRAPHY

Ayoub EM, Chun CSY: Nonsuppurative complications of group A streptococcal infection. *Adv Pediatr Infect Dis* 5:69–92, 1990.

Bisno AL: Group A streptococcal infections and acute rheumatic fever. *N Engl J Med* 325:783–793, 1991.

deShazo RD, Smith DL (eds): Primer on allergic and immunologic diseases. *JAMA* 268:20, 1992.

Frank MM, Austen KF, Claman HN, Unanue ER: *Sampter's Immunologic Diseases,* 5th ed. Boston, Little, Brown, 1994.

Harris ED: Rheumatoid arthritis: Pathophysiology and implications for therapy. *N Engl J Med* 322:1277–1289, 1990.

Middleton E, Reed CE, Ellis EF, et al: *Allergy: Principles and Practice,* 4th ed. St. Louis, Mosby Year Book, 1993.

Roitt I, Brostoff J, Male D: *Immunology,* 2nd ed. New York, Gower, 1989.

Chapter 10

Infectious Diseases

Peter J. Krause
Henry M. Feder, Jr.
Michael A. Gerber

I. INTRODUCTION

A. **Significance of infectious diseases.** Infectious diseases are the leading cause of morbidity in infants and children. Since the introduction of effective vaccines, the incidence of certain infections (e.g., polio, diphtheria, measles, mumps, rubella, pertussis, tetanus, *Haemophilus influenzae* type b) has been reduced dramatically; however, only smallpox has been eradicated worldwide. Other infectious diseases [e.g., hepatitis, shigellosis, Lyme disease, Rocky Mountain spotted fever, acquired immune deficiency syndrome (AIDS)] are on the rise. Antimicrobial compounds have markedly improved the prognosis associated with many infections, but the emergence of resistant strains has required the continued development of new antimicrobial compounds. Infectious diseases covered elsewhere in this text are listed in Table 10-1.

B. **Diagnosis of infectious diseases**

1. **Diagnostic criteria.** The diagnosis of infectious diseases in children is based on the **history and physical examination,** with the specific cause determined with the help of the microbiology laboratory. Certain **laboratory tests** (e.g., a complete blood count, erythrocyte sedimentation rate, radiologic studies, tissue histology, skin tests) may help to support or eliminate the diagnosis. **Confirmation of the etiologic agent** usually is made by culture, antigen detection, or antibody detection.

2. **Effective use of the microbiology laboratory.** Accurate microbiologic diagnosis of an infectious disease depends on appropriate specimen collection. To ensure the best result, it is important to sample the correct anatomic site before initiating antibiotics, to obtain an adequate quantity of material to culture, to avoid contamination, and to deliver the specimen in a prompt and appropriate manner to the laboratory.
   a. **Methods of organism identification**
      (1) **Microscopic examination** of specimens is performed with or without stains, depending on the nature of the organism.

TABLE 10-1. Infectious Diseases Covered in Other Chapters

Topic	Chapter	Section
Acute infectious diarrhea	11	V A
Acquired immune deficiency syndrome	9	II E
Genitourinary infections	5	IV
	14	VI
Hepatitis	11	IX C
Neonatal infections	6	V F
Tuberculosis	13	VIII A

(a) Unstained specimens. Organisms that have typical structural features (e.g., fungi, parasites) can be identified with an ordinary light microscope, without staining.

(b) Stained specimens. Special stains can be used to make organisms (or parts of organisms) more visible or identifiable with microscopic examination. An enormous variety of stains are available; two of the most commonly used are **Gram stain** (for classifying bacteria) and **acid-fast stain** (for identifying acid-fast microorganisms).

(c) ELISA (enzyme-linked immunosorbent assay). The ELISA can be used to detect antibody or antigen.

(d) Western blot. This procedure is used to detect specific antibodies against microbial pathogens.

(2) Immunologic methods are used to identify microbial antigens or antibodies in body fluid specimens or cultures.

(a) Immunofluorescence uses fluorescein-labeled antibody that is specific for a particular antigen. This method is also used for rapid detection of microbial antigens or antibodies in body fluid specimens or cultures.

(b) Agglutination tests serve to detect and quantitate agglutinins (i.e., antibodies that agglutinate cellular structures, such as bacteria). A common procedure is latex agglutination, in which latex beads coated with antibodies against specific bacteria are reacted with patient serum, cerebrospinal fluid (CSF), urine, and other body fluids. Agglutination tests are rapid and specific and do not require living organisms.

(3) Culture

(a) Identification of bacteria or fungi on solid media or in liquid media is accomplished by noting the pattern of growth in the type of media used, colony morphology, and biochemical characteristics.

(b) Identification of viruses usually requires the use of tissue culture. Characteristic alterations in the morphology of the infected cells in the tissue, hemagglutination or hemadsorption of red blood cells to infected cells, and binding of specific fluorescein-labeled antibody may be used to identify the etiologic agent.

(4) Polymerase chain reaction (PCR) is a newly developed method of identifying the DNA of a microorganism in tissue. PCR can be highly sensitive and specific, but care must be taken to avoid false-positive reactions due to laboratory contamination.

b. Evaluation of antimicrobial activity

(1) Antimicrobial susceptibility tests are used to determine the effects of antimicrobial agents on the growth of the microbial isolate. Susceptibility testing is indicated for bacterial isolates that are clinically significant and should not be performed on isolates that are part of the normal flora.

(a) Antimicrobial susceptibility often is expressed in terms of the concentration of antibiotic needed to inhibit the growth of the microorganism, or the **minimum inhibitory concentration (MIC)**. The lower the MIC, the more susceptible the organism.

(b) In some cases, the clinician requests both the MIC and the **minimum bactericidal concentration (MBC)** of an antimicrobial agent. (The MBC is the lowest concentration of the antibiotic that kills > 99.9% of the microbial isolate being tested.)

(c) Occasionally, combinations of antibiotics are studied to determine whether the combined agents have a greater or lesser effect than that of either agent alone.

(2) Serum bactericidal test is used to determine the effect of both the peak antibiotic level and the antimicrobial factors in the serum (e.g., antibody, complement) on the microbial isolate. Standard concentrations of serially diluted serum are reacted against a standard concentration of the causative organism to determine the lowest concentration of serum that kills the bacteria.

(3) **Tests for β-lactamase production** by staphylococci, *H. influenzae, Neisseria gonorrhoeae,* and other microorganisms are rapid and useful in treating infections due to these agents. Any organism that produces β-lactamase will be resistant to penicillin G and ampicillin.

C. **Antimicrobial therapy.** Treatment of infectious diseases primarily involves antimicrobial agents combined with supportive care. It is incumbent on any physician caring for children with infectious diseases to understand the antimicrobial spectrum, pharmacokinetics, and side effects of antimicrobial agents. A thorough understanding of supportive therapy also is necessary. Severe morbidity or death may result from inadequate supportive therapy, regardless of whether the appropriate antimicrobial agents are used. For example, a child with septic shock must have appropriate intravenous fluid management and cardiovascular and ventilatory support as well as appropriate antibiotic therapy to survive.

1. **Whether to begin antimicrobial therapy.** This is the initial therapeutic question in managing a patient with an infection, the answer to which is determined by several factors.
    a. **Diagnosis.** In general, the more severe the illness, the more important it is to begin antimicrobial therapy after appropriate microbial cultures have been obtained. For example, antimicrobial therapy always is begun for purulent meningitis, but may be withheld for pharyngitis until results of the throat culture are available.
    b. **Host defense factors.** Patients with underlying immunologic defects or deficiencies (e.g., newborns) who show signs of bacterial infection are more likely to be given antibiotics than are patients whose host defenses are intact.
    c. **Follow-up.** A child with suspected streptococcal pharyngitis who may not return for follow-up is more likely to be given penicillin than is a child who will return for follow-up.

2. **Antimicrobial choice.** Antimicrobial therapy is **empiric** if it is chosen on the basis of a probable clinical diagnosis and is **specific** if it is chosen on the basis of culture or antigen test results.
    a. **Antimicrobial activity** is the most important consideration in choosing an antibiotic. The spectrum should be broad enough to cover the likely pathogens if empiric therapy is begun, but should be as narrow as possible when a specific organism is being treated. New antibiotics are constantly being developed because microorganisms develop resistance to conventional antibiotics.
    b. **Toxicity and side effects.** There usually are several antibiotics to choose from when treating an infection. The antibiotic with the lowest toxicity is preferred.
    c. **Previous experience.** Antibiotics that have been shown to be efficacious for a long time are preferred to more recently introduced antibiotics.
    d. **Cost.** Antimicrobial therapy often is expensive. The least expensive antibiotic should be used when all other factors are equal. Because of the costs of preparing and infusing drugs, a single expensive antibiotic given intravenously may be more cost effective than a combination of two or more less expensive antibiotics.
    e. **Dosage and route.** For oral antibiotics, fewer doses each day may improve patient compliance. Pediatric dosages usually are based on body weight. Antibiotics given by mouth may allow for outpatient administration, whereas intravenous antibiotics are not as easily administered on an outpatient basis.

II. FEVER AND FEVER OF UNKNOWN ORIGIN

A. Definitions

1. **Fever** has no universally recognized definition. It is not uncommon for healthy children to have a rectal temperature of 100.4°F (38°C) in the afternoon or after exercise; thus, a practical definition of fever in children is a rectal temperature above 100.4°F (38°C).

Oral temperatures usually are about 1°F lower than rectal temperatures. Patients with a high temperature (> 106°F) are at increased risk for bacterial illness; however, viral infections may cause a temperature to be higher than 105°F.

2. **Fever of unknown origin** has been defined as an illness that persists for 3 or more weeks with an accompanying temperature above 101°F (38.4°C) and an uncertain diagnosis after a 1-week investigation in the hospital. Many children are admitted to the hospital with a relatively brief febrile illness without localizing findings on physical examination. It is more useful clinically to classify this fever syndrome as **fever without localizing signs**.

B. **Diagnosis.** Several general principles are important to consider when performing a workup on a child with fever of unknown origin or fever without localizing signs.

1. **The major illnesses that cause fever in children** are infectious diseases, collagen vascular diseases, malignancies, and inflammatory bowel disease. Infectious diseases are the most common cause of fever of unknown origin in children. Fever usually is not the only manifestation of illness in children with malignancies.

2. **The presence of fever must be documented.** Parents may exaggerate the actual temperature of their child, in some cases deliberately (factitious fever). The **erythrocyte sedimentation rate** usually is elevated in patients with fever and significant illness.

3. Most children with fever of unknown origin have **common illnesses with uncommon presentations**. The most common infectious causes of fever of unknown origin in children are tuberculosis, brucellosis, tularemia, salmonellosis, diseases due to rickettsiae or spirochetes, infectious mononucleosis, cytomegalic inclusion disease, and hepatitis.

4. **Continued observation** of the child, with repeated review of the history and physical examination and occasionally repeated laboratory tests, is important in helping to establish a specific diagnosis.

5. **Young children** (younger than 2 years) **with fever and no localizing findings are at higher risk for serious infection,** including bacteremia, than are older children. Consequently, these children should have at least a complete blood count, urinalysis, and blood culture as part of their workup. A febrile or hypothermic newborn often receives a **septic workup,** consisting of a lumbar puncture; blood, urine, and CSF cultures; and a chest radiograph.

C. **Therapy.** Neonates and children with underlying immunodeficiency who have fever without localizing signs generally are admitted to the hospital and begun on empiric antibiotic therapy while the results of the cultures are pending. The management of immunocompetent older patients with this problem is more variable. In general, it is better to withhold antibiotics until a definitive diagnosis is made.

III. BACTEREMIA AND SEPSIS

A. **Definitions**

1. **Bacteremia** is defined as the presence of bacteria in the blood. **Occult bacteremia** is a transient bacterial invasion of the bloodstream, without an obvious focus of infection.

2. **Sepsis** is a life-threatening bacterial invasion of the intravascular compartment, which may or may not be associated with a focus of infection.

B. **Occult bacteremia**

1. **Incidence and etiology.** Studies done in the 1960s showed that routine blood cultures in infants with febrile seizures often were positive for *Streptococcus pneumoniae*

but that most of these infants had no focus of infection and recovered without therapy. Subsequent studies have shown that occult pneumococcal bacteremia is not uncommon, with the greatest risk (5%–10%) occurring in infants between the ages of 6 months and 2 years who have a temperature above 102°F (38.9°C) and leukocytosis.

2. **Clinical features.** Signs and symptoms usually consist of a temperature of at least 102°F (39.8°C) and irritability without an obvious focus of infection. Febrile seizures have been associated with occult bacteremia.

3. **Diagnosis.** Laboratory workup consists of a white blood cell count (which usually exceeds 15,000/mm^3) and blood culture. Quantitative blood culture usually reveals a low titer of the causative microorganism (i.e., about 10 bacteria/ml).

4. **Therapy.** Occult pneumococcal bacteremia usually resolves spontaneously in 24 to 48 hours. Large controlled studies are needed to determine whether patients at greatest risk for occult bacteremia should be followed as outpatients without treatment or should be given empiric treatment with penicillin.

C. **Sepsis in infants and children**

1. **Incidence and etiology.** Sepsis is uncommon in children who are older than 3 months of age and immunologically normal. The most common causative agents are *Neisseria meningitidis* and *S. pneumoniae.* The incidence of sepsis and other illnesses due to *H. influenzae* type b is decreasing as a result of the development of *H. influenzae* type b vaccines.

2. **Clinical features.** Sepsis should be suspected in any previously healthy infant or child who develops a fever without an obvious focus of infection and appears ill. A petechial rash occurs frequently with sepsis due to *N. meningitidis.*

3. **Diagnosis.** Laboratory evaluation of an infant or child with suspected sepsis and no obvious focus of infection consists of white blood cell count (which usually exceeds 15,000/mm^3 and demonstrates a shift to the left), chest radiograph, urinalysis, blood and urine cultures, and lumbar puncture (if clinically indicated).

4. **Therapy** for suspected sepsis in a previously healthy patient older than 3 months of age usually consists of a third-generation cephalosporin.

D. **Sepsis in the immunocompromised patient.** Defects in immune function may be congenital or acquired (see Chapter 9) and include disorders of humoral immunity (antibody and complement defects), cellular immunity (neutrophil, monocyte, and lymphocyte defects), and structural immune mechanisms (e.g., compromised skin integrity, splenic dysfunction). One of the most commonly encountered immunocompromised patients is the patient with cancer whose neutrophil count has fallen below 500/mm^3 secondary to chemotherapy.

1. **Etiology.** Common causative agents include *Pseudomonas aeruginosa*, gram-negative enteric rods, and *Staphylococcus aureus. Staphylococcus epidermidis* is a common cause of sepsis in children with central venous or intraarterial catheters.

2. **Clinical features.** Fever may be the only manifestation of life-threatening sepsis in immunocompromised children. These patients must be examined carefully for a focus of infection, especially in the oral and rectal areas.

3. **Diagnosis.** Laboratory evaluation includes white blood cell count, chest radiograph, and cultures of the blood, urine, and skin.

4. **Therapy.** Empiric therapy usually consists of vancomycin and ceftazidime. Alternatively, oxacillin, an aminoglycoside (e.g., tobramycin), and an antipseudomonal penicillin (e.g., ticarcillin) can be used.

IV. CENTRAL NERVOUS SYSTEM INFECTIONS

A. **Meningitis** refers to any inflammation of the meninges. Most commonly, the term refers to an inflammation of the leptomeninges, which includes the arachnoid membrane, the sub-arachnoid space (including the CSF), and the pia mater covering the brain.

1. **Classification and etiology.** There are two major classifications of meningitis: bacterial and aseptic. These usually can be distinguished on the basis of CSF characteristics.
   a. In patients with **bacterial meningitis,** the CSF has an increased white cell count with a predominance of neutrophils, an increased protein level, and a lowered glucose level. The cause of bacterial meningitis varies with the age of the patient.
      (1) In **neonates,** the most common causes are group B streptococci and *Escherichia coli.*
      (2) In **infants and children,** the most common causes are *S. pneumoniae,* and *N. meningitidis.*
   b. In patients with **aseptic meningitis,** the CSF does not contain bacteria. It is character-ized by a mildly elevated white cell count with a predominance of mononuclear cells, a normal or mildly elevated protein level, and a normal glucose level. The cause of aseptic meningitis usually is viral. The most common viral causes of menin-gitis in infants and children are enteroviruses (e.g., coxsackieviruses, echoviruses) and mumps virus.

2. **Incidence.** Meningitis, particularly bacterial meningitis, is a serious infection in infants and children. The risk of a child having bacterial meningitis in the United States by age 5 years is approximately 1 in 2000.

3. **Clinical features.** The early signs and symptoms of meningitis are less specific in young infants than in older children. Generally, the clinical manifestations are more severe in bacterial meningitis than in viral meningitis.
   a. **Central nervous system involvement** manifests as severe headache, lethargy, confu-sion, irritability, seizures, vomiting, and a bulging fontanelle.
   b. **Meningeal involvement** manifests as neck or back pain and **Brudzinski sign** (i.e., neck flexion causes flexion of the legs) and **Kernig sign** (i.e., inability to extend the leg after the thigh is flexed to a right angle with the axis of the trunk). **Nuchal rigidity** is a sensitive sign in children older than 12 months with meningitis, but is less sensitive in children younger than 12 months of age.
   c. **Nonspecific features** include fever, poor feeding, and petechial lesions (most com-monly seen with meningitis due to *N. meningitidis*).

4. **Diagnosis.** Bacterial meningitis is a medical emergency. Diagnostic procedures must be carried out immediately, and therapy must be started promptly. The diagnosis is made on the basis of CSF findings after **lumbar puncture.** In rare cases, the CSF culture may be positive with all other parameters normal if a lumbar puncture is performed early in the course of illness. Unless the patient has been partially treated with antibiotics, bac-terial cultures of CSF are very reliable. In cases of viral meningitis, viral cultures of CSF are positive in less than half of patients.
   a. **Normal values for CSF** are shown in Table 10-2.

TABLE 10-2. Normal Values for Cerebrospinal Fluid

	Opening Pressure	White Blood Cell Count	PMNs (%)	Protein	Glucose (% of Serum)
Neonate	< 60 mm Hg	< 30	< 40%	< 180 mg/dl	> 50%
Infant/child	< 90 mm Hg	< 10	< 10%	< 50 mg/dl	> 50%

PMNs = polymorphonuclear cells.

TABLE 10-3. CSF Findings in Bacterial and Viral Meningitis

Parameter	Bacterial Meningitis	Viral Meningitis
CSF pressure	Increased	Increased
White blood cell count	100–10,000	10–500
White blood cell type	Predominantly PMN	Predominantly mononuclear
Protein content (mg/dl)	>> 40	> 40
Glucose content (mg/dl)	< 40 (< 50% blood glucose)	Normal
Gram stain/culture	Positive for bacteria	Negative
Latex agglutination	Positive for bacteria	Negative

CSF = cerebrospinal fluid; PMN = polymorphonuclear cell.

    b. CSF findings in bacterial and viral meningitis are given in Table 10-3.
    c. Contraindications to lumbar puncture. The decision to perform a lumbar puncture is based on clinical suspicion of bacterial meningitis. There are only a few contraindications to this procedure. They include:
        (1) Increased intracranial pressure due to a space-occupying lesion
        (2) Shock
        (3) Respiratory failure
        (4) Bleeding diathesis
        (5) Presence of bacterial skin lesion (e.g., cellulitis, abscess) at the lumbar puncture site

  5. Therapy for bacterial meningitis consists of antibiotics and supportive care.
    a. Antimicrobial therapy
        (1) Initial therapy (before identification of the causative organism) is based on patient age.
            (a) Neonates and infants younger than 2 months usually are given ampicillin and an aminoglycoside, or ampicillin and cefotaxime.
            (b) Infants and children older than 2 months usually are given cefotaxime or ceftriaxone.
        (2) The **duration of therapy** varies, but usually is 2–3 weeks in neonates and 1–2 weeks in older children.
    b. Supportive care is very important, and consists of:
        (1) Fluid restriction to minimize cerebral edema (generally, two-thirds of the daily maintenance requirement) and to treat inappropriate secretion of antidiuretic hormone
        (2) Maintenance of intravascular volume by rapid administration of intravenous fluids if meningitis is accompanied by shock (e.g., fulminant *N. meningitidis* meningitis)
        (3) Anticonvulsants if seizures occur
        (4) Assisted ventilation if respiratory failure occurs
        (5) Subdural taps for evacuation of extensive subdural effusions
    c. Corticosteroid therapy for *H. influenzae* type b meningitis has been shown to improve CSF findings and decrease the incidence of hearing loss and neurologic sequelae. Its use for children with pneumococcal and meningococcal meningitis is controversial.
    d. Follow-up care. Children who have had meningitis should have a complete neurologic evaluation at the time of their discharge from the hospital, including a vision test, a hearing test, and a formal developmental assessment. Periodic monitoring of neurologic and developmental status should be carried out for at least 2 years.

B. **Encephalitis** is an inflammation of the brain.

  1. Etiology. Acute encephalitis usually has a viral etiology, most commonly herpes simplex virus, arboviruses, and enteroviruses. The incidence of encephalitis due to common childhood infections such as measles and mumps has declined significantly with the increased use of vaccines.

a. **Herpes simplex virus** causes encephalitis year round and is the most common cause of sporadic acute encephalitis in the United States. Herpes simplex virus type 2 usually is the cause of encephalitis in neonates, whereas herpes simplex virus type 1 causes most cases of encephalitis in older children.

b. **Arboviruses** cause encephalitis outbreaks during the summer because these viruses are transmitted by insects (usually mosquitoes). Important arboviral causes of encephalitis in the United States include:

   (1) California encephalitis virus
   (2) St. Louis encephalitis virus
   (3) Eastern equine encephalitis virus
   (4) Western equine encephalitis virus

c. **Enteroviruses** (i.e., coxsackieviruses and echoviruses) cause encephalitis outbreaks during the summer.

d. **Viruses associated with childhood illnesses** (e.g., mumps, measles, varicella, rubella) may cause acute or postinfectious encephalitis. In postinfectious illness, the encephalitis is thought to be mediated primarily by immune mechanisms.

e. **Epstein-Barr virus** is a rare cause of encephalitis; occasionally, encephalitis may develop during infectious mononucleosis.

f. **Nonviral causes** of encephalitis include *Mycoplasma pneumoniae, Toxoplasma gondii, Bartonella henselae* (formerly known as *Rochalimaea henselae*), and *Borrelia burgdorferi.*

2. **Clinical features** of encephalitis vary widely in severity, but most commonly include the following symptoms.

   a. **Early signs and symptoms** are nonspecific and typical of acute systemic illness (e.g., fever, headache, vomiting, upper respiratory symptoms).

   b. **Neurologic signs and symptoms** develop abruptly. Most commonly, there is a decreased level of consciousness, which may range from confusion to deep coma. Seizures, paralysis, and abnormal reflexes also are common. Increased intracranial pressure can result in papilledema.

3. **Diagnosis.** A detailed medical history should be obtained, which should include an evaluation of all possible exposures to infected people, insects, or animals. In addition, the following laboratory tests commonly are used to confirm the diagnosis of encephalitis. Occasionally, these tests may reveal a specific infectious etiology.

   a. **Lumbar puncture and CSF examination** are essential.

      (1) **Typical CSF findings** in patients with viral encephalitis include:
         (a) Increased intracranial pressure
         (b) Variable pleocytosis (generally 10–500 cells/mm^3) with a predominance of mononuclear cells
         (c) Increased protein level (> 40 mg/dl)
         (d) Normal glucose level
      (2) In addition, the CSF should be examined directly for bacteria and fungi and cultured for bacteria, mycobacteria, fungi, and viruses.

   b. **Brain biopsy** may be performed to obtain tissue specimens for culture and rapid viral antigen tests. Although the diagnosis of herpes simplex encephalitis is best confirmed by brain biopsy, this procedure is seldom carried out in clinical practice. PCR for detection of herpes simplex in CSF is a promising new diagnostic technique.

   c. **Serologic tests** (e.g., hemagglutination inhibition, complement fixation, ELISA) may be used to detect viral antibodies. The diagnosis of arboviral encephalitis is best confirmed by serologic tests.

   d. **Electroencephalograms, computed tomography (CT), and brain scans** may reveal focal or generalized abnormalities in patients with encephalitis.

4. **Therapy**

   a. **Antimicrobial therapy**

      (1) **Acyclovir** is the drug of choice for treatment of herpes simplex and varicella-zoster encephalitis.

(2) There is no specific therapy for other types of viral encephalitis.
   b. Supportive care
   (1) Patients with encephalitis should be cared for in an **intensive care** unit, with close **cardiac monitoring** and placement of an **intracranial pressure transducer,** if intracranial pressure is moderately to severely increased.
   (2) Phenobarbital (5 mg/kg/24 hours) is given to prevent convulsions.
   (3) Severe cerebral edema can be decreased by the following methods:
      (a) Dexamethasone (0.5 mg/kg/24 hours), given parenterally
      (b) Mannitol (1.5–2.0 mg/kg/24 hours), given intravenously as a 20% solution
      (c) Furosemide (1–2 mg/kg), given intravenously every 6 hours

V. UPPER AIRWAY INFECTIONS

A. **Otitis media,** or inflammation of the middle ear, is one of the most common infections of childhood. The characteristic feature of otitis media is a bulging, erythematous tympanic membrane with impaired mobility. Otitis media is classified as acute or chronic. Otitis media that persists longer than several months is considered to be chronic. The pathologic process of chronic otitis media usually is well established before the onset of clinical complaints.

1. Etiology
   a. Bacteria are the primary agents of otitis media.
   (1) The **most common causes** in all age groups are *S. pneumoniae* (25%–40% of cases), unencapsulated strains of *H. influenzae* (15%–25% of cases), and *Moraxella catarrhalis* (12%–20% of cases). In addition, gram-negative bacilli cause about 20% of otitis media in neonates; however, these bacteria rarely are found in older children with otitis media.
   (2) **Less common causes** include group A streptococci (acute form), *S. aureus*, and *P. aeruginosa* (chronic form).
   b. Viruses are not important direct causes of otitis media. However, viral upper respiratory infections commonly result in obstruction of the eustachian tube, which allows bacteria to multiply in the middle ear space. In rare cases, respiratory syncytial virus, parainfluenza viruses, adenoviruses, and coxsackieviruses have been isolated from middle ear fluid.

2. Predisposing factors. The following factors are associated with an increased incidence of otitis media in childhood: otitis media occurring in the first 6 months of life, immunodeficiency, structural defects that impair eustachian tube function (e.g., cleft palate), day care attendance, and siblings with recurrent otitis media.

3. Clinical features of otitis media are variable and often nonspecific. Neonates and infants may be asymptomatic or may present with only nonspecific manifestations of illness (e.g., irritability, diarrhea, vomiting).
   a. Classic signs and symptoms of acute otitis media include pain in one or both ears and hearing loss. A discharge may be present.
   b. Common signs and symptoms of chronic otitis media include hearing impairment, perforation of the tympanic membrane, and a foul-smelling discharge from the ear canal (otorrhea). Ear pain and fever coincide with flare-ups of acute infection.
   c. Nonspecific signs and symptoms include fever, irritability, mild upper respiratory symptoms, vomiting, and diarrhea.

4. Diagnosis
   a. Otoscopy and tympanometry are used to provide the basis for a diagnosis of otitis media.
   (1) Bulging of the tympanic membrane, as evidenced by partial or total loss of the light reflex or bony landmarks, and diffuse erythema generally are accepted as

reliable indications of otitis media. Erythema can result from crying or fever and, by itself, does not establish the diagnosis.

    (2) Impaired mobility of the tympanic membrane is another diagnostic sign of otitis media, which can be assessed with a pneumatic otoscope.

    (3) Tympanic membrane compliance can be determined more objectively using a tympanometer.

  b. Needle aspiration and culture of the middle ear contents is the most reliable method for confirming the presence of infection and can be used to identify the causative agent. Only rarely is this procedure necessary, as in the case of a critically ill child or a child who fails to respond to standard antimicrobial therapy.

5. Therapy

  a. Acute otitis media

    (1) Initial treatment of acute otitis media is directed against the most commonly encountered bacteria, *S. pneumoniae* and *H. influenzae*. The drug of choice is amoxicillin, which usually is effective against both of these organisms.

    (2) If there is a poor response to initial therapy or the patient is allergic to penicillin or lives in an area where ampicillin-resistant strains of *H. influenzae* are common, **alternative antibiotic regimens** are used. Alternative antibiotics include amoxicillin–clavulanic acid, cefaclor, cefuroxime, cefixime, cefpodoxime, cefprozil, erythromycin–sulfisoxazole, loracarbef, or trimethoprim–sulfamethoxazole. Most clinical trials show no significant therapeutic differences among these drug regimens, but there are differences in cost, ease of administration, and side effects.

    (3) Patients who are not cured after a second course of antibiotics or who become severely ill may be considered for **tympanocentesis** to identify the offending pathogen so the most appropriate antibiotic can be used.

    (4) Tubes may be inserted through the tympanic membranes to promote drainage of the middle ear space. There are few controlled studies that demonstrate the efficacy of these procedures in the treatment of otitis media.

  b. Recurrent otitis media. Patients with recurrent otitis media may be placed on daily doses of an antibiotic such as sulfisoxazole for 3–6 months after the acute infection has cleared. **Sulfisoxazole or amoxicillin prophylaxis** has been shown to decrease the incidence of recurrent otitis media in controlled trials. Antibiotic prophylaxis usually is given to children with three or more episodes of otitis media in the previous 6 months, although the time of year and previous otitis history affect the decision to use antibiotic prophylaxis.

  c. Chronic otitis media

    (1) Chronic suppurative otitis media. The classic symptoms are otorrhea and hearing loss. The pathogens are usually mixed and commonly include *S. aureus*, *P. aeruginosa*, or both. Initial therapy with an oral antibiotic that is effective against staphylococci may be tried, but optimal therapy is based on middle ear cultures and may require intravenous antipseudomonal therapy.

    (2) Otitis media with effusion (OME). Chronic OME may be related to infection but also to such conditions as allergy and immunologic disorders. Treatment is controversial. Some studies suggest that a 2- to 4-week course of oral antibiotic may be effective. Placement of tympanostomy tubes is recommended in children with persistent middle ear effusion for more than 2–3 months that is unresponsive to antibiotic therapy. Oral antihistamine–decongestant preparations, nonsteroidal antiinflammatory drugs, and tonsillectomy or adenoidectomy do not appear to be effective therapy for OME.

B. **Otitis externa** (swimmer's ear) is inflammation of the outer ear canal, usually caused by *S. aureus*. Other causative organisms include *P. aeruginosa* and *E. coli*. There often is purulent drainage from the canal and slight pain. Therapy consists of local antibiotic ear drops and oral antibiotic.

C. **Sinusitis** is an inflammation of the mucous membrane lining the paranasal sinuses, which may be acute or chronic.

1. **Acute and chronic forms**
   a. **Acute sinusitis** may involve one or more sinuses. Inflammation of the ethmoid sinuses (**ethmoiditis**) is most common in children, because these are the only sinuses that are fully developed at birth. The maxillary sinuses also may be involved but are not clinically important until after 18 months of age. **Frontal sinusitis and sphenoidal sinusitis** are rare before 10 years of age, because these sinuses begin to develop after 6 years of age.
   b. **Chronic sinusitis** occurs after prolonged episodes of untreated or inadequately treated acute sinusitis that result in permanent changes in the mucosal lining of the sinus. Sterility no longer is maintained in the sinus. Although patients with chronic sinusitis may have acute infectious exacerbations, there is no evidence that chronic sinusitis is primarily an infectious problem.

2. **Predisposing factors.** Several conditions may predispose to sinusitis, the most common being viral upper respiratory infection, allergy (allergic rhinitis), and asthma. Other contributing factors include periodontal disease, rapid changes in altitude, swimming, trauma, exposure to tobacco smoke, and immunologic defects.

3. **Etiology.** Although sinusitis may be caused by a viral infection or an allergy, the clinician making the diagnosis of sinusitis primarily is concerned with bacterial infection.
   a. The **predominant microorganisms** recovered from both children and adults with acute sinusitis are the same organisms that cause acute otitis media, namely *S. pneumoniae*, unencapsulated strains of *H. influenzae*, and *M. catarrhalis*.
   b. *S. aureus* sometimes is cultured from sinus fluid of patients with acute sinusitis, but this organism is not a major cause of sinusitis.
   c. **Anaerobic organisms** are **uncommon** causes of acute sinusitis.

4. **Clinical features**
   a. **Common symptoms** of acute sinusitis in children older than 5 years are fever, facial pain, sore throat, and headache. In younger children, the most common symptoms are fever, purulent nasal discharge, and cough that persists longer than 7–10 days.
   b. **Suggestive signs** of acute sinusitis include periorbital swelling, localized tenderness to pressure, and malodorous breath.

5. **Diagnosis** of sinusitis is complicated by the fact that the mucous membrane of the paranasal sinuses is continuous with that of the nose. As a result, even a transient viral upper respiratory infection may cause sinus membrane swelling.
   a. **Radiography** is the most commonly used method for the diagnosis of acute sinusitis. The presence of air–fluid levels or complete opacification of the sinus cavity is strong evidence of acute bacterial sinusitis. In general, a sinus series is performed consisting of frontal, lateral, and Water projections. Although not routinely performed, CT scanning gives the best views of the sinuses.
   b. **Transillumination** of the frontal and maxillary sinuses may provide valuable information for the diagnosis of sinusitis in older children, but not in younger ones. Opacity of the sinus cavity suggests the presence of sinusitis, whereas normal light transmission suggests the absence of infection.
   c. **Sinus aspiration and culture** can identify the specific microbial etiology of sinusitis. Although sinus aspiration also provides the definitive diagnosis of sinusitis, it rarely is needed to confirm the diagnosis in children. Sinus aspiration usually is performed only in children with persistent symptoms or complications unresponsive to initial therapy.
      (1) When aspiration is used, a Gram stain and culture of the sinus aspirate usually are obtained, although a biopsy of the sinuses also can give useful information.
      (2) Swab cultures of the anterior nares, nasal vestibule, and throat are not reliable because they do not correlate well with cultures of sinus aspirates.

6. **Therapy**
   a. **Antimicrobial therapy**
      (1) **Initial treatment** of acute sinusitis is directed against the most common bacterial causes, *S. pneumoniae* and *H. influenzae*. The drug of choice, therefore, is amoxicillin.
      (2) An **alternative antibiotic regimen** should be given in the case of apparent antibiotic failure or in the case of a patient who is allergic to penicillin or who lives in an area where ampicillin-resistant strains of *H. influenzae* or *S. pneumoniae* are common. Alternatives include amoxicillin–clavulanic acid, cefaclor, cefuroxime, cefixime, cefpodoxime, cefprozil, erythromycin–sulfisoxazole, loracarbef, or trimethoprim–sulfamethoxazole.
   b. **Sinus irrigation or surgical drainage** of the sinuses is indicated in patients who do not respond to antimicrobial therapy and in those who have intraorbital or intracranial complications, such as orbital cellulitis, cavernous sinus thrombosis, meningitis, or brain abscess.
   c. **Supportive care**
      (1) **Nasal decongestants** may be helpful in the supportive care of patients with acute sinusitis. These may be administered locally (by drops or spray) or orally for shrinkage of the nasal mucosa. In addition, **saline drops** may be very helpful.
      (2) **Antihistamines** may be helpful in patients with associated allergic rhinitis. However, these agents may thicken purulent nasal secretions, thus inhibiting drainage.

D. **Infections of the oral cavity. Gingivitis and stomatitis** refer to inflammatory disease of the gingivae (gums) and oral mucosa, respectively. Combined inflammation of the gingivae and oral mucosa is termed gingivostomatitis. The following discussion is limited to clinically important examples of gingivitis and stomatitis that occur in infants and children, and excludes infections of the teeth and tongue.

1. **Necrotizing ulcerative gingivitis (Vincent disease, trench mouth)** consists of necrosis and ulceration of the interdental papillae.
   a. **Incidence.** This infection is most common in adults but may also occur in children.
   b. **Etiology and pathogenesis**
      (1) Necrotizing ulcerative gingivitis results from a decreased resistance of the gingivae to infection by normal oral flora. Subgingival plaque is present in large amounts and consists of a mixture of fusiform bacilli and spirochetes.
      (2) The infection begins in an area of the gum that is in contact with plaque (the interdental papillae) and results in the punched-out, eroded papillae and purulent, gray membrane characteristically seen in these patients.
   c. **Clinical features** include gingival pain, fever, malaise, and foul-smelling breath.
   d. **Therapy**
      (1) Oral irrigation with **oxidizing agents** relieves the pain associated with the infection.
      (2) **Antimicrobial therapy** (usually penicillin G) is effective against the infection and, along with oral irrigation, usually brings prompt relief.

2. **Aphthous stomatitis (canker sore)** is a common and often recurrent oral mucosal lesion. It consists of circular, shallow ulcers that are painful and may occur anywhere on the oral mucosa, particularly the freely movable (buccal) mucosa. The lesions may occur singly or in clusters, are covered by a gray membrane, and are surrounded by a raised border of inflammation.
   a. **Etiology.** The exact cause of aphthous stomatitis is not known, but several infectious agents have been suspected.
   b. **Clinical course and therapy.** Aphthous stomatitis is a self-limited infection that heals in 1–2 weeks without treatment, but tends to recur in susceptible individuals. Symptomatic therapy with saline mouthwash may be helpful in mild cases.

3. **Herpetic gingivostomatitis**
   a. **Incidence.** Herpetic gingivostomatitis is the most common type of gingivostomatitis in children. The first infection (primary infection) usually occurs within the first 5 years of life.

b. Etiology. Herpes simplex virus is the causative agent. Most cases are caused by herpes simplex virus type 1 rather than type 2.

c. Pathogenesis

(1) Primary infection affects the mouth and gums, whereas recurrent disease usually affects the lips (**herpes labialis**) and is less severe than the primary infection.

(2) Recurrent illness often is precipitated by emotional stress, exposure to the sun, or febrile illness (e.g., viral upper respiratory infection, pneumonia, meningitis). They are therefore also called sun blisters or fever blisters.

d. Clinical features. Primary herpetic gingivostomatitis causes painful, erythematous, edematous, and ulcerative lesions on the buccal mucosa, gums, and, sometimes, the hard palate and tongue. There usually is fever, often to a temperature of 105°F (40.6°C). The infection occurs after a 3- to 9-day incubation period, improves after 3–5 days, and usually resolves within 2 weeks.

e. Therapy. Cold foods (e.g., ice cream) and oral fluids should be given. Viscous xylocaine (2%) can provide some pain relief. The condition may be severe enough that a child refuses to eat or drink and requires intravenous rehydration in the hospital.

4. Herpangina. Although herpangina has been considered a specific febrile disease, the term is more appropriately used to refer to the characteristic oropharyngeal lesions noted as one of the protean manifestations of enteroviral infections. Herpangina can occur in association with meningitis, exanthems, and other clinical presentations of the enteroviruses. **Hand-foot-and-mouth disease** is another infectious disease caused by enteroviruses, which is characterized by vesicular lesions of the mouth, hands, and feet.

a. Etiology and incidence. Coxsackieviruses (types A and B) and echoviruses are the causative agents. Herpangina occurs almost exclusively in the summer and fall, when enteroviruses are prevalent.

b. Clinical features

(1) **Fever, sore throat, and pain on swallowing** are the hallmarks of herpangina. The fever is of sudden onset and may rise to 106°F (41.1°C). Headache, myalgia, and vomiting also may occur at the onset of the illness.

(2) The **characteristic lesions** are 1- to 2-mm vesicles and ulcers surrounded by an erythematous ring measuring up to 10 mm in diameter. The lesions occur in the posterior pharynx, including the anterior tonsillar pillars, soft palate, uvula, tonsils, and pharyngeal wall.

(3) The fever subsides in 2–4 days, but the ulcers may persist for a period of up to 1 week.

c. Therapy. No treatment is necessary other than prevention of dehydration and observation for signs of more severe enteroviral illness.

5. Candidal gingivostomatitis. "Thrush" is the term used to describe gingivostomatitis due to infection by *Candida* species, usually *Candida albicans.*

a. Incidence. Candidal gingivostomatitis is common in newborns. The condition usually clears by 3 months of age, except in severely debilitated infants. Oral antibiotic therapy may predispose an individual to thrush. When candidal gingivostomatitis occurs after infancy, a defect of cell-mediated immunity should be considered.

b. Clinical features. Grayish-white lesions occur on the buccal mucosa and dorsum of the tongue. Occasionally, the gingival mucosa and posterior pharynx may be involved. If a scraping from the affected area is Gram stained, yeast forms, and pseudohyphae are seen. Culture on blood agar will yield *Candida* organisms.

c. Therapy consists of administering a solution of **nystatin** orally four times daily for 1 week. Retreatment sometimes is necessary. **Clotrimazole troches** are an effective alternative.

E. **Streptococcal pharyngitis.** "Acute pharyngitis" refers to any of the numerous inflammatory conditions involving the pharynx. Most often it is caused by a virus and occurs as a component of a generalized upper respiratory infection (e.g., the common cold). However, the most clinically significant cause of acute pharyngitis is **group A β-hemolytic strepto-coccus**. Because penicillin is effective against streptococcal but not viral pharyngitis, it is important to recognize streptococcal pharyngitis so that its symptoms can be alleviated and its complications (see V E 5) can be prevented.

1. **Epidemiology.** Streptococcal pharyngitis is one of the most common respiratory infections of childhood. Although all age groups may be affected, the peak incidence occurs in children between the ages of 5 and 15 years. There is no sex or race predilection. The incidence of streptococcal pharyngitis is highest in the winter and early spring.

2. **Clinical features**
   a. **Symptoms** may vary widely from very mild to severe. In **older children** there is an abrupt onset of fever and sore throat accompanied by headache and malaise. **Younger children** may present with nausea, vomiting, and abdominal pain.
   b. **Physical signs** that may be seen in patients include:
      (1) Temperature higher than 101°F (38.4°C)
      (2) Tonsillar enlargement with exudate
      (3) Edema, erythema, and lymphoid hyperplasia of the pharynx
      (4) Tender anterior cervical lymph nodes and petechiae on the soft palate
      (5) Conjunctivitis, cough, hoarseness, and diarrhea, which suggest viral rather than streptococcal infection

3. **Diagnosis**
   a. **Differential diagnosis.** Acute pharyngitis may be caused by a variety of pathogens, most of which are viruses.
      (1) **Viruses** that can cause infections that mimic streptococcal sore throat include Epstein-Barr virus, adenovirus, herpes simplex virus, enterovirus, influenza virus, and parainfluenza virus.
      (2) **Other bacterial causes** of pharyngitis include *M. pneumoniae, N. gonorrhoeae, Arcanobacterium hemolyticum,* and other β-hemolytic streptococci (e.g., group C and group G streptococci).
   b. **Throat culture** is the primary method for the diagnosis of streptococcal pharyngitis and the most reliable means of differentiating streptococcal from viral pharyngitis. A swab is rubbed over the tonsils and posterior pharynx, with care taken to avoid the buccal mucosa and tongue, and the swab is rolled over a blood agar plate. Presumptive differentiation of group A from other hemolytic streptococci is made by the use of a bacitracin disk (group A disk). Group A hemolytic streptococci are sensitive (zone of inhibition), whereas relatively few other hemolytic streptococci are sensitive (no zone of inhibition) to bacitracin.
   c. **Rapid diagnostic tests** have been developed for office use, which involve the extraction of streptococcal antigens from throat swabs so that the antigens can be identified using immunologic methods such as enzyme immunoassay. Some of these commercial kits can secure the diagnosis within 10–60 minutes. In general, these tests are as specific but less sensitive and more expensive than throat cultures.

4. **Therapy**
   a. The **treatment of choice** for streptococcal pharyngitis is oral **penicillin V** (250 mg) given 3 times daily for 10 days. Noncompliant patients may be given a single intramuscular injection of benzathine penicillin G, which provides adequate penicillin levels for 10 days. The usual dose is 600,000 units for children weighing less than 60 pounds and 1,200,000 units for children weighing 60 pounds or more.
   b. Penicillin-allergic patients may be given any one of several **alternative antibiotics**.
      (1) Oral **erythromycin** is the favored alternative, given in the form of erythromycin estolate (30 mg/kg/day) or erythromycin ethylsuccinate (50 mg/kg/day).
      (2) Oral **cephalosporins,** such as cephalexin, also may be used to treat streptococcal pharyngitis, but are expensive and carry a 5%–10% risk of cross-reactivity in patients who are allergic to penicillin.

5. Complications

a. Streptococcal pharyngitis may give rise to several **suppurative complications,** including acute otitis media, acute sinusitis, peritonsillar cellulitis or abscess, retropharyngeal abscess, and suppurative cervical lymphadenitis.

b. Of even more importance, however, are the delayed **nonsuppurative complications** of streptococcal pharyngitis: acute rheumatic fever (see Chapter 9) and acute glomerulonephritis (see Chapter 14).

F. **Cervical adenitis** refers to inflammation and enlargement of the lymph nodes of the neck. Swollen and tender cervical lymph nodes are common in children. In many cases the illness is self-limited (as in cervical adenitis associated with a viral infection); however, in other cases the illness requires prompt and effective treatment.

1. **Etiology.** The etiologic agents of childhood cervical adenitis are highly varied. Most cases are related either to bacterial infection of the oral cavity or other areas of the head and neck (e.g., streptococcal pharyngitis) or to viral upper respiratory infection.

a. **Common agents.** The most frequently identified agents of childhood cervical adenitis are *S. aureus* and group A streptococci; in addition, group B streptococci are common causes in neonates. Studies also have implicated anaerobic bacteria, which may cause cervical adenitis alone or in combination with other bacteria.

b. **Less common agents**

(1) **Cat-scratch disease** primarily affects children and is an important cause of cervical adenitis. The causative organism has been identified as *B. henselae*. Transmission usually is by a cat scratch; occasionally, the skin injury results from the scratch of a dog or other animal, a splinter, or a thorn.

(2) Several species of **atypical mycobacteria** cause cervical adenitis in infants and young children. The most common of these are *Mycobacterium scrofulaceum* and *Mycobacterium avium-intracellulare*.

(3) **Other agents** of childhood cervical adenitis include:

(a) Epstein-Barr virus

(b) Measles

(c) Rubella

(d) *Mycobacterium tuberculosis*

(e) *Francisella tularensis*

(f) *Yersinia pestis*

(g) *Candida* species

(h) Histoplasmosis

(i) *T. gondii*

2. **Clinical features**

a. **General description.** Typically, a child with cervical adenitis presents with swollen, tender nodes in a single location of the neck, with reddening of the skin overlying the nodes. **Bilateral involvement** suggests a nonspecific or viral infection, which usually resolves spontaneously. **Unilateral involvement** with nodes that are more severely swollen (3–6 cm in diameter), tender, and warm suggests a pyogenic infection. Low-grade fever is an inconsistent finding.

b. In **cat-scratch disease,** which is unilateral, the involved nodes may be quite large and in 10%–25% of cases are suppurative. Low-grade fever and a transient maculopapular rash also may be noted.

c. In **atypical mycobacterial infection,** the cervical adenitis usually involves the submandibular or submaxillary nodes, is unilateral, and runs an indolent course. Fever and other systemic signs usually are absent.

3. **Diagnosis**

a. **Medical history and physical examination.** The medical history of a child with cervical adenitis should include information concerning exposure to individuals with tuberculosis, contact with pets (especially cats), recent upper respiratory infections, and the duration of the lymphadenopathy. All node sites should be examined, with dimensions noted. Liver and spleen size also should be noted.

b. Specific diagnosis of the cause of cervical adenitis usually is not attempted if the child has only slightly enlarged and minimally tender lymph nodes. A diagnostic workup is performed if the child has a moderate fever and systemic symptoms when first examined, if a large (> 3 cm) or fluctuant node is found, if findings suggest an unusual etiology, or if empiric antibiotic therapy has failed (see V F 4).

    (1) Needle aspiration, incision and drainage, or excision and biopsy are the most direct methods for the diagnosis of cervical adenitis. When appropriately performed, needle aspiration is a safe and accurate procedure. The aspirated material should be prepared for Gram stain, acid-fast stain, and culture.

    (2) A **tuberculin skin test** should be part of the diagnostic workup of all children with cervical adenitis, even if there has been no history of exposure to tuberculosis.

    (3) Serologic tests may help to identify viruses (e.g., Epstein-Barr virus), bacteria (e.g., *B. henselae*, *F. tularensis*), and protozoa (*T. gondii*).

    (4) Other diagnostic tests include:

        (a) Gram stain and culture of any primary focus of infection

        (b) Blood culture

        (c) Complete blood count

        (d) Chest radiograph

4. Therapy

    a. Cervical adenitis that is characterized by only **slight enlargement and minimal tenderness** of the lymph nodes is closely observed but otherwise untreated.

    b. Cervical adenitis that is characterized by **more severe enlargement and tenderness** usually is treated first with empiric antibiotic therapy for 10–14 days.

        (1) The **preferred agents** are penicillinase-resistant penicillins (e.g., **dicloxacillin, amoxicillin–clavulanate potassium**) or **clindamycin**.

        (2) Penicillin-allergic patients usually are given an **oral cephalosporin** or clindamycin.

    c. If there is a poor response to empiric therapy, a diagnostic workup is performed that may include **needle aspiration**. If a specific etiology is determined, appropriate therapy is as follows:

        (1) Cervical adenitis due to *S. aureus* or group A streptococci is treated with an oral antistaphylococcal agent or oral penicillin, respectively. Excision and drainage may be necessary in severe cases.

        (2) Cervical adenitis associated with cat-scratch disease usually is self-limited and requires only analgesics. Suppuration may occur and is managed with needle aspiration to remove pus. Antibiotic therapy may be considered in more severe cases, and might include trimethoprim–sulfamethoxazole orally or gentamicin parenterally, although efficacy of antibiotic therapy has not been demonstrated.

        (3) Cervical adenitis due to atypical mycobacteria is treated with excision and drainage of infected nodes. Antituberculous drug therapy alone usually is unsuccessful, although it may be used in addition to surgical excision.

G. **Acute infectious laryngitis** is common and usually occurs in association with the common cold and influenza. Infectious laryngitis is often included as part of the croup syndromes.

1. Etiology. Acute laryngitis is caused primarily by **viruses,** the most frequently implicated being adenovirus, influenza virus, and rhinovirus. In addition, acute laryngitis may be caused by *Streptococcus pyogenes.*

2. Clinical features. The illness usually is mild and does not cause respiratory distress, except in young infants. In rare cases (usually with diphtheria), subglottic obstruction can be significant and result in severe inspiratory stridor, dyspnea, and respiratory arrest.

3. Diagnosis of acute laryngitis usually is apparent from the clinical features of the illness. **Mirror examination** of the larynx reveals hyperemic and edematous mucosa. A specific diagnosis sometimes can be made with a **throat culture** for bacteria and viruses.

4. **Therapy.** Supportive measures include resting the voice and inhaling moistened air. Antimicrobial therapy is indicated for laryngitis due to group A β-hemolytic streptococci or *Corynebacterium diphtheriae*. For laryngitis due to *C. diphtheriae*, diphtheria antitoxin is administered in a single dose.

H. **Croup** is a general term used to describe several acute conditions (both infectious and noninfectious) involving the larynx and, to a lesser extent, the trachea and bronchi. Croup syndromes are characterized by a distinctively brassy cough combined with one or more of the following: hoarseness, inspiratory stridor, and signs of respiratory distress due to laryngeal obstruction. In clinical practice, the term "croup" usually is used to describe acute laryngotracheitis (viral croup) and acute spasmodic laryngitis (spasmodic croup) rather than epiglottitis or acute infectious laryngitis, although the latter two entities are also included under the formal definition of croup.

1. **Acute laryngotracheitis** is the most common of the clinical entities termed "croup."
   a. **Etiology.** Acute laryngotracheitis is caused primarily by respiratory viruses, most commonly, **parainfluenza virus**. Because of its viral etiology, this croup syndrome often is referred to as **viral croup**.
   b. **Clinical features.** Viral croup usually has a gradual onset and course. Symptoms often are worse at night and persist for several days.
      (1) Patients present initially with symptoms of **upper respiratory infection,** followed after several days by the characteristic **barking cough, inspiratory stridor, and respiratory distress**.
      (2) **Fever** often is low grade, but temperatures as high as 104°F (40°C) have been noted.
      (3) **Hoarseness and aphonia** are common.
   c. **Diagnosis** usually is apparent from the clinical features but can be aided by radiograph of the larynx, which reveals subglottic narrowing. An anteroposterior view of the neck shows the classic narrowing of the trachea ("church steeple" or "wine bottle" sign).
   d. **Therapy** for viral croup consists mainly of improving air exchange.
      (1) **Humidification**
         (a) **Home.** Patients with mild illness may be treated at home with humidified air from a hot shower or bath, hot steam from a vaporizer, or "cold steam" from a nebulizer. Respiratory distress may improve within minutes, but humidification should be continued until the cough subsides, which usually is after 2 or 3 days.
         (b) **Hospitalization.** Patients with moderate-to-severe illness should be hospitalized if any one of the following signs and symptoms is noted: cyanosis, decreased level of consciousness, progressive stridor, or a toxic appearance. Cold, humidified oxygen should be provided, and the patient should be observed closely in case emergency intubation is needed, but otherwise should be disturbed as little as possible. Arterial blood gas analysis is important to assess the adequacy of air exchange.
      (2) **Racemic epinephrine** (2.5% solution delivered by nebulizer) has been shown to improve air exchange in these patients. It should be used in moderately ill, hospitalized patients, and it may eliminate the need for intubation during the 24–48 hours when the illness is most severe.
      (3) **Corticosteroids** have been the subject of much debate but may be helpful in severe cases. Patients given **dexamethasone** (0.3–0.5 mg/kg given once and repeated in 2 hours) have had a shorter course of illness than those not given dexamethasone.
      (4) **Contraindications.** Sedatives, opiates, expectorants, bronchodilators, and antihistamines should not be given to these patients.

2. **Acute spasmodic laryngitis,** or spasmodic croup, refers to brief, repeated attacks of symptoms that are clinically similar to those of viral croup but less severe. Spasmodic croup occurs most often in children between 1 and 3 years old.
   a. **Etiology.** Spasmodic croup is believed to be caused by viruses, although important allergic and psychological factors probably contribute to the illness in some patients.

    b. Clinical features. Spasmodic croup is characterized by the sudden onset (usually at night) of croupy cough and respiratory stridor. The episodes usually last less than 1 day, but may recur several times per year.

    c. Therapy. Treatment at home with humidified air generally is sufficient for this illness.

3. Laryngotracheobronchitis, or bacterial tracheitis, is far less common than laryngotracheitis or acute spasmodic laryngitis, but is more severe and is often caused by a combination of a bacterial and respiratory viral pathogen. Severe tracheal obstruction with copious, thick secretions is common.

    a. Etiology. Laryngotracheobronchitis is caused by **parainfluenza or influenza viruses** and often a **bacterial coinfection,** including either *S. aureus, S. pyogenes, S. pneumoniae,* or *H. influenzae* type b.

    b. Clinical features. Laryngotracheobronchitis is usually similar in onset to laryngotracheitis but results in more serious illness.

    c. Therapy. Treatment is similar to that of tracheobronchitis, with the exclusion of steroids and racemic epinephrine and the inclusion of antibiotics. Intubation with vigorous suctioning of the airway to remove secretions is usually necessary.

I. **Acute epiglottitis** is a rapidly progressive infection of the epiglottis and contiguous structures that may cause life-threatening airway obstruction.

1. Etiology. Almost all cases of acute epiglottitis in children are caused by *H. influenzae* type b. The incidence of acute epiglottitis has markedly decreased owing to the use of the *H. influenzae* type b vaccine.

2. Clinical features. The abrupt onset of high fever, moderate-to-severe respiratory distress, and stridor in a child who is sitting forward with mouth open and drooling (because of the inability to swallow normally) are highly suggestive of acute epiglottitis.

3. Diagnosis

    a. Physical examination should be done quickly and with care to minimize anxiety. Even a slight increase in restlessness may cause complete obstruction of the airway by the swollen epiglottis. The diagnosis is based on finding a swollen, cherry-red epiglottis. It is essential to **visualize the epiglottis with a laryngoscope or bronchoscope in an operating room,** with complete cardiorespiratory support. Visualization of the epiglottis in other settings by depressing the tongue is contraindicated because of the possibility of inducing airway obstruction.

    b. Radiography. In patients with mild stridor who are not acutely ill, radiographs (lateral neck views) of the nasopharynx and upper airway are useful in determining whether epiglottitis is present.

    c. Culture of the epiglottis and blood should be obtained for identification of the causative organism and its antimicrobial susceptibility pattern.

    d. Immunologic tests. Rapid tests for *H. influenzae* type b antigen on serum or urine may be helpful.

    e. Differential diagnosis. The major differential consideration is acute laryngotracheobronchitis. Epiglottitis has a more abrupt onset and more severe symptoms, and the usual age range is 2–7 years compared with 3 months to 5 years for laryngotracheobronchitis. A complete blood count may be helpful for differentiating the two conditions: epiglottitis is characterized by leukocytosis with a marked shift to the left. Other differences between croup and epiglottitis are given in Table 10-4.

4. Therapy

    a. Ventilatory support. After visual confirmation of epiglottitis, the patient should be intubated and given ventilatory support until edema subsides, usually after several days.

    b. Intravenous antibiotic therapy is given for 7–10 days and is directed against *H. influenzae* type b. The agents of choice are ampicillin or a third-generation cephalosporin, depending on the sensitivity pattern of the causative organism.

    c. Contraindications. Racemic epinephrine and corticosteroids should not be given to these patients.

TABLE 10-4. Characteristics of Three Upper Airway Infections

Characteristic	Viral Croup and Spasmodic Croup	Bacterial Tracheitis	Epiglottitis
Etiology	Respiratory viruses, including parainfluenza viruses and influenza viruses	Respiratory viruses and bacteria, including *S. aureus, S. pyogenes, S. pneumoniae*	*Haemophilus influenzae* type b
Common age of occurrence	3 months–3 years	3 months–5 years	2–7 years
Clinical features			
Onset	Variable (12–48 hours)	Gradually progressive (12 hours–7 days)	Rapid (4–12 hours)
Fever	Variable (100°–105°F)	Variable (100°–105°F)	High (≥ 103°F)
Hoarseness and barking cough	Yes	Yes	No
Dysphagia	No	No	Yes
Course of obstruction	Variable progression	Variable progression, usually severe	Rapid progression
Lab findings			
Leukocyte count	Mildly elevated	Variable, possible increased band count	Usually markedly elevated with increased band forms
Roentgenogram	Subglottic narrowing on PA film	Subglottic narrowing on PA film; irregular soft tissue density within trachea on lateral film	Swollen epiglottis on lateral film
Treatment	Humidification, epinephrine, corticosteroid	Humidification, antibiotic, intubation	Antibiotic, intubation

PA = posteroanterior; *S. aureus* = *Staphylococcus aureus*; *S. pneumoniae* = *Streptococcus pneumoniae*; *S. pyogenes* = *Streptococcus pyogenes*.

J. **Mumps** is a highly contagious, acute viral disease, the most characteristic feature of which is painful enlargement of the salivary glands, primarily the parotid glands. The disease is benign and resolves spontaneously; 20%–40% of infections are subclinical.

1. **Epidemiology.** Mumps is found throughout the world and occurs year round, although epidemics are more frequent during the winter and spring. The disease is uncommon in infants younger than 1 year of age; the highest incidence is in school-age children.

2. **Etiology and pathogenesis**
   a. **Etiology.** Mumps is caused by a **paramyxovirus**—the mumps virus—of which only one serotype has been identified. Mumps virus has been isolated from the saliva, CSF, blood, urine, and infected tissues of patients with mumps.
   b. **Pathogenesis.** The virus is spread by direct contact, by airborne droplet nuclei, and by fomites that have been contaminated by saliva. Viral transmission usually occurs during the period 48 hours before to 7 days after the appearance of swollen salivary glands.

3. **Clinical features**
   a. The **incubation period** varies in length from 2–4 weeks but usually is 16–18 days. After the incubation period, a **prodrome** of fever, anorexia, headache, and malaise may occur but is uncommon.

    b. Within 1 day, the illness manifests as **pain and swelling in one or both parotid glands,** from the posterior border of the mandible forward and downward. Pain and erythema often occur at the opening of the parotid duct (Stensen duct).

        (1) The swelling usually **peaks in 1–3 days** and **then resolves over a 3- to 7-day period**.

        (2) Submandibular or sublingual gland swelling may accompany the parotitis but rarely is the only manifestation of disease.

    c. Fever usually is moderate, although temperatures may reach 104°F (40°C). Fever is absent in 20% of cases.

4. Diagnosis often can be made on the basis of known exposure to mumps combined with characteristic symptoms and physical signs. An elevated serum amylase level due to parotid involvement or pancreatitis is the most useful laboratory indicator in any patient with mumps.

    a. Definitive diagnosis requires either culture of the virus from the saliva, urine, CSF, or blood or demonstration of a significant rise in circulating mumps antibody from the acute to convalescent stage.

    b. Differential diagnosis includes acute parotiditis (due to coxsackie A virus infection or lymphocytic choriomeningitis), suppurative parotiditis (due to bacterial infection), recurrent parotiditis, and a salivary calculus.

5. Therapy for mumps is entirely symptomatic and supportive.

6. Prevention

    a. Passive prophylaxis with anti-mumps antibody has not been shown to be effective for preventing mumps or decreasing the incidence of complications.

    b. Active immunization with live attenuated mumps virus vaccine is effective for prevention of mumps and has few side effects (see Chapter 1).

7. Complications of mumps are uncommon and usually not severe.

    a. Meningoencephalitis is the most frequent complication in childhood, with clinical manifestations noted in about 10% of patients. Mumps is one of the most common causes of aseptic meningitis.

    b. Orchitis is rare in prepubescent boys but develops in 20%–30% of postpubertal men; it usually is unilateral. Symptoms usually occur about 8 days after parotiditis develops but may occur in the absence of salivary gland infection. Approximately 50% of infected testes show some degree of atrophy, but infertility is rare.

    c. Pancreatitis usually presents as epigastric pain and tenderness combined with fever, chills, and vomiting.

    d. Unilateral deafness occurs in 1 in 20,000 mumps patients. Hearing loss is complete and permanent. Bilateral nerve deafness due to mumps is rare.

    e. Other complications include oophoritis, nephritis, thyroiditis, myocarditis, arthritis, thrombocytopenic purpura, and mastitis.

K. **Infectious mononucleosis** is an acute infection characterized by fever, sore throat, lymphadenopathy, splenomegaly, atypical lymphocytosis, and the presence of heterophil antibody. Infectious mononucleosis most often affects adolescents and young adults.

1. Etiology. Infectious mononucleosis is caused by Epstein-Barr virus, a herpesvirus. Cytomegalovirus and *T. gondii* cause illnesses that are virtually indistinguishable from Epstein-Barr virus-induced mononucleosis.

2. Clinical features of infectious mononucleosis are highly variable, often being less severe in younger children than in older children, adolescents, or adults. A prodrome of malaise, fever, and headache may prevail for 3–7 days before the onset of more profound symptoms.

    a. Fever is invariably present and may last as long as 21 days. Temperature may reach as high as 104°F (40°C).

   b. Pharyngitis occurs in about 80% of patients with infectious mononucleosis and may
   be severe. Although group A streptococci may be cultured from these patients, the
   incidence of streptococcal pharyngitis in patients with infectious mononucleosis is
   not increased compared with otherwise healthy controls.
   c. Lymphadenopathy usually is generalized and most often involves the posterior cervical nodes. Other anatomic sites also may be affected.
   d. Splenomegaly is noted in most patients with infectious mononucleosis.
   e. Rash occurs in 10%–40% of patients overall, but it develops in almost all patients
   who are given ampicillin. The rash is maculopapular and generalized.
   f. Other clinical findings include fatigue, eyelid edema, abdominal pain, and, rarely,
   jaundice.

3. **Diagnosis.** Suggestive laboratory tests include a predominance of mononuclear cells on
   complete blood count (more than 50% mononuclear cells) and more than 10% atypical
   lymphocytes. Laboratory confirmation of infectious mononucleosis consists of positive
   serologic findings. Several serologic tests have been developed.
   a. The Paul-Bunnell-Davidsohn test is an extension of the classic Paul-Bunnell test for
   the heterophil antibody characteristic of infectious mononucleosis. **Heterophil antibodies** can react with antigens that are different from the antigens that induced their
   production.
      (1) Heterophil antibodies in **patients with infectious mononucleosis** cause sheep
      erythrocytes to agglutinate. The antibody can reach high titers.
      (2) Heterophil antibodies in **healthy individuals** and those with diseases other than
      infectious mononucleosis (e.g., serum sickness) may cause agglutination of
      sheep erythrocytes, but these antibodies are absorbed by guinea pig kidney cells,
      whereas those of patients with infectious mononucleosis are not.
   b. Commercial heterophile antibody kits (e.g., the Monospot test) are simple, rapid,
   and fairly sensitive. The tests usually are positive within the first week of infection
   and remain positive for several months. Only 80% of patients with Epstein-Barr virus
   infection have positive results. Also, for unknown reasons, children younger than
   5 years of age with Epstein-Barr virus infection often have false-negative results on
   Monospot testing.
   c. Antibodies to Epstein-Barr virus. Patients with infectious mononucleosis produce
   antibodies to various specific antigens, including Epstein-Barr viral capsid antigen
   (VCA), Epstein-Barr nuclear antigen (EBNA), and Epstein-Barr virus-induced early
   antigen (EA).
      (1) Antibodies to VCA [initially immunoglobulin M (IgM) followed by IgG] peak in
      the second or third week of illness and persist for life.
      (2) Antibodies to EA appear early in the course of illness and disappear 2–6 months
      later.
      (3) Antibodies to EBNA appear 3–6 months after the onset of infection and probably
      persist for life.

4. **Therapy.** In most cases, **rest** is the only treatment that is necessary; there is no specific
   drug therapy for infectious mononucleosis. Convalescence may take weeks to months
   and is relatively shorter in younger patients compared with older patients. **Corticosteroids** generally are used in patients with:
   a. Impending airway obstruction
   b. Severe thrombocytopenia
   c. Hemolytic anemia

5. **Complications**
   a. Splenic rupture, due either to trauma or occurring spontaneously, is a rare complication. Patients should be advised not to engage in any contact sports until they are
   fully recovered and splenomegaly has resolved.
   b. Airway obstruction due to tonsillar or pharyngeal hypertrophy also is rare. Treatment
   with corticosteroids often is effective, although tracheal intubation or tonsillectomy
   and adenoidectomy may be necessary in some cases.

c. Neurologic complications usually are self-limited and reversible and include aseptic meningitis, encephalitis, myelitis, peripheral neuropathies, and Guillain-Barré syndrome.

d. Icteric hepatitis occurs in about 5% of cases, whereas subclinical hepatitis occurs in about 20%–40%. Acute liver failure is rare.

e. Other rare complications include autoimmune hemolytic anemia, thrombocytopenia, neutropenia, acute renal failure, complete heart block, myositis, pericarditis, pneumonia, acrocyanosis, and immunologic disorders (e.g., impaired cell-mediated immunity, agammaglobulinemia).

VI. LOWER RESPIRATORY TRACT INFECTIONS

A. **Bronchiolitis** is an acute viral infection of the bronchioles.

1. **Epidemiology.** Bronchiolitis is a common lower respiratory tract illness of children younger than 2 years (owing to their small airways), with a peak incidence at 6 months of age. Most cases occur in the winter and early spring months.

2. **Etiology.** Over 50% of cases are caused by respiratory syncytial virus. Other causes include parainfluenza virus and adenovirus.

3. **Pathophysiology.** Bronchiolitis causes inflammation of bronchioles with narrowing of bronchial diameter leading to hyperinflation and atelectasis. Young infants with bronchiolar obstruction are more likely to have extensive atelectasis with increased hypoxia and respiratory distress than are older children.

4. **Clinical features**
   a. Symptoms
      (1) The onset of bronchiolitis is characterized by mild upper respiratory tract symptoms, which last several days and may be accompanied by a mild fever [temperature of 101°–102°F (38.3°–38.9°C)].
      (2) Lower respiratory tract involvement follows, with gradual development of respiratory distress (i.e., paroxysmal cough, wheezing, tachypnea, dyspnea) accompanied by irritability and decreased appetite.
   b. Physical signs of bronchiolitis include tachypnea, flaring of the alae nasi, and, occasionally, cyanosis. Rales and expiratory wheezes are characteristic. The liver may appear to be enlarged on palpation as a result of diaphragm depression due to hyperinflation of the lung.

5. **Diagnosis** of bronchiolitis usually is made on the basis of the history, physical examination, and classic, confirmatory radiographic findings including hyperinflation and occasional scattered areas of consolidation due to atelectasis. The white blood cell count and differential usually are within the normal range.
   a. Diagnosis of the specific agent of bronchiolitis can be made by rapid tests for viral antigen in the nasopharynx (especially, immunofluorescence for respiratory syncytial virus), viral cultures, or a rise in serum antibody titers.
   b. Differential diagnostic considerations include, most importantly, asthma as well as congestive heart failure, foreign body in the lung or trachea, pertussis, chlamydial infection, cystic fibrosis, and bacterial pneumonia.

6. **Therapy**
   a. Ribavirin is an antiviral agent that can be used for treatment of severe bronchiolitis and pneumonia due to respiratory syncytial virus. Ribavirin has been shown to improve arterial oxygen tension (Po_2) significantly and to shorten the course of the illness.
      (1) Indication. Ribavirin is indicated in hospitalized infants who have severe bronchiolitis due to respiratory syncytial virus or who are at high risk for severe bronchiolitis.

(2) Dosage. Ribavirin is given daily by aerosol over 12–20 hours per day for 3–5 days, depending on the patient's clinical course.

(3) Special care must be taken with the use of ribavirin for patients on ventilators to prevent precipitation of the drug within the ventilator. Constant monitoring of such patients is mandatory. **Pregnant health care workers should avoid caring for patients on ribavirin because of the remote possibility that the drug is a human teratogen.**

b. Hospitalization. In some children—especially infants with congenital heart disease, cystic fibrosis, bronchopulmonary dysplasia, or other underlying pulmonary disease—respiratory distress progresses rapidly and is severe enough to require that the patient be hospitalized with **assisted ventilation**. The mortality rate among these patients is much higher than in those with the usual case of bronchiolitis.

(1) Hospitalized infants are placed in an atmosphere of **cold, humidified oxygen** to relieve dyspnea and cyanosis. **Intravenous or oral fluids** are given to offset the dehydrating effects of tachypnea and anorexia.

(2) In young infants, especially premature infants, apnea may develop that usually is transient. Infants who require hospitalization often are placed on an **apnea monitor** until clinically improved and without episodes of apnea.

c. The overall **mortality rate** for bronchiolitis is **less than 1%**. In most cases, patients recover spontaneously after the first 48–72 hours of illness and do not require ribavirin therapy or hospitalization.

d. Contraindications. The use of sedatives and corticosteroids is not recommended.

B. **Pneumonia** is an inflammation of the lung parenchyma (i.e., the portion of the lower respiratory tract consisting of the respiratory bronchioles, alveolar ducts, alveolar sacs, and alveoli). There are numerous infectious causes of pneumonia, including viruses, bacteria, fungi, parasites, and rickettsiae. Although most cases of childhood pneumonia are caused by viruses, antibiotics are prescribed because the precise etiology usually is not determined.

1. Bacterial pneumonia
   a. Etiology
   (1) Common bacterial causes of pneumonia in children older than 3 months of age include *S. pneumoniae* and group A streptococcus. Group B streptococcus is a common pathogen in neonates.
   (2) Other bacterial causes of pneumonia in children include *S. aureus*, gram-negative enteric organisms, *Chlamydia trachomatis*, anaerobes (especially in patients at risk for aspiration), *H. influenzae* type b, and *M. tuberculosis*.
   b. Clinical features. The clinical presentation in older children (about 6 years old and older) is fairly classic and not unlike that noted in adults with pneumonia. The clinical presentation in infants and children younger than 6 years is somewhat variable.
   (1) Older children with bacterial pneumonia typically present first with mild upper respiratory tract symptoms (e.g., cough, rhinitis) followed by the abrupt onset of fever, tachypnea, chest pain, and shaking chills. Physical examination often reveals lateralizing chest signs, such as decreased breath sounds and rales on the affected side.
   (2) Younger children (i.e., < 6 years) with bacterial pneumonia may present with nonspecific manifestations of infection, including fever, malaise, gastrointestinal complaints, restlessness, apprehension, and chills. **Respiratory signs** may be minimal and include tachypnea, cough, grunting respirations, and flaring of the alae nasi. Signs of pneumonia also may be subtle in the young infant, with absence of rales and rhonchi.
   c. Diagnosis
   (1) Laboratory findings include a peripheral blood leukocytosis with a preponderance of neutrophils and dense, focal infiltration on chest radiograph.
   (2) Specific diagnosis can be made from culture or rapid testing of the blood, urine, alveolar fluid, or pleural fluid. Fluid may be obtained by lung biopsy, lung

puncture, thoracentesis, or bronchoscopy. Although Gram stain and culture of the sputum may help to identify the pathogen, sputum usually is difficult to obtain from children.

d. **Therapy.** There is no universally accepted antibiotic regimen for treatment of presumed bacterial pneumonia. In addition to the following general guidelines, such factors as age, severity of illness, presence of illness in the child's family, and results of laboratory studies must be considered when an antibiotic is chosen.

(1) **Neonates** with pneumonia should be hospitalized and initially treated intravenously either with ampicillin and an aminoglycoside (e.g., gentamicin) or with ampicillin and cefotaxime or ceftazidime. If there is reason to suspect staphylococcal infection, a penicillinase-resistant penicillin should be used in addition to these antibiotics. In addition, hospitalized infants should receive supportive care in the form of intravenous fluids, supplemental oxygen, ventilatory support, and chest physical therapy.

(2) **Children younger than 6 years** with mild-to-moderate illness can be observed closely at home and given oral amoxicillin. Children with more severe illness require hospitalization and intravenous cefuroxime, ceftriaxone, or oxacillin and ceftazidime.

(3) **Children older than 6 years** with mild-to-moderate illness are given oral penicillin or, if *M. pneumoniae* is the likely cause, erythromycin (see VI B 3). Children with severe illness are hospitalized and treated with intravenous cefuroxime, ceftriaxone, ceftazidime, or oxacillin and an aminoglycoside.

2. **Viral pneumonia**

a. **Etiology.** A virus is the most common cause of pneumonia in children. Respiratory syncytial virus is the most common viral etiology; other common causes include parainfluenza virus, adenovirus, and enterovirus. Less common causes of pneumonia in children include rhinovirus, influenza virus, and herpesvirus.

b. **Clinical features.** The clinical presentation of viral pneumonia, like that of bacterial pneumonia, begins with several days of rhinitis and cough followed by fever and more pronounced respiratory symptoms, such as dyspnea and intercostal retractions. In general, the symptoms of viral pneumonia are less fulminant than those of bacterial pneumonia, with lower fever and milder respiratory distress.

c. **Diagnosis**

(1) **Laboratory findings** include a preponderance of lymphocytes on complete blood count and diffuse, bilateral infiltrates on chest radiograph.

(2) **Specific diagnosis** can be made by rapid tests for viral antigen (e.g., immunofluorescence) and by culturing nasopharyngeal and rectal specimens for viruses.

d. **Therapy** for viral pneumonia at one time was limited to supportive care; however, the introduction of antiviral chemotherapy has allowed for specific therapy.

(1) **Antiviral therapy**

(a) **Ribavirin** (see VI A 6 a) is effective against both respiratory syncytial virus and influenza virus and should be used to treat severe pneumonia caused by either of these pathogens. It is administered by aerosol over a period of 5–7 days.

(b) Oral **amantadine** may shorten the course of influenza A infection.

(c) **Acyclovir** has been used to treat pneumonia caused by herpes simplex virus or varicella zoster virus. It is given by intravenous infusion over a period of 7–10 days.

(2) **Supportive care** includes administration of intravenous fluids and supplemental oxygen as well as ventilatory support and chest physical therapy.

3. **Other causes of pneumonia**

a. *M. pneumoniae* is the most common nonviral cause of pneumonia in children older than 6 years. The peak incidence of *M. pneumoniae* pneumonia is between the ages of 5 and 15 years.

(1) **Clinical features.** In general, *M. pneumoniae* pneumonia is less severe than traditional bacterial pneumonia and often is referred to as "walking pneumonia." Hospitalization rarely is necessary.

(a) The **onset of illness** is gradual; fever, headache, and malaise are experienced for 2–4 days before respiratory symptoms develop.

(b) **Symptoms.** A nonproductive cough is the characteristic respiratory symptom. Pharyngitis also is common.

(2) **Diagnosis**

(a) **Laboratory findings.** The complete blood count usually is negative, but leukocytosis with a shift to the left may be noted. The chest radiograph usually is interstitial in appearance but may be focal. Cold agglutinins usually are elevated (> 1:64) during the first week of illness, but may be negative in young children.

(b) **Specific diagnosis** is made by demonstration of a rise in antibody titer in convalescent-phase serum or by isolation of *M. pneumoniae* from sputum or throat culture.

(3) **Therapy. Erythromycin** is the drug of choice for treatment of *M. pneumoniae* pneumonia.

b. *Pneumocystis carinii* produces a progressive pneumonia in immunocompromised hosts, such as those with AIDS, congenital immunodeficiency, or immunosuppression caused by cancer or cancer chemotherapy.

(1) **Clinical features.** In infants, the disease usually begins as a mild illness with low-grade fever and cough but progresses to severe respiratory distress with cyanosis.

(2) **Diagnosis**

(a) The diagnosis is suggested by the typical clinical course and presentation and by a bilateral, generalized granular pattern on radiography.

(b) **Definitive diagnosis** is made by demonstration of *P. carinii* on specially stained smears from tracheal or bronchial washings, lung aspirates, or lung biopsy specimens.

(3) **Therapy. Trimethoprim–sulfamethoxazole** is the drug of choice for treatment of *P. carinii* pneumonia. An alternative choice is **pentamidine isoethionate**.

VII. EXANTHEMS are rashes that arise as cutaneous manifestations of infectious diseases.

A. **Measles (rubeola)** is an acute, highly contagious viral disease that occurs chiefly in young children living in densely populated areas.

1. **Epidemiology.** Although measles is becoming uncommon in developed countries where vaccine is used, it continues to be a major health problem worldwide. Measles persists as a sporadic problem in the United States, despite continued efforts to eradicate the disease.

2. **Etiology.** Measles is caused by a **paramyxovirus** (the measles virus), of which only one serotype has been identified.

3. **Clinical features.** The clinical course of measles has three stages.
   a. An **incubation period** extends for 8–12 days after initial exposure to the virus; signs and symptoms are absent during this stage.
   b. A **prodrome** follows, consisting of malaise, fever [temperatures up to 105°F (40.6°C)], cough, coryza, conjunctivitis, and photophobia. Within 2 or 3 days after the onset of symptoms, **Koplik spots** (small, irregular red spots with central gray or bluish-white specks) appear on the buccal mucosa.
   c. An **erythematous maculopapular rash** erupts about 5 days after the onset of symptoms. The rash begins on the head and spreads downward, lasting about 4–5 days and then resolving from the head downward.

4. **Diagnosis** usually can be made on the basis of observed characteristic clinical findings. A fourfold or greater rise in hemagglutination inhibition antibodies over 2 or 3 weeks confirms the diagnosis.

5. **Therapy** mainly is supportive. Ribavirin has been given to severely affected or immuno-compromised children with measles, but no controlled trials have been conducted. Vitamin A supplementation should be considered for patients 6 months to 2 years of age who are hospitalized with measles and its complications, or for patients who have measles, who are not receiving vitamin A, and who have any of the following risk factors:
   a. Immunodeficiency
   b. Ophthalmologic evidence of vitamin A deficiency
   c. Impaired intestinal absorption
   d. Moderate to severe malnutrition
   e. Recent immigration from areas where high mortality rates from measles have been observed

6. **Prevention**
   a. A **live attenuated vaccine** given alone or as part of the measles, mumps, and rubella (MMR) or measles and rubella vaccines is highly effective in preventing measles (see Chapter 1). It may provide protection if given within 72 hours of measles exposure.
   b. **Immunoglobulin** can be given to modify or prevent measles in a susceptible person if given within 6 days of exposure.

7. **Complications** are rare but may occur, especially in malnourished (especially vitamin A-deficient) or immunocompromised children. Measles complications include pneumonia, encephalitis, subacute sclerosing panencephalitis, pericarditis, and hepatitis. The mortality rate is low in healthy children, but may exceed 10% in malnourished children living in poor and crowded environments.

B. **Rubella (German measles)** is a viral disease that usually is innocuous when acquired postnatally; however, it can have devastating effects when a fetus is infected transplacentally during maternal infection. Before the development of a rubella vaccine in 1969, rubella was the most important cause of congenital infection, resulting in thousands of fetal deaths, premature deliveries, and children born with congenital defects.

1. **Etiology.** Rubella is caused by rubella virus, an RNA virus that is classified as a **togavirus** based on its biochemical and morphologic properties.

2. **Clinical features**
   a. **Postnatal rubella.** Clinical manifestations are absent in many cases of rubella.
      (1) An **incubation period** of 12–23 days is followed by a prodrome of malaise, fever, and anorexia in adults. There is no prodrome in children.
      (2) Several days after the onset of symptoms, posterior auricular, cervical, and sub-occipital **lymphadenopathy** develops, followed by the appearance of a **maculo-papular rash**. The rash begins on the face and then becomes generalized; it seldom lasts longer than 5 days. Fever may accompany the rash on the first day, and then resolve.
   b. **Congenital rubella** most commonly results in deafness, cataracts, glaucoma, congenital heart disease, and mental retardation, but numerous other defects have been described. Some complications, such as a progressive encephalopathy, do not become apparent until the child is older. The risk of congenital defects increases the earlier in pregnancy that the disease occurs.
      (1) **Disease at 1–3 months' gestation** is associated with a 30%–60% risk of multiple congenital defects and spontaneous abortion.
      (2) **Disease at 4 months' gestation** is associated with a 10% risk of a single defect.
      (3) **Disease at 5–9 months' gestation** occasionally is associated with a single defect.

3. **Diagnosis**
   a. **Definitive diagnosis** of rubella requires either virus isolation or serologic confirmation.
      (1) **Virus isolation** can be performed in specialized laboratories, but it is difficult and time consuming.

        (2) Confirmation. The diagnosis usually is confirmed by a fourfold or greater rise in titer of **hemagglutination inhibition or complement-fixing antibodies.** Congenital rubella also can be diagnosed in the neonatal period by the presence of a positive IgM antibody to rubella virus in the newborn's serum; **increased IgM titer** indicates recent rubella infection of the fetus, because IgM does not cross the placenta.

    b. Differential diagnosis. The diagnosis of rubella is difficult because the symptoms often are mild and may be confused with those of enteroviral infections, roseola, toxoplasmosis, infectious mononucleosis, mild measles, and scarlet fever.

4. Therapy and prevention

    a. Therapy. Postnatal rubella usually is mild and self-limited, requiring no treatment. Treatment of congenital rubella is supportive.

    b. Prevention of rubella is effected by a live attenuated vaccine, which usually is given at age 15 months as part of the MMR vaccine.

C. **Roseola infantum (exanthem subitum)** is a common, acute disease of infants and young children, which is caused by human herpesvirus 6.

1. Clinical features

    a. Onset. The illness usually begins with an **abrupt fever** characterized by temperatures of 103°–106°F (39.5°–41.2°C). The fever persists for 1–5 days, although the child appears well and has no physical findings to explain the fever.

    b. The temperature usually returns to normal by the third or fourth day of illness, and a **macular or maculopapular rash** appears on the trunk and spreads peripherally. The rash often resolves within 24 hours.

    c. Initially, the **leukocyte count** may be as high as 20,000/mm^3, with a shift to the left. By the second day of illness, leukopenia and neutropenia are noted.

2. Therapy. Most cases are benign and self-limited. No treatment is available to shorten the course of the illness or to prevent it.

3. Complications are uncommon, although febrile convulsions may occur. The prognosis generally is good.

D. **Erythema infectiosum (fifth disease)** is a mild, self-limited systemic illness accompanied by a distinctive rash. It occurs primarily in epidemics involving children, although adults infrequently are affected.

1. Etiology. Parvovirus B-19 is the cause of the illness.

2. Clinical features

    a. Usually there is no prodrome, and fever may be absent or only low grade. Systemic symptoms, especially recurrent arthralgias, occur more frequently in adults.

    b. The **rash progresses through three stages.**

        (1) The rash begins as a marked **erythema of the cheeks,** which gives a "slapped cheek" appearance.

        (2) An **erythematous maculopapular rash** then involves the arms and spreads to the trunk and legs, producing a reticular pattern.

        (3) The third stage lasts 2–3 weeks but may persist for several months, with low-grade fever. This stage is characterized by fluctuations in the severity of the rash with environmental changes.

3. Therapy consists of supportive measures and, for chronic infection that may develop in immunocompromised patients, intravenous immunoglobulin.

4. Complications (e.g., arthritis, hemolytic anemia, encephalopathy) are rare. Parvovirus B-19 infection during pregnancy can cause fetal hydrops and death. The risk of miscarriage is less than 10% after proven maternal infection in the first half of pregnancy, and may be negligible in the second half.

E. **Varicella and zoster** are two different infectious diseases caused by **varicella-zoster virus**.

1. **Definitions**
   a. **Varicella (chickenpox)** is a highly contagious disease, occurring primarily in children younger than 10 years of age. It usually is a mild, self-limited disease in otherwise healthy children but may be a severe or even fatal illness in immunocompromised children.
   b. **Zoster (shingles)** represents a reactivation of varicella infection, occurring predominantly in adults who previously had varicella and who have circulating antibodies. Although zoster occurs in children, it is uncommon in those younger than 10 years of age. Zoster is an acute infection characterized by crops of vesicles confined to a dermatome and often accompanied by pain in the affected dermatome.

2. **Clinical features**
   a. **Varicella**
      (1) After an **incubation period** ranging from 10–21 days (usually 14–16 days), a prodrome begins, consisting of mild fever, malaise, anorexia, and, occasionally, a scarlatiniform or morbilliform rash.
      (2) The **characteristic pruritic rash** begins the following day, appearing first on the trunk and spreading peripherally.
         (a) The rash begins as red papules and develops rapidly into clear "teardrop" vesicles that are about 1–2 mm in diameter on an erythematous base. The vesicles become cloudy, breaking down into thin ulcerative lesions that crust before healing.
         (b) The lesions occur in widely scattered "crops," so that several stages of the lesions usually are present at the same time. Vesicles may occur on mucous membranes.
      (3) The **severity of the illness** ranges from a few lesions associated with a low-grade fever, to hundreds of lesions associated with temperatures up to 105°F (40.6°C), to fatal disseminated disease in immunocompromised children. In most children, it manifests as a generalized rash with mild fever and mild systemic symptoms.
      (4) **Infectious period.** Patients are infectious beginning approximately 24 hours before the appearance of the rash until all lesions are crusted, which usually occurs 1 week after the onset of the rash.
   b. **Zoster**
      (1) **Onset.** Attacks of zoster may begin with pain along the affected sensory nerve, accompanied by fever and malaise, although these symptoms are more common in adults than in children.
      (2) A vesicular eruption similar to the vesicular form of varicella then appears in a dermatome area and, in most cases, clears in 7–14 days. The rash may last as long as 4 weeks, however, with pain persisting for weeks or months.
      (3) The lesions are infectious if there is direct contact.

3. **Diagnosis of both varicella and zoster** usually is obvious from the clinical presentation.
   a. If the diagnosis is unclear, a **Tzanck test** should be performed on scrapings taken from the base of a vesicle, early in the course of illness. The demonstration of multinucleated giant cells with intranuclear inclusions indicates varicella, zoster, or herpes simplex infection.
   b. The **definitive diagnosis** is made by positive culture from a vesicular scraping or by demonstration of a fourfold rise in antibody titer between acute and convalescent sera.

4. **Therapy**
   a. **Uncomplicated cases of varicella** are treated with an antipruritic medication and daily bathing to reduce secondary bacterial infection.
   b. **Immunocompromised children** (e.g., those with AIDS or leukemia and those on immunosuppressive drugs) who have not had varicella and who are exposed to someone with the disease should receive **prophylaxis with varicella-zoster immune globulin** within 96 hours of exposure and be observed closely. Immunocompromised

patients with varicella or disseminated zoster should be **treated with intravenous acyclovir**.

   c. Oral acyclovir is given to adolescents and adults with increased risk of serious disease. To be effective, acyclovir must be given within 24 hours of the onset of rash and should be continued for 5 days.

5. Prevention is now possible. Studies of a varicella vaccine indicate that it is effective for healthy children and for children with malignancies (see Chapter 1).

6. Complications

   a. The **most common** complications of a varicella-zoster infection include encephalopathy, cerebellitis, Guillain-Barré syndrome, aseptic meningitis, pneumonia, hepatitis, thrombocytopenic purpura, purpura fulminans, cellulitis, abscess formation, and arthritis.

   b. Progressive varicella (with meningoencephalitis, pneumonia, and hepatitis) occurs in immunocompromised children and is associated with a mortality rate of approximately 20%.

   c. Maternal varicella during the first trimester may be associated with congenital malformations in 1%–2% of cases.

F. | **Scarlet fever** is an acute illness characterized by fever, pharyngitis, and an erythematous rash. Scarlet fever is rare in infancy. It can occur more than once in a single patient.

1. Etiology. Scarlet fever results from infection with group A streptococcal strains that produce erythrogenic toxin. The disease usually is associated with pharyngeal infections but, in rare cases, follows streptococcal infections at other sites (e.g., wound infections, impetigo).

2. Clinical features

   a. The **characteristic rash** is erythematous, finely punctate, and blanches with pressure. It appears initially on the trunk and becomes generalized within a few hours to several days. The face is flushed with circumoral pallor, and there is increased erythema in the skin folds (Pastia lines). The skin may feel rough, similar to sandpaper. The skin rash fades over 1 week followed by desquamation, which may last for several weeks.

   b. A **strawberry tongue** (rough, erythematous, swollen tongue) and pharyngeal erythema with exudate may be present.

3. Diagnosis is made on the basis of the clinical presentation and the isolation of group A streptococci on throat culture.

4. Therapy for scarlet fever is the same as that for streptococcal pharyngitis, consisting of 10 days of orally administered penicillin.

5. Complications. Both suppurative (e.g., cellulitis) and nonsuppurative (e.g., rheumatic fever) complications can occur with scarlet fever, just as with streptococcal pharyngitis (see V E).

G. | **Rocky Mountain spotted fever** is an acute febrile illness characterized by the sudden onset of fever, headache, myalgia, mental confusion, and rash. The disease may be severe, leading to shock and death in 5%–7% of patients, even with appropriate antimicrobial therapy.

1. Etiology and epidemiology

   a. Rocky Mountain spotted fever is a **tick-borne illness** caused by *Rickettsia rickettsii*, which is widespread in the United States but most predominant in the eastern coastal and southeastern states.

   b. The principal **vectors** of Rocky Mountain spotted fever are *Dermacentor andersoni*, which is the **wood tick** that is found in the West and is most active during the spring, and *Dermacentor variabilis*, which is the **dog tick** that is found in the East and is most active during the summer.

   c. Almost two thirds of the cases of Rocky Mountain spotted fever occur in patients who are younger than 15 years of age.

2. Clinical features
   a. The clinical onset of Rocky Mountain spotted fever is abrupt and follows an incubation period that averages about 7 days (usually 2–8 days after an infected tick bite).
   Typical initial presentations include:
   (1) Fever, which lasts 2–3 weeks in untreated patients
   (2) Chills
   (3) Headache, which is generalized and severe
   (4) Signs of meningoencephalitis (e.g., irritability, confusion, delirium)
   (5) Myalgia, especially of the gastrocnemius
   (6) Conjunctivitis with photophobia
   (7) Nonpitting edema, which may be profuse
   b. A **characteristic rash** develops on the third to fifth day of illness. The lesions begin as
   rose-colored, blanching macules on the hands, wrists, feet, and ankles, which spread
   to involve the entire body. The rash then becomes more **papular, petechial, and
   eventually purpuric** if treatment is delayed.

3. Diagnosis is made primarily on the basis of clinical appearance and history (a history
   of tick bite exists in 60%–85% of cases). Isolation of the organism is difficult and
   dangerous; serologic confirmation generally takes 7–10 days and may be delayed
   for 5 or more weeks if antibiotics are begun early. If a specialized laboratory is available, rapid diagnosis can be made using immunofluorescence of a skin biopsy
   specimen.

4. Therapy
   a. Antibiotic therapy includes either chloramphenicol or tetracycline given until
   2–3 days after the temperature returns to normal (usually a course of 5–7 days).
   Tetracycline is given only to children older than 8 years of age.
   b. Supportive therapy is essential for patients with serious illness, such as those with
   shock.

5. Prevention is best achieved by avoidance of tick-infested areas and by prompt removal
   of a tick. Ticks should be removed with forceps applied to the head, so that the contents
   of the tick are not squeezed into the skin.

6. Complications of Rocky Mountain spotted fever include focal neurologic deficits,
   coma, renal failure, disseminated intravascular coagulation, gangrene of the distal
   extremities and scrotum, pneumonia, and shock possibly leading to death.

VIII. OTHER DISORDERS WITH CUTANEOUS MANIFESTATIONS

A. **Lyme disease** is a multisystem inflammatory disease that primarily affects the skin, joints,
and nervous system.

1. Epidemiology. Lyme disease is the most common vector-borne disease in the United
   States. It has been reported in 47 states, but there are three major foci in the northeast,
   upper midwest, and northwest United States. Lyme disease is transmitted to humans
   through the bite of an ixodid tick. It is rapidly increasing in incidence and is spreading
   into new areas.

2. Etiology. Lyme disease is caused by the spirochete *B. burgdorferi*. The white-footed
   mouse is the major reservoir for *B. burgdorferi* in the northeastern and midwestern
   United States.

3. Clinical features
   a. Early, localized infection is characterized by an expanding erythematous annular
   skin lesion (erythema migrans), fever, headache, fatigue, arthralgias, myalgias, neck
   pain, and back pain.

b. **Early, disseminated infection** is characterized by multiple erythema migrans, aseptic meningitis, cranial neuropathies (especially of the facial nerve), radiculoneuritis, and heart block.

c. **Late, persistent infection** is characterized by asymmetrical, pauciarticular arthritis (especially of the knee), polyneuropathy, and encephalopathy.

4. **Diagnosis** is made by the presence of erythema migrans in a patient in an endemic area. In the absence of erythema migrans, the diagnosis is based on the presence of clinical findings consistent with Lyme disease and laboratory evidence (usually based on serologic tests) of an infection with *B. burgdorferi*.

5. **Therapy.** Oral antibiotic therapy (doxycycline, amoxicillin) is effective for early, localized infection, mild cardiac disease, facial nerve palsy, and arthritis. Intravenous antibiotic therapy (ceftriaxone, penicillin G) is recommended for more serious central nervous system disease, more serious cardiac disease, and for patients with arthritis who have not responded to oral antibiotic therapy.

6. **Complications.** With appropriate antibiotic therapy, the long-term outcome is excellent regardless of the stage of disease at which it is initiated. In a very small proportion of patients, chronic arthritis or chronic neurologic disease may develop despite appropriate antibiotic therapy.

B. **Kawasaki disease** is a generalized vasculitis of unknown etiology that is a leading cause of acquired heart disease in children in the United States.

1. **Epidemiology.** About 80% of patients are younger than 4 years of age, and the disease is unusual after 8 years of age. Less than 2% of patients have recurrences. Children of Asian ancestry have the highest incidence. The greatest number of cases are in the winter and spring, and epidemics have been reported. Person-to-person transmission has not been documented.

2. **Etiology.** The etiology remains unknown. Clinical and epidemiologic characteristics suggest an infectious agent. Infection may lead to an immune-mediated disease in certain genetically predisposed children.

3. **Clinical features.** The diagnosis is established by the presence of fever and at least four of the five other principal clinical criteria without other explanations for the illness (Table 10-5). Other clinical and laboratory findings are associated with Kawasaki disease (Table 10-6).

4. **Diagnosis.** No specific diagnostic test is available.

5. **Therapy.** High doses of aspirin are given during the acute phase for the antiinflammatory effect. After the child is afebrile, low doses of aspirin are given for the antithrombotic effect. Intravenous gamma globulin given within the first 10 days of illness can significantly reduce the risk of coronary artery abnormalities. Aspirin may need to be temporarily withheld if influenzae or varicella develop while the child is being treated for Kawasaki disease to prevent the development of Reye syndrome.

TABLE 10-5. Principal Diagnostic Criteria for Kawasaki Disease

Fever of at least 5 days' duration

Presence of four of the following:
- Changes in extremities
- Polymorphous exanthem
- Bilateral conjunctival injection
- Changes in the lips and oral cavity
- Cervical lymphadenopathy

Exclusion of other diseases with similar findings

TABLE 10-6. Associated Features of Kawasaki Disease

Clinical Findings	Laboratory Findings
Extreme irritability	Neutrophilia with immature forms
Arthralgia, arthritis	Elevated ESR
Aseptic meningitis	Positive C-reactive protein
Cardiac disease	Thrombocytosis
Hepatic dysfunction	Proteinuria
Hydrops of gallbladder	Sterile pyuria
Diarrhea	Elevated serum transaminases
Otitis media	
Pneumonitis	

ESR = erythrocyte sedimentation rate.

6. **Complications.** Kawasaki disease is usually self-limited, but coronary artery abnormalities, including aneurysms, develop in 20% of untreated patients. Fatalities are unusual and occur with myocardial infarctions secondary to thrombosis within a coronary artery aneurysm.

IX. CARDIAC INFECTIONS

A. **Infective endocarditis** is an inflammatory disorder, mainly of the cardiac valves, that results from infection by any of several types of microorganisms, including bacteria, fungi, and rickettsiae.

1. **Etiology**
   a. **Viridans streptococcus** (α-hemolytic streptococcus) is the most common cause of infective endocarditis in children. However, this etiologic agent has decreased in importance since the introduction of antimicrobial therapy.
   b. **S. aureus and S. epidermidis** have become progressively more important causes of infective endocarditis.
   c. **Enterococcus,** which is a common cause of infective endocarditis in adults, rarely is implicated in childhood disease.

2. **Epidemiology.** Pediatric patients who are at greatest risk for infective endocarditis include those with congenital heart disease, those with acquired valvular heart disease (e.g., rheumatic carditis), and those with prosthetic valves.
   a. Infective endocarditis is a rare disease in children without underlying heart conditions, although adolescent drug abusers and children with central venous or arterial lines demonstrate an increased risk for the disease.
   b. The relatively good oral hygiene and condition of the heart in children may explain the lower incidence of infective endocarditis in children compared with adults.

3. **Pathogenesis**
   a. Endocarditis develops when a jet of blood, turbulence, or trauma leads to **cardiac endothelial damage,** which serves as the nidus for bacterial infection. In most cases, **oral bacteria,** which intermittently invade the bloodstream, infect the damaged endothelium.
   b. **Vegetations** consisting primarily of fibrin, platelet aggregations, and bacterial masses form on the valve leaflet. They may be single or multiple and range in size from a few millimeters to several centimeters. Pieces of the vegetations may break off and cause embolization (e.g., splinter hemorrhages, Roth spots).

4. **Clinical features**
   a. **Early manifestations.** Infants and children with early infective endocarditis may be nearly free of symptoms, with fatigue sometimes the only manifestation of disease.

Fever, malaise, and weakness are common. The classic signs of endocarditis (e.g., splinter hemorrhages, changing heart murmurs) are not always evident. Other signs that may occur include cardiomegaly, splenomegaly, petechiae, weight loss, and clubbing of the fingers.

    b. Late manifestations of infective endocarditis classically include such lesions as **Roth spots** (retinal hemorrhages with clear centers), **Janeway lesions** (flat, painless hemorrhagic macules on the hands or feet), and **Osler nodes** (pea-sized painful nodules, usually on the fingers). These infrequently occur in appropriately treated patients.

5. Diagnosis

    a. Laboratory findings. The erythrocyte sedimentation rate usually is elevated but may be normal early in the course of the illness. The leukocyte count may be normal or elevated. Microscopic hematuria may occur.

    b. Blood cultures are critical for the diagnosis of infective endocarditis, and identify the causative agent in more than 90% of cases. It rarely is necessary to obtain more than four cultures, but at least three blood cultures should be obtained during the first 24 hours of hospitalization.

    c. Two-dimensional echocardiography is helpful for establishing the presence and location of vegetations. About half of all patients tested have vegetations on echocardiography.

6. Therapy. When untreated, this infection is almost uniformly fatal.

    a. Antibiotic therapy should be provided in a patient with suspected endocarditis after an etiology is established (usually by blood culture). In very ill patients, antibiotic therapy generally is initiated when the diagnosis is suspected and immediately after blood cultures have been obtained. **Intravenous antibiotics** are given for 4 weeks, except for patients with staphylococcal endocarditis or for those with an artificial valve, in whom 6 weeks of therapy is preferred.

        (1) Initial therapy usually consists of **ampicillin plus gentamicin,** unless staphylococci are suspected, in which case **oxacillin or vancomycin and gentamicin** are given.

        (2) It is **important that the MBC is determined,** because peak antibiotic levels in the serum must exceed the MBC for successful therapy.

        (3) A **serum bactericidal (Schlicter) test** is recommended to document adequate antibiotic therapy. The dosage usually is adjusted to achieve a peak serum bactericidal titer of at least 1:8 against the causative pathogen.

    b. Surgical intervention (for removal of vegetations or valve replacement) may be required for patients who fail to respond to medical treatment.

7. Complications of infective endocarditis must be anticipated and, with early intervention, may be minimized or even prevented. Important sequelae of infective endocarditis include:

    a. Emboli to the brain, lungs, coronary arteries, or any peripheral artery

    b. Mycotic aneurysms, which are infected aneurysms of the arterial vessels in the brain

    c. Congestive heart failure, which usually results from valvular dysfunction

    d. Local cardiac abscesses, which can present as aneurysm or persistent fever

    e. Drug reactions

    f. Autoimmune phenomena (e.g., nephritis, arthritis)

    g. Depression, which can occur as a result of the prolonged hospitalization

B. **Myocarditis** is an infection of the myocardium (i.e., the muscle of the heart). It occurs infrequently in children.

1. Etiology. Most cases of myocarditis are caused by enteroviruses, predominantly coxsackie B virus and echovirus. Important bacterial causes include *C. diphtheriae* and *Salmonella typhi*.

2. Clinical features include fever, congestive heart failure, and arrhythmias. The electrocardiogram is abnormal, with ST segment depression and T wave inversion.

3. Therapy for patients with viral myocarditis is supportive.

C. **Pericarditis** is an inflammation of the pericardium (i.e., the fibrous sac that contains the heart).

1. **Etiology.** The most common causes of pericarditis are bacteria, especially *S. aureus*, and viruses, especially coxsackie B virus, echovirus, influenza virus, and adenovirus. Other causes include fungi and *M. tuberculosis*.

2. **Clinical features**
   a. **Left shoulder pain and back pain,** which decrease when the patient is sitting, are characteristic of pericarditis. Fever, tachypnea, tachycardia, cough, and decreased heart sounds due to pericardial fluid and pericardial friction rub also are common.
   b. **It is important to recognize significant pericardial fluid accumulation,** which can lead to cardiac tamponade. Signs of tamponade include neck vein distention on inspiration and paradoxic pulse. The essential features of paradoxic pulse are a greater-than-normal inspiratory decrease in arterial blood pressure and an absence of the normal inspiratory fall in venous pressure.

3. **Diagnosis**
   a. **Electrocardiographic findings** with pericarditis include a low-voltage QRS complex, ST segment changes, and T wave inversion.
   b. **Chest radiography** reveals a rapidly increasing cardiothoracic ratio without increasing pulmonary vascular markings.
   c. **Echocardiography** allows an estimate of the amount of pericardial fluid, although false-negative results may be obtained.

4. **Therapy** for severe cases of pericarditis involving cardiac tamponade consists of pericardial drainage and supportive measures, such as the administration of oxygen and isoproterenol. Prolonged antibiotic therapy is given for cases of pericarditis due to bacteria.

X. SKIN, JOINT, AND BONE INFECTIONS

A. **Skin infections**

1. **Impetigo** is a common, contagious skin infection in infants and children, which is characterized by pustular, crusted, or bullous lesions. It occurs more frequently in warm, humid weather and is transmitted from child to child by direct contact.
   a. **Etiology.** The primary causes of impetigo in children are group A β-hemolytic streptococcus (*S. pyogenes*) and *S. aureus*. In past years, *S. aureus* was the etiologic agent in roughly 10% of cases, mostly in newborns and young infants. Recent studies suggest that *S. aureus* is increasing in importance as a cause of impetigo. Occasionally, both agents can be identified.
   b. **Clinical features**
      (1) **Lesions**
         (a) The lesions of **vesicopustular impetigo** begin as papules that progress to vesicles and then to painless pustules measuring about 5 mm in diameter, with a thin erythematous rim. The pustules rupture, revealing a honey-like exudate, which then forms a crust over a shallow ulcerated base. Although previously considered to be caused by group A β-hemolytic streptococcus, *S. aureus* has been increasingly cultured from such lesions.
         (b) The lesions of **bullous impetigo** begin as red macules that progress to bullous (fluid-filled) eruptions on an erythematous base. These lesions range from a few millimeters to a few centimeters in diameter. After the bullae rupture, a clear, thin, varnish-like coating forms over the denuded area. Bullous impetigo usually is associated with *S. aureus* infection.
      (2) **Local adenopathy** is common with streptococcal impetigo.
      (3) **Fever** seldom occurs, even with extensive superficial impetigo.

   c. **Diagnosis** is made by Gram stain and positive culture of specimens obtained from the base of pustular or ulcerated lesions or of fluid obtained from bullous lesions.
   d. **Therapy.** Until recently, impetigo was treated with oral antibiotics. A new topical therapy, mupirocin, has been found to be effective. It may be considered for use in children with mild impetigo.
      (1) Oral **penicillin V** (250 mg 3 or 4 times daily for 10 days) is the treatment of choice for more severe streptococcal impetigo.
      (2) Oral **dicloxacillin or cephalexin** is indicated for staphylococcal impetigo. Cephalexin suspension is more palatable than dicloxacillin, which has a bitter taste.

2. **Cellulitis** is a localized, acute inflammation of the skin and subcutaneous tissue characterized by erythema and warmth. The location of the infection is important because it may arise from underlying osteomyelitis, septic arthritis, sinusitis, or deep wound infection.
   a. **Etiology and clinical features.** Most cellulitis in children is caused by group A β-hemolytic streptococcus or *S. aureus.*
      (1) Trauma-related cellulitis. Cellulitis that occurs after some form of skin trauma (e.g., wound, burn, surgery) usually is caused by group A streptococcus or *S. aureus.*
         (a) Erysipelas refers to an acute infection of the skin and superficial subcutaneous tissues, which is characterized by a sharply demarcated, firm, raised border. Group A streptococcus is the predominant cause.
         (b) Local trauma, with or without marked cellulitis, may give rise to **lymphangitis,** which presents as a thin line of redness from the point of trauma to the draining regional node. Group A streptococcus, again, is the primary cause.
      (2) Cellulitis unrelated to trauma. Cellulitis that occurs in a child who is younger than 2 years, without evidence of trauma, may be caused by *H. influenzae* type b or *S. pneumoniae.* Cellulitis of the face (e.g., buccal or periorbital cellulitis) often is caused by *H. influenzae* type b. Other causes include group A β-hemolytic streptococcus and *S. aureus.*
   b. **Diagnosis**
      (1) Blood cultures are sometimes positive for group A β-hemolytic streptococcus, *S. aureus,* or *H. influenzae* type b in cellulitis.
      (2) Aspiration of material from the leading edge or center of the cellulitis and culture may yield the etiologic agent.
      (3) Culture of material that has drained from a wound associated with cellulitis is helpful for defining etiology.
   c. **Therapy.** Children with cellulitis usually are hospitalized and given parenteral antibiotics, such as oxacillin, cefazolin, or ceftriaxone, which are effective against the likely pathogens.

3. **Abscess** represents a deeper skin infection than cellulitis; in addition, it contains pus.
   a. **Etiology.** Abscesses usually are caused by *S. aureus* or group A streptococcus.
   b. **Therapy.** Treatment of superficial abscesses consists of warm compresses until the abscesses become fluctuant. Surgical drainage is necessary if spontaneous drainage has not occurred. Appropriate antibiotics are indicated.

B. **Septic arthritis** occurs when bacteria from the circulation enter the joint space. It also may occur from direct implantation of bacteria from an osteomyelitis or penetrating trauma. Septic arthritis may cause destruction of articular cartilage because of a lack of normal nutrients in the synovial fluid or as a result of purulent exudate and increased pressure in the joint space. The joints usually involved are the knee (40%), hip (20%), ankle (15%), elbow (15%), wrist (5%), and shoulder (5%).

1. **Etiology.** Blood cultures are positive in up to 50% of patients with septic arthritis.
   a. **Neonates.** Group B streptococcus, *S. aureus,* and enteric gram-negative rods are the most common pathogens in this age group.

b. Older children. *S. aureus* is the most common pathogen. Other causes include group A streptococcus, *S. pneumoniae*, *N. meningitidis*, and (now uncommonly) *H. influenzae* type b. *N. gonorrhoeae* causes septic arthritis in adolescents.

2. **Clinical features.** In most children, the affected joint is warm, swollen, and very painful when moved. Septic arthritis in a young infant may present simply as fever and poorly localized pain in the affected extremity. **Signs and symptoms** associated with a septic hip often are subtle and, in an infant, may be limited to a limp or a fixed, flexed hip.

3. **Diagnosis**
   a. **Synovial fluid analysis.** Joint aspiration is necessary for the diagnosis of septic arthritis, and it has the additional benefit of decreasing pressure in the joint space. Gram stain, culture, white blood cell count, and protein and glucose concentrations of the synovial fluid are obtained.
   b. **Laboratory findings.** The peripheral white blood cell count usually is elevated, with a shift to the left, and the erythrocyte sedimentation rate usually is increased.
   c. **Imaging results.** Radiographs frequently show widening of the joint space. A gallium scan shows increased uptake of gallium in the involved joint.
   d. **Differential diagnosis** of septic arthritis includes other causes of monoarticular arthritis, including *M. pneumoniae, M. tuberculosis, C. albicans,* Lyme disease, toxic synovitis, trauma, juvenile rheumatoid arthritis, and Reiter syndrome.

4. **Therapy**
   a. **Antibiotic therapy** initially should consist of broad-spectrum, parenteral antibiotics to treat the likely pathogens (i.e., oxacillin for children older than 6 years of age; ceftriaxone or oxacillin for children younger than 6 years of age). Antibiotics should be continued for a minimum of 3 weeks. In some cases, subsequent high-dose oral therapy can be substituted for parenteral therapy.
   b. **Drainage of the joint space** by needle aspiration or surgical excision is important to remove inflammatory material. Septic arthritis of the hip requires immediate surgical drainage, because the blood supply of the femoral head may be compromised, which carries the risk of serious sequelae.

C. **Osteomyelitis** refers to inflammation of the bone. Osteomyelitis in children occurs most frequently in the long bones of the lower extremities and, to a lesser extent, of the upper extremities.

1. **Etiology**
   a. **Staphylococci and streptococci** account for more than 90% of bacterial isolates in childhood osteomyelitis.
   b. *Salmonella* species are common pathogens in patients with sickle cell anemia.
   c. *P. aeruginosa* is a common pathogen in patients with puncture wounds of the foot.

2. **Pathogenesis.** The tortuous course of the nutrient vessels in bone cause bacteria to be trapped in the metaphysis. The metaphysis is located between the epiphysis (growth plate) and the diaphysis (shaft of the bone). The epiphyseal plate prevents infection from entering the joint space in older children, but not in neonates. Joint infection secondary to osteomyelitis may occur in the shoulder and hip as a result of the synovial membrane inserting distally to the epiphysis, allowing bacteria to spread directly from the metaphysis to the joint space.

3. **Clinical features**
   a. In **young infants,** fever may be the only manifestation of osteomyelitis.
   b. Fever and localized bone tenderness are the most common symptoms in **older children**. Local swelling, redness, warmth, and, rarely, suppuration may occur subsequently.
   c. There is a **history of minor trauma** in about half of the cases.

4. **Diagnosis**
   a. **Hematologic findings**
      (1) The **white blood cell count and erythrocyte sedimentation rate** usually are elevated. The erythrocyte sedimentation rate is useful for monitoring therapy.
      (2) **Blood cultures** are positive in approximately 50% of the cases.
   b. **Imaging results**
      (1) A **bone scan** usually is positive 24 hours after symptoms begin and provides strong evidence of osteomyelitis.
      (2) **Radiographs** do not become positive until 10–12 days after the onset of symptoms.
      (3) **Magnetic resonance imaging or CT scans** are more specific than a radiograph but usually are not performed unless the diagnosis is questionable or a patient has a prolonged or difficult clinical course.

5. **Therapy**
   a. **Aspiration** of the affected site is desirable to recover the causative organism and to determine whether an abscess is present, which would require surgical drainage. Aspiration and drainage are essential if a bone abscess or an unusual organism (e.g., *P. aeruginosa* from a puncture wound) is suspected.
   b. **Antibiotic therapy** initially should consist of a parenteral antistaphylococcal antibiotic (e.g., oxacillin), unless a gram-negative organism is suspected. Appropriate antibiotic therapy is continued for a minimum of 4 weeks. In some cases, an oral antibiotic can be substituted after 1 week of parenteral antibiotics.
   c. **Surgical drainage** is necessary in addition to antibiotics for successful treatment of bone abscess.

XI. INFESTATIONS AND COMMON PARASITIC INFECTIONS

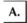 **Lice.** Three types of lice infest humans: head lice, body lice, and crab lice. Head lice and body lice are quite similar in body structure and range from 2–4 mm in length. Crab lice are 1–2 mm in length and bear a striking resemblance to crabs, with widespread pincers.

1. **Head lice.** The head louse (*Pediculus humanis* var. *capitis*) is a common problem in preschool and elementary school children. Head lice usually are confined to the fine hair of the head; they rarely infest clothing. Head lice are most common in the winter, they usually are not the result of poor hygiene, and they are not more common in children with long hair. They are spread by direct contact. The female louse lays eggs (nits) on hair close to the scalp, and as the hair grows, the eggs dry.
   a. **Clinical features.** Pruritus and a macular rash on the scalp occur. Head lice sometimes cause no signs or symptoms.
   b. **Diagnosis.** The discovery of nits and, less commonly, live lice usually is made by a child's parent or teacher.
   c. **Therapy.** Four effective shampoo therapies are available for head lice: **permethrin, malathion, pyrethrin,** and **lindane.** (The latter drug should be used with caution in very young children because of its potential for causing neurotoxicity.) A second shampooing should be done 7 days after the first application to kill hatching progeny. The lice live for only a short time on inanimate objects. Thus, washing of all clothing and bed linens is not necessary.

2. **Body lice.** The body louse (*P. humanis* var. *corporis*) lives on the body and on clothing. Body lice are not endemic to the United States. They may carry typhus, trench fever, and relapsing fever.

3. **Crab lice.** The crab louse (*Phthirus pubis*) lives in pubic hair and, in rare cases, can infest hair other than pubic hair, such as eyelashes.
   a. **Clinical features.** Crab lice usually are asymptomatic but can cause local pruritus and a macular rash.
   b. **Treatment** consists of local application of pyrethrin or lindane.

B. **Scabies** is caused by a round mite that is 0.4 mm long and has four sets of legs. It is spread by direct contact.

1. **Clinical features.** Scabies causes an intensely pruritic rash with pustules and burrows. The rash can be generalized or have a focal distribution; it is especially common in intertriginous areas (e.g., the folds between the fingers and toes).

2. **Diagnosis.** Scrapings of the burrows with mineral oil can reveal the mites. However, this procedure often produces negative results, and the diagnosis usually relies on demonstration of the characteristic rash.

3. **Therapy** consists of permethrin (treatment of choice), crotamiton (cream or lotion), sulfur ointment in petrolatum, benzyl benzoate, or lindane.

C. **Giardiasis.** *Giardia lamblia* is a parasite that is a common cause of diarrhea. It is spread from person to person or can be acquired from animal contact or from contaminated water.

1. **Clinical features.** Diarrhea due to *G. lamblia* is characterized by watery stools without blood, mucus, eosinophils, or leukocytes. Fever is absent. A prolonged course of diarrhea accompanied by excessive abdominal gas is characteristic of giardiasis.

2. **Diagnosis** most commonly is made by identification of the parasite (trophozoite or cyst) in formed or unformed stool. The parasite also can be recovered from the duodenum if a string is passed, by mouth, into the duodenum (string test).

3. **Therapy**
   a. **Quinacrine** is the drug of choice for treatment of giardiasis in children. Alternatives are metronidazole and furazolidone (a liquid preparation).
   b. The finding of *G. lamblia* eggs in the stool of an asymptomatic patient is not an indication for therapy. They are commonly identified in infants who attend day care centers.

D. **Enterobiasis,** or **pinworm infestation,** is a common infection in children caused by *Enterobius vermicularis*. The eggs of *E. vermicularis* are passed on hands, clothing, and house dust. Gravid females migrate at night to the perianal region to deposit their eggs.

1. **Clinical features.** Although many symptoms have been associated with pinworm infection, the only well documented symptom is perianal pruritus.

2. **Diagnosis.** Eggs can be detected by pressing adhesive cellophane tape against the perianal region in the morning. Adult worms may be seen by direct inspection.

3. **Therapy.** Mebendazole, 100 mg in a single oral dose, usually is sufficient therapy.

E. **Ascariasis,** or **roundworm infestation,** is caused by *Ascaris lumbricoides*. Ascariasis is a very common infection, especially in preschool and younger children.

1. **Life cycle**
   a. **Eggs** are found in the soil, and humans are infected by contact with the soil. The eggs are ingested and hatch in the intestine, where they become larvae.
   b. The **larvae** penetrate the intestine, enter the venules or lymphatics, and subsequently reach the lungs, where they mature.
   c. **Mature roundworms** then migrate up the bronchioles into the pharynx, where they are swallowed and finally pass into the small intestine, and the cycle is repeated.
   d. The **adult worm** is 25–30 cm in length.

2. **Clinical features**
   a. Most patients are asymptomatic. Abdominal pain may occur with heavy infection.
   b. Pulmonary symptoms are rare and result from large numbers of larvae passing through the lungs, causing cough, blood-stained sputum, eosinophilia, and pulmonary infiltrates.

3. **Diagnosis.** Worms that appear like long, pink, earthworms are seen in the stool. Eggs are found in the stool and can be identified microscopically.

4. **Therapy.** Pyrantel pamoate in a single dose is curative in 80%–90% of cases. The drug is well tolerated. Mebendazole and piperazine citrate also are effective.

BIBLIOGRAPHY

Committee on Infectious Diseases, American Academy of Pediatrics: *Report of the Committee on Infectious Diseases*, 23rd ed. Elk Grove Village, IL, American Academy of Pediatrics, 1994.

Feigin RD, Cherry JD (eds): *Textbook of Pediatric Infectious Diseases*, 3rd ed. Philadelphia, WB Saunders, 1992.

Mandell GL, Douglas RG, Dolin R (eds): *Principles and Practice of Infectious Diseases*, 4th ed. New York, Churchill-Livingstone, 1995.

Moffet HL: *Pediatric Infectious Diseases: A Problem-Oriented Approach*, 3rd ed. Philadelphia, JB Lippincott, 1989.

Remington JS, Klein JO (eds): *Infectious Diseases of the Fetus and Newborn Infant*, 4th ed. Philadelphia, WB Saunders, 1995.

DIRECTIONS: Each of the numbered items or incomplete statements in this section is followed by answers or by completions of the statement. Select the ONE lettered answer or completion that is BEST in each case.

1. A 1-year-old boy is brought to the emergency room with a 10-hour history of fever and listlessness. Physical examination reveals a lethargic child with a temperature of 103°F, a respiratory rate of 35, blood pressure of 60/30, a full fontanelle, and a petechial rash. The most appropriate initial action is

(A) blood culture and lumbar puncture
(B) Gram stain of the petechiae
(C) blood culture and administration of intravenous fluids and antibiotics
(D) administration of corticosteroids
(E) examination of the fundi

2. A 6-year-old girl presents with a nonsuppurative and moderately tender anterior cervical lymph node that measures 2 cm × 4 cm. What is the most appropriate initial therapy?

(A) Amoxicillin
(B) Dicloxacillin
(C) Erythromycin
(D) Penicillin
(E) Incision and drainage

3. A previously healthy 13-year-old boy has a mild pneumonia characterized by a nonproductive cough. The most appropriate therapy is

(A) cephalexin
(B) amoxicillin
(C) erythromycin
(D) penicillin
(E) trimethoprim–sulfamethoxazole

4. A 3-month-old infant with bronchopulmonary dysplasia is admitted to a hospital with fever, wheezing, and respiratory distress. A chest radiograph shows hyperinflation and extensive bilateral, interstitial infiltrates. The complete blood count is negative, and a rapid test for respiratory syncytial virus is positive. Blood cultures are obtained. The most appropriate therapy is

(A) intravenous ampicillin
(B) intravenous ceftriaxone
(C) oral amoxicillin
(D) ribavirin
(E) close observation without use of antibiotic or antiviral agents

5. A 2-year-old child is noted to have an erythematous, bulging right tympanic membrane. The two most likely bacterial causes of this illness are

(A) *Streptococcus pyogenes* and *Staphylococcus aureus*
(B) *Haemophilus influenzae* and *S. aureus*
(C) *H. influenzae* and *Streptococcus pneumoniae*
(D) *S. pneumoniae* and *S. aureus*
(E) *Moraxella catarrhalis* and *S. pyogenes*

6. A 4-year-old boy presents with a low-grade fever, headache, and nasal discharge. Sinusitis is suspected but transillumination of the sinuses and a throat culture are nondiagnostic. A sinus radiograph shows bilateral maxillary sinus membrane swelling. The most accurate statement regarding the diagnosis of sinusitis in this child is

(A) his symptoms are not typical of acute sinusitis in young children
(B) transillumination of the sinuses seldom provides valuable information for the diagnosis of sinusitis in older children
(C) swab cultures of the throat are usually reliable for the diagnosis of sinusitis
(D) evidence of bilateral maxillary sinus membrane swelling on radiography confirms the diagnosis of acute bacterial sinusitis
(E) sinus puncture seldom is needed to confirm the diagnosis of sinusitis

DIRECTIONS: Each set of matching questions in this section consists of a list of four to twenty-six lettered options (some of which may be in figures) followed by several items. For each numbered item, select the ONE lettered option that is most closely associated with it. To avoid spending too much time on matching sets with large numbers of options, it is generally advisable to begin each set by reading the list of options. Then, for each item in the set, try to generate the correct answer and locate it in the option list, rather than evaluating each option individually. Each lettered option may be selected once, more than once, or not at all.

Questions 7–10

For each description of a patient with a rash, select the proper diagnosis.

(A) Measles
(B) Rubella
(C) Erythema infectiosum
(D) Varicella
(E) Rocky Mountain spotted fever

7. A 7-year-old child develops conjunctivitis and a maculopapular rash that begins on the head and spreads downward

8. A 4-year-old child develops a rash that begins as a marked erythema of the cheeks

9. A 3-year-old child develops a vesicular rash that appears in crops

10. A 12-year-old child is seen in the emergency room for a petechial rash that begins on the wrists and ankles

ANSWERS AND EXPLANATIONS

1. The answer is C *[IV A 4 c, 5 a (1) (b), b (2)].* The most appropriate initial action is blood culture and administration of intravenous fluids and antibiotics. This patient presents with classic findings of meningococcal sepsis and meningitis. Although the diagnosis of meningitis and the microbiologic etiology of the illness can be established by examination of cerebrospinal fluid (CSF), a lumbar puncture should be deferred until the patient's condition is stabilized. The blood pressure indicates that the child is in shock. Initial efforts, therefore, should focus on maintaining intravascular volume by the intravenous administration of fluids. Intravenous antibiotics also should be administered promptly (preferably after a blood culture is obtained), and, in this case, an appropriate choice would be a third-generation cephalosporin.

2. The answer is B *[V F 4 b].* The most appropriate initial therapy would be administration of dicloxacillin. Inflammation and enlargement of the lymph nodes of the neck, or cervical adenitis, is a common problem in children. Appropriate treatment of cervical adenitis depends on the causative microorganism and the presence or absence of pus. Initial therapy for a nonsuppurative node of moderate size and tenderness usually consists of an oral antistaphylococcal antibiotic (e.g., dicloxacillin) for treatment of *Staphylococcus aureus* and group A streptococcus, which are the most likely causative organisms. Erythromycin would be a logical choice in a penicillin-allergic child, but it is not as effective against *S. aureus* as dicloxacillin. Neither amoxicillin nor penicillin usually is effective against *S. aureus*. Incision and drainage are indicated only when the nodes contain pus.

3. The answer is C *[VI B 1 d (3), 3 a (3)].* The most appropriate treatment is erythromycin. The most common nonviral causes of pneumonia in children who are older than 6 years of age are *Mycoplasma pneumoniae* and *Streptococcus pneumoniae*. Pneumonia due to *M. pneumoniae* usually is milder than that due to traditional bacteria, with a gradual onset of illness that is characterized by fever, headache, malaise, and a nonproductive cough. The clinical picture described in the question, therefore, is consistent with *M. pneumoniae* pneumonia, for which the treatment of choice is erythromycin. Cephalexin, amoxicillin, penicillin, and trimethoprim–sulfamethoxazole would be effective treatment for *S. pneumoniae* pneumonia but not for *M. pneumoniae* pneumonia.

4. The answer is D *[VI A 6 a].* The most appropriate treatment is administration of ribavirin. This infant has evidence of severe bronchiolitis, pneumonia, and respiratory syncytial infection, all of which are conditions that call for treatment with aerosolized ribavirin. Bronchiolitis is an acute viral infection of the bronchioles, which is common in infants younger than 2 years of age. Clinical features include cough, wheezing, tachypnea, and dyspnea. Hyperinflation of the lungs typically is evident on chest radiography. Complete blood cell count often is negative, reflecting a viral etiology. Over 50% of cases are caused by respiratory syncytial virus, which is identified by rapid immunofluorescence. In most cases, patients recover spontaneously and do not require hospitalization or specific therapy. However, severe infection is more common among children with underlying pulmonary disease (e.g., bronchopulmonary dysplasia). In such cases, hospitalization is necessary and therapy includes oxygen, fluids, and possibly intubation with assisted ventilation. Aerosolized ribavirin is indicated for severe infection due to respiratory syncytial virus.

5. The answer is C *[V A 1 a (1)].* The most likely bacterial causes of the illness described are *Haemophilus influenzae* and *Streptococcus pneumoniae*. This child presents with otitis media, which is one of the most common infections of childhood. The characteristic feature of otitis media is a bulging, erythematous tympanic membrane with impaired mobility. Bacteria are the primary agents of otitis media. The most common causes in all age groups are *S. pneumoniae* (25%–40% of cases) and unencapsulated *H. influenzae* (15%–25% of cases). Less common causes include group A streptococcus, *Moraxella catarrhalis*, and, for chronic otitis media, *Staphylococcus aureus* and *Pseudomonas aeruginosa*.

6. The answer is E *[V C 5].* Sinus puncture is infrequently needed to confirm the diagnosis of sinusitis. Transillumination of the sinuses often provides valuable information for the diagnosis of sinusitis. Swab cultures of the throat are not usually reliable for diagnosis of sinusitis. Because the mucous membrane of the paranasal sinuses is continuous with that of the nose, even transient viral upper respiratory infections may cause sinus membrane swelling, which appears as hazy densities on sinus radiography. A unilateral air–fluid level or complete opacification of a sinus cavity strongly suggests acute bacterial sinusitis. For this reason, sinus radiographs should be reviewed with an experienced radiologist.

7–10. The answers are: 7-A *[VII A 3 c],* **8-C** *[VII D 2 b],* **9-D** *[VII E 2 a (2)],* **10-E** *[VII G 2 b].* The characteristic rash of measles begins on the head and spreads down the body, becoming generalized. It is erythematous and maculopapular but becomes confluent as it progresses. The rash lasts 4 or 5 days and then resolves from the head downward. Cough, coryza, and conjunctivitis are characteristic findings early in the course of this illness.

The rash of erythema infectiosum begins as a marked erythema of the cheeks, which gives a "slapped cheek" appearance. An erythematous, maculopapular rash then appears on the extremities and often has a lace-like appearance. It may be morbilliform, confluent, or annular. The rash often disappears and recurs, seemingly with fluctuations in environmental conditions.

The characteristic, pruritic rash of varicella usually appears first on the trunk and then becomes generalized. The rash begins as erythematous papules and progresses rapidly to vesicles that are 1–2 mm in diameter, which subsequently crust. The lesions occur in "crops," so that different stages of the rash are present simultaneously.

The rash of Rocky Mountain spotted fever initially appears on the hands, wrists, feet, and ankles and spreads to involve the skin of the rest of the body. The lesions are macular, 1–4 mm in diameter, and rose-colored, but they can become petechial and then purpuric if treatment is delayed.

Chapter 11

Gastrointestinal Diseases

William R. Treem
Jeffrey S. Hyams

I. **INTRODUCTION.** Gastrointestinal problems represent the second most common reason, after respiratory infection, for seeking medical care. The differential diagnosis and treatment of routine gastrointestinal symptoms in children (e.g., abdominal pain, vomiting, diarrhea) are often quite different from those in adults. At times, gastrointestinal symptoms may represent a nonspecific manifestation of serious infections such as pneumonia, meningitis, or pyelonephritis. The limited ability of the young child to describe his or her symptoms may make diagnosis more difficult. Subtle alterations in gastrointestinal function may adversely affect growth while causing minimal symptoms. Only careful examination of the child's growth curve may alert the physician to the possibility of underlying gastrointestinal disease.

II. **DISORDERS OF THE ESOPHAGUS**

A. **Gastroesophageal reflux** is the most common esophageal problem in infants. Some degree of gastroesophageal reflux occurs in otherwise healthy adults and children, but it occurs in up to 50% of young infants. Physiologic gastroesophageal reflux is regarded as a manifestation of a developmental variation in gastrointestinal motility that resolves as the infant matures. All pediatricians and parents have witnessed the regurgitation of small amounts of formula by healthy babies after feedings. **When this regurgitation is unusually severe, persists beyond 18 months of age, or is associated with complications, it is deemed pathologic** and warrants appropriate diagnostic testing and medical or surgical management.

1. **Pathophysiology.** Many factors contribute to the maintenance of the antireflux barrier, including an increased intrinsic basal tone of the lower esophageal sphincter (LES).
   a. **LES pressure.** Low resting tone of the LES is associated with reflux in a small group of children, primarily those who are neurologically impaired or who have some other underlying cause of esophageal dysfunction (e.g., a large hiatal hernia, a collagen vascular disease, a previous repair of a tracheoesophageal fistula or esophageal atresia). More commonly, however, LES pressure is normal in infants with gastroesophageal reflux. Thus, the concept of transient relaxations of the LES at inappropriate moments or a failure of adaptation of the LES to increases in intragastric pressure (created by crying, straining at stool, diaper changes, or positional changes) has been invoked to explain gastroesophageal reflux.
   b. **Other contributing factors** include:
      (1) Delayed gastric emptying
      (2) Impaired esophageal motility (decreased esophageal clearance of refluxate)
      (3) Gastric distention and increased intragastric pressure
      (4) Loss of extrinsic mechanical factors that maintain the antireflux barrier, such as the crural diaphragm and the cardioesophageal angle of His (oblique angle at which the esophagus enters the stomach)

2. **Clinical features**
   a. **Vomiting** may occur soon after or up to several hours after a feeding. The vomiting, which is usually effortless and painless, is often described as multiple episodes of

small amounts of curdled formula rolling out of the mouth. Occasionally, vomiting may be forceful and may be confused with symptoms of pyloric stenosis.

(1) In the older child, a tendency to vomit easily, heartburn, dysphagia, rumination, halitosis, and even loss of dental enamel may occur.

(2) The vomiting is always nonbilious and only rarely contains blood.

(3) Underlying diseases or conditions associated with gastroesophageal reflux include progressive systemic sclerosis (scleroderma), mixed connective tissue disease, cystic fibrosis, Down syndrome, myotonic dystrophy, and tracheo-esophageal fistula.

b. Complications. Persistent gastroesophageal reflux can lead to a number of complications (Table 11-1).

3. Diagnosis. The diagnosis of gastroesophageal reflux is based on the history, physical examination, and exclusion of anatomic abnormalities that may predispose to the clinical features of reflux. The following tests are necessary only when the diagnosis is in doubt or when the presentation is dominated by one of the complications of gastroesophageal reflux and a causal link between reflux and that complication (e.g., apnea, bronchospasm) is sought.

a. Barium swallow and upper gastrointestinal radiograph has high false-negative and false-positive rates, which diminish its usefulness; however, it is the best test for eliminating other anatomic causes of vomiting.

b. Prolonged esophageal pH monitoring is the best test for assessing gastroesophageal reflux. This 18- to 24-hour study should be reserved for patients presenting with apnea, bronchospasm, or failure to thrive in whom reflux is suspected as the underlying cause.

c. Radionuclide scanning. Gastroesophageal reflux may be detected and gastric emptying may be quantitated by adding technetium 99m (^{99m}Tc) to formula or milk and scanning.

d. Esophageal manometry is used to measure resting LES pressure, the response of the LES to a swallow, peristalsis in the body of the esophagus, and functioning of the upper esophageal sphincter.

e. Endoscopy with esophageal biopsy. Endoscopy allows direct visualization of esophageal mucosa, and biopsies may show microscopic evidence of esophagitis, even if the mucosa appears grossly normal.

4. Therapy

a. Simple measures. Most infants with gastroesophageal reflux can be treated conservatively with simple measures while awaiting maturation of upper gastrointestinal motility and resolution of symptoms.

TABLE 11-1. Complications of Gastroesophageal Reflux

Complication	Symptom
Peptic esophagitis	Heartburn, subxiphoid and chest pain, sore throat, excessive crying, decreased oral intake, feeding aversion, belching, dysphagia, failure to thrive, hematemesis, anemia, iron deficiency, occult blood in the stools
Esophageal stricture	Dysphagia, food impaction, vomiting of undigested food, drooling
Barrett's esophagus (metaplastic changes in the normal esophageal squamous epithelium)	Similar to esophagitis or stricture, can lead to adenocarcinoma of esophagus
Failure to thrive	Anorexia, excessive vomiting
Aspiration	Apnea, cyanosis, choking, laryngitis, pneumonia.
Bronchoconstriction	Cough, nocturnal cough, wheezing
Rumination	Gagging, mouthing, reswallowing

(1) Positioning
  (a) Infants should be positioned with the mattress of the crib elevated 20 degrees for sleep. The infant seat has not been shown to be useful in preventing reflux and may even be harmful if the infant slumps down in the seat with his knees pressing against his abdomen. Other positions that increase intraabdominal pressure, such as diaper changes with the infant on his back and his legs up, also may provoke reflux episodes.
  (b) Older children should sleep with the head of the bed elevated.
(2) Dietary changes
  (a) Size and frequency of meals
    (i) Infants. Frequent, smaller feedings of formula thickened with 2 tsp/oz of cereal may aid infants with gastroesophageal reflux. Thickening the formula has not been conclusively proven to be useful, and may provoke more coughing.
    (ii) Older children should eat smaller, more frequent meals and abstain from eating for at least 1 hour before bedtime.
  (b) Fatty foods, alcohol, chocolate, and caffeine-containing liquids may aggravate reflux and should be eliminated. Whey protein-predominant and lower-fat, higher-carbohydrate formulas may empty out of the stomach faster than casein protein-predominant formulas or those with a high long-chain triglyceride content.
  (c) Changing formulas is discouraged because it sends mixed messages about potential food allergy. Cow's milk and soy protein allergy are distinct entities and should be suspected only if the vomiting is accompanied by diarrhea, heme-positive stool, an eczematoid rash, and a strong family history of allergy, asthma, or eczema.
b. Medication. Drug intervention is reserved for patients whose emesis has persisted without improvement after 12 months of age, patients whose emesis has worsened between 6 and 12 months of age, and patients in whom complications have developed at any age (Table 11-2).
c. Surgery is indicated for patients who have failed medical therapy, patients with life-threatening or severely debilitating complications, and patients with esophageal stricture or Barrett esophagus.

TABLE 11-2. Pharmacologic Therapy of Gastroesophageal Reflux

Class	Drug	Mechanism	Dose
Antacid	Numerous	Neutralizes gastric acid	0.5 ml/kg/dose 1 hour postprandial
H_2-receptor antagonist	Cimetidine Ranitidine Famotidine	Blocks histamine receptor on parietal cell	10 mg/kg/dose qid 2 mg/kg/dose tid 0.4 mg/kg/dose bid
Proton-pump inhibitor	Omeprazole	Blocks H^+-K^+-ATPase pump in parietal cell membrane	20 mg every 12 hours (adult dose)
Prokinetic agents	Bethanechol	Cholinergic stimulation increases LES tone	0.2 mg/kg/dose tid
	Metoclopramide	Dopamine antagonist increases LES tone, promotes gastric emptying	0.2 mg/kg/dose tid–qid
	Cisapride	Cholinergic stimulation increases LES tone, promotes gastric emptying	0.2–0.3 mg/kg/dose tid–qid
	Erythromycin	Motilin agonist	20 mg/kg/day divided tid

bid = twice daily; LES = lower esophageal sphincter; qid = four times daily; tid = three times daily.

(1) Procedure. Surgical procedures are designed to reestablish esophagogastric competence. The most commonly used procedure is the **Nissen fundoplication,** during which part of the gastric fundus is wrapped around the distal esophagus to create a high-pressure zone to resist gastroesophageal reflux.

(2) Side effects (e.g., gastric distention, dysphagia, diarrhea) may occur, but usually are transient.

    (a) In severely neurologically impaired children with spastic cerebral palsy, the incidence of complications after Nissen fundoplication is increased—especially retching, abdominal distention, herniation of the wrapped stomach above the diaphragm, and loosening of the plicated stomach with subsequent incompetence of the wrap.

    (b) A scan that demonstrates delayed gastric emptying before surgery in such patients dictates consideration of a pyloroplasty along with the fundoplication to prevent some of these complications.

d. Adjunctive nutritional therapy consists of constant nasogastric, gastrostomy tube, or nasojejunal tube feedings at a regulated rate, either around-the-clock or for 8–12 hours overnight. This is particularly useful in infants with failure to thrive who are not tolerating intermittent small-volume feedings by mouth. Adjunctive nutritional therapy offers the advantage of providing high-calorie formulas in a small, steady volume during sleep, when reflux usually is markedly decreased.

B. **Achalasia.** Primary disorders of esophageal motility—other than those contributing to gastroesophageal reflux—are rare. The most common of these is achalasia, which is a disorder of unknown etiology characterized by lack of esophageal peristalsis and failure of a hypertonic LES to relax adequately with swallowing.

1. Clinical features. Most children with achalasia are older than 5 years of age at the time of presentation, although the disorder has been reported in infants.

a. Dysphagia for both solid and liquid foods is the cardinal symptom.

b. Other symptoms include slow eating, regurgitation of undigested food, weight loss, substernal pain, and respiratory symptoms such as nocturnal cough due to aspiration of esophageal contents.

2. Diagnosis

a. Barium swallow usually demonstrates a widened, tortuous esophagus with a narrowed distal "beak." Sometimes, even on a plain film, an air–fluid level in the esophagus may be seen.

b. Esophageal manometry is necessary to document lack of peristalsis, an abnormally high LES pressure, and incomplete LES relaxation with swallowing.

c. Endoscopy is used to exclude other causes of distal esophageal disease.

3. Therapy. Although medical therapy (i.e., calcium channel blockers) may occasionally improve symptoms, disruption of the LES by pneumatic dilatation or surgery usually is required.

C. **Structural abnormalities**

1. Tracheoesophageal fistula

a. Clinical features. A congenital tracheoesophageal fistula may not cause difficulty until the child is several months of age or older, if it is not associated with esophageal atresia. Under this circumstance, however, the child may present with coughing, especially with feedings, and with recurrent pneumonia due to aspiration.

b. Diagnosis. To detect this H-type tracheoesophageal fistula, the radiologist must ensure that the esophagus is adequately distended on barium swallow.

c. Therapy is surgical ligation of the lesion. Postsurgical complications include esophageal stricture formation, reformation of the tracheoesophageal fistula, and chronic gastroesophageal reflux.

2. **Congenital strictures** usually occur at the junction of the middle and distal thirds of the esophagus and result in dysphagia. This lesion must be differentiated from the more common peptic stricture due to gastroesophageal reflux or strictures secondary to caustic ingestions. **Congenital webs** present in a similar manner. **Epidermolysis bullosa** is associated with the formation of esophageal strictures.

D. **Esophageal damage by exogenous agents**

1. **Caustic agents** are common accidentally ingested materials in children. Strong alkali solutions (e.g., lye) used as drain cleaners are most dangerous. Less damaging are ammonia cleaning solutions, bleaches, and dishwasher detergents. Acids and caustic liquids tend to cause more damage to the stomach than to the esophagus. The early presence or absence of oral burns or dysphagia does not predict the presence or degree of esophageal damage from caustic agents.

   a. **Clinical features**
      (1) **Acute.** There may be burns of the hands, face, and oral cavity; local pain; drooling; dysphagia, stridor, or dyspnea; abdominal and chest pain; and shock if there is mediastinal penetration.
      (2) **Chronic.** Stricture formation may develop 2–4 weeks after ingestion and cause persistent dysphagia.

   b. **Diagnosis**
      (1) A **chest radiograph** can detect evidence of perforation and mediastinitis.
      (2) **Endoscopy** should be performed within 24 hours to document esophagitis or gastritis and the extent of the damage.
      (3) A **barium swallow** is performed 1–2 weeks after ingestion and sequentially to detect and note progression of stricture.

   c. **Therapy**
      (1) No attempt should be made to induce vomiting or to neutralize the caustic agent.
      (2) **Water or other neutral fluids** may be administered carefully to dilute the caustic agent initially.
      (3) **Intravenous fluids** are necessary.
      (4) The cardiorespiratory status should be monitored carefully.
      (5) The use of corticosteroids to prevent stricture formation is controversial, but they are contraindicated if there has been perforation.
      (6) Antibiotics may be administered, particularly if there is suspicion of perforation or if corticosteroids have been administered.
      (7) Repetitive esophageal dilatation or even reconstructive surgery may be needed.

2. **Foreign bodies.** The esophagus is the most difficult portion of the gastrointestinal tract to navigate, and objects that lodge in the esophagus should be expeditiously removed so that respiratory complications and esophageal ulceration and perforation do not occur. Coins are the most common esophageal foreign bodies in children.

   a. **Children** with esophageal foreign bodies will not always have symptoms of dysphagia, drooling, or chest discomfort.
   b. Occasionally, **infants** will present with stridor due to compression of the trachea, even though they are still able to swallow formula or breast milk.
   c. If there is clinical suspicion, a chest radiograph should be taken to rule out a radiopaque foreign body, or a barium swallow to outline a radiolucent one.

III. **DISORDERS OF THE STOMACH**

A. **Pyloric stenosis**

1. **Epidemiology.** Pyloric stenosis is an important cause of gastric outlet obstruction and vomiting in approximately 1 in every 500 infants. It frequently affects more than one child in a family, with a male-to-female ratio of 4:1.

2. **Symptoms** usually begin between 2 and 4 weeks of age, although in 5% of cases they are present shortly after birth.

3. **Clinical features**
   a. **Projectile nonbilious vomiting** is the cardinal feature and is seen in virtually all patients.
   b. **Constipation and poor weight gain** may be observed when the diagnosis is delayed.
   c. Although metabolic alkalosis is commonly seen secondary to the persistent vomiting, normal serum electrolytes never exclude a diagnosis of pyloric stenosis.

4. **Diagnosis**
   a. The palpation of a firm, mobile, nontender, olive-shaped **mass** in the right hypochondrium or epigastrium in the appropriate clinical setting confirms the diagnosis.
   b. Visible **peristaltic waves** traveling from left to right across the abdomen may be seen.
   c. If a pyloric mass cannot be palpated, ultrasonographic or radiographic evaluation should be performed.

5. **Therapy.** Pyloromyotomy is the preferred surgical approach once fluid and electrolyte abnormalities have been adequately corrected.

B. **Gastritis** is frequently associated with peptic ulcer disease in children. The gram-negative bacillus *Helicobacter pylori* may be an important contributing factor to gastric inflammation. Other causes may include allergies, aspirin, alcohol, nonsteroidal antiinflammatory agents, corrosive ingestions, vasculitis, Crohn disease, viral infection, and radiation.

1. **Clinical features** include abdominal pain and tenderness (usually epigastric), nausea, vomiting, and, occasionally, overt bleeding.

2. **Diagnosis** of gastritis may be difficult because a barium study of the stomach usually is unrevealing in this disorder. If the clinical picture warrants investigation (i.e., if there is severe pain, bleeding, or persistent vomiting), endoscopy can be performed. Antral gastritis with nodularity is frequently seen in *H. pylori* infection.
   a. Specific histochemical stains or a rapid urease test on biopsy tissue can be performed to identify *H. pylori*.
   b. Serologic studies may also reveal infection with *H. pylori*.

3. **Therapy**
   a. If the gastritis is secondary to ingestion of aspirin or another drug, that medication should be discontinued and a brief (1- to 2-week) course of antacids or an H_2-blocker should be initiated.
   b. If significant idiopathic gastritis is found grossly or on biopsy, a minimum 6-week course of an H_2-blocker is indicated. If *H. pylori* is identified, treatment with a combination of omeprazole (1 mg/kg/day; maximum 40 mg) and amoxicillin (30 mg/kg/day in 3 doses) for 2 weeks is currently the treatment of choice.

C. **Peptic ulcer disease.** In children younger than 6 years of age, ulcers are found with equal frequency in boys and girls, a gastric location is as common as a duodenal one, and a precipitating event (e.g., drugs, stress) is common. In children older than 6 years of age, ulcers are most frequently found in boys and are more common in the duodenum.

1. **Clinical features**
   a. In **neonates,** bleeding and perforation from a gastric ulcer usually are the first indications that an ulcer is present. These infants usually have other underlying problems, such as sepsis or respiratory distress. Rarely, peptic ulceration may be observed in otherwise healthy-appearing neonates.
   b. **Older infants and toddlers** frequently present with vomiting and poor eating. Bleeding also is common and is seen with equal frequency in primary (idiopathic) and secondary (e.g., stress) ulcers.
   c. In **older children,** pain becomes a more important feature and may persist for some time before the child receives medical attention. Although many patients have

"classic" ulcer pain relieved by eating, it is not uncommon for some children to claim that eating makes their pain worse. Either overt or occult bleeding is seen in about half of school-age children with ulcer disease.

2. **Diagnosis.** Endoscopic evaluation of the upper gastrointestinal tract is preferred because of its superior sensitivity in detecting pathology compared to contrast radiography. Endoscopy also allows for tissue biopsy and evaluation of patterns of inflammation (e.g., allergic versus peptic) and possible infection (e.g., *H. pylori*).

3. **Therapy.** If the ulcer is thought to be secondary to an underlying illness, the predisposing factors must be addressed. The management of the ulcer itself has historically been directed against gastric acid, either through neutralization (via antacids) or suppression of secretion (via H_2-receptor antagonists). The goal of either modality is the maintenance of gastric pH at or above 5. New, possibly cytoprotective, agents (e.g., sucralfate) are being evaluated for treatment of ulcers. Documented *H. pylori* infection should be treated as discussed previously.

   a. **Medications**
      (1) **Antacids.** In the acutely ill patient, antacids can be administered either orally or through a nasogastric tube at a dose of 0.5 ml/kg every 1–2 hours.
      (2) **H_2-receptor antagonists.** Ranitidine (3 mg/kg every 12 hours orally, 1–1.5 mg/kg every 8 hours intravenously) and cimetidine (10 mg/kg every 6 hours orally or intravenously) have been used in the pediatric population. Because ranitidine does not inhibit the cytochrome P_{450} hepatic enzyme system as does cimetidine, its use may be preferred when additional medications are being used.

   b. **Duration of therapy.** A minimum 6-week course of therapy is recommended. Thirty to fifty percent of children with primary peptic ulcers suffer at least one recurrence. The recurrence rate is especially high in adolescents.

   c. **Dietary restrictions** probably are unnecessary, although elimination of substances that increase gastric acid secretion (e.g., alcohol, caffeine) is advisable.

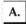 **IV.** **GASTROINTESTINAL HEMORRHAGE.** Bleeding from the gastrointestinal tract is a common and, occasionally, life-threatening condition in infants and children. Usually, a careful history and physical examination, as well as consideration of the patient's age, will suggest the most likely etiologies (Table 11-3). However, attempts to make a specific diagnosis should be made only after the patient's cardiovascular status has been adequately stabilized.

A. **Diagnosis.** The diagnostic approach in the patient with suspected gastrointestinal bleeding involves three sequential steps.

1. **Did the patient actually bleed?**
   a. Food coloring can cause vomit and stools to turn red, and bismuth and iron may make stools black.
   b. Confirmation of the presence of heme protein is done with a **guaiac test**.

2. **Did the bleeding originate in the upper or the lower tract?**
   a. Hematemesis suggests a site proximal to the ligament of Treitz.
   b. If the clinical picture is unclear, **gastric aspiration** should be performed.
      (1) A gastric aspirate positive for blood is highly specific for upper tract bleeding.
      (2) A negative aspirate suggests lower tract bleeding but cannot exclude an upper tract source that has stopped bleeding or a duodenal lesion with no reflux of blood back into the stomach.

3. **What is the specific source of the bleeding?** A variety of noninvasive and invasive techniques may identify the source of the bleeding.
   a. **Radiologic evaluation**
      (1) A **plain film of the abdomen** may exclude bowel obstruction and free intraabdominal gas.

TABLE 11-3. Differential Diagnosis of Gastrointestinal Bleeding in Children by Likely Symptom and Age at Presentation

Symptom	Infant	Child (2–12 Years)	Adolescent (> 12 Years)
Hematemesis	Swallowed maternal blood Peptic esophagitis Mallory-Weiss tear Gastritis Gastric ulcer Duodenal ulcer Gastric, duodenal duplication	Epistaxis Peptic esophagitis Caustic ingestion Mallory-Weiss tear Esophageal varices Gastritis Gastric ulcer Duodenal ulcer Hereditary hemorrhagic telangiectasia Hemobilia Henoch-Schönlein purpura	Esophageal ulcer Peptic esophagitis Mallory-Weiss tear Esophageal varices Gastric ulcer Gastritis Duodenal ulcer Hereditary hemorrhagic telangiectasia Hemobilia Leiomyoma (sarcoma) Henoch-Schönlein purpura
Painless melena	Duodenal ulcer Duodenal duplication Ileal duplication Meckel diverticulum Gastric heterotopia*	Duodenal ulcer Duodenal duplication Ileal duplication Meckel diverticulum Gastric heterotopia	Duodenal ulcer Leiomyoma (sarcoma)
Melena with pain, obstruction, peritonitis, perforation	Necrotizing enterocolitis Intussusception‡ Volvulus	Duodenal ulcer Hemobilia† Intussusception‡ Volvulus Ileal ulcer (isolated)	Duodenal ulcer Hemobilia Crohn disease (ileal ulcer)
Hematochezia with crampy abdominal pain	Infectious colitis Pseudomembranous colitis Eosinophilic colitis Hirschsprung enterocolitis	Infectious colitis Pseudomembranous colitis Ulcerative colitis Granulomatous (Crohn) colitis Hemolytic–uremic syndrome Henoch-Schönlein purpura Lymphonodular hyperplasia	Infectious colitis Pseudomembranous colitis Ulcerative colitis Granulomatous (Crohn) colitis Hemolytic uremic syndrome Henoch-Schönlein purpura
Hematochezia without diarrhea or abdominal pain	Anal fissure Eosinophilic colitis Rectal gastric mucosa Heterotopia Colonic hemangiomas	Anal fissure Solitary rectal ulcer Juvenile polyp Lymphonodular hyperplasia	Anal fissure Hemorrhoid Solitary rectal ulcer Colonic arteriovenous malformation

Reprinted with permission from Treem WR. Gastrointestinal bleeding in children. *Gastrointest Endosc Clin North Am* 4:75, 1994.
*Ectopic gastric tissue in jejunum or ileum without a Meckel diverticulum.
†Hemobilia often accompanied by vomiting, right upper quadrant abdominal pain.
‡Classic "currant jelly" stool.

(2) Barium studies are contraindicated in the actively bleeding child because they usually are insensitive and will make other diagnostic tests difficult. A **barium enema** may be the first diagnostic test if intussusception (see VII A 3) is suspected.

(3) Bleeding scans involving injection of ^{99m}Tc pertechnetate-labeled red blood cells may detect very slow rates of bleeding. ^{99m}Tc pertechnetate injected intravenously may detect ectopic gastric mucosa in the case of Meckel diverticulum.

(4) Angiography may be used to detect bleeding sites in more difficult cases.

b. Endoscopy

(1) In up to 90% of patients with upper tract bleeding, **esophagogastroduodenoscopy** detects the site of hemorrhage.

(2) Sigmoidoscopy should be the first diagnostic study in patients with suspected colonic bleeding. Abnormal colonic mucosa will immediately alert the clinician to an infectious or other type of inflammatory process (e.g., ulcerative colitis) or possibly identify a structural lesion (e.g., a polyp).

(3) If inspection of the entire colon is indicated, **colonoscopy** may be performed.

B. | **Therapy**

1. Cardiovascular resuscitation should be vigorous in the presence of orthostatic hypotension.

a. With massive bleeding, whole blood (or a combination of packed cells and fresh frozen plasma) should be given to maintain intravascular volume. Once bleeding has stopped, packed cells alone may be given.

b. Vitamin K (1 mg per year of age, up to 10 mg), platelets, and plasma should be given as needed to correct any coagulopathy.

2. Treatment of upper tract lesions

a. Mucosal lesions of the upper tract should be treated with antacids or H_2-receptor antagonists.

b. Esophageal varices may be treated with a variety of techniques, including the following.

(1) Vasopressin infusion may be used to decrease splanchnic blood flow. A bolus of 0.3 units/kg up to a maximum of 20 units is given over 20 minutes, followed by a continuous infusion of 0.2–0.4 units/1.73 ml/minute. Recent studies suggest that octreotide, a somatostatin analogue (1–2 µg/kg bolus, then 1 µg/kg/hour), may be as effective as vasopressin but with fewer side effects.

(2) Variceal obliteration may be accomplished by direct variceal injection of a sclerosant solution, such as 5% morrhuate sodium. Ligation by banding is now being done in some patients.

(3) Transjugular intrahepatic portosystemic stent is a new angiographic technique in which a stent is placed within the liver through hepatic parenchyma to connect intrahepatic branches of the portal vein and hepatic veins.

(4) Surgery to decompress the portal system can be performed, but with the emergence of nonoperative techniques, it is being used less frequently.

3. Treatment of lower tract lesions depends on the specific lesions causing the bleeding (e.g., surgery is used for Meckel diverticulum).

V. **DIARRHEAL DISORDERS**

A. | **Acute infectious diarrhea** remains a leading cause of morbidity and mortality throughout the world.

1. Diarrhea as a result of bacterial pathogens (e.g., *Escherichia coli*, *Campylobacter jejuni*, and *Salmonella*, *Shigella*, and *Yersinia* species)

a. Pathogenic mechanisms

(1) Toxin production (e.g., *Vibrio cholerae*)

(2) Adherence to the intestinal mucosa with a local cytopathic effect (e.g., entero-adherent *E. coli*)

(3) Invasion (e.g., *Shigella* sp)

(4) Other (enterohemorrhagic *E. coli*)

b. Clinical features. Bacterial diarrhea may present as either a cholera-like picture caused by bacterial toxins, or a dysentery-like picture with bloody stools associated with invasive bacteria.

c. Diagnosis depends on isolation of the particular organism by stool culture. A Gram stain of the stool may reveal leukocytes, and this usually is indicative of an invasive pathogen.

d. Therapy with antibiotics is not always needed.

(1) *Salmonella* gastroenteritis should not be treated with antibiotics unless it is accompanied by septicemia, because it may prolong fecal excretion of this organism.

(2) If symptoms associated with other bacterial pathogens have abated by the time of diagnosis, treatment usually is unnecessary.

(3) Drugs that slow intestinal motility (e.g., diphenoxylate hydrochloride, loperamide) should never be used in cases of bacterial diarrhea.

2. Diarrhea as a result of viral pathogens

a. Rotavirus is the primary viral pathogen associated with diarrhea in children. It is a 70-nm, double-stranded, segmented RNA virus.

(1) Epidemiology. Rotavirus is found worldwide, generally in children from 6 months to 2 years of age, and is most common during the cooler months of the year.

(2) Pathogenesis. Rotavirus infects and destroys only the mature villous cells of the small intestine, not small intestinal crypt cells or colonic epithelial cells. Functionally immature crypt cells predominate, and abnormalities in electrolyte and carbohydrate absorption ensue.

(3) Clinical features are seen after a 48- to 72-hour incubation period and include a predictable sequence of fever, vomiting, and subsequent diarrhea. Upper respiratory symptoms are common.

(4) Diagnosis. Specific diagnosis can be made with a commercially available enzyme-linked immunosorbent assay kit.

(5) Therapy is supportive, and oral rehydration usually is successful. Lactose intolerance is seen in approximately 50% of infants suffering rotavirus infection, and may last for several weeks.

b. Norwalk agent, a 27-nm virus, is the prototype of a larger group of viruses that are associated with outbreaks of gastroenteritis. It is found more commonly in older children than in infants. After a 48-hour incubation period, vomiting, diarrhea, or both may be seen. Therapy is supportive and similar to that for rotavirus infection.

c. Enteric adenovirus (serotypes 40 and 41) has been increasingly recognized as a cause of diarrhea in young children. Clinically, this infection resembles that seen with rotavirus, although the diarrhea may last somewhat longer (mean duration, 5–6 days). Infection is seen year-round.

3. Diarrhea as a result of protozoal pathogens

a. *Giardia lamblia* is a protozoan parasite that occurs either in active trophozoite form in the small bowel or as cysts, which is the form more commonly identified in feces.

(1) Epidemiology. Ingestion of water contaminated with *G. lamblia* cysts is the usual mode of spread, but venereal transmission has also been described.

(2) Pathogenesis. Significant intestinal epithelial cell injury usually is seen.

(3) Clinical features. One to three weeks after ingestion, affected individuals experience cramping, abdominal distention, flatulence, and diarrhea. Many individuals may remain asymptomatic.

(4) Diagnosis is made by careful examination of several fresh stool specimens for trophozoites or cysts. Rarely, duodenal intubation with tissue biopsy and fluid sampling may be required.

(5) Therapy. Several drugs may be used for a 1-week course, including metronidazole, quinacrine, and furazolidone. Transient lactose malabsorption is common.

b. *Entamoeba histolytica* may also exist in either a trophozoite or cyst form.

   (1) Epidemiology. Transmission is by the fecal–oral route and is associated with the ingestion of cysts. Infection is most common in areas with poor sanitation. Venereal transmission also is possible.

   (2) Pathogenesis. Trophozoites of *E. histolytica* invade colonic epithelium and exert a cytopathic effect.

   (3) Clinical features. Patients with dysenteric colitis have fever, numerous bloody stools, and cramping. Extraintestinal spread is common and may result in formation of a hepatic abscess.

   (4) Diagnosis. Trophozoites of *E. histolytica* can be identified by stool examination. Serologic testing occasionally is useful.

   (5) Therapy is drug treatment with metronidazole.

c. Cryptosporidium is a coccidian parasite.

   (1) Epidemiology. Infection usually is via the fecal–oral route, with many human infections being zoonotic (acquired from animals).

   (2) The **pathogenesis** of diarrhea is not known.

   (3) Clinical features. Asymptomatic carriers have been described, but more commonly a profuse, watery diarrhea is present. In immunocompetent individuals, the diarrhea is self-limited, whereas in immunocompromised hosts the infection may be fatal.

   (4) Therapy. Effective therapy for cryptosporidial infection is not available.

B. **Food-associated diarrhea**

1. Protein sensitivity

a. Celiac disease, also called **gluten-sensitive enteropathy,** is an important cause of chronic diarrhea in children.

   (1) Pathogenesis. Gliadin, a wheat protein, contains the substance that damages the small intestine. Surface epithelial cells are destroyed, the villi become blunted or flat, and the crypts hypertrophy. Brush border enzyme levels are greatly decreased.

   (2) Clinical features. Most children show symptoms between 9 and 24 months of age.
      (a) Diarrhea
      (b) Failure to thrive
      (c) Vomiting
      (d) Abdominal distention
      (e) Irritability
      (f) Short stature, iron-resistant anemia, and rickets (older children)

   (3) Diagnosis. Serologic screening for celiac disease with anti-gliadin, anti-endomysial, and anti-reticulin antibodies is now common. If positive, a small bowel biopsy is performed. Demonstration of villous atrophy and crypt hyperplasia is consistent with the diagnosis.

   (4) Therapy for gluten-sensitive enteropathy is the provision of a gluten-free diet. Restriction of lactose as well as vitamin and iron supplementation may be necessary for several weeks to months as the small intestinal mucosa heals. Anti-gliadin antibody levels should fall with a gluten-free diet, and rise on rechallenge. Repeat biopsy is now performed only rarely.

b. Cow's milk and soy protein intolerance (allergic enterocolitis)

   (1) Pathogenesis. The precise mode by which these dietary proteins may cause disease is unknown. Sensitization may occur de novo (i.e., without any known precipitating event) or after a bout of acute infectious enteritis. Variable mucosal abnormalities may be found in the stomach, small bowel, and colon. Thirty percent of infants who are sensitive to cow's milk protein also are sensitive to soy protein.

   (2) Clinical features. Most symptoms develop in the first 3 months of life.
      (a) Vomiting and diarrhea are most commonly seen and, in rare cases, may persist for weeks to months.

        (b) Rectal bleeding may be seen if allergic colitis is present.

        (c) Edema secondary to excessive enteric protein loss may be dramatic and often is associated with anemia.

        (d) Rhinorrhea, wheezing, and eczema occasionally may be seen and frequently are accompanied by eosinophilia and an elevated serum immunoglobulin E level. Anaphylaxis rarely is observed, but may be life threatening.

    (3) Diagnosis usually is made empirically once symptoms resolve after elimination of the suspected dietary antigen.

    (4) Therapy. Elimination of the offending dietary antigen usually is curative, although severely affected infants may take weeks to months to recover and may require intravenous alimentation until the intestinal mucosa heals.

  c. Breast milk allergy

    (1) Pathogenesis. Some infants appear to react to antigenic material ingested via breast milk. At times this material appears to reflect the maternal diet, and cow's milk protein fractions have been isolated from breast milk. At other times, maternal dietary features appear unimportant.

    (2) Clinical features usually develop in the first several weeks of life and include:

      (a) Diarrhea (frequently bloody)

      (b) Vomiting

      (c) Irritability

    (3) Diagnosis is based on the dietary history and exclusion of infectious agents. Rectal biopsy may reveal an intense eosinophilic infiltrate.

    (4) Therapy. Initial treatment is restriction of maternal ingestion of cow's milk protein. If this is not successful, or if the infant's symptoms are severe, provision of a protein hydrolysate formula is indicated.

  d. Other food-induced small bowel disturbances have been associated with goat's milk, eggs, fish, beef, and poultry.

2. Carbohydrate intolerance is a very common cause of diarrhea in childhood.

  a. Pathogenesis. Dietary carbohydrate is processed by several enzymes, beginning with amylase (which metabolizes starch) and ending with the brush border enzymes lactase, sucrase, isomaltase, and glucoamylase. Any process—congenital or acquired—that diminishes the activities of these enzymes may lead to carbohydrate malabsorption.

  b. Clinical features. Diarrhea, vomiting, flatulence, borborygmus, and cramping may be present; however, blood is not seen in the stool.

  c. Diagnosis

    (1) Breath hydrogen testing is the most accurate diagnostic test.

    (2) Stool pH and examination of stool for reducing substances (e.g., lactose, glucose, fructose) are less helpful in making the diagnosis, but a stool pH less than 5 and the presence of reducing substances suggest carbohydrate malabsorption.

    (3) Intestinal biopsy with direct assay of brush border enzyme activity rarely is needed.

  d. Therapy is restriction of the offending carbohydrate. Lactase enzyme now is commercially available and may be ingested along with lactose-containing foods to lessen symptoms. Yogurt and aged cheeses may be well tolerated even by lactose-intolerant individuals. If lactose restriction is severe and prolonged, calcium supplementation is needed.

C. **Intractable diarrhea of infancy** is an uncommon problem but one that may have life-threatening consequences. Multiple disease states may be responsible for this clinical entity (Table 11-4).

1. Pathogenesis. Some infants have a specific defect in pancreatic, hepatic, or intestinal function, which can readily explain the cause of their diarrhea. Unfortunately, a significant number of infants with intractable diarrhea have no readily identifiable underlying disease.

TABLE 11-4. Causes of Intractable Diarrhea

Congenital enzymatic/transport defects
  Glucose–galactose malabsorption
  Chloridorrhea
  Primary bile acid malabsorption
  Enterokinase deficiency
  Acrodermatitis enteropathica

Secretory tumors

Infection
  Enteroadherent *Escherichia coli*
  Bacterial overgrowth

Hirschsprung enterocolitis

Immunodeficiency

Congenital microvillous inclusion disease

Pancreatic insufficiency
  Cystic fibrosis
  Shwachman-Diamond syndrome
  Lipase deficiency

Iatrogenic
  Laxatives
  Sorbitol

a. Current knowledge suggests that some children may suffer a **series of important pathogenetic events,** which include:
  (1) Mucosal injury of the small bowel caused by an unrecognized infection or allergy
  (2) Malnutrition, which results from the malabsorption associated with the intestinal mucosal injury
  (3) Delayed healing of the mucosal injury and depressed immunity, which result from the malnutrition
b. Others appear to suffer intestinal injury on an autoimmune basis.

2. Clinical features
  a. Diarrhea is severe and often persists even when the patient is given nothing by mouth (secretory diarrhea).
  b. Vomiting is common.
  c. Fluid, electrolyte, and enteric protein losses may be excessive, resulting in dehydration, acidosis, hyponatremia, hypokalemia, hypoalbuminemia, and edema.
  d. Severe failure to thrive is evident.

3. Diagnosis. A systematic approach to diagnose readily treatable conditions must be made. This includes:
  a. Culture of stool, urine, and blood
  b. Stool examination for blood, leukocytes, pH, reducing sugars, ova, and parasites
  c. Assessment of renal and hepatic function
  d. Sweat test for cystic fibrosis
  e. Immunologic evaluation
  f. Small intestinal biopsy and sigmoidoscopy
  g. Radiologic evaluation (e.g., upper gastrointestinal series, barium enema)

4. Therapy. If the underlying condition permits specific treatment, that treatment should be given. In most cases of idiopathic intractable diarrhea, the primary treatment is nutritional support.
  a. Central venous hyperalimentation frequently is required and should be instituted early to reverse the patient's severely catabolic state.
  b. Elemental formulas are required when enteric nutrition is initiated. These usually need to be given slowly by continuous infusion through a nasogastric tube.

D. **Chronic nonspecific diarrhea,** or **irritable bowel syndrome,** is the most common cause of chronic diarrhea in otherwise healthy children.

1. **Pathogenesis.** Although the precise pathogenesis of chronic nonspecific diarrhea is unknown, alterations in gastrointestinal motility are thought to be of primary importance. A number of additional factors have been noted to increase symptoms, including:
   a. Chilled foods or fluids
   b. Excessive fluid intake, especially of fruit juices
   c. A low-fat, high-carbohydrate diet
   d. Stress and anxiety

2. **Clinical features.** Chronic nonspecific diarrhea usually manifests between 9 and 36 months of age.
   a. Diarrhea is variable in severity and may occur up to six times each day. Occasionally, normal or even hard stools are seen.
   b. Undigested food (particularly vegetables) and mucus frequently are observed in the stools.
   c. Abdominal cramping may be present.
   d. Activity and appetite usually are normal, and growth generally is unaffected.

3. **Diagnosis** is based on a compatible clinical history and the exclusion of other disorders (e.g., carbohydrate malabsorption, chronic infection).

4. **Therapy.** Frequently, no treatment other than parental reassurance is needed. Symptoms usually resolve spontaneously by 3–4 years of age. Specific measures that can be of help include:
   a. Decreasing fluid intake, particularly fruit juices, and providing high-fat foods to slow gastric emptying
   b. Increasing fiber intake through the use of bulking agents
   c. Pharmacologic intervention, although rarely required, including the use of cholestyramine and loperamide

VI. INFLAMMATORY BOWEL DISEASE (IBD) is a generic term usually used to refer to two chronic disorders of intestinal inflammation—**ulcerative colitis** and **Crohn disease.**

A. **Epidemiology.** Recent studies suggest a modest increase in the incidence of Crohn disease and perhaps a mild decrease in the incidence of ulcerative colitis over the past decade. Up to 30% of newly diagnosed cases of IBD occur in individuals younger than 20 years of age.

B. **Pathogenesis.** A number of genetic and environmental factors may be contributory.

1. **Immunologic.** A variety of immunologic abnormalities have been noted in patients with IBD, including anti-colon antibodies, anti-neutrophil cytoplasmic antibodies, and lymphocytes cytotoxic to intestinal cells. It is not clear whether these phenomena are primary or secondary. The factors that control the normal "physiologic" inflammation in the intestine may be abnormal in patients with IBD.

2. **Infectious.** No infectious agent has been reproducibly isolated and thought to be causative in patients with IBD.

3. **Psychological.** Despite numerous theories regarding the so-called colitis personality, no consistent psychological abnormalities have been found preceding disease onset in patients with IBD.

4. **Multifactorial.** It is likely that a variety of factors as detailed above are important. Genetic predisposition to IBD may be a crucial factor.

C. **Pathologic and clinical features** (Table 11-5)

TABLE 11-5. Comparative Pathologic and Clinical Features of Ulcerative Colitis and Crohn Disease

	Ulcerative Colitis	Crohn Disease
Location	Colon only Proctitis Left-sided Pancolititis	Mouth to anus 60% Ileocolonic 30% Small bowel 10% Colonic
Histology	Mucosal inflammation Diffuse involvement Crypt abscesses Crypt distortion	Transmural inflammation Skip areas Aphthoid lesions Fissuring ulceration Granuloma Fibrosis
Clinical features		
Diarrhea	++ → ++++	0 → ++++
Rectal bleeding	++ → ++++	0 → ++++
Abdominal pain	0 → ++	++ → ++++
Abdominal mass	0	0 → ++++
Weight loss	0 → +	+ → ++++
Short stature	0 → +	0 → ++++
Perirectal disease	0	0 → ++++
Carcinoma risk	+ → ++++	0 → +

Extraintestinal manifestations
(ulcerative colitis, Crohn disease)
Arthritis
Ankylosing spondylitis
Erythema nodosum
Pyoderma gangrenosum
Uveitis/episcleritis
Stomatitis
Sclerosing cholangitis

D. **Diagnosis.** In the presence of symptoms consistent with a diagnosis of IBD, hematologic, biochemical, radiologic, and endoscopic studies may be performed (Table 11-6).

E. **Differential diagnosis.** A number of conditions may present with signs and symptoms suggestive of idiopathic IBD, including:

1. Appendicitis

2. Enteric infection (e.g., *Helicobacter, Salmonella, Shigella, Yersinia, Entamoeba* species)

3. Pseudomembranous colitis (antibiotic-associated diarrhea) secondary to *Clostridium difficile* infection

4. Hemolytic–uremic syndrome

5. Henoch-Schönlein purpura

6. Radiation enterocolitis

7. Eosinophilic gastroenteritis

F. **Therapy**

1. Medication
   a. Sulfasalazine is the mainstay of treatment in mild-to-moderate cases of ulcerative colitis and Crohn disease involving the colon. It has no efficacy in Crohn disease

TABLE 11-6. Laboratory Findings to Establish a Diagnosis of Inflammatory Bowel Disease

Hematologic
  Anemia
  Bandemia
  Thrombocytopenia
Biochemical
  Iron deficiency
  Hypoalbuminemia
  Elevated serum aminotransferases (10%)
Radiographic
  Decreased colonic haustrations (UC)
  Nodularity (CD)
  Skip areas (CD)
  String sign (CD)
  Fistula (CD)
Endoscopy
  Granularity
  Friability
  Loss of vascular pattern
  Aphthoid lesions (CD)
  Cobblestoning

CD = Crohn disease; UC = ulcerative colitis.

involving the small bowel. In patients who are allergic to sulfasalazine, **5-aminosalicylate** (the active moiety) can be administered orally (mesalamine, 30–50 mg/kg/day) or as an enema preparation.

b. Corticosteroids remain the most efficacious therapy, particularly in severe disease and in Crohn disease involving the small bowel. Because daily corticosteroid therapy can inhibit growth, attempts should be made to wean to alternate-day therapy when possible.

c. Metronidazole currently is used to treat severe perirectal fistulae in patients with Crohn disease.

d. 6-Mercaptopurine is used in patients with severe Crohn disease who are dependent on high doses of corticosteroids. It may permit reduction of the steroid dosage.

e. Cyclosporine may be efficacious for the short-term treatment of severe ulcerative colitis.

f. Diphenoxylate and loperamide may be used for symptomatic relief but never in the presence of severe symptoms.

2. **Nutrition**
   a. Anorexia and increased nutrient losses through stool are common in children with inflammatory bowel disease, so **adequate calories and protein** are essential. A variety of techniques may be used and often are effective in reversing growth retardation, including:
   (1) Oral supplements
   (2) Nasogastric tube feedings
   (3) Central venous hyperalimentation
   b. Vitamin and mineral (particularly iron) supplementation may be required.

3. **Surgery**
   a. Ulcerative colitis
      (1) Indications
         (a) Fulminant colitis with severe blood loss or toxic megacolon
         (b) Intractable disease with a high-dose steroid requirement, steroid toxicity, growth failure, or invalidism
         (c) Colonic dysplasia

(2) Procedure. Ileoanal–endorectal pull-through procedures after colectomy and mucosal proctectomy are the methods of choice and eliminate the need for a permanent ileostomy.

b. Crohn disease

(1) Indications

(a) Hemorrhage

(b) Obstruction

(c) Perforation

(d) Intractability

(e) Severe fistula formation

(f) Ureteral obstruction

(g) Growth retardation (if medical measures are unsuccessful)

(2) Procedure. In general, a conservative approach is warranted because removal of the diseased bowel is not curative in Crohn disease. After segmental resection, recurrence rates of about 50% have been reported.

VII. ABDOMINAL PAIN

A. Acute pain

1. **Approach to the patient** with acute abdominal pain. The most urgent consideration in evaluating a child with acute abdominal pain is to determine whether there is an underlying cause requiring surgery. Most causes of abdominal pain in children do not require surgical treatment, although such causes of pain are more common in children younger than 2 years of age. Sources of pain outside the abdominal cavity (e.g., lower lobe pneumonia) must be considered in the evaluation.

   a. Important causes of abdominal pain **possibly requiring surgery** (the acute abdomen)

   (1) Intestinal obstruction due to malrotation and volvulus, intussusception, strangulated hernia, or adhesions

   (2) Appendicitis, Meckel diverticulum, or an abdominal abscess

   (3) Toxic megacolon

   (4) Perforated duodenal ulcer or perforation of intestine secondary to another process

   (5) Cholecystitis

   (6) Rupture of the spleen or other organ due to trauma

   b. Clinical features suggesting a cause **requiring surgery**

   (1) Vomiting, especially if it is bilious or feculent

   (2) Sudden onset of abdominal distention

   (3) Absent bowel sounds or high-pitched sounds suggestive of intestinal obstruction

   (4) Abdominal signs of peritonitis (e.g., rigidity, guarding, rebound tenderness)

   c. Important causes of acute abdominal pain **not requiring surgery**

   (1) Enteritis; colitis of any cause

   (2) Henoch-Schönlein purpura, hemolytic–uremic syndrome, and other types of vasculitis

   (3) Fecal impaction

   (4) Hepatitis

   (5) Pancreatitis

   (6) Vasoocclusive crisis of sickle cell anemia

   (7) Primary peritonitis

   (8) Mesenteric adenitis

   (9) Urinary tract infection or urinary calculi

   (10) Extraabdominal causes (e.g., pneumonia, osteomyelitis, acute neurologic processes)

   (11) Unusual causes [e.g., porphyria, familial Mediterranean fever, diabetic ketoacidosis, lead poisoning, Kawasaki disease (gallbladder hydrops)]

2. Appendicitis is the most common indication for acute abdominal surgery in childhood. Appendicitis occurs more frequently in children between 10 and 15 years of age. Less than 10% of patients are younger than 5 years of age.

   a. Pathogenesis. Bacterial invasion of the appendix occurs, especially if the lumen is obstructed by a fecalith, parasite, or lymph node.

   b. Clinical features

   (1) Classically, fever, vomiting, anorexia, and diffuse periumbilical pain develop. Subsequently, pain and abdominal tenderness localize to the right lower quadrant as the parietal peritoneum becomes involved.

   (2) The incidence of perforation and diffuse peritonitis is high, especially in a child younger than 2 years of age, when diagnosis may be delayed.

   (3) Atypical presentations are common in childhood.

   (4) Certain bacterial infections (e.g., *C. jejuni, Yersinia* sp) may be associated with right lower quadrant pain and tenderness, and may mimic appendicitis.

   c. Diagnosis of appendicitis should be established clinically by history and by a physical examination (including a rectal examination to detect tenderness or a mass). Laboratory tests may help confirm the diagnosis.

   (1) The white blood cell count is only moderately elevated in uncomplicated appendicitis.

   (2) A plain film of the abdomen may demonstrate a fecalith or other nonspecific abnormalities.

   (3) Occasionally, a barium enema may be useful.

   d. Therapy. When the diagnosis of appendicitis cannot be ruled out after a period of close observation, laparotomy and appendectomy are indicated.

   e. Prognosis. The mortality rate is very low unless perforation has occurred.

3. Intussusception is the invagination of one part of the intestine into another. It is one of the most common causes of intestinal obstruction in infancy.

   a. Pathogenesis. Most intussusceptions are ileocolic.

   (1) In patients beyond the neonatal period but younger than the age of 2 years (the period of peak incidence), no lead point of the intussusception is typically found. A previous viral infection may cause hypertrophy of the Peyer patches or mesenteric nodes, which are hypothesized to play a role in intussusception.

   (2) A specific lead point is identified in only about 5% of cases, but it should be sought in neonates or in children older than 5 years of age. Recognizable causes of the intussusception include Meckel diverticulum, an intestinal polyp, lymphoma, or a foreign body. Meckel diverticulum usually presents as melena unassociated with abdominal pain or intussusception.

   (3) As a result of impaired venous return, the affected bowel may swell, become ischemic and necrotic, and perforate.

   b. Clinical features

   (1) Bouts of **irritability** and **colicky pain** start suddenly. **Vomiting** is common. **Rectal bleeding** may occur but only rarely in the form of the classic "currant jelly" stools (i.e., stools containing red blood and mucus).

   (2) The degree of **lethargy** demonstrated by the child may be striking. At times the prominent presenting feature may be "altered consciousness."

   (3) A **tubular mass** is palpable in about half of the patients.

   c. Diagnosis

   (1) A plain abdominal film may show a paucity of gas in the right lower quadrant or evidence of obstruction.

   (2) A barium enema demonstrates a **coiled-spring appearance** to the bowel, which is diagnostic.

   d. Therapy

   (1) Hydrostatic reduction by careful barium enema performed by an experienced radiologist is successful in about 75% of cases. Peritoneal signs or the presence of peritoneal free air are an absolute contraindication to this procedure.

   (2) Surgery is indicated when hydrostatic reduction is inappropriate or unsuccessful.

e. Prognosis. The immediate recurrence rate is about 15%. When a specific lead point is present, the recurrence rate is higher.

B. **Chronic pain.** Chronic abdominal pain is a frequent problem in children (see Chapter 3 VI). Most often, no specific cause can be documented. Two particularly vexing problems are infantile colic and irritable bowel syndrome.

1. **Infantile colic** is observed in up to 15% of otherwise healthy newborns.
   a. Pathogenesis. The cause of infantile colic remains unknown. Postulated important factors have included abnormal mother–infant interaction, protein allergy, hormonal imbalances, and increased sensitivity to colonic distention.
   b. Clinical features of infantile colic include:
      (1) Pulling up of legs during paroxysms, often with a change in facial color to bright red
      (2) Difficulty with defecation despite soft stools
      (3) Inconsolability
   c. Diagnosis
      (1) A clinical diagnosis is based on a characteristic history and a negative physical examination.
      (2) Other causes of irritability (e.g., protein allergy, hernia, gastroesophageal reflux) must be excluded.
   d. Therapy. Parental support is the mainstay of therapy. Rocking machines or increased dietary fiber may be helpful.
   e. Prognosis. In over 80% of cases, symptoms abate by 4–5 months of age.

2. **Irritable bowel syndrome** may represent the most common cause of chronic abdominal pain, yet it is probably the least characterized.
   a. Pathogenesis. The precise pathogenesis of irritable bowel is unknown, but abnormal intestinal (primarily colonic) motility has been described. In addition, increased sensitivity to colonic distention appears to be common in these patients.
   b. Clinical features
      (1) **Abdominal cramping** is a cardinal feature of irritable bowel syndrome and may be described in virtually any part of the abdomen. It frequently is paroxysmal and severe.
      (2) **Stool consistency** may frequently vary from hard to loose.
      (3) **Nausea, diaphoresis, and lightheadedness** occasionally are seen.
      (4) **Anxiety** often provokes an attack.
   c. Diagnosis
      (1) A clinical diagnosis is based on a characteristic history and a negative physical examination.
      (2) Other disorders (e.g., lactose intolerance, inflammatory bowel disease, giardiasis) must be excluded.
   d. Therapy consists of:
      (1) **Reassurance** that the symptoms, although they are frequent, do not suggest a life-threatening disease
      (2) **Dietary fiber supplementation**
      (3) **Anticholinergic medications** (e.g., dicyclomine)
      (4) **Psychotherapy** (if stress frequently exacerbates symptoms)
   e. Prognosis. Little is known about the natural history of irritable bowel syndrome in children, although clinical experience suggests that the problem may persist for intervals of months to years.

VIII. **CONSTIPATION** can be defined as a decrease in the frequency or fluidity of bowel movements. Fewer than three bowel movements per week is considered abnormal. Most constipated children have no underlying disorder, and treatment can be directed solely at the symptom. Formal evaluation is reserved for cases beginning at birth and those that are intractable to standard symptomatic treatment.

A. Pathogenesis

1. Functional or simple constipation occurs in the **absence of an organic cause**. In an otherwise healthy child, constipation may result simply from an episode of painful defecation, difficulties during the period of toilet training, inattention to the urge to defecate because of involvement in other activities, or discomfort with toilet facilities in school. Frequently, a family history of constipation may be elicited. Inadequate fiber in the diet also may play a role.

2. **Specific causes**
   a. **Structural lesions,** including anal fissure, anterior ectopic anus, stenosis of the bowel, inflammatory proctitis, and extrinsic lesions causing bowel obstruction
   b. **Neuromuscular disorders,** such as spinal cord defects, disorders of smooth muscle, and Hirschsprung disease (see VIII E)
   c. **Medications,** particularly opiates and anticholinergic agents
   d. **Metabolic causes,** including hypothyroidism, hypercalcemia, hypokalemia, uremia, pregnancy, and disorders causing dehydration
   e. **Toxins,** particularly chronic lead intoxication
   f. **Infection** with *Clostridium botulinum* in infants (infant botulism)

B. Clinical features

1. **Pattern of defecation.** A detailed history of the pattern of defecation may be difficult to obtain. Even a history of regular bowel movements does not exclude constipation if evacuation is incomplete. In a child with large stools, stool-withholding behavior may be misinterpreted as an attempt to defecate.

2. **Accompanying symptoms** include pain, abdominal distention, and flatulence. Occasional symptoms include rectal bleeding, poor appetite, enuresis, and a history of urinary tract infection. Rectal prolapse may rarely be seen with defecation.

3. **Encopresis.** In cases of long-standing constipation, children may become incontinent of liquid stool and be thought to have diarrhea. This "overflow incontinence" is called encopresis and is present in more than 50% of children with long-standing constipation (see Chapter 4 II B).

C. Diagnosis

1. Physical examination of the abdomen may reveal **distention** or **palpable fecal masses**. The perianal area should be examined for congenital or acquired abnormalities, including trauma. Digital rectal examination is necessary to evaluate the sphincter and estimate the amount of stool in the ampulla.

2. When no underlying disorder is identified by history and physical examination, a favorable response to treatment supports the diagnosis of **functional constipation**.

3. **Treatment failure** or **relapse** should prompt investigation of an underlying disorder with appropriate radiographic and laboratory studies.

D. Therapy for functional constipation. An individualized, multifaceted treatment program should be designed.

1. **Medications** are continued until a regular pattern of defecation is established and then are slowly tapered.
   a. In **infants,** short-term or intermittent treatment with glycerin suppositories may be rewarding. Excessive milk or cow's milk protein formula (i.e., more than 32 oz/day) should be avoided, and juices such as apple or pear juice may be helpful. Extra fiber in the form of barley malt extracts or methylcellulose also may help.
   b. In **older children,** mineral oil or mild laxatives such as senna derivatives commonly are used.

    c. In cases of **severe constipation,** a period of aggressive treatment including enemas (otherwise to be avoided) may be required.

    d. A balanced **polyethylene glycol–electrolyte solution** administered by the oral or nasogastric route is safe, prompt, and effective in cleansing the bowel and may avoid prolonged use of enemas or the need for manual disimpaction.

2. Other measures

    a. High-fiber diet and fiber supplements

    b. Reinforcement of regular toilet use

    c. Psychological evaluation, which may be necessary to address emotional factors resulting in voluntary withholding

E. **Hirschsprung disease** is an uncommon developmental disorder (incidence is 1 in 5000) resulting in constipation.

1. Pathogenesis. In children with Hirschsprung disease, progenitor cells destined to become the ganglion cells of the submucosal and myenteric plexuses fail to complete their distal bowel migration in the colon. As a result, the abnormally innervated distal colon remains tonically contracted and obstructs the flow of feces. In approximately 75% of cases, the aganglionic segment is limited to the rectosigmoid, but the entire colon may be involved.

2. Clinical features

    a. In most cases, the onset of symptoms occurs in the first month and the diagnosis is made in the first 3 months of life. The neonate classically has delayed passage of meconium and then shows evidence of obstruction with poor feeding, bilious vomiting, and abdominal distention. Bloody diarrhea, sepsis, and shock are possible.

    b. In the **older child,** failure to thrive and persistent abdominal distention may be seen, as well as intermittent bouts of intestinal obstruction. Enterocolitis with bloody diarrhea may also occur.

3. Diagnosis

    a. Rectal examination may reveal a narrowed high-pressure zone in continuity with the sphincter, and stool may not be palpable.

    b. Plain-film radiographs may show gaseous distention of proximal bowel but no gas or feces in the rectum.

    c. Barium enema may demonstrate a transition zone between the narrowed abnormal distal segment and the dilated normal proximal bowel.

    d. Anal manometry demonstrates failure of the internal anal sphincter automatically to relax with balloon distention of the rectum.

    e. A **rectal biopsy** revealing no ganglion cells and hypertrophied nerve trunks is necessary for the diagnosis.

4. Therapy. Initial treatment usually is a diverting colostomy. Subsequently, at 6 months or 1 year of age, the aganglionic segment is removed and the remaining colon is anastomosed to the anorectal region.

IX. LIVER DISEASE

A. **General principles.** Certain unique aspects of liver disease in infancy and childhood must be considered before specific hepatic disorders can be evaluated.

1. Estimation of liver size. In healthy children younger than 2 years of age, both the liver and spleen are usually palpable below the costal margins owing to the relatively large size of these organs at this age. Standards have been established for liver span as measured by percussion in the midclavicular line in older children.

2. Reaction to hepatic injury in infancy. Jaundice is the most important manifestation of a variety of hepatic insults in infancy. **Hypoglycemia** occurs early in the course of hepatic injury.

3. **Key elements of the history**
   a. The **family history** is especially important in the consideration of metabolic liver disease.
   b. Illness or exposure during pregnancy may suggest a vertically transmitted (i.e., from mother to infant) **infectious cause** of hepatitis.
   c. A **dietary history** is crucial in the diagnosis of hepatic disease resulting from the failure to metabolize galactose or fructose.

4. **Diagnostic tests.** The serum alkaline phosphatase level usually is elevated in children with obstructive or inflammatory hepatic lesions. Care must be used, however, in the interpretation of the concentration in infancy and adolescence. Because of rapid growth at these ages, the level of serum alkaline phosphatase from bone is elevated, and other enzymes, such as γ-glutamyl transpeptidase (GGT), must be used to evaluate cholestasis.

B. **Neonatal obstructive jaundice.** Direct hyperbilirubinemia in the neonate is never "physiologic," and therefore should always be thoroughly investigated. Direct hyperbilirubinemia is defined as a direct bilirubin greater than 2 mg/dl or greater than 20% of the total bilirubin (see also Chapter 6 V C).

1. **Differential diagnosis** (Table 11-7). Direct hyperbilirubinemia in the neonate is a medical emergency and must be expeditiously investigated to avoid severe permanent liver damage. The key distinction in the neonatal period is between intrahepatic and extrahepatic causes of direct hyperbilirubinemia. Extrahepatic causes require prompt surgical therapy to relieve obstruction and reconstitute bile flow from the liver. Certain intrahepatic metabolic causes can be effectively treated by dietary therapy, and some intrahepatic infectious causes can be specifically treated with antimicrobial agents.
   a. **Tests for specific causes of neonatal cholestasis**
      (1) **Serum tests,** including total and direct bilirubin, aminotransferase and GGT levels, complete blood count, titers of TORCH organisms (see Chapter 8 II B), Venereal Disease Research Laboratory (VDRL), hepatitis B surface antigen (HBsAg), α_1-antitrypsin level and phenotyping, amino acids, blood culture (if clinically indicated), serum albumin, prothrombin time, and partial thromboplastin time
      (2) **Urine tests,** including urinalysis, reducing substances, urine culture, and organic and amino acids
      (3) **Sweat test**
      (4) **Abdominal ultrasound** to rule out a choledochal cyst or common duct stone

TABLE 11-7. Causes of Direct Hyperbilirubinemia with Cholestasis (Obstructive Jaundice in the Infant)

| Extrahepatic Causes | Intrahepatic Causes | | |
	Infectious	Metabolic	Miscellaneous
Biliary atresia	Cytomegalovirus	Galactosemia	Neonatal hepatitis
Choledochal cyst	Toxoplasmosis	Hereditary fructose	Alagille syndrome
Common duct stenosis	Rubella	intolerance	Byler disease
Common duct stone	Herpes virus	α_1-Antitrypsin deficiency	Zellweger syndrome
Obstructing tumor	Coxsackie virus	Cystic fibrosis	Trisomy (17, 18, 21)
Bile/mucus plug	Echovirus	Niemann-Pick disease	Hypopituitarism
Spontaneous perforation of common duct	Syphilis	Gaucher disease	Hepatic hemangiomatosis
	Hepatitis B	Glycogen storage	TPN-induced cholestasis
	Epstein-Barr virus	disease	
	Urinary tract infection		

TPN = total parenteral nutrition.

     (5) Radionuclide biliary imaging to document patency of the extrahepatic biliary system

     (6) Liver biopsy

  b. Differentiation of intrahepatic and extrahepatic idiopathic causes (Table 11-8)

    (1) Often, the tests for neonatal cholestasis reveal no specific etiology. In fact, neonatal hepatitis and biliary atresia are the most common causes of persistent direct hyperbilirubinemia. No serum test (including aminotransferases, GGT, bilirubin, α-fetoprotein, or lipoprotein X) reliably distinguishes between these two entities. Further testing is directed at distinguishing these two entities, including percutaneous liver biopsy, which can reliably differentiate more than 90% of the time, when read by an experienced pediatric hepatologist or pathologist.

    (2) In spite of testing, it is occasionally necessary to perform a laparotomy and intraoperative cholangiography to delineate accurately the presence or absence of the extrahepatic biliary system.

2. Therapy

  a. Neonatal hepatitis. The treatment for neonatal hepatitis and for other causes of prolonged intrahepatic cholestasis is supportive. It includes:

    (1) Administration of ursodeoxycholic acid, a secondary bile acid, to increase bile flow and reduce hypercholesterolemia.

    (2) Fat-soluble vitamin (A, D, E, K) supplementation

    (3) Supplementation of the diet with medium-chain triglycerides that do not require bile acids for assimilation

    (4) Use of cholestyramine, a bile acid-binding resin, and antihistamines to combat pruritus

  b. Biliary atresia

    (1) Surgical management. In less than 20% of patients, there are identifiable proximal hepatic bile ducts that can be anastomosed to the bowel. In most patients, a portoenterostomy must be created between the cut surface of the liver at the porta hepatis and the bowel (Kasai procedure).

TABLE 11-8. Features of Intrahepatic and Extrahepatic Neonatal Obstructive Disease

Feature	Intrahepatic Causes	Extrahepatic Causes
Clinical		
Gestation	Premature	Full term
	SGA	AGA
Family history	15%–20%	None
Appearance	Ill	Well
Stool color	Intermittent acholic	Acholic
Organomegaly	Hepatosplenomegaly	Splenomegaly later
Liver texture	Soft	Firm to hard
Anomalies	Peripheral pulmonic stenosis	Polysplenia
	Vertebral anomalies	Malrotation of gut
	Posterior embryotoxon	
Laboratory		
GGT	< 10 × normal	> 10 × normal
Ultrasound	Gallbladder	No gallbladder or small
Hepatobiliary scan	Excretion into bowel	No excretion
Liver biopsy		
Bile ducts	Normal or decreased	Proliferating
Fibrosis	Minimal	Established, portal
Giant cells	Often	25% of the time
Cholestasis	Yes	Yes
Other	Hepatocellular necrosis	Bile plugs, bile lakes
	Lobular disarray	

AGA = appropriate for gestational age; GGT = γ-glutamyl transpeptidase; SGA = small for gestational age.

    (2) Timing of operation. Successful drainage of the biliary tract occurs most fre-
quently when the operation is performed before the infant is 60 days old
(approximately 8 weeks).

    (3) Complications of surgery include failure to establish bile flow, loss of bile flow
due to further injury to bile ducts, and ascending cholangitis.

3. Prognosis

a. Neonatal hepatitis

    (1) In most patients, the cholestasis resolves over the first year of life with no sequelae.

    (2) A few infants develop progressive liver disease and cirrhosis, with its complica-
tion of ascites, portal hypertension, esophageal varices, and liver failure. These
children may be candidates for liver transplantation.

b. Biliary atresia

    (1) Without surgical correction, biliary cirrhosis and its complications supervene,
and most patients die in the first 2 years of life.

    (2) After successful portoenterostomy, with normalization of serum bilirubin, the
5-year survival rate is 60%–90%.

    (3) Liver transplantation now is showing promise as treatment for patients with bil-
iary atresia for whom attempts at corrective surgery fail. The 5-year survival rate
for liver transplant recipients having biliary atresia is approximately 70%.

C. | **Acute viral hepatitis** (Table 11-9)

1. Diagnosis (Table 11-10). Typically, children with acute viral hepatitis have elevated
serum aminotransferase levels (sometimes to more than 2000 U/L), although most cases
are anicteric. In severe cases, hepatic synthesis of clotting factors may be affected, with
resulting prolongation of the prothrombin time.

a. Hepatitis A (infectious hepatitis). The diagnosis of acute hepatitis A is established by
the finding of hepatitis A antibodies of the immunoglobulin M (IgM) class (IgM antibody is present for 1–3 months; IgG antibody is longer lasting).

b. Hepatitis B (serum hepatitis)

    (1) The standard marker for hepatitis B is the presence of HBsAg. The presence of
antibodies directed against HBsAg (anti-HBs) usually indicates immunity.

    (2) IgG antibodies directed against hepatitis B core antigen (anti-HBc) may indicate
acute infection, chronic infection, or past infection. IgM antibodies against
HBcAg (anti-HBc IgM) are more indicative of acute infection.

    (3) Hepatitis B e antigen (HBeAg) is a marker of viral replication and infectivity and
chronic infection if it is present for more than 2 months. Its presence almost
guarantees transmission of hepatitis B virus (HBV) from mother to infant.

c. Hepatitis C (transfusion-related hepatitis). Both recombinant immunoblot and
enzyme-linked assays for circulating viral antibodies to hepatitis C virus (HCV) have
been developed. Reverse polymerase chain reaction to detect HCV RNA in the
serum or liver is the most sensitive marker of infection with HCV.

    (1) Anti-HCV antibody is a marker for hepatitis C, not for immunity. Its appearance
may be delayed for up to 6–12 months after infection if the first-generation tests
for anti-HCV are used. With the newer assays (second and third generation),
HCV infection can usually be detected within 3 months of the time of exposure.

    (2) Anti-HCV antibody persists in chronic hepatitis C but eventually disappears after
recovery from acute hepatitis C.

d. Hepatitis D (delta hepatitis)

    (1) Delta antigen in the serum is only briefly detectable (first 2 weeks of the disease).
Antibodies to delta virus (anti-HDV) become detectable in more than 90% of
cases within 3–8 weeks of acute hepatitis D.

    (2) The highest titers of anti-HDV are found in patients with chronic hepatitis D.

2. Therapy. No specific therapy exists for acute viral hepatitis. Strict bed rest is not necessary, but vigorous activity should be avoided.

TABLE 11-9. Comparison of Viral Hepatitis Types A, B, C, D, and E in the United States

	Hepatitis A	Hepatitis B	Hepatitis C	Hepatitis D	Hepatitis E
Virus	RNA	DNA	RNA	Defective RNA*	RNA
Age group	Primarily young	All ages	All ages	All ages	All ages, primarily 15–40 years
Onset	Abrupt	Insidious	Insidious	Insidious, fulminant	Abrupt
Incubation	21–42 days	50–180 days	42–56 days	Variable†	30–45 days
Transmission					
Feces	+	−	−	−	+
Water, food	+	−	−	+	+
Semen	−	+	?	+	−
Saliva	−	+	+	+	−
Transfusion	−	+	+	+	−
Needlestick	−	+	+	+	−
Drug abuse	−	+	+	+	−
Dialysis	−	+	+	+	−
Sexual contact	+	+	+	+	
Household contact	+	−	−	−	+
Mother–infant	−	+	+	+	−
Secondary cases	10%–20%	Rare	Rare	Rare	2.5%
Prevalence	5%–10%	> 2%	0.6%	1%–10% of HBV	Rare
Symptoms					
Anorexia	Common	Common	Common	Common	Common
Nausea, vomiting	Common	Common	Common	Uncommon	Common
Fever	Common before jaundice	Uncommon	Uncommon	Uncommon	Common
Jaundice	Uncommon in children	More common	Uncommon	More common	Uncommon
Rash, arthritis	Rare	Common	Rare	Rare	Rare
Outcome					
Severity	Mild	Mild to severe	Intermediate	Mild to severe	Mild to severe
Mortality	Low (< 1%)	Low (1%–3%)	Low (1%–3%)	Low–moderate	High (pregnant women ≤ 20%)
Chronic hepatitis	No	Yes (5%–10%)	Yes (30%–50%)	Yes	No
Chronic carrier	No	Yes	Yes	Yes	No
Liver cancer	No	Yes	Yes	?	No

*Replicates and causes hepatitis only in patients who concurrently are infected with hepatitis B virus (HBV).
†Incubation period typical of hepatitis B if infection with delta virus is simultaneous. Incubation period short (35 days) if hepatitis D is superimposed on chronic HBV carrier state.

TABLE 11-10. Understanding Serology in Viral Hepatitis

Hepatitis Marker	Abbreviation	Meaning
A antibody (IgM)	Anti-HAV (IgM)	Recent hepatitis A infection
B surface antigen	HbsAg	Infection with HBV (acute or chronic)
B surface antibody	anti-HBs	Clinical recovery from HBV (protective)
B core antibody	anti-HBc	Active HBV infection (acute–chronic)
	anti-HBc (IgM)	Active HBV infection
B e antigen	HBeAg	Active HBV infection, high infectivity (> 6–8 weeks suggests chronic carrier)
B e antibody	anti-HBe	Resolving infection
B virus DNA	HBV DNA	Active HBV infection (high levels of infectivity)
C virus RNA	HCV RNA	Transfusion-related non-A, non-B is detectable in serum or liver by PCR; confirms infection with HCV
C virus antibody	anti-HCV	Present in acute and chronic infection (not protective—up to 12 months to seroconvert)
Delta antigen	HD Ag	Acute HDV infection
Delta antibody	anti-HDV	Exposure to HDV; may transmit infection

PCR = polymerase chain reaction.

3. **Prognosis.** The prognosis is excellent for full recovery from nonfulminant hepatitis A. Chronic active or chronic persistent hepatitis develop in 5% of patients with hepatitis B.

4. **Prevention**
   a. **Hepatitis A.** Family members, children, and staff exposed at day care centers, as well as their sexual contacts, should receive immune globulin (0.02 ml/kg) within 2 weeks of contact. A formalin-inactivated vaccine is still being tested but appears to be extremely effective at preventing infection with hepatitis A in endemic areas.
   b. **Hepatitis B**
      (1) **Hepatitis B immune globulin (HBIG).** People who have had sexual, percutaneous, or mucosal exposure should receive HBIG (0.06 ml/kg) plus full vaccination. The dose of HBIG should be repeated in 1 month.
      (2) **Hepatitis B vaccine** is a recombinant yeast-derived vaccine, is effective in infants as well as in older children, and has few side effects. The vaccine is recommended for residents and staff of institutions for the retarded, family contacts of chronic carriers, and other high-risk populations, including all health care workers engaged in patient care or in contact with laboratory specimens from patients, seronegative homosexual men, intravenous drug abusers, prisoners, dialysis patients, and recipients of high-risk blood products (e.g., hemophiliacs).
      (3) **Prophylaxis in infants.** All infants born in the United States should be immunized against hepatitis B (see Chapter 1). Infants of women who are serum HBsAg positive in the third trimester of pregnancy, especially if they are also HBeAg positive, should also receive 0.5 ml HBIG within 12 hours of birth. With the proper and timely administration of HBIG and hepatitis B vaccine, 90% of the cases of chronic HBV infection that would have resulted from perinatal transmission can be prevented.
      (4) **Postexposure prophylaxis.** Hepatitis B vaccine is also recommended for sexual contacts of HBsAg-positive individuals, those exposed to HBsAg-positive blood via needlestick exposure, and individuals infused with high-risk blood products. Accelerated induction of protective antibody levels may be facilitated by an accelerated vaccine schedule of injections at 0, 2, and 6 weeks postexposure.
      (5) **Booster doses.** Antibodies to HBsAg (anti-HBs) that are generated by exposure to the vaccine appear to diminish with time. Long-term studies of children and

adults indicate protection against chronic HBV infection for 10 years or more, even though anti-HBs concentrations may become low. At present, routine booster doses of vaccine are not recommended, except for people continuously exposed to hepatitis B (e.g., health care workers) and for immunocompromised patients (e.g., hemodialysis patients, those with human immunodeficiency virus infection).

D. **Fulminant hepatitis** is severe acute hepatitis resulting in progressive liver failure and hepatic encephalopathy.

1. Etiology
  a. Viral infection. Fulminant hepatitis may follow any of the hepatitis viral infections described earlier. **Hepatitis A** is the most common cause of fulminant hepatitis in children reported from underdeveloped countries. **Hepatitis B** is an uncommon cause but is usually seen in infants of HBsAg-positive, anti-HBe–positive mothers, or in children exposed to blood products from donors with that same serologic profile. **Delta hepatitis** infection superimposed on chronic hepatitis B may convert a stable or chronic persistent hepatitis B patient to one with severe chronic active or even fulminant hepatitis. **Hepatitis E** is particularly virulent in pregnant women, causing fulminant hepatitis in approximately 20% of cases. Other important viral causes of fulminant hepatitis in infancy include echovirus, herpes virus, cytomegalovirus, and Epstein-Barr virus.
  b. Metabolic causes. Tyrosinemia, galactosemia, hereditary fructose intolerance, neonatal iron-storage liver disease, α_1-antitrypsin deficiency, Zellweger syndrome, and disorders of fatty acid oxidation in the neonate may lead to fulminant hepatic failure. Wilson disease, α_1-antitrypsin deficiency, cystic fibrosis, Niemann-Pick disease, and glycogen storage disease (type IV) may lead to this condition in the older child.
  c. Hepatotoxic drugs can cause fulminant hepatic failure by overdosage (e.g., acetaminophen), through a genetic proclivity to slow metabolism (e.g., isoniazid), or through an idiosyncratic hypersensitivity reaction to a normal dose of the drug (e.g., halothane, phenytoin). In some patients, valproic acid is converted to toxic metabolites, which disrupt various intramitochondrial pathways resulting in hyperammonemia, hypoglycemia, and hepatic steatosis and failure.
  d. Plant toxins also have been implicated (e.g., *Amanita phalloides* mushrooms).

2. Clinical features
  a. Early symptoms include persistent anorexia and fever, progressive jaundice, and mental status changes.
  b. On sequential **physical examinations,** a shrinking liver size despite a worsening clinical status may be noted, as may be hyperventilation and the development of ascites.
  c. Laboratory tests reflect hepatic failure, indicated by vitamin K-resistant coagulopathy, hypoglycemia, hypokalemia, hypoalbuminemia, low blood urea nitrogen, low cholesterol, and high blood ammonia levels.
  d. Central nervous system signs. Agitation, stupor, and eventually coma with diffuse slowing of activity on electroencephalogram are seen.

3. Complications
  a. Gastrointestinal bleeding
  b. Secondary bacterial or fungal infection
  c. Renal dysfunction
  d. Increased intracranial pressure (ICP)

4. Therapy. The use of sedatives (especially benzodiazepines) and barbiturates should be avoided.
  a. Supportive care consists of:
    (1) Maintenance of fluid and electrolyte balance with correction of hyponatremia and hypokalemia

      (2) Correction of hypoglycemia, hypokalemia, and hypophosphatemia

      (3) Administration of H_2-receptor antagonists to prevent upper gastrointestinal bleeding and the use of fresh frozen plasma to correct clotting abnormalities when there is clinical evidence of bleeding

      (4) Endotracheal intubation and assisted ventilation as required by deepening coma and to hyperventilate the patient to reduce cerebral blood flow and ICP.

      (5) Treatment of ICP, including ICP monitoring and the use of mannitol

  b. Measures to minimize encephalopathy. Treatment involves measures to lower serum ammonia levels by decreasing protein available as substrate and eliminating ammonia-producing bacteria in the bowel, including:

      (1) Restriction of oral and intravenous protein

      (2) Use of cathartics

      (3) Oral or nasogastric administration of neomycin or lactulose

  c. Heroic measures. Interventions such as plasmapheresis, exchange transfusion, charcoal hemoperfusion, and dialysis alone have not improved survival rates. However, as adjunctive measures to stabilize and maintain a patient before liver transplantation, they appear to have a definite role.

  d. Liver transplantation. Children with fulminant hepatic failure have been transplanted with a 50%–60% survival rate. This compares favorably with the 20%–40% survival rate previously obtained with intensive conservative management.

E.   **Chronic hepatitis** can be defined as an inflammatory process of the liver lasting longer than 6 months. The distinction between chronic persistent and chronic active hepatitis is made pathologically.

  1. Chronic persistent hepatitis

    a. Pathology. The inflammatory reaction is limited to the portal zone, and there is little or no fibrosis.

    b. Etiology. Chronic persistent hepatitis is usually the result of persistent hepatitis B, hepatitis C, or some other unknown virus.

    c. Clinical features. Malaise or anorexia, which fails to resolve after a bout of acute hepatitis, is common. There may be mild hepatomegaly.

    d. Laboratory findings. Usually, the only abnormality is a mild elevation of the serum aminotransferase levels.

    e. Prognosis. The prognosis for complete resolution without treatment is very good. Only rarely is there progression to chronic active hepatitis.

  2. Chronic active hepatitis

    a. Pathology. The inflammatory reaction is not limited to the portal area, and fibrosis may occur in areas of necrosis.

    b. Etiology. In addition to viral infection, chronic active hepatitis may be caused by drugs or associated with Wilson disease or inflammatory bowel disease. Some cases are idiopathic or ascribed to autoimmune mechanisms.

    c. Clinical features. Almost all patients have jaundice and hepatosplenomegaly. Ascites, digital clubbing, cutaneous stigmata of chronic liver disease (spider angioma, prominent abdominal wall venous pattern), and arthritis or glomerulonephritis also may occur.

    d. Laboratory findings

      (1) The serum bilirubin level is elevated but is usually less than 5 mg/dl. The serum aminotransferase levels are typically elevated at least 10-fold. Of the plasma proteins, serum albumin is low and gamma globulin is elevated. The erythrocyte sedimentation rate is likewise increased.

      (2) About 25% of patients have detectable levels of serum HBsAg. Serum HBsAg-negative patients may have antinuclear antibodies, anti-smooth muscle antibodies, anti-liver–kidney microsomal antibodies, or other serologic evidence of autoimmune disease. It is important to test for anti-HCV or HCV RNA in the serum to rule out hepatitis C as a cause.

      (3) Hypersplenism may result in anemia, leukopenia, and thrombocytopenia.

e. Therapy and prognosis

(1) Until recently, there was no effective therapy for HBsAg-positive or anti-HCV–positive patients with chronic hepatitis.

(a) **Hepatitis B.** Treatment with recombinant interferon-α, either alone or after a brief course of prednisone, results in a disappearance of viral markers of replication and infectivity and normalization of aminotransferases in approximately 50% of patients with chronic hepatitis B. Long-term follow-up reveals that some of these patients relapse after therapy, but about one third of patients treated achieve a sustained response.

(b) For patients with **hepatitis C,** the initial response is equivalent but the relapse rate is very high.

(2) About 75% of HBsAg-negative, anti-HCV–negative patients (presumed autoimmune chronic active hepatitis) have a biochemical response to prednisone or a combination of prednisone and azathioprine. The 5-year survival rate is approximately 70%.

(3) **Liver transplantation** may be necessary in patients in whom cirrhosis develops, with its attendant complications (e.g., portal hypertension, esophageal varices, ascites, liver failure).

F. **Metabolic liver disease.** The metabolic diseases affecting liver function are numerous and varied in presentation. For example, α_1-antitrypsin deficiency can present in neonates as cholestasis and in the older child as cirrhosis. The remainder of this section focuses on two metabolic liver diseases of particular importance to the pediatrician: namely, α_1-antitrypsin deficiency and Wilson disease.

1. α_1-Antitrypsin deficiency

a. Pathogenesis

(1) α_1-Antitrypsin is a **serum protease inhibitor** synthesized in the liver. Codominant alleles dictate the type and concentration of α_1-antitrypsin inherited.

(2) **Deficiency** of α_1-antitrypsin results from homozygous inheritance of the z-type α_1-antitrypsin gene. This results in low serum α_1-antitrypsin levels and an abnormally slow-moving protein (PiZZ protein) on acid–starch electrophoresis compared with the normal protein.

(3) **Liver disease** results from a defect in secretion of the PiZZ protein and accumulation of abnormal α_1-antitrypsin in hepatocytes.

b. Clinical features

(1) About 5%–10% of PiZZ individuals have neonatal cholestasis. Jaundice resolves in most cases. Occasionally, severe disease causes death in the **first year of life**. Breast-feeding in early infancy appears to confer some protection against liver damage owing to inherent antiproteases in human breast milk.

(2) **Older infants and children** may present with failure to thrive, hepatomegaly, or cirrhosis.

(3) In the **adolescent and adult,** the deficiency may cause early pulmonary disease (emphysema), cirrhosis, and hepatocellular carcinoma.

c. Diagnosis

(1) There are **low serum levels of α_1-antitrypsin** (usually less than 100 mg/dl) and an abnormal protein phenotype (PiZZ).

(2) Liver biopsy shows characteristic eosinophilic cytoplasmic granules in periportal hepatocytes.

2. Wilson disease (see also Chapter 18 IX B 1) is a treatable autosomal recessive disorder that should be considered in the differential diagnosis of any liver disease in the school-age child.

a. Pathogenesis. Organ damage is the result of toxicity from copper deposition. Although levels of the copper-binding protein ceruloplasmin are low in 95% of patients, the exact mechanism underlying Wilson disease is not known.

b. Clinical features. Wilson disease has many unusual modes of presentation, and there often is a delay in diagnosis.

    (1) Liver disease is the primary mode of presentation in pediatric patients. Liver disease rarely is clinically evident before 5 years of age. The presentation may include an episode of acute hepatitis, fulminant hepatitis, chronic hepatitis, or cirrhosis.

    (2) Neurologic symptoms (e.g., tremor, dysarthria, loss of fine motor control, seizures) usually occur when the child is older than 10 years of age. Personality changes may be striking.

    (3) Coombs-negative hemolytic anemia occurs.

    (4) There is **renal involvement,** usually a Fanconi-like syndrome.

    (5) Corneal deposition of copper causes the formation of characteristic Kayser-Fleischer rings.

c. Diagnosis

    (1) Kayser-Fleischer rings are pathognomonic when present (a slit lamp may be required to see them).

    (2) The **ceruloplasmin level usually is low** in Wilson disease, but it may be low in other disorders as well. A level exceeding 30 mg/dl excludes Wilson disease.

    (3) Patients with Wilson disease have elevated urinary copper excretion (> 100 μg/24 hours).

    (4) Quantification of liver copper by biopsy demonstrates levels greater than 250 μg/g dry weight.

    (5) Studies of incorporation of radioactive copper into ceruloplasmin occasionally are necessary if other tests fail to distinguish Wilson disease from other disorders with elevated concentrations of hepatic copper and urine copper excretion.

d. Therapy

    (1) Dietary restrictions. Chocolate, nuts, shellfish, mushrooms, and other foods rich in copper should be avoided.

    (2) Life-long treatment with chelating agents is necessary. Such agents include D-penicillamine, trientine (if penicillamine is not tolerated), and oral zinc (to reduce intestinal copper absorption and help maintain negative copper balance).

e. Prognosis. The prognosis is excellent with early treatment. However, fulminant hepatitis continues to be associated with a poor prognosis.

G. **Reye syndrome** is characterized by encephalopathy and acute liver dysfunction, with fatty infiltration of the liver and kidney in individuals who are usually between 2 and 16 years of age. The incidence has dropped dramatically in the last 8 years, corresponding to the association of the disease with aspirin ingestion and subsequent warnings.

1. Etiology

    a. Reye syndrome may follow a viral infection, typically influenza or varicella.

    b. Rarely, it has been associated with toxins, including aflatoxin B_1 (from a fungus) and hypoglycin A (from unripe akee fruit).

2. Pathophysiology. A basic defect in energy metabolism on a cellular level exists. Electron micrographs demonstrate a derangement of mitochondria.

3. Clinical features

    a. After an apparent viral illness, vomiting develops.

    b. Subsequently, mental status changes occur (e.g., confusion and agitation, then stupor and coma).

    c. Infants may have seizures or apneic episodes.

4. Diagnosis

    a. Serum tests. Serum aminotransferase levels always are elevated. Serum ammonia levels usually are elevated, and the prothrombin time is prolonged. The bilirubin is usually less than 3 mg/dl.

    b. Liver biopsy reveals microvesicular fat but no acute inflammatory reaction. Oil Red-O staining of the liver biopsy specimen may be necessary to recognize the microvesicular fat in hepatocytes.

c. Differential diagnosis

    (1) Other causes of central nervous system dysfunction (e.g., meningitis, toxic ingestion) must be excluded.

    (2) Inborn errors of metabolism, including urea cycle defects and defects in fatty acid oxidation, can be confused with Reye syndrome, particularly in infants and young children.

5. Therapy for Reye syndrome is supportive. Increased ICP must be monitored and treated aggressively.

6. Prognosis. The overall fatality rate is approximately 20%. Rapid progression to deeper levels of coma and an ammonia level greater than 300 mg/dl imply a poor prognosis.

H. | **Liver transplantation.** Orthotopic liver transplantation has become the accepted therapy for end-stage liver disease and metabolic liver disease in children. More than 500 pediatric liver transplants were performed in the United States in the 1980s.

1. Major indications for liver transplantation in children include:
    a. Biliary atresia (particularly after an unsuccessful Kasai procedure)
    b. α_1-Antitrypsin deficiency
    c. Tyrosinemia, Wilson disease, and other inborn errors of metabolism
    d. Cryptogenic cirrhosis and chronic active hepatitis
    e. Fulminant hepatitis

2. Postoperative management. Chronic immunosuppression with cyclosporine, prednisone, and azathioprine is necessary to prevent rejection.

3. Prognosis. Five-year survival rates are approximately 70%.

4. Long-term complications of liver transplantation and chronic immunosuppression include:
    a. Nephrotoxicity and hypertension
    b. Susceptibility to infection, including viral (e.g., Epstein-Barr virus, cytomegalovirus), *Pneumocystis carinii*, bacterial, and fungal infections
    c. Biliary strictures, obstruction, or leak
    d. Predisposition to malignancy, especially lymphoma and lymphoproliferative syndromes
    e. Growth impairment if high doses of corticosteroids are required

X. DISORDERS OF THE PANCREAS

A. | **Pancreatic insufficiency**

1. Cystic fibrosis is the major cause of pancreatic insufficiency in the United States, Canada, and western Europe. The general aspects of cystic fibrosis and its pulmonary complications are discussed in Chapter 13 IV. The following discussion focuses on pancreatic insufficiency and other gastrointestinal manifestations of cystic fibrosis.

a. Pancreatic disease due to cystic fibrosis

    (1) Pancreatic insufficiency. Of patients with cystic fibrosis, 85%–90% have evidence of exocrine pancreatic dysfunction.

        (a) Pathogenesis. Abnormally viscid pancreatic secretions lead to plugging of ducts and eventual autodigestion of ducts and acinar tissue.

        (b) Clinical features

            (i) Malnutrition and failure to thrive may begin in the first few months of life.

            (ii) Steatorrhea occurs, and stools are bulky, foul-smelling, and pale and greasy in appearance.

            (iii) Complications due to malabsorption of fat-soluble vitamins or calcium may occur (e.g., hemorrhagic diathesis, rickets, neurologic abnormalities).

            (c) Diagnosis is made on the basis of the following:
                (i) Quantitative determination of fecal fat excretion
                (ii) Duodenal intubation and pancreozymin–secretin stimulation to assay enzymes and bicarbonate produced by the pancreas
                (iii) New tests using artificial substrates of pancreatic enzymes
            (d) Therapy (see Chapter 13) consists of:
                (i) Pancreatic extracts given before meals to supplement enzyme activity
                (ii) A balanced but high-caloric diet
        (2) Pancreatitis may recur in some patients who retain some pancreatic exocrine function.
      b. Other gastrointestinal and hepatic disorders associated with cystic fibrosis
        (1) Meconium ileus presenting with neonatal intestinal obstruction due to abnormal meconium [see Chapter 13 IV C 2 c (1)]
        (2) Intestinal impaction in older children (distal intestinal obstruction syndrome)
        (3) Intussusception
        (4) Rectal prolapse
        (5) Liver disease, including neonatal cholestatic syndrome, fatty liver, and focal biliary fibrosis (in older children), which may progress to biliary cirrhosis
        (6) Abnormal gallbladder function and cholelithiasis

   2. Other conditions associated with pancreatic insufficiency include:
      a. Malnutrition, which is the most common cause of childhood pancreatic insufficiency worldwide
      b. Shwachman-Diamond syndrome (pancreatic insufficiency and bone marrow dysfunction)
      c. Isolated enzyme defects

B. | Pancreatitis

   1. Etiology. A variety of factors may lead to activation of pancreatic enzymes, causing autodigestion and inflammation of the pancreas. Such factors include:
      a. Abdominal trauma (or surgery)
      b. Infections (e.g., mumps and other viruses, mycoplasmas)
      c. Biliary obstruction
      d. Congenital anomalies of the pancreatic ducts (e.g., pancreas divisum)
      e. Drugs
      f. Systemic diseases (e.g., collagen vascular disease, hyperlipidemia, hypercalcemia)
      g. Cystic fibrosis
      h. Penetrating duodenal ulcer
      i. Metabolic abnormalities (e.g., organic acidemias)
      j. Unidentified factors (30% of cases are idiopathic, some of these factors may be familial)

   2. Clinical features
      a. More than 75% of patients have **epigastric pain,** which may radiate to the back and is frequently exacerbated by eating.
      b. Nausea and vomiting are common.
      c. On examination, the abdomen is **slightly distended** and is **tender** on palpation. Bowel sounds are diminished.
      d. Severe cases may result in **shock.**

   3. Diagnosis
      a. The serum amylase and lipase levels are usually elevated. However, normal values do not exclude the diagnosis.
      b. Abdominal ultrasound may demonstrate pancreatic edema in some cases.

   4. Complications include:
      a. Hypocalcemia
      b. Hyperglycemia

    c. Pseudocyst formation, which occurs in 5% of patients and is heralded by an epigastric mass and recurrent pain (pseudocysts are easily detected and monitored by ultrasound)

    d. Pancreatic phlegmon, with a potential for secondary bacterial infection and abscess formation

    e. Peritonitis

5. Therapy is aimed at minimizing pancreatic stimulation and includes:

    a. Nothing by mouth

    b. Nasogastric suction for patients with persistent vomiting secondary to ileus

    c. Administration of adequate intravenous fluids and electrolytes with appropriate hemodynamic monitoring of patients with severe cases

    d. Meperidine for pain

    e. With recovery, gradual introduction of a high-carbohydrate, low-fat diet

    f. Surgical drainage, which eventually may be needed for pseudocysts

6. Prognosis

    a. Fulminant hemorrhagic pancreatitis has a high mortality rate.

    b. Episodes may recur if the cause is not identified and remedied.

BIBLIOGRAPHY

Balistreri WF: Acute and chronic viral hepatitis. In *Liver Disease in Children.* Edited by Suchy F. St. Louis, Mosby, 1994, pp 460–509.

Drumm B, Rhoads JM, Stringer DA, et al: Peptic ulcer disease in children: Etiology, clinical findings, and clinical course. *Pediatrics* 82:410–414, 1988.

Hyams J, Leichtner A, Schwartz A: Recent advances in the diagnosis and treatment of gastrointestinal hemorrhage in infants and children. *J Pediatr* 106:1–9, 1985.

Murray MS: Constipation. In *Pediatric Gastrointestinal Disease: Pathophysiology, Diagnosis, Management.* Edited by Walker W, Durie P, Hamilton J, et al. Philadelphia, BC Decker, 1991, pp 90–110.

Orenstein SR: Gastroesophageal reflux. In *Pediatric Gastrointestinal Disease: Pathophysiology, Diagnosis, Management.* Edited by Wyllie R, Hyams JS. Philadelphia, WB Saunders, 1993, pp 337–369.

Podolsky DK: Inflammatory bowel disease. *N Engl J Med* 325:928–937, 1008–1016, 1991.

Treem WR: Jaundice. In *Pediatric Primary Care: A Problem-Oriented Approach,* 2nd ed. Edited by Schwartz W, Charney EB, Curry TA, Ludwig S. Chicago, Year Book, 1990, pp 257–266.

DIRECTIONS: Each of the numbered items or incomplete statements in this section is followed by answers or by completions of the statement. Select the ONE lettered answer or completion that is BEST in each case.

1. A 28-month-old boy presents with increasing irritability, decreased appetite, and an episode of vomiting with streaks of red blood in the emesis. He underwent repair of a tracheoesophageal fistula and esophageal atresia in his first year of life. The physical examination is unremarkable. The patient swallows barium, and there is no evidence of an esophageal stricture at the level of the prior esophageal anastomosis. Which of the following diagnoses is most likely in this child?

(A) Gastric ulcer
(B) Esophageal varices
(C) Peptic esophagitis
(D) An unknown caustic ingestion
(E) Achalasia

2. A severely mentally retarded 12-year-old boy with cerebral palsy and a seizure disorder is brought to your office from his residential home because of an inability to swallow solids and increased vomiting, choking, and gagging. Before this visit, he had been on a regular diet but is now able to take only pureed foods. His physical examination is unremarkable, but his initial laboratory data show a hematocrit of 31%; a mean corpuscular volume of 67, with a normal white blood cell and platelet count, and stool that is positive for occult blood. Which of the following tests is most appropriate for discovering this child's problem?

(A) Hemoglobin electrophoresis followed by a bone marrow examination
(B) Prolonged intraesophageal pH probe and gastric emptying scan
(C) Esophageal and anal manometry
(D) Barium swallow (upper gastrointestinal series) and upper gastrointestinal endoscopy
(E) Iron and total iron-binding capacity

3. An 11-month-old female infant is admitted for the third time with wheezing without fever or coryza. The mother relates that the first episode occurred at 2 months of age and that each of the episodes has started abruptly. She has noted some nocturnal cough on the nights before the admissions. The baby is growing and gaining weight on a cow's milk protein formula, and although she did a lot of spitting earlier, now seems to be resolving this problem. There is no family history of hay fever, asthma, or eczema. On each of the two prior occasions, the child has partially responded to bronchodilator therapy, but has continued to wheeze mildly in between episodes. Physical examination is unremarkable except for some coarse rhonchi bilaterally and expiratory wheezing. The stool is negative for occult blood and the complete blood count does not show peripheral eosinophilia. The chest radiograph shows mild hyperinflation of both lung fields but no infiltrates. The most likely explanation for these recurrent bouts of wheezing is

(A) gastroesophageal reflux
(B) cow's milk protein allergy
(C) aspirated foreign body
(D) tracheoesophageal fistula
(E) cystic fibrosis

4. A 3-year-old child is brought to the emergency department after being found with a lye-containing, hair-straightening cream on his hands, face, and lips. He is crying, drooling, and has erythematous patches noted on his lips, buccal mucosa, and soft palate. Although frightened, he does not appear to be in respiratory distress and has no stridor. His mother has given him water to drink before coming to the emergency department. Which of the following actions is most appropriate?

(A) Perform an immediate barium swallow
(B) Induce vomiting
(C) Prepare the child for an upper gastrointestinal endoscopy within 12–24 hours
(D) Order an immediate chest radiograph
(E) Give a bolus of intravenous corticosteroids

5. A 4-month-old male infant is admitted to the intensive care unit with bloody diarrhea, vomiting, fever, and shock. He had been breast-fed and was doing well, until his 2-month check-up, when his mother noted that he was having only one bowel movement every 5–7 days. One week before admission, he was noted to be distended, and his usual postprandial spit-up turned to intermittent, frank vomiting. After not having a bowel movement for 10 days, the infant began having loose, frequent, mucus-filled bowel movements, which turned bloody 1 day before admission. After bloody diarrhea and frequent bilious vomiting for 24 hours, he was admitted with a sunken anterior fontanelle, cool extremities, poor perfusion, and a markedly distended abdomen. His temperature was 103.1° F. A complete blood count showed a white blood cell count of 2300 with 58 polymorphonuclear leukocytes, 30 bands, and 2 metamyelocytes; his platelet count was 64,000. A flat plate of his abdomen showed markedly distended air-filled loops of intestine, including both small intestine and colon. Which of the following diagnoses is the most likely cause of this infant's sepsis and shock?

(A) Enterocolitis secondary to Hirschsprung disease
(B) *Salmonella* enterocolitis
(C) Hemolytic–uremic syndrome
(D) Intussusception
(E) A mid-gut volvulus

6. An 8-week-old male infant presents with jaundice. He was born a full-term, appropriate for gestational age infant who went home on day 5 of life, after spending 2 days undergoing phototherapy for a total bilirubin of 13.8 mg/dl. His bilirubin when discharged was 9.5 mg/dl. At the 2-week check-up, the infant was still jaundiced, but the jaundice was attributed to breast-feeding. Weight gain was appropriate. The infant next returned at 2 months of age. By then, the jaundice had deepened, the stools were noted to be pale green or clay colored, and the urine was dark. Although the infant had grown and still appeared vigorous, the liver was enlarged with a firm, sharp edge, and the spleen was palpable 3 cm below the left costal margin. Laboratory tests revealed total bilirubin of 14.5 mg/dl, direct bilirubin of 8.8 mg/dl, aspartate aminotransferase was 243 IU/L, alanine aminotransferase was 184 IU/L, γ-glutamyl transferase was 487 IU/L (normal is up to 40 IU/L), and reducing sugars were absent from the urine. An abdominal ultrasound showed a small gallbladder, no gallstones, no choledochal cysts, and no dilated intrahepatic bile ducts. A radionuclide biliary imaging study showed concentration in the liver but no excretion into the gallbladder or small intestine. Which of the following steps is most appropriate?

(A) Stop breast-feeding, send the baby home, and recheck the bilirubin in 4 weeks
(B) Check the hepatitis B serologies of the infant and the mother
(C) Test the serum for α_1-antitrypsin deficiency and await the results
(D) Check the prothrombin and partial thromboplastin times; if they are normal, perform an immediate percutaneous liver biopsy
(E) Test the serum for galactose-1-uridyl transferase, which is the defective enzyme in galactosemia

7. A 9-month-old Vietnamese girl adopted at 4 months of age is referred to a pediatrician by her family physician because of elevated liver enzymes. The infant has been well, has never received a blood transfusion, is growing well, is not jaundiced, and has no palpable liver or spleen. Her aspartate aminotransferase level is 84 IU/L, her alanine aminotransferase level is 66 IU/L, her bilirubin is normal, and her γ-glutamyl transferase level is 55 U/L (normal is 0–45 U/L). There is no accompanying medical history from Vietnam and no information about the biologic parents. Tests most likely to yield valuable information about the etiology of this infant's elevated aminotransferases include which of the following?

(A) Anti-hepatitis C virus (HCV) and HCV RNA
(B) Anti-hepatitis A virus (HAV) immunoglobulin M (IgM)
(C) Serum copper and ceruloplasmin
(D) Sweat test
(E) Hepatitis B surface antigen (HBsAg), anti-hepatitis B surface antigen (anti-HBs), anti-hepatitis B core antigen (anti-HBc) IgM

8. A sexually active 17-year-old boy comes to the clinic asking for a test for acquired immune deficiency syndrome (AIDS). On further questioning, he admits to being sexually promiscuous and to having intercourse with multiple partners in the last 6 months. He vehemently denies intravenous drug use but does say that he "hangs out" with several girls who use intravenous drugs. One of his previous sexual partners recently became ill and was diagnosed with acute hepatitis B. In addition to testing this adolescent for hepatitis B and hepatitis C, the physician should take which of the following actions?

(A) Give hepatitis B immune globulin (HBIG) and initiate the hepatitis B vaccine series immediately
(B) Screen for elevations in aminotransferases and follow the patient's liver enzymes for the next 6 months
(C) Test the patient for human immunodeficiency virus and inform him of the results
(D) Give HBIG alone
(E) Wait for all the serology results before deciding whether to give immunoprophylaxis

9. A 4-week-old male infant presents with a 2-week history of increasing vomiting and poor weight gain. The vomiting, often projectile in nature, has persisted despite multiple formula changes. Blood-tinged emesis has been noted for the past 24 hours. Stools have been firm and passed every other day. Physical examination reveals a thin, irritable infant with a flat abdomen. A firm, olive-shaped mass is noted in the right hypochondrium. Which of the following laboratory studies should be performed first?

(A) Radiograph of the abdomen
(B) Abdominal ultrasound
(C) Upper gastrointestinal contrast radiography
(D) Serum electrolyte evaluation
(E) Complete blood count

10. A 15-year-old girl presents with recent persistent epigastric abdominal pain and vomiting. She states that the pain is burning in nature and is made worse by eating. It awakens her from her sleep. She has lost 5 pounds. No hematemesis or melena have been noted. She takes ibuprofen for menstrual cramps. Family history is positive for peptic disease. Upper gastrointestinal endoscopy reveals diffuse nodular antral gastritis but no ulceration.

In this patient, gastric antral mucosal biopsies most likely reveal which of the following results?

(A) Intense eosinophilic infiltration
(B) Granuloma
(C) Gram-negative curved bacilli
(D) Vasculitis
(E) G-cell hyperplasia

DIRECTIONS: This set of matching questions consists of a list of five lettered options followed by four numbered items. For each numbered item, select the ONE lettered option that is most closely associated with it. Each lettered option may be selected once, more than once, or not at all.

Questions 11–14

For each clinical presentation of lower gastrointestinal bleeding, select the most likely diagnosis.

(A) Eosinophilic colitis
(B) Hemolytic–uremic syndrome
(C) Ulcerative colitis
(D) Juvenile polyps
(E) Meckel diverticulum

11. A 6-year-old with streaks of bright red blood on the side of normal-formed stool and drops of bright red blood in the toilet, but no complaints of abdominal or rectal pain

12. A 3-year-old with bloody diarrhea, crampy abdominal pain, a low hematocrit, and a low platelet count

13. A 6-week-old with scant streaks of red blood mixed with normal stool

14. An 18-month-old with large amounts of melanotic stool who is anemic and in shock but has no history of diarrhea

1. The answer is C *[II A 2; Table 11-1).* Children who have undergone repair of tracheo-esophageal fistula and esophageal atresia all have some degree of gastroesophageal reflux. If not prophylactically treated, many of them will have complications of gastroesophageal reflux, especially peptic esophagitis secondary to chronic reflux. The occurrence of this problem is often signaled by nonspecific signs (e.g., irritability, anorexia, failure to thrive), than by more specific findings (e.g., vomiting, hematemesis, iron-deficiency anemia, and occult blood in the stool). Toddlers do not complain of such classic symptoms as heartburn, dysphagia, or chest pain. Chronic vomiting is not always present before the discovery of peptic esophagitis.

Of the other choices, only gastric ulcer and caustic ingestion may be associated with blood-streaked emesis. Esophageal varices bleed more profusely. Caustic ingestions can result in the above symptoms, but they would be acute and often associated with drooling, inability to swallow, and oropharyngeal burns. Gastric ulcers can cause these symptoms, but in the setting of tracheoesophageal fistula repair, one should always be aware of chronic gastroesophageal reflux as a long-term complication.

2. The answer is D *[II A 3].* This child has an esophageal stricture most likely caused by chronic peptic esophagitis secondary to gastroesophageal reflux. Children with severe spasticity and neurologic handicaps are at greater risk for chronic unremitting gastroesophageal reflux and the development of significant complications associated with reflux. The barium swallow is the best test for outlining the anatomy of the esophagus and defining both the tightness and location of the stricture. Peptic strictures tend to be in the distal third of the esophagus, close to the gastroesophageal junction. An upper gastrointestinal endoscopy with biopsy is important both to document the expected findings in peptic esophagitis and to rule out other causes of esophagitis and stricture. It is also used to ascertain whether the patient has developed the histologic changes consistent with Barrett esophagus. The metaplastic change seen with Barrett esophagus increases the risk of adenocarcinoma of the esophagus and usually indicates the need for consideration of antireflux surgery. A prolonged intraesophageal pH probe is a very useful test to document chronic gastroesopha-

geal reflux. However, acid may not reflux above a tight stricture, and the probe may not easily pass below the stricture. Esophageal manometry is the procedure of choice when trying to diagnose a primary motility disorder of the esophagus such as achalasia.

3. The answer is A *[II A 2; Table 11-1].* Typical features of reflux-induced bronchospasm are: (1) young age at onset; (2) abrupt onset of wheezing without environmental triggers such as cold, exercise, or viral infection; (3) no family history of atopy; (4) nocturnal cough, which may signal reflux with microaspiration of stomach contents; and (5) poor or incomplete response to bronchodilators. The chest radiograph may show only nonspecific changes of bronchospasm because microaspiration of stomach contents often results in little or no pulmonary parenchymal inflammatory changes. Also, the bronchospasm may be mediated by increased vagal tone secondary to acidification of the distal esophagus and not necessarily by direct contact of the refluxate with the bronchi. At 11 months of age, pulmonary parenchymal disease and lung infiltrates would be expected in children with tracheoesophageal fistula (where the wheezing and coughing should be related to feeding) as well as with cystic fibrosis. In addition, the lack of diarrhea and the adequate growth mitigate against cystic fibrosis. A previously aspirated foreign body should have resulted in atelectasis or bronchopneumonia and asymmetric findings in both the examination and the chest radiograph. Cow's milk protein allergy might be expected to be found in a child with a strong family history of allergy, heme-positive stools, eczema, peripheral eosinophilia, and chronic vomiting and diarrhea.

4. The answer is C *[II D 1].* The most important piece of information needed in any case of ingestion of caustic material is the presence and extent of mucosal burns to the upper gastrointestinal tract, particularly the esophagus. This can be reliably obtained only by performing an upper gastrointestinal endoscopy. The absence of burns in the mouth or oropharynx should not exclude performing this examination, because patients can have esophageal mucosal burns without face, lip, or oropharyngeal pathology. The presence and degree of esophageal and gastric mucosal damage dictates the management, including whether the patient is allowed to drink or eat, whether the patient needs parenteral nutrition, and whether treatment with corticosteroids or antibiotics is considered. The decision as to whether a follow-up barium study is necessary to screen for the possibility of stricture formation can be made when the presence and degree of mucosal damage is determined. Vomiting should never be induced in patients who ingested a caustic substance. Diluting the caustic substance with water is a good idea, but then endoscopy must be delayed until the stomach is empty. A barium study is not an appropriate initial examination, but may be useful several weeks later to determine whether there is stricture formation. A chest radiograph is important if an esophageal perforation and mediastinitis are suspected.

5. The answer is A *[VIII E].* Although there is a wide range of normal frequency of bowel movements in breast-fed infants, one bowel movement every 5–7 days is considered outside the range of normal and should raise suspicions of a gastrointestinal problem. Infants with Hirschsprung disease may escape detection for several months or years if the segment of aganglionic bowel is relatively short. The most drastic presentation of Hirschsprung disease in infancy is with enterocolitis and sepsis, as exemplified by this infant. Sepsis is most likely the result of chronic stasis and bacterial overgrowth in the distended, functionally obstructed colon, with seeding of the blood with enteric flora. The abdominal radiographs in this case could be consistent with either an ileus or a low (colonic) gastrointestinal obstruction.

Salmonella enterocolitis can present with bloody diarrhea, sepsis, and shock in infants but would not account for the previous abnormal infrequent bowel movements or abdominal distention noted in this infant. Both intussusception and mid-gut volvulus might present with bilious vomiting, distention, sepsis, and shock, but should show a pattern of small-bowel obstruction, which does not include a dilated colon on the abdominal plain film. Hemolytic–uremic syndrome can present with bloody diarrhea and thrombocytopenia, but rarely with septic shock, and rarely in an infant this age.

6. The answer is D *[IX B; Table 11-7].* Direct hyperbilirubinemia in an infant is a medical emergency and must be investigated without delay because of the possibility of an obstructive biliary tract lesion, such as biliary atresia

or a choledochal cyst. If bile flow from the liver to the intestine is not reestablished by 8 weeks of age, the damage may already be extensive and the liver may already be cirrhotic. Infants with biliary atresia may have a rudimentary gallbladder not in continuity with the liver or intestine, and thus the presence of a gallbladder seen on the ultrasound does not rule out biliary atresia. The nonexcreting biliary imaging scan does not automatically make the diagnosis of biliary atresia, because severe intrahepatic cholestatic lesions (e.g., Alagille syndrome) and α_1-antitrypsin deficiency may occasionally result in the absence of biliary excretion of the radionuclide. A liver biopsy should distinguish between intrahepatic and extrahepatic cholestasis by either the paucity or proliferation of bile duct elements and other findings. If the biopsy shows bile duct proliferation, suggesting an obstructive lesion such as biliary atresia, an immediate exploration, intraoperative cholangiogram, and a procedure to reestablish biliary continuity with the bowel should be performed.

Breast milk jaundice causes indirect hyperbilirubinemia. Hepatitis B is rarely evident in an infant this young and would not cause acholic stools. Because this patient is a medical emergency, waiting for the results of the α_1-antitrypsin test cannot delay the investigation of the possibility of biliary atresia. The urine being negative for reducing substances while the infant is consuming lactose-containing human milk makes the possibility of galactosemia highly unlikely.

7. The answer is E *[IX C; Tables 11-9, 11-10].* Hepatitis B is endemic in Asia, and approximately 75%–90% of infants born to mothers in endemic areas acquire hepatitis B at the time of birth or soon thereafter. Most of these infants progress to having chronic infection with hepatitis B. Usually, these infants are anicteric and asymptomatic, except for persistent mild elevations in aminotransferases. The presence of hepatitis B surface antigen (HBsAg) and anti-hepatitis B core antigen (anti-HBc) immunoglobulin M (IgM) defines an acute infection with hepatitis B. The lack of anti-hepatitis B surface antigen (anti-HBs) and the presence of hepatitis B e antigen (HBeAg) in a 9-month-old infant suggest acquisition of the virus perinatally and persistence of viral replication with no effective immune response to clear the virus.

Acute hepatitis A [signalled by the presence of anti-hepatitis A virus (HAV) IgM] is also commonly an anicteric infection in children but often presents with other symptoms of acute infection, including fever, coryza, vomiting, diarrhea, and more elevated aminotransferases. Hepatitis C can be vertically transmitted from mother to infant, but the likelihood of the infant acquiring hepatitis C from an infected mother is very low. Also, this infant has not received a blood transfusion, which is one of the prime methods of transmission of hepatitis C in the United States. Hepatitis E is also a common infection in Asia, but it is very rare in the United States. Its incubation period is short and the baby has been in this country too long to be showing signs of hepatitis E contracted in Vietnam. Wilson disease does not present until later in life, so obtaining serum levels of copper and ceruloplasmin is not appropriate. Cystic fibrosis can rarely cause liver enzyme abnormalities in infants, but is a more cholestatic lesion with elevations of the bilirubin and γ-glutamyl transferase.

8. The answer is A *[IX C 4]*. With multiple sexual partners, many of whom may be in a high-risk group for hepatitis B, and recent sexual exposure to someone with acute hepatitis B, there is a high likelihood that this patient has acquired hepatitis B. Postexposure prophylaxis with hepatitis B immune globulin (HBIG) and hepatitis B vaccine has proven effective at modifying the infection and preventing the development of the chronic carrier state. Accelerated induction of protective antibody levels may be facilitated by an accelerated vaccine schedule. There is no decrease in the acquisition of effective immunity by giving HBIG and the first dose of vaccine simultaneously. There is no danger in giving the vaccine to a person who is already hepatitis B surface antigen (HBsAg)-positive. Giving HBIG alone may ameliorate the infection but may not prevent the development of chronic hepatitis B. This adolescent is in a high-risk group and needs to receive the hepatitis B vaccine regardless of whether he has already been exposed, so there is no rationale for waiting to get the results of testing before starting the vaccine series. Likewise, the sooner HBIG is given after exposure, the more effective it is, so there is no valid reason to wait.

9. The answer is D *[III A]*. The history and physical examination are classic for a diagnosis of hypertrophic pyloric stenosis. In this setting, the most important consideration is the patient's fluid and electrolyte status because

severe abnormalities may occasionally be seen. Hypochloremic metabolic alkalosis is most common, and initial therapy, preceding surgical correction, must include normalization of serum electrolytes. Hematemesis is seen in many infants with pyloric stenosis, and usually results from a superficial gastritis. It rarely is of hemodynamic consequence. Confirmation of the diagnosis can readily be made in most cases with an abdominal ultrasound, which reveals a thickened and elongated pyloric channel. Radiograph of the abdomen may reveal a distended, air-filled stomach. Contrast radiography reveals an elongated pyloric channel with delayed gastric emptying.

10. The answer is C *[III B]*. Infection with *Helicobacter pylori* is now know to be common in adolescents with gastritis. Nodularity and inflammation in the gastric antrum are usually seen. The nodularity appears to result from lymphoid hyperplasia. Antral gastritis in infants may be associated with eosinophilic infiltration in the setting of eosinophilic gastroenteritis. Mucosal granuloma may be seen in gastroduodenal Crohn disease. Vasculitis is associated with disorders such as Henoch-Schönlein purpura. G-cell hyperplasia (gastrin-producing cells) is a rare finding in children with refractory peptic inflammation who have increased gastric acid secretion.

11–14. The answers are: 11-D, 12-B, 13-A, 14-E *[IV A; Table 11-3]*. The differential diagnosis of lower gastrointestinal bleeding in children depends on the child's age, the color and amount of blood, the presence or absence of diarrhea, and the presence or absence of abdominal pain or signs of peritonitis and a surgical abdomen. Certain disease entities presenting with lower gastrointestinal bleeding are almost always confined to particular age groups. Eosinophilic colitis is usually a manifestation of cow's milk or soy protein allergy seen in infants younger than 6 months of age. Ulcerative colitis rarely presents in children younger than 3 years of age. Juvenile polyps usually present between 2 and 12 years of age, whereas the bleeding associated with Meckel diverticulum is usually first manifest when the patient is younger than 2 years of age.

The color and amount of blood are also characteristic of several of these lesions. Both eosinophilic colitis and juvenile polyps give rise to scant amounts of streaks of bright red blood. Most juvenile polyps are solitary and found in the rectosigmoid, and thus the blood seen is still red. In contrast, bleeding from a Meckel diverticulum located in the terminal ileum is usually copious and melanotic (purple clots).

The presence or absence of diarrhea in the history of a child with lower gastrointestinal bleeding is extremely important. Both ulcerative colitis and hemolytic–uremic syndrome present with abdominal cramps, tenesmus, and bloody, mucusy diarrhea. The bleeding from eosinophilic colitis and juvenile polyps is usually seen in the presence of otherwise normal stools.

Whether the child is sick or has signs of peritonitis or bowel obstruction is also a key element in evaluating the patient with lower gastrointestinal bleeding. Children with intussusception or volvulus, both of which can be accompanied by the passage of blood via the rectum, usually appear ill and have physical signs such as vomiting, abdominal distention, high-pitched or decreased bowel sounds, or even peritoneal signs. Patients with ulcerative colitis and hemolytic–uremic syndrome often appear pale, ill, and have diffuse abdominal tenderness. In contrast, patients with eosinophilic colitis and juvenile polyps almost always look well and have no significant physical signs.

The 6-year-old has a juvenile polyp. Hemorrhoids are very unusual in children. Anal fissures are common but are often associated with anorectal pain and constipation. The 3-year-old with bloody diarrhea could have ulcerative colitis, but he is young and has a low platelet count. Because platelets are acute-phase reactants, they are often elevated or at least normal in ulcerative colitis, and rarely decreased. In contrast, a low platelet count is an early sign of the intravascular coagulation and hemolysis that accompanies hemolytic–uremic syndrome. The 6-week-old has eosinophilic colitis. The other common cause of this presentation in a young infant is anal fissures. The 18-month-old with melanotic stool, anemia, and shock has a Meckel diverticulum until proven otherwise. Other rare possibilities include a colonic arteriovenous malformation, an isolated ileal ulcer, or a duodenal ulcer.

Chapter 12

Cardiovascular Diseases

Leon Chameides
Daniel J. Diana
Harris B. Leopold

I. EVALUATION OF THE CARDIOVASCULAR SYSTEM

A. History

1. **Cyanosis**
   a. **Peripheral cyanosis** (i.e., bluish discoloration around the mouth and over the eyelids but not of the mucous membranes) is normal in infants.
   b. Cyanosis of the mucous membranes is diagnostic of a right-to-left shunt; it may be present only with exertion.

2. A history of shortness of breath, exercise intolerance, dyspnea on exertion, feeding difficulty in infants, and disturbances in growth may be due to abnormal cardiac function.

3. **Familial disorders.** Some cardiovascular problems (e.g., hyperlipidemia, hypertension) may be familial. Some congenital heart abnormalities (e.g., atrial septal defect, aortic valve disease) have been described in multiple family members.

4. **Chest pain** is common in the pediatric age-group, particularly in adolescents, but is **rarely of cardiac origin**. Analysis of specific features (e.g., quality, distribution, relationship to level of activity) helps to distinguish anginal pain from pain due to more benign causes.

B. Physical examination

1. **General observations**
   a. **Subnormal weight** gain as compared to normal growth curves may indicate the presence of cardiac disease.
   b. **Cyanosis** and **clubbing** of the fingers and toes are diagnostic features of a right-to-left shunt. Cyanosis should always be confirmed by pulse oximetry and arterial blood gas analysis and, when present in a newborn, should be considered an urgent problem. Desaturation of **pulmonary** origin can usually be improved with oxygen administration, whereas desaturation of **cardiac** origin does not respond to oxygen.
   c. Signs pointing to a **syndrome** or **genetic disorder** that includes congenital heart disease as one of its components should be looked for in the general examination (Table 12-1).

2. **Pulses.** The presence and quality of peripheral pulses should be noted. It is important to palpate both brachial (or radial) arteries simultaneously for timing and volume. If both are of equal volume, a brachial (or radial) and femoral artery should be palpated simultaneously to rule out coarctation of the aorta. The quality and timing of the femoral pulse should be noted; the pulse may appear delayed if the arteries are filled via collateral vessels.

3. **Blood pressure** should be measured over the brachial and popliteal arteries with a cuff that has a bladder approximately two-thirds the size of the extremity and that completely covers its circumference. The diastolic pressure is recorded at the disappearance of the Korotkoff sounds.

TABLE 12-1. Cardiovascular Manifestations of Selected Congenital Disorders

Disorder	Cardiovascular Manifestation
Marfan syndrome	Aortic aneurysm, aortic valve insufficiency, mitral valve prolapse and regurgitation
Glycogen storage disease	Hypertrophic cardiomyopathy
Down syndrome	Endocardial cushion defect
Turner syndrome	Aortic coarctation
Noonan syndrome	Pulmonary valve stenosis, aortic valve stenosis
Williams syndrome	Supravalvular aortic stenosis
Trisomy 18 syndrome	Ventricular septal defect
Rubella syndrome	Patent ductus arteriosus

4. **Precordial palpation.** A thrill or "palpable murmur" defines an area of maximal turbulence. A diffuse impulse in the parasternal region (heave) may indicate right ventricular enlargement.

5. **Cardiac auscultation**
   a. **Heart sounds** (Figure 12-1)
      (1) The **first heart sound (S_1)** may be single or split.
      (2) The **second heart sound (S_2)** is split during inspiration; abnormally wide splitting occurs with right ventricular overload, right ventricular conduction delay, and prolonged right ventricular emptying (Table 12-2).
         (a) The **pulmonary component** of S_2 is accentuated in pulmonary hypertension.
         (b) The **aortic component** of S_2 is accentuated in systemic hypertension or if the aortic valve is close to the chest wall, as in transposition of the great arteries.
      (3) A **third heart sound (S_3)** is usually normal in children but may represent a pathologic condition if associated with other abnormal findings.
      (4) A **fourth heart sound (S_4)** is always abnormal in children.

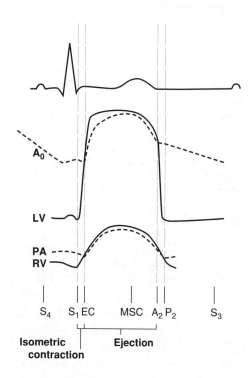

S_4 S_1 EC   MSC $A_2 P_2$ S_3

Isometric contraction | **Ejection**

FIGURE 12-1. Relationship of the electrocardiogram, heart sounds, and pressures in the aorta (A_o), left ventricle (*LV*), pulmonary artery (*PA*), and right ventricle (*RV*). *EC* = ejection click; *MSC* = midsystolic click.

TABLE 12-2. Abnormally Wide Splitting of the Second Heart Sound (S₂)

Mechanism	Diagnosis
Increased right ventricular pressure	Pulmonary valve stenosis
Increased right ventricular volume	Atrial septal defect Anomalous pulmonary venous return Pulmonary valve regurgitation Ventricular septal defect
Right ventricular conduction delay	Right bundle branch block
Premature left ventricular emptying	Mitral valve regurgitation Ventricular septal defect

> **b. Clicks**
> > **(1) Ejection clicks** occur shortly after S_1; they originate from the opening of a stenotic but mobile semilunar valve or from sudden distention of an enlarged or hypertensive pulmonary artery.
> > **(2) Mid- or late-systolic clicks** indicate prolapse of the mitral or tricuspid valve.
> **c. Murmurs**
> > **(1) Functional murmurs** (i.e., physiologic sounds of turbulence) are almost universally present at some time during childhood and are often characteristic of a particular age-group (Table 12-3; see also Chapter 1).
> > **(2) Pathologic murmurs** may occur during systole or diastole.
> > > **(a) Systolic murmurs**
> > > > **(i)** Murmurs beginning with S_1 are called regurgitant murmurs. They are caused by insufficiency of and regurgitation through the atrioventricular (AV) valves or by left-to-right flow through a ventricular septal defect. Regurgitant murmurs that extend through systole are referred to as pansystolic (or holosystolic) murmurs.
> > > > **(ii)** Murmurs that begin immediately after isovolumic contraction are referred to as ejection murmurs; they coincide with opening of the semilunar valves. Ejection murmurs may be caused by right or left ventricular outflow obstruction but may be functional.
> > > > **(iii)** Murmurs that begin late in systole are characteristic of mitral valve prolapse.
> > > **(b) Diastolic murmurs** beginning with S_2 are caused by semilunar valve regurgitation; those beginning in mid-diastole are caused by increased flow across one of the AV valves or AV valve stenosis.

C. **Laboratory evaluation**

> **1. Chest x-ray** permits evaluation of the location of the heart and abdominal organs (see III), the size of the heart, and whether the pulmonary vasculature is normal, diminished, or increased. Evaluation of the pulmonary vasculature is especially important in arriving at a differential diagnosis of cyanosis in the newborn (Table 12-4).

TABLE 12-3. Functional Murmurs

Murmur	Approximate Age	Timing	Origin
Peripheral pulmonary stenosis (PPS)	Newborn	Systolic ejection	Bifurcation of pulmonary artery
Vibratory (Still's)	3–8 years	Systolic ejection	Unknown
Carotid bruit	3–8 years	Systolic ejection	Carotid artery
Venous hum	3–8 years	Continuous	Jugular vein and superior vena cava
Pulmonary flow	6–18 years	Systolic ejection	Pulmonary valve

TABLE 12-4. Chest X-ray in Newborns with Desaturation (Cyanosis) Based on the Appearance of Pulmonary Vascularity

Increased or Normal Pulmonary Blood Flow	Diminished Pulmonary Blood Flow
Transposition of great arteries	Tricuspid atresia
Total anomalous pulmonary veins	Pulmonary valve atresia with intact ventricular septum
Truncus arteriosus	Pulmonary valve atresia with ventricular septal defect
	Truncus arteriosus

2. The **electrocardiogram (ECG)** permits diagnosis of cardiac rhythm, reflects anatomic changes (e.g., ventricular or atrial hypertrophy) that develop in patients with cardiac disease, and indicates the presence of myocardial ischemia.

3. The **echocardiogram** permits a systematic evaluation of cardiac structure and function. Direction and velocity of flow are visualized with color flow mapping, thus permitting visualization of shunt direction and valve regurgitation. Continuous flow Doppler permits estimation of pressure gradients across valves.

4. **Cardiac catheterization** allows measurement of intracardiac and intravascular pressures and determination of pressure gradients across the cardiac valves.
   a. **Blood analysis of oxygen content and saturation** permits detection of the presence and size of left-to-right and right-to-left shunts, measurement of cardiac output, and calculation of systemic and pulmonary vascular resistances.
   b. **Selective angiography** permits the visualization of cardiac and vascular anatomy.
   c. **Therapeutic catheter interventions** include balloon atrial septostomy, balloon angioplasty of stenotic valves and vessels, and, in selected cases, occlusion of communications such as shunts and collateral arteries.

II. FETAL AND NEONATAL CIRCULATION.
Patency of three structures—the foramen ovale, ductus arteriosus, and ductus venosus—is a critical feature of the cardiovascular anatomy and physiology of the fetus.

A. **Normal physiology** (see also Chapter 6)

1. **Fetal circulation** (see also Chapter 6)
   a. Fetal blood is oxygenated in the **placenta** and then enters the umbilical vein.
      (1) One portion of the oxygenated blood perfuses the liver and proceeds to the inferior vena cava via the hepatic veins.
      (2) Another portion enters the ductus venosus, which empties directly into the inferior vena cava.
   b. Together with venous return from the lower part of the body, this blood flows into the **right atrium**.
      (1) Approximately one third is shunted, via the foramen ovale, to the left atrium, left ventricle, and ascending aorta.
      (2) The remainder joins the venous return from the upper part of the body and enters the right ventricle and pulmonary artery. A small portion (< 10%) of this blood enters the lungs, and the remainder, because of high pulmonary vascular resistance and low systemic vascular resistance, crosses the ductus arteriosus to the descending aorta.

2. **Transition to neonatal circulation** (see also Chapter 6)
   a. At birth, the infant's first breaths cause an increase in arterial oxygen tension (PO_2); this lowers pulmonary vascular resistance, resulting in increased pulmonary blood flow. The increased pulmonary venous return to the left atrium causes the pressure to rise, resulting in **functional closure of the foramen ovale**.
   b. Systemic vascular resistance is increased by the elimination of the low-resistance vascular circuit of the placenta at birth.

    c. Closure of the ductus arteriosus occurs shortly after birth, first functionally and then anatomically.

    d. The neonatal circulation, with the ventricles working in series, is thus established.

  3. Normal changes in pulmonary vascular resistance. Pulmonary vascular resistance is inversely related to the diameter of the small pulmonary arterioles.

    a. In the fetus, high pulmonary vascular resistance is maintained by constriction of the muscular tunica media of these arterioles.

    b. The arterioles begin to dilate after birth, and the tunica media gradually atrophies. (In the average adult, cardiac output can increase fourfold without causing an increase in pulmonary artery pressure.)

B. | **Abnormalities of the pulmonary circulation**

  1. Persistent pulmonary hypertension of the newborn. Pulmonary vascular resistance can remain high after birth if constriction of the arteriolar lumina by a pathologic process occurs (e.g., due to hypoxemia, acidosis, or some unidentified factor). The resultant pulmonary hypertension leads to right-to-left shunting at the ductus or foramen ovale.

  2. Other arteriolar abnormalities

    a. Anatomic changes. If stimuli to pulmonary arteriolar constriction, such as pulmonary or venous hypertension, continue into infancy, the media remains thickened instead of atrophying with age. Progressive pathologic changes may develop in a small number of infants and children, including cellular intimal proliferation, fibrosis of the intima and media, angioma formation, and arteriolitis.

    b. Physiologic changes. A rise in pulmonary vascular resistance causes a diminution in left-to-right shunting (e.g., through a patent ductus or ventricular septal defect) and then, as pulmonary vascular resistance surpasses systemic resistance, a reversal of the shunt. Once fibrosis of the arterioles occurs, the process is irreversible. The combination of an irreversibly high pulmonary vascular resistance (culminating in pulmonary vascular obstructive disease) and a right-to-left shunt is known as the **Eisenmenger reaction**.

III. POSITION OF CARDIAC STRUCTURES

A. | **Cardiac position (situs).** Cardiac situs is best determined by examining the chest x-ray. Note should be made of the position of the stomach and the liver, and whether there is viscerocardiac concordance (i.e., levocardia with abdominal situs solitus or dextrocardia with abdominal situs inversus) or discordance (i.e., levocardia with abdominal situs inversus or dextrocardia with abdominal situs solitus). In viscerocardiac discordance, there is a high incidence of congenital heart disease.

  1. In **levocardia,** the apex of the heart points to the left (situs solitus, or usual site).

  2. In **dextrocardia,** the apex of the heart points to the right.

B. | **Abdominal viscera and atria** (Figure 12-2)

  1. In **situs solitus,** the liver is on the right and the stomach is on the left. The right atrium usually is on the same side as the liver.

  2. In **situs inversus,** there is a mirror-image arrangement of the abdominal organs: the liver is on the left and the stomach on the right. The right atrium usually is located on the left.

  3. In **situs ambiguous,** the visceral situs is uncertain; the liver is midline without a dominant lobe. This represents a group of abnormalities known as **heterotaxia;** the body consists of two right sides (**asplenia syndrome**) or two left sides (**polysplenia syndrome**). Complex congenital heart disease is usually present.

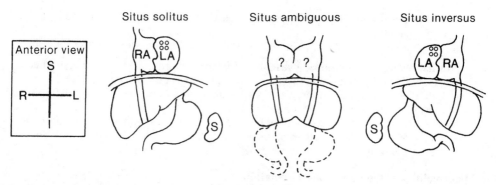

FIGURE 12-2. Visceroatrial situs. *S* = superior; *I* = inferior; *R* = right; *L* = left; *RA* = right atrium; *LA* = left atrium; *S* = spleen. (Adapted with permission from Paul MH: Transposition of the great arteries. In *Heart Disease in Infants, Children, and Adolescents.* Edited by Moss AJ, Adams FH. Baltimore, Williams & Wilkins, 1968, p 529.)

C. **Ventricles** (Figure 12-3). In the embryonic formation of the heart, the cardiac tube usually loops to the right (**dextro-,** or **D-**), so that the right ventricle, derived from the bulbus cordis, develops to the right of the left ventricle. If the tube loops to the left (**levo-,** or **L-**), ventricular inversion results. Position of the ventricles is best evaluated by echocardiography or by angiography.

D. **Great arteries** (Figure 12-4). The pulmonary valve is normally anterior and to the left of the aortic valve (see Figure 12-4B). The usual cardiac looping in **situs inversus** is an L-loop (ventricular inversion), and the corresponding great artery arrangement places the pulmonary valve anterior and to the right of the aortic valve (see Figure 12-4C). In both the D- and the L-ventricular loop, the great arteries can be transposed.

1. When the great arteries are transposed in a **D-ventricular loop,** the most common (> 90%) arrangement of the great arteries is **D-transposition,** where the aortic valve is anterior and to the right of the pulmonary valve (see Figure 12-4A); the right ventricular conus is subaortic.

2. When the great arteries are transposed in an **L-ventricular loop** (ventricular inversion), the most common (> 90%) great artery arrangement is **L-transposition,** where the aortic valve is anterior and to the left of the pulmonary valve (see Figure 12-4D); the right ventricular conus is subaortic.

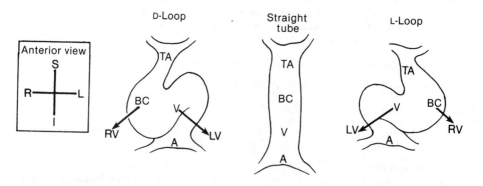

FIGURE 12-3. Cardiac looping. *S* = superior; *I* = inferior; *R* = right; *L* = left; *TA* = truncus arteriosus; *BC* = bulbus cordis; *V* = ventricle; *A* = atrium; *RV* = right ventricle; *LV* = left ventricle. (Adapted with permission from Paul MH: Transposition of the great arteries. In *Heart Disease in Infants, Children, and Adolescents.* Edited by Moss AJ, Adams FH. Baltimore, Williams & Wilkins, 1968, p 529.)

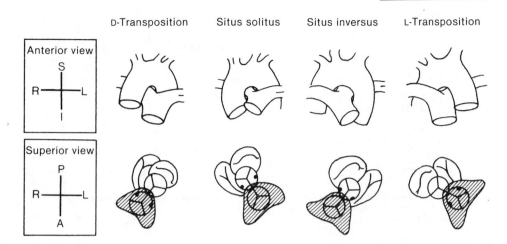

FIGURE 12-4. Relationships between the great arteries and the semilunar (i.e., aortic and pulmonary) and atrioventricular (i.e., mitral and tricuspid) valves. *Crosshatching* indicates distal conal myocardium. *S* = superior; *I* = inferior; *R* = right; *L* = left; *P* = posterior; *A* = anterior. (Adapted with permission from Paul MH: Transposition of the great arteries. In *Heart Disease in Infants, Children, and Adolescents.* Edited by Moss AJ, Adams FH. Baltimore, Williams & Wilkins, 1968, p 529.)

E. **Notation** codes are a useful shorthand method of describing the various anatomic configurations. The first letter (**S** or **I** for solitus or inversus) describes the abdominal situs and therefore the location of the right atrium; the second letter (**D** or **L**) describes the ventricular looping and therefore the location of the ventricles; the third letter (**D** or **L**) describes the location of the great arteries. For example, **SDD** denotes situs solitus (the right atrium probably is on the right), a D-ventricular loop (the right ventricle is on the right), and a D-transposition of the great arteries.

IV. CONGENITAL STRUCTURAL DISORDERS

A. **General considerations**

1. **Etiology**
   a. The cause of congenital heart disease is usually unknown in individual cases; evidence points to a **multifactorial etiology,** with the insult probably occurring in the first 8 weeks of gestation.
   b. Most congenital heart lesions are **sporadic**. However, their incidence is slightly higher in families that include one member with such an abnormality; there are families with several affected members.
   c. Congenital heart disease has been associated with several **teratogenic factors**.
      (1) **Medications** that are known or suspected cardiovascular teratogens include thalidomide, folic acid antagonists, dextroamphetamine, anticonvulsants, lithium, and estrogens.
      (2) **Excessive maternal alcohol ingestion** has been associated with the development of congenital heart defects.
      (3) **Maternal infection.** Antenatal **rubella** has proven to be teratogenic. There is also evidence that maternal **cytomegalovirus** and **coxsackievirus** infections may cause congenital cardiovascular abnormalities.

2. **Clinical considerations**
   a. Congenital heart disease is a **component of several syndromes** (see Table 12-1; see also Chapter 8).

TABLE 12-5. Initial Regimen of Endocarditis Prophylaxis

Drug	Weight Range	Dose*
Amoxicillin	< 15 kg	750 mg
	15–30 kg	1500 mg
	> 30 kg	3000 mg
Erythromycin ethylsuccinate[†]	< 30 kg	20 mg/kg
	> 30 kg	800 mg
Erythromycin stearate[†]	< 30 kg	20 mg/kg
	> 30 kg	1000 mg
Clindamycin[†]	< 30 kg	10 mg/kg
	> 30 kg	300 mg

*For second dose, administer one half the initial dose 6 hours after initial dose.
[†]For penicillin-allergic patients.

    b. Children with turbulent cardiac abnormalities (high-pressure or low-pressure flow) are susceptible to the development of **subacute bacterial endocarditis** whenever transient bacteremia is likely (e.g., with dental procedures or with surgery involving the respiratory, gastrointestinal, or genitourinary tract). Children with such abnormalities undergoing surgical procedures likely to cause a bacteremia (especially dental procedures) should receive antibiotic prophylaxis (Table 12-5).

B. **Atrial septal defect (ASD)**

    1. Description. ASD (persistent patency of the interatrial septum) can occur high in the septum [**sinus venosus defect** (Figure 12-5A)], in the midportion [**ostium secundum defect** (Figure 12-5B)], and low in the septum primum [**ostium primum defect** (Figure 12-5C), also known as **partial endocardial cushion defect**]. In ostium primum atrial septal defect, the **anterior leaflet** of the **mitral valve** is often **cleft** and **incompetent**.

    2. Pathophysiology. Greater right than left ventricular compliance and low pulmonary vascular resistance result in a left-to-right shunt at the atrial level, thus increasing flow across the tricuspid and pulmonary valves. As a result, the right ventricle and the pulmonary artery are usually enlarged.

    3. Clinical features. Symptoms can include slow weight gain and frequent lower respiratory infections, but most commonly children with ASD are asymptomatic.

    4. Diagnosis
        a. Physical examination. The precordium is hyperdynamic, and a right ventricular heave is present. A systolic ejection murmur in the pulmonic area and a mid-diastolic rumble in the lower right sternal area reflect the increased flow across the pulmonary and tricuspid valves. S_2 is widely and constantly split.
        b. Laboratory evaluation
            (1) Chest x-ray. The heart and main pulmonary artery segment are enlarged; pulmonary vascularity is increased.
            (2) ECG. Right-axis deviation often is seen in secundum defects. The hallmark of a primum defect is an extreme left-axis deviation. Right ventricular hypertrophy is represented by an rsR' in the right precordial leads.
            (3) Echocardiogram. The right ventricle is enlarged, and the septum often moves in a paradoxical fashion. The defect usually can be visualized on a two-dimensional study. Color flow mapping demonstrates the direction of flow as well as mitral valve anatomy and competence.
            (4) Cardiac catheterization is usually not necessary for diagnosis. If it is performed, the presence and size of a left-to-right shunt are indicated by an increase in oxygen saturation at the atrial level. Pressure in the pulmonary artery is normal

or slightly elevated, and a small pressure gradient may be present across the pulmonary valve. Severe pulmonary hypertension is rare in children. Mitral regurgitation often is found in ostium primum defects.

5. **Therapy**
   a. **Medical management.** Bacterial endocarditis prophylaxis is not necessary in secundum defects but is indicated in primum defects if mitral valve regurgitation is present.
   b. **Surgical closure** of both secundum and primum defects can be accomplished with minimal risk. In the future, selected secundum atrial defects may be closed with a device in the catheterization laboratory.

C. Ventricular septal defect (VSD)

1. **Description** (see Figure 12-5). VSD (persistent patency of the interventricular septum) is the most common congenital heart disorder, accounting for 26% of all congenital cardiac lesions. A VSD may be single or multiple and may be found anywhere along the septum; it is most common in the membranomuscular portion. Inflow VSDs, also called **endocardial cushion defects,** often have associated abnormalities of the tricuspid and mitral valves and are most commonly seen in children with **Down syndrome**.

2. **Pathophysiology**
   a. In small defects, the size of the shunt is determined by resistance at the defect; small defects result in small shunts. If the defect is large, both the size and direction of the shunt are determined by the relative resistances in the pulmonary and systemic circuits.
   b. As long as pulmonary vascular resistance is lower than systemic vascular resistance, the shunt is left-to-right. If pulmonary vascular resistance rises above systemic vascular resistance, the shunt reverses.
   c. Large defects tend to result in pulmonary hypertension, whereas in small defects pulmonary vascular dynamics remain normal.
   d. The size of the left atrium and left ventricle is directly proportional to the size of the left-to-right shunt. Right ventricular enlargement occurs only when pulmonary vascular resistance increases.
   e. Pulmonary hypertension may lead to the development of pulmonary vascular obstructive disease (Eisenmenger reaction) and reversal of the shunt.

3. **Clinical features.** Symptoms are related to the size of the shunt.
   a. If the defect is small, no symptoms are present. Many of the small defects close spontaneously.

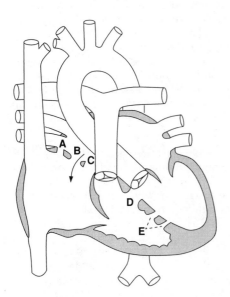

FIGURE 12-5. Anatomy of atrial and ventricular septal defects. *A* = sinus venosus atrial defect; *B* = ostium secundum atrial defect; *C* = ostium primum atrial defect; *D* = membranous ventricular defect; *E* = muscular ventricular defect.

  b. If the defect is large and pulmonary vascular resistance is not significantly elevated (large left-to-right shunt), growth failure, congestive heart failure, and repeated lower respiratory infections usually occur, most commonly beginning at 1–2 months of age.

  c. If the defect is large and pulmonary vascular resistance is very high (i.e., Eisenmenger reaction), shortness of breath, dyspnea on exertion, chest pain, and cyanosis may occur. Irreversible pulmonary vascular obstructive disease is uncommon below two years of age.

4. Diagnosis

  a. Physical examination

    (1) A left-to-right shunt produces turbulence during isovolumic contraction, and the murmur therefore begins with S_1 and ends in midsystole in small defects, and extends to S_2 in large left-to-right shunts. The murmur is harsh and is best heard at the midsternal or lower left sternal border. In large left-to-right shunts, a mid-diastolic rumble of relative mitral stenosis is also heard.

    (2) As pulmonary vascular resistance increases, and the left-to-right shunt decreases, the mid-diastolic murmur disappears, the systolic murmur becomes shorter, and the pulmonary component of S_2 increases in intensity.

    (3) In the presence of pulmonary vascular obstructive disease, a right ventricular heave, ejection click, short systolic ejection murmur, diastolic murmur of pulmonary valve insufficiency, and a loud S_2 are heard.

  b. Laboratory evaluation

    (1) Chest x-ray

      (a) In small defects, the chest x-ray may be normal or show mild cardiomegaly and a slight increase in pulmonary vascularity.

      (b) In large left-to-right shunts, cardiomegaly, increased pulmonary vascularity, and enlargement of the left atrium and left ventricle are seen. As a rule, the size of the heart is directly proportional to the magnitude of the left-to-right shunt. As pulmonary vascular resistance rises and the left-to-right shunt decreases, the heart and the distal pulmonary arteries become smaller but the proximal pulmonary arteries enlarge.

    (2) ECG

      (a) In small defects, the ECG is normal.

      (b) In large left-to-right shunts, left atrial, left ventricular, or biventricular hypertrophy is seen. Right ventricular hypertrophy predominates when pulmonary vascular resistance is high. An extreme left axis deviation is characteristic of VSDs in the endocardial cushion region.

    (3) Echocardiogram. Chamber size can be determined and moderate to large defects can be identified with a two-dimensional study. Color flow mapping can localize defects that are too small for two-dimensional resolution. Continuous-wave Doppler allows estimation of right ventricular and pulmonary artery pressures.

    (4) Cardiac catheterization. Measurement of intracardiac and intravascular oxygen content defines the magnitude and direction of shunting. Pulmonary arterial pressure can be measured and pulmonary and systemic vascular resistances calculated. Left ventricular angiography defines the interventricular septum and can show the size as well as the number of defects.

5. Therapy

  a. Medical management. Bacterial endocarditis prophylaxis (see Table 12-5) is indicated. Congestive heart failure is treated with digoxin, diuretics, and afterload reducing medications.

  b. Surgical management. A large VSD should be repaired before pulmonary vascular changes become irreversible. Small defects do not require surgical repair.

D. | **Patent ductus arteriosus (PDA)**

  1. Description. The ductus arteriosus connects the pulmonary artery and the descending aorta in the fetus and normally closes shortly after birth. Patency of the ductus constitutes approximately 10% of congenital heart defects; patency is especially common in very low–birth-weight babies with pulmonary disease.

2. **Pathophysiology**
   a. The **direction of flow** through a large PDA depends on the relative resistances in the pulmonary and systemic circuits. As long as the former is lower than the latter, a left-to-right shunt is present. If pulmonary vascular resistance rises above systemic vascular resistance, a right-to-left shunt develops.
   b. The **size of the shunt** depends on the size of the PDA and the relative resistances in the pulmonary and systemic circuits. The left atrium and left ventricle enlarge in direct proportion to the magnitude of the left-to-right shunt. If the PDA is large, pulmonary vascular obstructive disease (Eisenmenger reaction) can develop. The right ventricle enlarges with the development of an increase in the pulmonary vascular resistance. If the PDA is small, its size limits the left-to-right shunt, and pulmonary vascular disease does not develop.

3. **Clinical features.** Symptoms are related to the size of the defect and the direction of flow. A small PDA causes no symptoms. A large PDA with a large left-to-right shunt may result in congestive heart failure, slowed growth, and repeated lower respiratory tract infections. Even small left-to-right shunts may cause severe compromise in low–birth-weight infants with pulmonary disease. Reversal of flow as a result of high pulmonary vascular resistance causes shortness of breath, dyspnea on exertion, and cyanosis.

4. **Diagnosis**
   a. **Physical examination**
      (1) Pulse volume is related to the pulse pressure, which in turn is related to the volume of the left-to-right shunt. If the flow is small, pulses are normal. In a large shunt, bounding pulses, representing an aortic diastolic runoff, are palpated.
      (2) The murmur is continuous: It begins after S_1, peaks with S_2, and trails off in diastole. If pulmonary vascular resistance rises, first the diastolic murmur and subsequently the systolic murmur become softer and shorter, and S_2 increases in intensity.
   b. **Laboratory evaluation**
      (1) **Chest x-ray.** Heart size, pulmonary vascularity, and left atrial and left ventricular size are all directly related to the magnitude of the left-to-right shunt. In a small PDA, the x-ray may be normal. If the PDA and left-to-right shunt are large, cardiomegaly and left heart enlargement are pronounced.
      (2) **ECG.** The ECG is normal if the PDA is small. Left ventricular or biventricular hypertrophy is seen if the left-to-right shunt is large. Right ventricular hypertrophy predominates in the presence of increased pulmonary vascular resistance.
      (3) **Echocardiogram.** The PDA sometimes can be visualized on a two-dimensional study. Doppler ultrasonography shows diastolic turbulence in the pulmonary artery and diastolic runoff in the aorta. Color flow mapping demonstrates the direction of flow. If the shunt is large, the left atrium and ventricle are enlarged.
      (4) **Cardiac catheterization** is not usually necessary for diagnosis, but, if performed, will show a step-up in pulmonary arterial oxygen saturation and the pulmonary artery pressure. The ductus often can be traversed with the catheter, and angiography with selective injection in the descending aorta shows the ductal anatomy.

5. **Therapy**
   a. **Medical management.** Bacterial endocarditis prophylaxis (see Table 12-5) is necessary as long as the ductus remains patent. Indomethacin is often effective in closing a PDA in the preterm newborn infant.
   b. **Surgical management.** Division or ligation of the ductus is curative. Ductal closure may be achieved in the catheterization laboratory, and in selected cases may become the preferred method of therapy in the future.

E. | **Ductus-dependent lesions** are those abnormalities in which either the systemic or pulmonary blood flow depends on patency of the ductus arteriosus.

1. **Ductus-dependent systemic flow lesions.** In this group of lesions, systemic blood flow depends on ductal patency. Symptoms and clinical findings are remarkably similar, despite anatomic differences, because they result from interruption of systemic flow when the ductus begins to narrow.

   a. **Hypoplastic left-heart syndrome**

      (1) **Description.** This syndrome is a continuum of anomalies characterized by underdevelopment of the aortic root, aortic valve, left ventricle, and mitral valve. The aortic valve is usually atretic; mitral valve atresia is common. The ascending aorta often measures only a few millimeters, and a coarctation is often present. The right atrium and right ventricle are dilated.

      (2) **Pathophysiology.** Because there is no antegrade aortic flow, perfusion of the ascending aorta and its branches (coronary, cerebral) depends on ductal patency. Systemic and pulmonary venous return mix at the atrial level (i.e., there is an obligatory left-to-right atrial shunt). Because pulmonary vascular resistance is high, flow is directed through the ductus to the aorta, with retrograde coronary artery perfusion. Closure of the ductus arteriosus interrupts flow to the vital organs.

      (3) **Clinical features.** Symptoms, usually evident in the first few days of life, of severe congestive heart failure, shock, and progressive acidosis occur as the ductus arteriosus closes.

      (4) **Diagnosis**

         (a) **Physical examination.** Poor systemic perfusion (shock) is characterized by mottling of the skin, weak or absent peripheral pulses, tachypnea, dyspnea, grunting, and agonal respirations. Hepatomegaly, diffuse rales, a gallop rhythm with a loud S_2, and a nonspecific systolic murmur are additional findings.

         (b) **Laboratory evaluation**

            (i) **Chest x-ray** shows cardiomegaly and pulmonary vascular congestion or edema.

            (ii) **ECG** is often normal for age and is not helpful for diagnosis.

            (iii) **Echocardiogram** is diagnostic; it shows the configuration and size of the various structures. The left ventricle is either absent or is tiny, the ascending aorta measures 2–3 mm, and the mitral valve is atretic. Doppler ultrasonography and color flow mapping define the left-to-right atrial flow and right-to-left ductal flow.

      (5) **Therapy**

         (a) **Medical management** is palliative and is directed at preserving systemic perfusion; the ductus is opened and patency maintained by an infusion of prostaglandin E_1 (PGE_1). In addition, ventilatory support is provided and acidosis is corrected.

         (b) **Surgical management.** Corrective surgery is not feasible.

            (i) **The Norwood procedure** has allowed some children to survive infancy. The first stage involves anastomosis of the main pulmonary artery to the hypoplastic aorta, ligation of the distal main pulmonary artery, creation of a shunt between a systemic and pulmonary artery, and creation of an ASD. The second stage is a **modified Fontan operation** in which systemic venous return is directed to the pulmonary arteries.

            (ii) Another proposed alternative is neonatal **cardiac transplantation**.

   b. **Coarctation of the aorta** (Figure 12-6)

      (1) **Description.** The constriction of the aorta is almost invariably located at the junction of the ductus arteriosus with the aortic arch, just distal to the subclavian artery. The constriction may be discrete or diffuse and usually is associated with isthmic narrowing and a contraductal shelf. Coarctation may be associated with PDA (66%), VSD (30%), and aortic valve abnormalities (often a bicuspid valve).

      (2) **Pathophysiology.** As the ductus constricts in the neonatal period, obstruction increases at the coarctation site, thus causing increased left ventricular afterload.

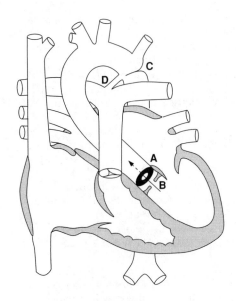

FIGURE 12-6. Anatomy of coarctation of the aorta, aortic valve stenosis, and discrete subvalve stenosis. The ductus arteriosus is patent. *A* = aortic valve stenosis; *B* = discrete subaortic stenosis; *C* = coarctation of the aorta; *D* = patent ductus arteriosus.

If the coarctation is severe and there has been insufficient time for the development of collateral vessels or left ventricular hypertrophy to accommodate this increase in afterload, left ventricular dysfunction with symptoms of congestive heart failure present in the neonatal period.

- **(3) Clinical features.** Symptoms are those of low cardiac output and congestive heart failure (e.g., irritability, lethargy, poor feeding, growth failure).
- **(4) Diagnosis**
    - **(a) Physical examination** reveals signs of low cardiac output and poor peripheral perfusion. Findings include ashen color, skin mottling, decreased or absent lower extremity pulses, gallop rhythm, single loud S_2, a nonspecific and often low-pitched systolic murmur, and hepatomegaly. Differential cyanosis in the presence of a patent ductus is usually difficult to recognize.
    - **(b) Laboratory evaluation**
        - **(i) Chest x-ray** in the symptomatic infant shows cardiomegaly and pulmonary congestion.
        - **(ii) ECG** often shows right ventricular hypertrophy with strain.
        - **(iii) Echocardiogram** is critical in defining the anatomy, localizing the coarctation, and demonstrating associated anomalies. Doppler ultrasonography allows estimation of a pressure gradient, and color flow mapping defines patency and direction of flow through the ductus.
        - **(iv) Cardiac catheterization** with angiography allows definition of the coarctation, associated anomalies, and size of the aorta.
- **(5) Therapy**
    - **(a) Medical management.** In the newborn with shock, therapy is directed at unloading the left ventricle and improving systemic flow by infusing PGE_1 to dilate the ductus arteriosus. In addition, inotropic agents may be given to improve left ventricular function, diuretics are given to decrease preload, and acidosis is treated.
    - **(b) Surgical management.** The obstruction is relieved surgically (see IV I 5 b). Restenosis at the surgical site is not uncommon.
- **c. Critical aortic stenosis**
    - **(1) Description.** Isolated aortic valve stenosis does not usually cause symptoms in infancy unless it is critical, in which case signs and symptoms of congestive heart failure and shock due to poor systemic perfusion occur. The aortic valve tissue is usually rigid and thickened with varying degrees of commissural fusion. The valve most often is bicuspid but may be unicuspid with an eccentric, small

opening. Annular hypoplasia may be present; often, left ventricular hypoplasia and endocardial fibroelastosis are also found.

(2) **Pathophysiology.** The small opening causes severe left ventricular obstruction and an increase in ventricular systolic as well as end-diastolic pressures. Decreased myocardial perfusion during diastole may result in myocardial ischemia and dysfunction. Tissue perfusion may remain adequate as long as the ductus remains patent, but symptoms of low output and tissue ischemia develop when the ductus begins to close.

(3) **Clinical features.** Symptoms are those of low cardiac output, shock, and congestive heart failure and include lethargy, irritability, poor feeding, and varying degrees of respiratory failure.

(4) **Diagnosis**

(a) **Physical examination.** Infants have poor skin perfusion characterized by mottling and ashen color. Peripheral pulses are weak or absent. Auscultation may reveal an ejection click and a systolic ejection murmur, but these may be absent if cardiac output is sufficiently depressed. The liver is enlarged, and there are signs of pulmonary venous congestion (e.g., tachypnea, dyspnea, rales).

(b) **Laboratory evaluation**

(i) **Chest x-ray** findings include cardiomegaly and pulmonary congestion.

(ii) **ECG** may show right ventricular hypertrophy, left ventricular hypertrophy, or evidence of myocardial ischemia.

(iii) **Echocardiogram** is diagnostic. The site of the lesion, the degree of obstruction, and the size and function of the left ventricle all can be determined. Pressure gradient across the aortic valve can be calculated by continuous-wave Doppler but may be misleadingly low in the presence of a very low cardiac output.

(iv) At **cardiac catheterization,** the pressure gradient can be measured, but the low cardiac output may underestimate the degree of obstruction. The major benefit of angiography is the definition of associated arch anomalies.

(5) **Therapy**

(a) **Medical management.** Hemodynamic stabilization is achieved by reopening the ductus arteriosus with PGE_1 infusion, using inotropic agents and diuretics, and correcting acid–base imbalances. Balloon angioplasty of the aortic valve can be lifesaving, but it may be difficult to pass the dilating catheter across the narrow orifice.

(b) **Surgical management.** Aortic valvotomy under direct vision may be achieved but is associated with a high mortality rate.

2. **Ductus-dependent pulmonary flow lesions.** In this group of lesions, pulmonary blood flow depends on ductal patency. Symptoms and clinical findings are remarkably similar, despite anatomic differences, because they result from diminution of pulmonary blood flow as the ductus closes.

a. **Hypoplastic right-heart syndromes**

(1) **Description of types**

(a) **Pulmonary atresia with intact ventricular septum**

(i) In 80% of cases, the pulmonary valve alone is involved and forms an imperforate membrane; in 20% of cases there is associated infundibular hypoplasia or atresia.

(ii) Right ventricular development is variable, ranging from normal (10%) to extremely hypoplastic (50%).

(iii) A patent foramen ovale or true ASD is present.

(b) **Tricuspid atresia** is characterized by atresia of the tricuspid orifice (which is often identifiable only as a dimple), accompanied by a patent foramen ovale or true ASD. Three major types are:

(i) Atresia with normally related great arteries, with or without VSD (70%)

    (ii) Atresia with D-transposition of the great arteries and VSD (23%)

    (iii) Atresia with L-transposition of the great arteries (7%)

(2) Pathophysiology. In both pulmonary atresia with intact ventricular septum and tricuspid atresia, a right-to-left atrial shunt is obligatory, with mixing of systemic and pulmonary venous return. Pulmonary blood flow depends on patency of the ductus and, in tricuspid atresia, on the size of the VSD (if present) and associated ventricular outflow obstruction.

(3) Clinical features. Severe cyanosis not relieved by inhaled oxygen is present in the neonatal period and is inversely related to the pulmonary blood flow.

(4) Diagnosis

    (a) Physical examination. A variable degree of desaturation is present.

        (i) In **pulmonary atresia with intact ventricular septum,** a single S_2 is present, and a continuous murmur of a PDA or a regurgitant murmur of tricuspid insufficiency, or both, may be heard.

        (ii) Findings in **tricuspid atresia** are more variable and depend on the size of the VSD and on pulmonary blood flow. If pulmonary blood flow is minimal, the VSD is very small, or associated pulmonary atresia is present, the findings may be identical to those in pulmonary atresia with intact ventricular septum. If the VSD is large and pulmonary blood flow is increased, signs of congestive heart failure and a harsh VSD murmur prevail.

    (b) Laboratory evaluation

        (i) Chest x-ray shows diminished pulmonary vascular markings (see Table 12-4); heart size is variable.

        (ii) ECG in both pulmonary and tricuspid atresia shows right atrial enlargement and decreased forces over the right ventricle. Left-axis deviation is seen in tricuspid atresia.

        (iii) Echocardiogram is diagnostic and demonstrates the anatomic defect. Color flow mapping demonstrates the direction of blood flow and presence of a PDA. Right ventricular pressure can be estimated by continuous-wave Doppler evaluation.

        (iv) Cardiac catheterization and angiography confirm the anatomy and allow quantification of pulmonary blood flow. In pulmonary atresia with intact ventricular septum, right ventricular pressure may be suprasystemic.

(5) Therapy

    (a) Medical management. PGE_1 infusion maintains patency of the ductus, thereby preserving pulmonary blood flow, and should be urgently instituted. At cardiac catheterization, a balloon atrial septostomy is performed if the atrial communication is inadequate.

    (b) Surgical management. Initially, the aim is to maintain adequate pulmonary blood flow via a systemic artery-to-pulmonary artery shunt. The most commonly performed shunt is the **modified Blalock-Taussig shunt,** which involves the interposition of a tubular Gore-Tex® graft between the subclavian and pulmonary arteries. In addition, in pulmonary atresia with intact ventricular septum, a pulmonary valvotomy is performed, if the size of the right ventricle is adequate, to decompress the right ventricle and allow for its future growth.

b. Pulmonary atresia with VSD

    (1) Description. This defect is the extreme expression of tetralogy of Fallot (see IV F), with atresia of the right ventricular outflow and a large ventricular septal defect. The pulmonary arteries are often hypoplastic.

    (2) Pathophysiology. Pulmonary blood flow depends on a PDA or on collateral flow to the pulmonary arteries. A ventricular right-to-left shunt is obligatory.

    (3) Clinical features. Severe cyanosis not relieved by inhaled oxygen is present and is inversely related to pulmonary blood flow.

    (4) Diagnosis

        (a) Physical examination. A right ventricular heave may be present. S_2 is single, and a continuous murmur of the ductus or collateral vessels may be heard.

      (b) Laboratory evaluation
- **(i) Chest x-ray** reveals diminished pulmonary vascular markings (see Table 12-4), a concavity in the area of the pulmonary artery, and normal heart size. A right aortic arch is often present.
- **(ii) ECG** shows right-axis deviation and normal neonatal right ventricular forces.
- **(iii) Echocardiogram** is diagnostic and demonstrates the anatomic defects. Color flow mapping shows no antegrade flow across the pulmonary valve, the right-to-left ventricular shunt, and the left-to-right ductal flow. The right ventricular pressure can be estimated using continuous-wave Doppler evaluation.
- **(iv)** At **cardiac catheterization,** right and left ventricular pressures are equal. Angiography demonstrates the anatomy, including the source and adequacy of pulmonary blood flow and size of the pulmonary arteries.

(5) Therapy
- **(a) Medical management.** PGE$_1$ infusion machine maintains patency of the ductus and preserves pulmonary blood flow. It should be started as soon as desaturation is detected.
- **(b) Surgical management.** The initial aim is to ensure adequate pulmonary blood flow by creating a systemic artery-to-pulmonary artery shunt [see IV E 2 a (5) (b)]. At a somewhat older age, complete correction is performed by closing the VSD and interposing a graft between the right ventricle and the pulmonary artery.

F. **Tetralogy of Fallot** (Figure 12-7)

1. **Description.** This is the most common cyanotic congenital cardiac abnormality, accounting for approximately 10% of all congenital cardiac lesions.
   - **a.** The primary lesion appears to involve underdevelopment of the infundibulum, which leads to:
     - **(1)** Variable right ventricular outflow tract obstruction (pulmonary stenosis)
     - **(2)** Dextroposition of the aorta (override of the ventricular septum)
     - **(3)** VSD
     - **(4)** Right ventricular hypertrophy
   - **b.** A **right aortic arch** is not uncommon, and a varying degree of hypoplasia of the pulmonary arteries is often present.

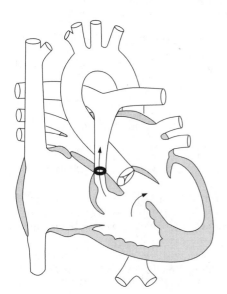

FIGURE 12-7. Anatomy of tetralogy of Fallot. The pulmonary annulus is hypoplastic and the aorta straddles the ventricular septum. *Arrows* indicate the usual direction of flow.

2. **Pathophysiology.** Of the four components of tetralogy of Fallot, only the VSD and the right ventricular outflow obstruction are physiologically important. This combination equalizes right and left ventricular pressures; the magnitude of the right-to-left shunt depends on the degree of right ventricular obstruction.

3. **Clinical features.** Major manifestations reflect the degree of hypoxemia, which is governed by the severity of right ventricular outflow obstruction. Signs include cyanosis, squatting posture, hyperpnea, and dyspnea on exertion. Hypoxemic spells consist of irritability, hyperpnea, increasing cyanosis, and syncope. These spells are often paroxysmal, may be fatal, and are not necessarily related to the severity of the obstruction.

4. **Diagnosis**
   a. **Physical examination**
      (1) Cyanosis is variable and sometimes may be absent (acyanotic tetralogy).
      (2) Digital clubbing and hyperpnea at rest are directly related to the degree of cyanosis.
      (3) A right ventricular heave is present, S_2 often is single, and a harsh systolic ejection murmur is heard along the sternal border; its length and loudness are inversely proportional to the degree of outflow obstruction.
   b. **Laboratory evaluation**
      (1) **Chest x-ray.** The heart size is normal. The apex is uptilted, and a concavity is noted in the pulmonary segment, giving the heart the appearance of a boot. The pulmonary vascular markings are diminished according to the severity of outflow obstruction (see Table 12-4). The aortic arch is right-sided in 25%–30% of cases.
      (2) **ECG** shows right-axis deviation and right ventricular hypertrophy.
      (3) The two-dimensional **echocardiogram** is diagnostic; it demonstrates the location and size of the VSD, the outflow obstruction, the size of the pulmonary annulus, and the degree of aortic override. Doppler analysis makes it possible to estimate the right ventricular outflow pressure gradient, and color flow mapping demonstrates the direction of flow through the VSD.
      (4) **Cardiac catheterization** is useful in measuring the degree of desaturation and the pressures in the ventricles and aorta. Angiography is used to evaluate the pulmonary and coronary arteries, the ventricular septal defect, and the nature of the right ventricular outflow obstruction.

5. **Therapy**
   a. **Medical management**
      (1) Bacterial endocarditis prophylaxis is necessary. Oral hygiene must be maintained.
      (2) Hypoxemic spells are treated by placing the child in a knee-chest position to increase systemic vascular resistance and to diminish right-to-left shunting. Morphine sulfate is given to depress the respiratory center, and oxygen is administered. α-Adrenergic agonists (e.g., phenylephrine) and β receptor blocking agents (e.g., propranolol) are also useful.
   b. **Surgical management**
      (1) **Palliative** surgery. A temporary increase in pulmonary blood flow can be obtained by the creation of a systemic artery-to-pulmonary artery shunt [see IV E 2 a (5) (b)].
      (2) **Corrective** surgery consists of closing the VSD and resecting the right ventricular outflow obstruction, and, if necessary, enlarging the area with a patch.

G. | **Persistent truncus arteriosus**

1. **Description.** A rare abnormality accounting for 1%–4% of congenital cardiac defects, persistent truncus arteriosus results when conotruncal septation does not proceed normally. A single trunk exits from the heart, and there is a large VSD. Anatomic classification is based on the exit site of the pulmonary arteries from the trunk. In the most common type, a short main pulmonary artery segment originates from the trunk. Truncal valve anatomy is variable; the valve often is stenotic or insufficient. A right aortic arch is present in 25% of cases.

2. **Pathophysiology.** Pulmonary and systemic venous return is ejected into the common trunk. Pulmonary blood flow is determined by the size of the pulmonary arteries, the presence of pulmonary artery stenosis, and the pulmonary vascular resistance.

3. **Clinical features.** Symptoms depend on the magnitude of pulmonary blood flow and truncal valve integrity.
   a. Early in life, the high pulmonary vascular resistance limits pulmonary blood flow. Cyanosis may occur without decompensation, unless significant truncal valve insufficiency is present.
   b. As the pulmonary vascular resistance falls, there is an increase in pulmonary blood flow, leading to symptoms of congestive heart failure (e.g., failure to thrive, irritability, poor feeding, tachypnea, dyspnea).

4. **Diagnosis**
   a. **Physical examination**
      (1) If pulmonary blood flow is very high, physical findings may mimic those of a large PDA with congestive heart failure.
      (2) If pulmonary blood flow is meager, the findings may be similar to those seen in severe tetralogy of Fallot.
      (3) An ejection click and, if truncal valve insufficiency is present, a diastolic murmur may be heard.
   b. **Laboratory evaluation**
      (1) **Chest x-ray.** Heart size is directly related to pulmonary blood flow. The main pulmonary artery segment is concave, and a right aortic arch may be seen. Pulmonary vascularity is usually increased but may be diminished, depending on the size and origin of the pulmonary arteries (see Table 12-4).
      (2) **ECG** reveals biventricular hypertrophy and left atrial enlargement if pulmonary blood flow is increased. If pulmonary blood flow is decreased, right ventricular hypertrophy is seen.
      (3) **Echocardiogram** is diagnostic, permitting visualization of the VSD and the origin of the pulmonary arteries. Doppler ultrasonography and color flow mapping demonstrate truncal valve stenosis or insufficiency.
      (4) **Cardiac catheterization** and angiography are useful in confirming the diagnosis and visualizing the pulmonary arteries. Pressure in the ventricles is equalized, and pulmonary vascular resistance can be calculated.

5. **Therapy**
   a. **Medical management** involves treatment of congestive heart failure.
   b. **Surgical management.** Correction is accomplished by closing the VSD so that the trunk is included in the left ventricle, and by interposing a conduit between the right ventricle and the pulmonary arteries, which are disconnected from the trunk.

H. **Aortic valve and discrete subaortic stenosis**

1. **Description**
   a. In **aortic valve stenosis,** the valve tissue is thickened, and often bicuspid, with a single fused commissure and an eccentric orifice.
   b. In **discrete subaortic stenosis,** a membranous diaphragm or fibrous ring encircles the left ventricular outflow tract just beneath the base of the aortic valve.

2. **Pathophysiology.** The pressure gradient between the left ventricle and aorta during systolic ejection is directly proportional to the square of the blood flow. Left ventricular end-diastolic pressure may be elevated if left ventricular function is impaired or if hypertrophy is severe enough to reduce compliance.

3. **Clinical features.** Symptoms are often absent, even if obstruction is fairly severe. When they occur, symptoms are related to diminished cardiac reserve (fatigability and exertional dyspnea) or to inadequate coronary blood flow to meet the needs of the hypertrophied left ventricle (angina). Syncope—due to inability of the left ventricle to increase output to maintain cerebral blood flow—may occur with exercise.

4. **Diagnosis**
   a. **Physical examination**
      (1) A harsh systolic ejection murmur is heard at the right base and, in aortic valve stenosis, is preceded by an ejection click that is heard best at the lower left sternal border.
      (2) A systolic thrill is often felt in the jugular notch, and a diastolic murmur of aortic regurgitation, heard best at the mid-left sternal border, is a finding in both valve and discrete subvalve stenosis.
   b. **Laboratory evaluation**
      (1) **Chest x-ray.** Poststenotic dilatation of the ascending aorta is present in aortic valve, but not subvalve, stenosis.
      (2) The **ECG** may show left ventricular hypertrophy, but correlation with the severity of the stenosis is lacking. Left ventricular ischemia, shown by ST depression and T-wave inversion, is indicative of severe stenosis, but its absence does not exclude it.
      (3) **Echocardiogram.** The lesion and degree of hypertrophy are demonstrated by a two-dimensional study. Doppler ultrasonography can estimate the pressure gradient and the presence of aortic valve insufficiency. Aortic valve area can be calculated.
      (4) With **cardiac catheterization,** the site and degree of obstruction may be assessed, and the valve area calculated.

5. **Therapy**
   a. **Medical management**
      (1) Bacterial endocarditis prophylaxis (see Table 12-5) is indicated. Avoidance of competitive sports in all but the mildest cases is usually recommended.
      (2) Balloon angioplasty of the aortic valve can decrease the severity of stenosis and significantly diminish the transvalve gradient. Angioplasty has not been found effective in relieving discrete subaortic stenosis.
   b. **Surgical management**
      (1) In selected patients with **aortic valve stenosis,** open valvotomy or aortic valve replacement must be performed.
      (2) In **discrete subvalvular stenosis,** treatment consists of resection of the subaortic membrane; recurrence of obstruction is not uncommon.

I. **Coarctation of the aorta** (see Figure 12-6)

1. **Description.** Coarctation of the aorta accounts for 8% of congenital heart defects. It is twice as common in boys as it is in girls. When it occurs in a girl, Turner syndrome must be considered (see Chapter 8). The obstruction is usually located in the descending aorta, just opposite the ligamentum arteriosum. It may coexist with tubular hypoplasia of the aortic arch. The aortic valve is bicuspid in more than 50% of cases. Mitral valve abnormalities (stenosis, regurgitation, or both) may be present.

2. **Pathophysiology.** Coarctation represents a mechanical obstruction between the proximal and distal aorta. The proximal aortic pressure and left ventricular afterload are elevated, whereas the distal aortic pressure is low. Collateral vessels, usually involving the internal mammary and the intercostal arteries, develop in response to the pressure differential.

3. **Clinical features.** Congestive heart failure develops in infancy in approximately 10% of cases (see IV E 1 b). Most children are asymptomatic; leg cramps, headaches, and chest pain occur only rarely.

4. **Diagnosis**
   a. **Physical examination**
      (1) Signs typically seen in the older infant include weak, delayed, or absent femoral pulses compared to upper extremity pulses, upper extremity hypertension, and blood pressure differential between the arm and leg. These signs may not be present in the newborn whose ductus arteriosus is patent.

(2) Flow across the coarctation or via collateral vessels may produce a systolic ejection murmur heard at the apex, left sternal border, and interscapular area. Collateral pulsations may be palpable around the scapula in older patients. If the aortic valve is bicuspid, an ejection click is heard.

b. Laboratory evaluation

(1) Chest x-ray. In older children, soft tissue densities consisting of the aortic knob and the dilated descending aorta may form a "3"; the same structures indent the barium-filled esophagus to form an "E". Notching of the fourth through eighth ribs, caused by erosion from collateral vessels, may be seen in children older than 5 years of age.

(2) ECG may be normal or show left ventricular hypertrophy.

(3) Echocardiogram. The coarctation may be visualized from the suprasternal notch approach. Left ventricular function and associated abnormalities may be evaluated.

(4) Cardiac catheterization. The aortic pressure gradient can be measured. Aortography allows visualization of the lesion and evaluation of the collateral vessels.

5. Therapy

a. Medical management

(1) Bacterial endocarditis prophylaxis (see Table 12-5) is indicated, and treatment of hypertension may be necessary.

(2) The coarctation can be dilated with balloon angioplasty, but long-term follow-up data are currently not available. Balloon angioplasty is the procedure of choice for the treatment of restenosis of the coarctation after its surgical correction.

b. Surgical management. Surgical repair is accomplished in one of several ways: resection with end-to-end anastomosis, subclavian flap angioplasty, patch repair, and graft repair.

J. Pulmonary stenosis

1. Description. Pulmonary stenosis accounts for 5%–8% of congenital heart defects. The pulmonary commissures are fused and the valve is domed and has a small central or eccentric opening; there is poststenotic dilatation of the main pulmonary artery. The pulmonary valve is occasionally bicuspid and is dysplastic in 10% of cases.

2. Pathophysiology. To maintain cardiac output, right ventricular pressure rises. In severe stenosis, right ventricular end-diastolic pressure may also increase. A consequent increase in right atrial pressure may open the foramen ovale and cause a right-to-left shunt.

3. Clinical features. Most patients are asymptomatic. Severe to critical pulmonary stenosis may cause exertional dyspnea, fatigability, and exertional chest pain. Congestive heart failure is unusual except in infants with critical stenosis.

4. Diagnosis

a. Physical examination

(1) An ejection click, the loudness of which varies with respiration, and a harsh systolic ejection murmur are present at the upper left sternal border.

(2) In moderately severe stenosis, a thrill and right ventricular heave are palpable, the pulmonary component of S_2 is diminished, the ejection click merges with S_1, and the murmur becomes longer and louder.

(3) If the stenosis is critical, cyanosis and an S_4 gallop may be found.

b. Laboratory evaluation

(1) Chest x-ray. Heart size and pulmonary vascularity usually are normal, but the pulmonary artery segment is prominent because of poststenotic dilatation. In critical stenosis, cardiomegaly and diminished pulmonary blood flow may be seen.

(2) ECG. The degree of right-axis deviation and right ventricular hypertrophy correlates well with right ventricular pressure and, therefore, with severity of the stenosis. An R wave of 20 mm or greater in lead V_1 or a positive T wave is indicative of systemic right ventricular pressure.

(3) **Echocardiogram.** Findings depend on the degree of stenosis. Right ventricular hypertrophy, dilatation, doming of the pulmonary valve, and poststenotic dilatation of the pulmonary artery can be seen. The integrity of the interatrial septum can be assessed. Doppler ultrasonography estimates the transvalvular gradient.

(4) **Cardiac catheterization.** Right ventricular function, anatomy of the pulmonary valve, and the transvalve gradient can be accurately assessed. In mild stenosis, right ventricular pressure is less than 50% of systemic pressure; in moderate stenosis, it is 50%–80% of systemic pressure; and in severe stenosis, it is greater than 80% of systemic pressure.

5. **Therapy**
   a. **Medical management.** Bacterial endocarditis prophylaxis (see Table 12-5) is necessary. Percutaneous balloon angioplasty of the pulmonary valve may be performed at the time of cardiac catheterization.
   b. **Surgical management.** Surgical resection of the pulmonary valve is reserved for those patients in whom balloon angioplasty has failed, including patients with dysplastic valves.

K. D-**Transposition of the great arteries** (Figure 12-8)

1. **Description.** This lesion, also known as **simple transposition,** accounts for 5% of congenital heart defects and is more common in boys than in girls. The anatomy is as follows: The aorta arises from the right ventricle anteriorly and to the right of the pulmonary artery, which arises posteriorly from the left ventricle. Associated abnormalities may include VSD, PDA, pulmonary stenosis, or a combination of these.

2. **Pathophysiology.** Systemic (unoxygenated) blood is recirculated through the body, and pulmonary venous (oxygenated) blood is recirculated through the lungs. A lesion that allows mixing of the systemic and pulmonary circulations (e.g., ASD, VSD, PDA) is necessary for survival.

3. **Clinical features.** Cyanosis is present from birth, the degree varying with the associated mixing lesion.

4. **Diagnosis**
   a. **Physical examination.** Intense cyanosis is noted in the absence of mixing lesions. In addition, a right ventricular heave and a single loud S_2 are usually found, and a soft flow murmur may be heard.

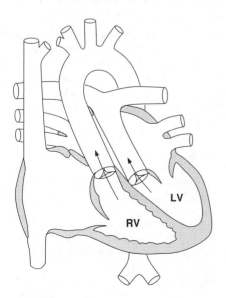

FIGURE 12-8. Anatomy of D-transposition of the great arteries. *Arrows* indicate the usual direction of flow. *RV* = right ventricle; *LV* = left ventricle.

b. Laboratory evaluation

(1) Chest x-ray. Pulmonary vascularity is increased or may be normal (see Table 12-4). Slight cardiomegaly and a narrow base produced by the anterior–posterior arrangement of the great arteries give the heart the shape of an egg on its side.

(2) Arterial blood gas analysis shows severe hypoxemia (Po_2 is often in the low 20s); increasing the ambient Fio_2 to 100% does not significantly alter the arterial Po_2.

(3) ECG is normal in the newborn.

(4) Echocardiogram shows the anterior–posterior arrangement of the great arteries and the chamber from which they originate, the normal anatomy of the ventricles, and the presence of associated abnormalities. Color flow mapping shows the direction of flow through associated abnormalities.

(5) Cardiac catheterization. Right ventricular pressure is systemic. Left ventricular pressure may be systemic in the newborn but decreases with a decline in pulmonary vascular resistance. Angiography confirms the anatomy and indicates the direction of blood flow. Balloon atrial septostomy (**Rashkind procedure**) allows the creation of an ASD, through which the mixing of oxygenated and deoxygenated blood can occur.

5. Therapy

a. Medical management. Creation of an ASD by balloon atrial septostomy may be life-saving. Correction of acidosis, hypoglycemia, and hypocalcemia in the neonatal period improves myocardial function.

b. Surgical management. The current procedure of choice is the **arterial switch procedure** with **coronary artery reimplantation,** which must be performed in the neonatal period and involves moving the arteries, but not the valves, into their "normal" position. Two atrial switch procedures, the **Senning** and the **Mustard** procedures, have been used in the past.

L. **ʟ-Transposition of the great arteries**

1. Description. ʟ-Transposition of the great arteries accounts for less than 1% of all congenital heart disease. The anatomy is as follows: The great arteries are transposed, with the aortic valve anterior to and to the left of the pulmonary valve. In 98% of cases, the bulboventricular loop has developed to the left, leading to inversion of the ventricles. The anatomic right ventricle is on the left, and the anatomic left ventricle is on the right (SLL). The AV valves are also inverted; the mitral valve leads into the anatomic left ventricle and the tricuspid valve into the anatomic right ventricle. Atrial position is unaffected. Associated abnormalities are common and may include AV conduction block, VSD, pulmonary stenosis, and left-sided AV (i.e., tricuspid) valve insufficiency.

2. Pathophysiology. The combination of transposition of the great arteries and inversion of the ventricles leads to a physiologically corrected circulation. (This lesion has also been called **"corrected" transposition**.) Systemic venous return flows via the mitral valve to the right-sided left ventricle and is ejected into a posterior pulmonary trunk; pulmonary venous return flows via the tricuspid valve to the left-sided right ventricle and from there to the anterior aorta. This "corrected" circulation may be altered by associated defects.

3. Clinical features. Symptoms reflect the associated defects.

a. A large VSD produces symptoms of a large left-to-right shunt, including congestive heart failure in infants.

b. Severe pulmonary valve or subvalve stenosis associated with a VSD produces symptoms of a right-to-left shunt (i.e., cyanosis, dyspnea), similar to those seen in tetralogy of Fallot.

c. Left-sided (tricuspid) valve regurgitation may produce tachypnea, dyspnea, cough, and other signs of pulmonary venous congestion.

d. Complete heart block may be associated with syncope and clinical evidence of low cardiac output.

4. Diagnosis

a. Physical examination

(1) In the absence of associated defects, the only physical finding that gives a hint of the underlying lesion is a loud single S_2.

(2) If a VSD is present, the findings are similar to those noted in IV C 4 a.

(3) When severe pulmonary stenosis is associated with a large VSD, the findings are those of tetralogy of Fallot (see IV F 4 a).

(4) Left atrioventricular valve (tricuspid valve) insufficiency is indistinguishable from severe mitral valve regurgitation.

b. Laboratory evaluation

(1) Chest x-ray

(a) Because the left heart border is formed by the ascending aorta, it is straight or slightly convex.

(b) Cardiomegaly, pulmonary hyperflow, and left atrial enlargement are seen in the presence of a large VSD.

(c) If severe pulmonary stenosis coexists with a VSD, the heart size is normal, and pulmonary vascularity is diminished.

(d) Severe left-sided AV valve regurgitation results in an enlarged left atrium and evidence of pulmonary venous congestion.

(2) ECG. Inversion of the septum causes reversal of initial depolarization, indicated by deep Q waves in leads II, III, and aVf and in the right precordial leads. Varying degrees of AV block may be seen.

(3) Echocardiogram demonstrates ventricular structure, great vessel location, and associated defects. Color flow mapping indicates AV valve regurgitation and direction of flow through a VSD, and Doppler ultrasonography estimates the severity of pulmonary stenosis.

(4) Cardiac catheterization. In the absence of associated abnormalities, right-sided left ventricular pressure is low, and left-sided right ventricular pressure is systemic. Oxygen saturations and pressures are modified by associated defects, which are accurately delineated by angiography.

5. Therapy

a. Medical management is determined by the presence of associated cardiac defects. Measures include treatment of congestive heart failure and conduction disturbances as well as implementation of bacterial endocarditis prophylaxis (see Table 12-5).

b. Surgical management

(1) Palliative systemic artery–pulmonary artery shunts relieve cyanosis produced by diminished pulmonary blood flow associated with VSD and severe pulmonary stenosis.

(2) Pacemaker implantation in symptomatic bradycardia, surgical repair of VSD and pulmonary stenosis, and annuloplasty or replacement of a severely regurgitant left-sided AV valve also are surgically feasible.

M. Abnormalities of the pulmonary veins

1. Total anomalous pulmonary venous return

a. Description. In this defect, the pulmonary veins are not incorporated into the left atrium. Instead, they carry oxygenated blood to the right atrium either directly or indirectly via venous channels. There are four possible routes:

(1) Supracardiac (50% of cases)—the pulmonary veins enter the innominate vein and thence to the superior vena cava or directly to the superior vena cava

(2) Cardiac (20% of cases)—the pulmonary veins enter into the coronary sinus or directly into the right atrium

(3) Infracardiac, also known as **infradiaphragmatic** (20% of cases)—the pulmonary veins drain into the portal or hepatic vein and thence into the inferior vena cava

(4) Mixed (10% of cases)—pulmonary venous blood returns to the heart via a combination of the above routes

b. Pathophysiology

(1) There is an obligatory right-to-left shunt, usually via a stretched foramen ovale or an ASD. The magnitude of pulmonary blood flow is inversely related to the pulmonary venous resistance.

(2) High resistance to pulmonary venous flow may exist in all types but is most common in the infracardiac type.

(a) If obstruction is severe, the pressure in the pulmonary veins and arteries is high, pulmonary blood flow is low, and systemic arterial blood is markedly desaturated.

(b) If there is no obstruction, pulmonary blood flow is high, pressures are only mildly elevated, and arterial blood is only mildly desaturated.

c. Clinical features. Symptoms depend on the degree of pulmonary venous obstruction. In severe obstruction, the classic presentation is that of an intensely cyanotic newborn with tachypnea and dyspnea. If no obstruction is present, desaturation may be subclinical, and symptoms are those of pulmonary hyperflow.

d. Diagnosis

(1) Physical examination

(a) If pulmonary venous flow is obstructed, there is a right ventricular heave and a loud, narrowly split S_2, a gallop rhythm, but usually no murmur.

(b) If pulmonary venous flow is unobstructed, the findings are similar to those of a high-flow ASD, including a prominent and active precordium with a right ventricular heave, clinical cardiomegaly, wide and fixed split S_2 with a loud pulmonary component, systolic ejection murmur at the upper left sternal border with wide radiation, and mid-diastolic rumble at the lower left sternal border.

(2) Laboratory evaluation

(a) **Chest x-ray.** Cardiomegaly with increased pulmonary blood flow is present in unobstructed anomalous pulmonary venous return. In the supracardiac type, the base of the heart may appear widened by dilated veins, and the entire silhouette may have a "snowman" or "figure 8" appearance. In obstructed venous return, the heart size is normal, and diffuse pulmonary edema may be difficult to distinguish from hyaline membrane disease.

(b) **ECG** indicates right-axis deviation and right ventricular hypertrophy.

(c) **Echocardiogram.** The right side of the heart and the pulmonary artery are enlarged; left-sided structures may be relatively small. The pulmonary veins do not enter the left atrium. The coronary sinus may be enlarged if the veins drain into it; in the infracardiac type, the common pulmonary vein may be seen behind the left atrium with the communicating vein traversing the diaphragm. Such anomalies can be subtle and easily missed. Color flow mapping is helpful in highlighting the pulmonary veins and evaluating the direction of flow.

(d) **Cardiac catheterization.** Because of mixing, oxygen saturation is similar in all chambers and arteries. Saturation is highest if sampling is performed near the drainage site of the pulmonary veins. Pulmonary artery pressure is proportional to the degree of pulmonary venous obstruction. Pulmonary arteriography defines the pulmonary venous drainage.

e. Therapy

(1) Medical management. Congestive heart failure is treated. If pulmonary edema is present, mechanical ventilation may be necessary.

(2) Surgical management. Surgical redirection of the pulmonary veins into the left atrium can be accomplished in all four types.

2. Partial anomalous venous return

a. Description. In this defect, most of the pulmonary veins drain normally into the left atrium, but one or several veins drain abnormally. Most frequently, the right upper pulmonary vein drains into the superior vena cava. A sinus venosus ASD often coexists with this anomaly.

b. Pathophysiology. There is a left-to-right shunt, similar to that seen in ASD.

c. Clinical features (see IV B 3)

d. Diagnosis (see IV B 4 for discussion of typical findings on physical examination, chest x-ray, and ECG)

    (1) Echocardiogram. A sinus venosus ASD may be seen, and occasionally, the anomalous pulmonary vein can be identified. Color flow mapping helps define the abnormal pulmonary vein and often highlights it.

    (2) Cardiac catheterization [see also IV B 4 b (4)]. Cardiac catheterization is not necessary if the echocardiogram is diagnostic. If performed, the anomalous vein can often be entered. Selective pulmonary artery angiography may be needed to identify the anomalous pulmonary vein.

e. Therapy

    (1) Medical management (see IV B 5 a)

    (2) Surgical management. The anomalous pulmonary vein can be surgically redirected into the left atrium at the time of closure of the ASD.

V. ACQUIRED STRUCTURAL DISORDERS

A. **Rheumatic heart disease** (see also Chapter 9) is a result of single or multiple episodes of acute rheumatic fever. **Mitral valve insufficiency** is the most common lesion, followed by **aortic valve insufficiency. Mitral valve stenosis** is less common and usually is the end result of multiple attacks of acute rheumatic fever. Least common is **aortic valve stenosis**. The tricuspid and pulmonary valves are virtually never affected. Symptoms are proportional to the degree of valve damage. Daily penicillin prophylaxis for patients who have had an episode of acute rheumatic fever are mandatory to prevent recurrent episodes and increased valve damage.

B. **Kawasaki disease** (see also Chapter 10). Cardiac effects may include pericarditis, myocarditis, and transient rhythm disturbances. However, it is the development of **coronary artery aneurysms,** with their potential for occlusion or rupture, that makes the disease potentially life threatening. Coronary artery aneurysms develop during the subacute phase (eleventh to twenty-fifth day) in about 30% of cases, but regress in most patients. Early therapy with gamma globulin decreases the incidence of coronary artery aneurysms. Low-dose salicylate therapy lessens the likelihood of aneurysm occlusion. Echocardiography is used to assess ventricular function and to visualize pericardial fluid and coronary artery aneurysms.

C. **Endocarditis** (see also Chapter 10) usually occurs on the low-pressure side of a turbulence-producing lesion (e.g., VSD, semilunar valve stenosis, AV valve regurgitation, semilunar valve regurgitation). It does not usually occur with abnormalities that do not produce turbulence (e.g., ASD). Bacterial endocarditis prophylaxis includes good dental hygiene and preventive dental care; antibiotic prophylaxis (see Table 12-5) should be instituted when the potential for bacteremia exists in children with turbulent cardiac defects.

D. **Coronary artery disease** is rare in childhood, but the atherosclerotic process appears to begin early in life. There is evidence that progression of atherosclerosis is adversely influenced by genetic factors (e.g., familial hypercholesterolemia; see Chapter 17) and lifestyle (e.g., cigarette smoking, high-cholesterol, high–saturated-fat diet). Because many lifetime habits are formed during childhood, an opportunity exists to influence young people to adopt healthful ones.

VI. FUNCTIONAL HEART DISORDERS

A. **Myocarditis** (inflammation of the myocardium) is most commonly of **infectious** etiology (see also Chapter 10). **Noninfectious** inflammatory lesions are primarily associated with collagen vascular diseases. Some patients may be asymptomatic, and the diagnosis is made only by observing changes in the ST segment and T wave on serial ECGs. Others may manifest signs of congestive heart failure, low cardiac output, or rhythm disturbances. Myocardial inflammation can be acutely fatal or progress to congestive cardiomyopathy and chronic congestive heart failure. Anticongestive therapy is usually necessary and myocardial biopsy can help guide initial therapy with antiinflammatory agents (steroids). Cardiac transplantation may be necessary for patients with chronic and unremitting myocardial failure.

B. Cardiomyopathy

1. **Congestive cardiomyopathy**
   a. **Description.** Congestive, or **dilated,** cardiomyopathy is characterized by myocardial dysfunction and ventricular dilatation. Although it usually is a primary disorder, it may be associated with neuromuscular disease (e.g., Duchenne muscular dystrophy) or result from drug toxicity (e.g., doxorubicin).
   b. **Pathophysiology.** Failure of the left ventricle causes an increase in end-diastolic volume, which results in increases in left atrial, pulmonary venous, and pulmonary capillary pressures. Mitral valve regurgitation may result from papillary muscle dysfunction or from severe dilatation of the valve annulus.
   c. **Clinical features.** Initially, dyspnea on exertion is present. As left ventricular failure progresses, small increases in left ventricular volume occur, followed by a marked increase in pulmonary capillary pressure. This results in orthopnea, paroxysmal nocturnal dyspnea, and bronchospasm. Eventually, right heart failure, characterized by dependent edema, occurs.
   d. **Diagnosis**
      (1) **Physical examination** depends on the stage of the disease but may include tachypnea, tachycardia, a right ventricular heave, prominent second pulmonary sound, gallop rhythm, and murmurs of mitral or tricuspid valve regurgitation. In advanced stages, blood pressure may be low and pulse pressure narrow; pulsus alternans may be present.
      (2) **Laboratory evaluation**
         (a) **Chest x-ray** may show cardiomegaly, an enlarged left atrium, pulmonary venous congestion, and pleural effusions.
         (b) **ECG** defines rhythm disturbances. Left ventricular hypertrophy as well as nonspecific ST segment and T-wave changes may be present.
         (c) Left ventricular **function** can be assessed by **echocardiography, radionuclide studies,** and if necessary, **cardiac catheterization**. Myocardial biopsy may be helpful in defining the pathologic process.
   e. **Therapy** is directed at improving left ventricular function with inotropic agents and at unloading the left ventricle with vasodilators. Preload is decreased with diuretics, and antiarrhythmic medications are used to control potentially fatal rhythm disturbances. In the event of clinical deterioration, cardiac transplantation may be needed.

2. **Hypertrophic cardiomyopathy**
   a. **Description.** This disorder, also known as **idiopathic hypertrophic subaortic stenosis** and **hypertrophic obstructive cardiomyopathy,** is an autosomal dominant genetic disorder with a high degree of penetrance, but can also be sporadic. The septum is thickened out of proportion to the left free ventricular wall, which may also be thickened.
   b. **Pathophysiology.** In the thickened, stiff left ventricle, systolic function is well preserved, but diastolic function is compromised. Thickening of the septum may result in left ventricular outflow obstruction and abnormal motion of the mitral valve. This abnormal motion may result in mitral regurgitation.
   c. **Clinical features.** Symptoms include dyspnea on exertion, because of an inability to increase significantly cardiac output with exercise; chest pain, due to myocardial ischemia; and syncope. Death may result from rhythm disturbances.
   d. **Diagnosis**
      (1) **Physical examination.** The pulse often is biferious (double peaked) because ejection is interrupted by septal obstruction. A forceful left ventricular impulse

may be present, and an S_3 or S_4 may be audible at the apex. Murmurs of left ventricular outflow obstruction or mitral regurgitation may be heard. Decreasing left ventricular volume (Valsalva maneuver, standing) increases left ventricular outflow obstruction, and with it the intensity of the murmur.

    (2) Laboratory evaluation

        (a) ECG often shows left-axis deviation, left ventricular hypertrophy, ST segment depression and T-wave inversion. Rhythm disturbances are best defined by Holter monitoring.

        (b) Echocardiogram is diagnostic. Measurement of the septum and the free wall of the left ventricle demonstrates the asymmetric hypertrophy of the former. In addition, the small diastolic left ventricular cavity size and the anterior motion of the mitral valve in systole can be demonstrated. Doppler ultrasound and color flow mapping allow evaluation of mitral valve regurgitation and estimation of the left ventricular outflow gradient.

  e. Therapy is aimed at preventing fatal arrhythmias and decreasing the stiffness of the left ventricle with negative inotropic medications (calcium channel blocking and β-adrenergic blocking agents). Avoidance of competitive sports is recommended because of the risk of sudden death with exertion. Ventricular pacing may prove helpful by decreasing the left ventricular outflow gradient and therefore the left ventricular mass.

VII. RHYTHM ABNORMALITIES (see also Chapter 7)

A. **Premature beats** may originate from either the atrium or ventricle.

  1. Premature atrial beats (Figure 12-9A) are characterized by an abnormally shaped P wave that occurs prematurely, a normal QRS complex, and no compensatory pause. Premature atrial beats are common and are usually benign.

  2. Premature ventricular beats (Figure 12-9B) are characterized by a wide QRS complex, a lack of a relationship between the P and QRS waves, an inverted T wave, and a compensatory pause. Premature ventricular beats are usually benign, unless they are multiform, increase with exercise, or are associated with a prolonged QT interval or with cardiomyopathy.

B. **Supraventricular tachycardia (SVT)** is the most common symptomatic arrhythmia in the pediatric age-group, is usually caused by a reentrant mechanism, is often paroxysmal, and may occur at any age, including in the fetus and newborn. A bypass tract (concealed or evident on the ECG) is sometimes one path of the reentry circuit. The ECG manifestation of the most common bypass tract is the **Wolff-Parkinson-White syndrome,** which consists of a short P-R interval, and a wide QRS with a slurred upstroke (delta wave) [Figure 12-9C].

  1. During a paroxysm of SVT, the R-R interval is uniform and the heart rate is usually around 160 beats per minute in adolescents, and may be as high as 300 beats per minute in infants (Figure 12-9D). Hemodynamic consequences depend on the heart rate, the age of the child, and the presence of underlying heart disease. In infants with very rapid rates, especially if they have heart disease, symptoms of low cardiac output may develop.

  2. Therapy of SVT includes vagal maneuvers, intravenous adenosine, digoxin, or β-blocking agents. Infants in imminent danger of cardiovascular collapse should be treated with synchronized electric cardioversion. If the paroxysms of tachyarrhythmia are difficult to control, radiofrequency ablation of the bypass tract eliminates the reentry circuit.

A

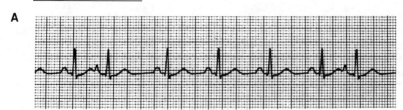

B

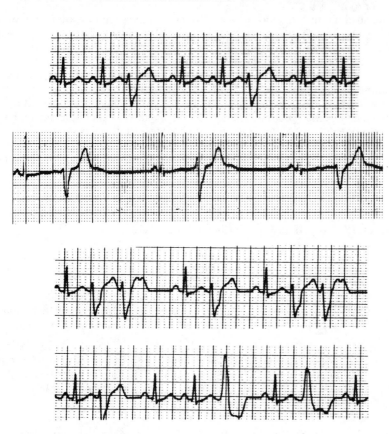

C

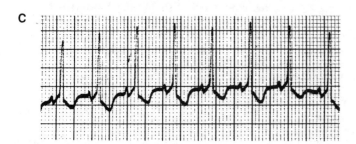

FIGURE 12-9. (*A*) Premature atrial beats. In the second and seventh beat, the P waves and P-R intervals are different from other beats. QRS waves are the same. (*B*) Premature ventricular beats. The *first strip* shows two similar premature ventricular beats (uniform). In the *second strip,* each premature beat is coupled with a normal beat (bigeminy). The *third strip* shows two consecutive premature ventricular beats (couplets). The *fourth strip* shows three different premature ventricular beats (multiform). (*C*) Wolff-Parkinson-White conduction disturbance. (*D*) Supraventricular tachycardia in an infant (*top*) at a rate of 240 beats per minute and in an adolescent (*bottom*) at a rate of 160 beats per minute. (*E*) Congenital complete heart block. The atrial rate is 140 beats per minute and the ventricular rate is 45 beats per minute.

D

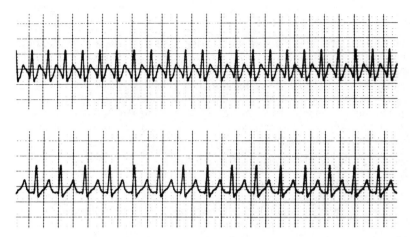

E

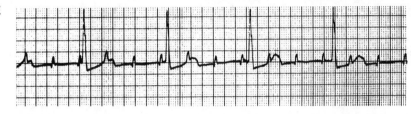

FIGURE 12-9. (*cont.*)

 C. In **complete heart block** (Figure 12-9E), there is loss of conduction from the atria to the ventricles. The ensuing idioventricular rhythm is slower than normal. Congenital heart block may be caused by maternal Ro antibodies formed in mothers with collagen vascular diseases that cross the placenta early in pregnancy and produce fibrosis of the conduction system. The pathophysiology and clinical symptoms of congenital complete heart block are related to the level of the block. The lower the level of the block, the slower the heart rate and the greater the symptoms of inadequate cardiac output. In symptomatic patients, therapy involves pacemaker implantation.

VIII. NEUROCARDIOGENIC SYNCOPE

A. **Definition.** Neurocardiogenic syncope is a temporary loss of consciousness caused by cerebral hypoperfusion.

B. **Pathophysiology.** An orthostatic stimulus causes venous pooling, estimated to be 300–800 ml in adults, that results in decreased cardiac output and blood pressure. Cerebral perfusion is usually preserved by tachycardia and vasoconstriction resulting from a reflex stimulus originating in the aortic arch, carotid body, and cardiac chambers. Neurocardiogenic syncope occurs if this reflex is interrupted by another reflex that originates in the cardiac chambers as a response to a hypercontractile state of the ventricles. The sudden withdrawal of the excitatory sympathetic tone and an increase in parasympathetic tone cause peripheral vasodilation, bradycardia, and cerebral hypoperfusion. The abnormal reflex is relaxed when the patient becomes horizontal.

C. Diagnosis

1. **History** is the single most important method of diagnosis because laboratory studies are usually negative. Syncope almost always occurs while standing or sitting, and is often immediately preceded by an anxiety-provoking or fearful event. There is often a **prodrome** that may include dizziness, light-headedness, loss of vision, or a feeling of impending loss of consciousness. Equally important is the absence of palpitations, which helps to rule out a tachyarrhythmia as a cause of the syncope. During the syncope there is pallor, and few postictal symptoms are present. The syncope itself is of short duration, usually not more than a few minutes.

2. **Physical examination.** No abnormalities are detectable.

3. **Laboratory evaluations.** Neurocardiogenic syncope is a clinical diagnosis. Laboratory evaluations are useful only to rule out other causes of syncope.
   a. **ECG** is characteristically normal. It is helpful in ruling out the prolonged Q-T interval syndrome and preexcitation. It may be helpful in the diagnosis of hypertrophic cardiomyopathy.
   b. **Chest x-ray** is normal and usually not helpful.
   c. **Echocardiogram** is normal in neurocardiogenic syncope but is helpful in ruling out other diagnoses, especially hypertrophic cardiomyopathy.
   d. The usefulness of reproducing the syncope with **head-up tilt table** testing is controversial because of the many false-positive and false-negative results and the lack of reproducibility. Some consider the test useful in confusing circumstances.

D. Therapy

1. Avoidance of hypovolemia is often sufficient to prevent syncope.

2. Fluorohydrocortisone, a safe, mild salt- and water-retaining hormone, is useful to help prevent hypovolemia.

3. Metoprolol has been found to be clinically safe and effective. Its exact mechanism of action is unknown, but it is theorized that it blunts the hypercontractile state or blocks sensitization of the C-fibers to catecholamines.

Bibliography

Emmanouilides GC, Riemenschneider TA, Allen HD, Gutgesell HP (eds): *Moss and Adams Heart Disease in Infants, Children, and Adolescents Including the Fetus and Young Adults,* 5th ed. Baltimore, Williams & Wilkins, 1994.

Fyler DC (ed): *Nadas' Pediatric Cardiology.* St. Louis, Mosby-Yearbook, 1992.

Gessner IH, Victoria BE (eds): *Pediatric Cardiology: A Problem Oriented Approach.* Philadelphia, WB Saunders, 1993.

Moller JH, Neal WA: *Fetal, Neonatal, and Infant Cardiac Disease.* Norwalk, CT, Appleton & Lange, 1990.

Park MK: *The Pediatric Cardiology Handbook.* St. Louis, Mosby-Yearbook, 1991.

DIRECTIONS: Each of the numbered items or incomplete statements in this section is followed by answers or by completions of the statement. Select the ONE lettered answer or completion that is BEST in each case.

1. A 2-year-old, active, asymptomatic boy is examined by a physician for the first time. His blood pressure is 130/86 in the right arm with a barely palpable right femoral pulse. The most likely finding in the remainder of the physical exam is

(A) pale, bluish discoloration of the lower extremities
(B) rib notching on chest x-ray
(C) an ejection click of a bicuspid aortic valve
(D) a normal left femoral pulse

2. A 5-year-old girl has a small ventricular septal defect (VSD). Her growth and development are normal and she has normal activity levels. Which of the following is a true statement?

(A) Her electrocardiogram demonstrates left atrial enlargement due to the left-to-right shunt
(B) She does not need endocarditis prophylaxis before dental work because the shunt is small
(C) Her pulmonary vascular resistance is increased
(D) The ventricular septal defect may close spontaneously

3. A healthy and asymptomatic 7-year-old boy is found to have an irregular heart rhythm on a preschool evaluation. Physical examination, electrocardiogram, and chest x-ray are normal. A Holter monitor shows single uniform ventricular premature beats. Which one of the following statements is true about this patient?

(A) He should be restricted from participating in gym class
(B) His echocardiogram will probably show myocardial dysfunction
(C) An exercise stress test will probably demonstrate normal exercise duration with suppression of the ectopy during exercise
(D) There is a high probability that he will develop ventricular tachycardia

4. A cyanotic infant has a ductus-dependent congenital heart defect with decreased pulmonary flow and good systemic blood flow. Which of the following belongs to this category of congenital heart defects?

(A) Hypoplastic left heart syndrome
(B) Pulmonary atresia with intact ventricular septum
(C) Total anomalous pulmonary venous return
(D) D-Transposition of the great arteries

DIRECTIONS: Each of the numbered items or incomplete statements in this section is negatively phrased, as indicated by a capitalized word such as NOT, LEAST, or EXCEPT. Select the ONE lettered answer or completion that is BEST in each case.

5. A 10-year-old boy presents with chest pain and dyspnea on exertion. Family history reveals that his mother died of a "cardiac problem." On physical examination, there is a murmur of left ventricular outflow obstruction that increases with a Valsalva maneuver. The electrocardiogram shows left ventricular hypertrophy and ST segment changes, and the echocardiogram is diagnostic for hypertrophic cardiomyopathy. Appropriate therapeutic measures include all of the following EXCEPT

(A) digoxin to increase left ventricular function
(B) restriction from weightlifting
(C) calcium channel blockers
(D) β-adrenergic blocking agents

6. A newborn is noted to be cyanotic in the first few hours of life. She is comfortable and in no respiratory distress. The remainder of her physical examination is remarkable only for a single second heart sound. By echocardiography, D-transposition of the great arteries is diagnosed. All of the following statements regarding D-transposition of the great arteries are true EXCEPT

(A) the aortic valve is to the right of the pulmonary artery
(B) the aortic valve is posterior to the pulmonary valve
(C) the right ventricular pressure is elevated
(D) a balloon atrial septostomy should be performed to improve systemic oxygenation

DIRECTIONS: Each set of matching questions in this section consists of a list of four to twenty-six lettered options (some of which may be in figures) followed by several numbered items. For each numbered item, select the ONE lettered option that is most closely associated with it. To avoid spending too much time on matching sets with large numbers of options, it is generally advisable to begin each set by reading the list of options. Then, for each item in the set, try to generate the correct answer and locate it in the option list, rather than evaluating each option individually. Each lettered option may be selected once, more than once, or not at all.

Questions 7–10

Match each pathophysiologic feature described below with the congenital cardiac defect it best characterizes.

(A) Hypoplastic left-heart syndrome
(B) Persistent truncus arteriosus
(C) Tricuspid atresia
(D) Pulmonary atresia with ventricular septal defect
(E) Critical aortic stenosis

7. An obligatory right-to-left atrial shunt

8. Ductus-dependent systemic flow with an obligatory left-to-right atrial shunt

9. Ductus-dependent pulmonary flow with an obligatory right-to-left ventricular shunt.

10. Symptoms primarily related to pulmonary artery size and pulmonary vascular resistance.

1. The answer is C *[IV E 1 b]*. A bicuspid aortic valve is commonly associated with a coarctation of the aorta. Blood flow to the aorta distal to the coarctation is supplied by collaterals carrying saturated blood, and the lower extremities should therefore not be discolored. Rib notching does not usually appear on chest x-ray until approximately 6 years of age. Both right and left femoral pulses are distal to the coarctation, and both should be diminished.

2. The answer is D *[IV C 3 a]*. Ventricular septal defects (VSDs) can close spontaneously at any age in childhood. The small left-to-right shunt through a small VSD does not produce left atrial enlargement. Patients with a small VSD should obtain antibiotic prophylaxis before dental work regardless of the size of the shunt. The resistance to pulmonary blood flow through a small VSD is at the level of the VSD, and the pulmonary vascular resistance is normal.

3. The answer is C *[VII A 2]*. Patients with single ventricular premature beats with an otherwise normal history, physical examination, and supporting laboratory tests normally have suppression of the ectopy with exercise. There is no need to restrict their activity. The echocardiogram is usually normal with normal myocardial function. They are not at risk for development of ventricular tachycardia.

4. The answer is B *[IV E 2 a (1) (a)]*. Pulmonary atresia with intact ventricular septum is a ductus-dependent pulmonary flow lesion. There is an obligatory right-to-left atrial shunt. Hypoplastic left-heart syndrome is a ductus-dependent systemic flow lesion. Total anomalous pulmonary venous return is characterized by desaturation, which can be severe and is proportional to the degree of pulmonary venous obstruction. D-Transposition of the great arteries often has marked cyanosis that may improve with ductal patency but is characterized by increased pulmonary blood flow.

5. The answer is A *[VI B 2]*. Digoxin can increase the left ventricular outflow obstruction in hypertrophic cardiomyopathy, and should not be used. Fatal arrhythmias can occur during exercise, and therefore patients should be restricted from performing aerobic as well as isometric exercise. Calcium channel blockers and β-adrenergic blocking agents can decrease the stiffness of the left ventricle and have been helpful in some patients.

6. The answer is B *[III D 1]*. In D-transposition of the great arteries, the aortic valve is anterior and to the right of the pulmonary valve, which is posterior and to the left. The right ventricle is the systemic ventricle, and therefore the right ventricular pressure is elevated. A balloon atrial septostomy allows for bidirectional mixing at the atrial level and improves systemic oxygenation.

7–10. The answers are: 7-C *[IV E 2 a (1) (b)]*, **8-A** *[IV E 1 a]*, **9-D** *[IV E 2 b]*, **10-B** *[IV G]*. A right-to-left atrial shunt is obligatory in tricuspid atresia and in pulmonary atresia with intact ventricular septum.

In hypoplastic left heart-syndrome with aortic and mitral valve atresia, there is no forward flow across the left side of the heart, and pulmonary venous return must cross the atrial septum from left atrium to right atrium. In critical aortic stenosis, systemic blood flow is ductus-dependent, but a left-to-right atrial shunt is not obligatory, although it is often present.

In pulmonary atresia with ventricular septal defect, pulmonary blood flow is ductus-dependent and a right-to-left ventricular shunt is obligatory.

In persistent truncus arteriosus, conotruncal septation does not proceed normally, resulting in a single arterial vessel arising from the heart. Symptoms depend on the pulmonary blood flow, and are therefore related to the size of the pulmonary arteries and the pulmonary vascular resistance.

Chapter 13

Pulmonary Diseases
Michelle M. Cloutier

I. GENERAL PRINCIPLES OF PULMONARY DISEASE IN CHILDREN

A. **Lung development**

1. **Prenatal lung development** (see also Chapter 6)
   a. The **lung bud** arises as a pouch from the primitive foregut at 22–26 days' gestation. The **bronchial tree** develops between 5 and 16 weeks' gestation by continuous budding and branching of the airways. Airway branching ends at 16 weeks; further growth occurs by an increase in diameter and length but not by an increase in airway number.
   b. Insults to the lung before 16 weeks' gestation decrease both airway number and subsequent alveolar growth and number. Insults after 16 weeks affect only alveolar number and growth.

2. **Postnatal lung development.** Approximately 60 million primitive alveoli exist at birth. The lung grows most rapidly in alveolar number during the first 2 years. The growth rate decreases thereafter, until the adult number of approximately 375 million alveoli is reached at age 8–12 years.

B. **Common pathologic features of pulmonary disease.** Of the 69 million children younger than age 17 years in the United States, 23% (15.9 million) have chronic disease, and 16% (11 million) have chronic pulmonary disease.

1. **Underlying pathologic process.** Most lung diseases in children are classified as obstructive or restrictive.
   a. **Obstruction** (i.e., airway narrowing) may be caused by intraluminal secretions, edema or inflammation of the airway wall, hypertrophy or contraction of the bronchial smooth muscle, or extrinsic compression.
   b. **Restriction** [i.e., impaired lung expansion (volume)] may be caused by decreased lung compliance (stiff lungs), atelectasis or pneumothorax causing lung collapse, neuromuscular disease, or disorders of the chest wall.

2. **Pathophysiology**
   a. **Hypoxemia** (i.e., deficient oxygenation of blood) most commonly is caused by ventilation–perfusion abnormalities but also may be the result of intracardiac or intrapulmonary shunts, diffusion problems, or hypoventilation.
   b. **Hypercapnia** (i.e., excess carbon dioxide in blood) most commonly is caused by primary hypoventilation (due to upper airway obstruction, neuromuscular weakness, or central nervous system depression), but also may be seen with increased lower airway obstructive disease and associated ventilation–perfusion mismatch, shunts, and impaired diffusion.

3. **Pathogenic factors**
   a. The **small airways** of the child result in high airway resistance and put the child at great risk for development of obstructive lung disease. Boys are affected more frequently and more severely than girls, in part because the peripheral airways in boys younger than age 5 years are smaller than those in girls.
   b. The young child lacks **specific immunity** (organism-specific antibody) and is relatively defenseless against invading microorganisms.
   c. In children, most pulmonary disease has a **single cause,** whereas in adults, pulmonary disease is apt to be multifactorial in etiology.

C. **Evaluation of pulmonary disease**

1. **History.** Many pulmonary diseases are missed or misdiagnosed. Therefore, a careful history should be obtained, focusing on the following questions.
   a. **Is the disorder acute, chronic, or recurrent?** The physician must determine whether the condition is acute and self-limited, chronic (i.e., with symptoms occurring daily for more than 4 weeks), or recurrent (i.e., with disease-free intervals). With chronic or recurrent disorders, the parents may not remember each episode clearly, but they usually can recall—in reasonably good detail—the first time the problem arose.
   b. **Is the disorder immediately or eventually life threatening?**
      (1) Cyanosis, respiratory distress, or severe stridor—regardless of cause—indicate severe difficulty and the need for immediate action.
      (2) Problems such as progressive weight loss or a progressive pulmonary opacification imply a serious long-term outlook.
   c. **What are the symptoms?** Specific pulmonary symptoms should be sought, such as:
      (1) The presence of a cough and its characteristics
      (2) Labored or noisy breathing and its interference with activities
      (3) The presence of wheezing, chest pain, sputum production, or foul breath
   d. **What factors affect the severity of symptoms?** It is important to identify factors that improve or worsen symptoms. Reactive airway disease is suggested when symptoms are exacerbated by changes in weather, viral infections (e.g., common colds), exercise, laughing or crying, or exposure to allergens.
   e. **Have any tests been performed?** The physician should determine which tests have been performed, where they were given, and what the results were.
   f. **Have any treatments been given?** Parents should be asked about the types of therapy the child has previously received, the dosages used, the duration of therapy, and the response of symptoms to treatment.
   g. **Is there a family history of pulmonary disease?** A family history of a similar problem or of any type of respiratory disease should be identified.

2. **Physical examination**
   a. **Respiratory rate** (Table 13-1) is the best indicator of pulmonary function in young infants. However, the respiratory rate is influenced by activity when the child is awake. Therefore, the most reliable and reproducible rate is the sleeping respiratory rate.
   b. **Effort of breathing** is a guide to pulmonary dysfunction.
      (1) **Grunting** is a sign of loss of lung volume. It is frequently heard in neonatal respiratory distress syndrome and pulmonary edema. In older children, it is frequently a sign of chest pain and suggests an acute pneumonic process with pleural involvement.
      (2) **Chest retractions**
         (a) **Intercostal retractions** are a sign of increased lung stiffness or increased work of breathing due to airway obstruction.
         (b) **Subcostal retractions** are a sign of hyperinflation and a flattened diaphragm due to small airway obstruction.

TABLE 13-1. Normal Respiratory Rates in Children

Age	Breaths/Minute
Newborn	30–75
6–12 months	22–31
1–2 years	17–23
2–4 years	16–25
4–10 years	13–23
10–14 years	13–19

(3) **Flaring of the alae nasi** (dilated nostrils) is a sign of increased airway resistance.

(4) **Head-bobbing** is a sign of dyspnea in an exhausted or sleeping infant; the head bobs forward owing to neck flexion with each inspiration.

c. **Breath sounds** also are informative.

(1) **Crackles** are heard primarily on inspiration. The sound is produced by the opening of small airways that closed on the previous breath.

(2) **Wheezing** is produced by partial airway obstruction. It usually is expiratory in origin but can be inspiratory when the airway obstruction is fixed and rigid, as in airway edema. Wheezing usually is a sign of asthma, but it can occur in any pulmonary disease when the airflow is through a sufficiently narrowed orifice.

(3) **Stridor** is a harsh, primarily inspiratory sound produced by laryngeal or tracheal obstruction to breathing.

(4) **Rales** is a broad term that can mean any abnormal breath sound. The term is used less now than in the past.

(5) **Rhonchi** are sonorous sounds produced by secretions in large airways.

d. **Anatomic changes** of significance include the following:

(1) **Clubbing of the fingers** is caused by lifting of the nail base by tissue proliferation on the dorsal surface of the terminal phalanx.

(a) As a sign of pulmonary disease in children, clubbing most often is caused by cystic fibrosis. Pulmonary abscess, empyema, some neoplasms, and, occasionally, bronchiectasis not associated with cystic fibrosis also can produce clubbing.

(b) Nonpulmonary causes of clubbing include congenital cyanotic heart disease, subacute bacterial endocarditis, biliary cirrhosis, chronic ulcerative colitis, and regional enteritis.

(2) **A change in tracheal position** is useful in detecting a mediastinal shift and an inequality between the two sides of the chest, suggesting a pneumothorax or atelectasis.

(3) **A change in thoracic configuration.** A **barrel-chest deformity** suggests hyperinflation and overdistention of the lungs due to chronic airway obstruction.

3. **Laboratory studies**

a. **Imaging procedures**

(1) **Chest x-ray** is indicated if pulmonary disease is suspected. An x-ray of the sinuses may be helpful in sinus disease. Neck films can sometimes help in upper airway obstruction.

(2) **Fluoroscopy** is useful for dynamic studies (e.g., to evaluate diaphragmatic movements or the cause of stridor) and for guiding invasive procedures (e.g., thoracentesis).

(3) **Ultrasonography** can be used instead of fluoroscopy when evaluating diaphragmatic motility, confirming pleural effusion, and guiding thoracentesis.

(4) **Contrast studies** of value include barium swallow, bronchogram, pulmonary arteriogram, and thoracic aortogram.

(5) **Radionuclide lung scans** are valuable in the evaluation of pulmonary ventilation and perfusion.

(6) **Computed tomography (CT) scanning** of the chest is useful in differentiating among pulmonary lesions that cannot be distinguished on chest x-ray (e.g., to differentiate a collapsed lung from a mediastinal mass or pleural fluid from a consolidated lung). Chest CT scanning may also show the extent of cystic lesions and bronchiectasis not visualized on routine chest x-rays.

b. **Pulmonary function tests** are used to evaluate obstructive, restrictive, and diffusion abnormalities in pulmonary function. They cannot diagnose specific diseases.

(1) **Commonly used tests** in children are **spirometry, flow–volume curves,** and **lung volumes**.

(a) Tests can be performed before and after inhalation of a bronchodilating agent (to determine whether abnormalities are reversible) or before and after exercise (as a challenge to elicit airway obstruction). Exercise testing is also used to evaluate cardiopulmonary fitness.

(b) Testing requires a child who can cooperate by taking a deep breath to total lung capacity and then exhaling completely. Therefore, the tests cannot be performed in most children younger than age 7 years, in most retarded children, or in children with tracheostomies.

(2) In **obstructive lung disease,** the following test results are seen.

(a) Peak expiratory flow rate (PEFR) and V_{max25} (flow rate at which 25% of the vital capacity has been exhaled), which depend on effort, are reduced in the presence of large airway obstruction.

(b) V_{max75} (flow rate at which 75% of the vital capacity has been exhaled) and FEF_{25-75} [average flow rate over the middle (25%–75%) portion of the vital capacity], which are effort independent, are reduced in the presence of small airway obstruction.

(c) Lung volumes such as residual volume (RV; volume of air left in the lung after a maximal exhalation) are increased and indicative of small airway obstruction and air trapping. Total lung capacity (TLC) is increased but not to the same extent as RV; therefore, the RV/TLC ratio is increased.

(d) The forced vital capacity (FVC) is preserved until obstruction is moderately severe, whereas the FEV1 (forced expiratory volume in 1 second) is reduced with mild to moderate obstruction; this results in a decreased FEV1/FVC ratio.

(3) In **restrictive lung disease,** the following features are seen on testing.

(a) Flow rates are well preserved until restriction is severe, and the shape of the flow–volume curve is normal.

(b) FVC is reduced in proportion to the decrease in FEV1; this results in a normal FEV1/FVC ratio.

(c) Lung volumes are decreased but TLC is decreased out of proportion to RV, resulting in an increased RV/TLC ratio.

(4) **Less commonly used tests** in children include maximal voluntary ventilation, diffusing capacity of the lung (D_LCO), and closing volume.

(5) Examples of different types of lung disorders are listed in Table 13-2 by pulmonary function.

c. Blood gas analysis

(1) Arterial oxygen tension (Po_2) is a sensitive indicator of overall pulmonary function. The arterial Po_2 in combination with arterial carbon dioxide tension (Pco_2) provides information about the adequacy of alveolar gas exchange.

(2) Capillary pH and Pco_2. Obtaining a sample of arterial blood may be difficult [e.g., in neonates with respiratory distress syndrome (hyaline membrane disease)]. In such cases, an alternative is to determine the pH and Pco_2 of capillary blood and to monitor oxygen saturation by pulse oximetry.

(3) Pulse oximetry is a noninvasive technique that uses the principle of differential light absorption spectra for saturated oxyhemoglobin compared to reduced hemoglobin to record oxygen saturation.

TABLE 13-2. Types of Pulmonary Disorders in Children

Obstructive Lung Disorders	Restrictive Lung Disorders	Diffusion Defects
Asthma	Interstitial pulmonary fibrosis	Pulmonary edema
Cystic fibrosis	Acute pneumothorax	Pulmonary embolism
Emphysema	Pleural effusion	Anemia
Foreign body	Duchenne muscular dystrophy	*Pneumocystis carinii* infection
Pneumonia	Respiratory distress syndrome	Drug induced (particularly
Drowning	Guillain-Barré syndrome	chemotherapeutic drugs such
Tumors	Hypersensitivity pneumonitis	as bleomycin, cyclophospha-
	Obesity	mide, methotrexate)

d. Tests for specific situations
  (1) In children suspected of having **asthma,** helpful tests include serum immunoglobulin E (IgE) level, the presence of eosinophils in a nasal smear, and total circulating eosinophil level. Antigen-specific IgE levels in serum can also be determined.
  (2) In children suspected of having **cystic fibrosis,** sweat testing for chloride levels is diagnostic (see IV D 1).
  (3) In children suspected of having **immunodeficiency disorders** (a number of which present as chronic lung disease), immunoglobulin levels and IgG subclass levels can be determined (see Chapter 9).
  (4) Serum drug levels can be useful for assessing the **adequacy of drug therapy** (e.g., with theophylline).
  (5) In infants who have had a significant episode of **apnea,** who are siblings or half-siblings of children who have died from **sudden infant death syndrome (SIDS),** who are **unstable, premature infants,** or who have **unexplained bradycardia,** pneumography may be helpful.
    (a) In this study, heart rate and rhythm and respiratory pattern are recorded during sleep or over a 12-hour period. Pneumography can be combined with other monitoring procedures, such as oxygen saturation, pH probe monitoring, or electroencephalography.
    (b) Pneumograms can help to distinguish between apnea and periodic breathing. They can also identify various cardiac arrhythmias, including heart rate lability and bradycardia.
e. Endoscopic procedures
  (1) **Laryngoscopy** is useful in patients with stridor or laryngeal disorders. Older children may often be examined indirectly by mirror, but infants may require direct laryngoscopy under sedation or general anesthesia.
  (2) **Bronchoscopy** may be performed as either a flexible or rigid technique.
    (a) **Flexible bronchoscopy** is useful for dynamic airway studies in patients with stridor or airway obstruction and for obtaining culture specimens. It is performed under local sedation and can be done on an outpatient basis.
    (b) **Rigid bronchoscopy** is used in foreign body removal and other airway surgery. It requires general anesthesia and usually is performed by a surgeon.
f. Thoracentesis is used to obtain pleural fluid for culture and analysis.

II. ACUTE RESPIRATORY FAILURE

A. **Definition.** Respiratory failure (pulmonary insufficiency) exists when the patient has hypoxemia (i.e., arterial Po_2 below 50 mm Hg) while breathing 50% oxygen, with or without associated hypercapnia (i.e., arterial Pco_2 above 50 mm Hg).

B. **Etiology.** Acute respiratory failure can be caused by many disorders. Classifying the possible causes helps to pinpoint the underlying pathophysiology and, thus, to direct appropriate management in an individual case. Representative examples of the many causes are shown in Table 13-3.

C. **Clinical features.** See Table 13-4.

D. **Therapy** depends on the degree of hypoxemia, the arterial Pco_2 and pH values, and the underlying pathophysiology. Ultimate recovery requires correction of the underlying cause of respiratory failure.

  1. Oxygenation should be at the lowest concentration of oxygen that will provide an adequate arterial Po_2 (above 60 mm Hg). Too high an oxygen concentration can cause pulmonary edema, atelectasis, or, in neonates, retinopathy of prematurity. Intubation may be necessary to provide continuous positive airway pressure for refractory hypoxemia.

TABLE 13-3. Causes of Acute Respiratory Failure in Children

Obstructive disorders
  Upper airway obstruction
    Anomalies
      Choanal atresia, Pierre Robin syndrome, laryngeal webs, subglottic stenosis, vascular rings
    Aspiration of gastric secretions or a foreign body
    Infections (epiglottitis, peritonsillar or retropharyngeal abscess)
    Allergic laryngospasm
    Growths (tumors, cysts, tonsillar and adenoidal hypertrophy)

  Lower airway obstruction
    Anomalies (bronchomalacia, lobar emphysema)
    Aspiration (due to tracheoesophageal fistula, pharyngeal incoordination)
    Infection (pertussis, bronchiolitis, pneumonia)
    Inflammation and bronchospasm (asthma, bronchopulmonary dysplasia)

Restrictive disorders of the lung parenchyma
  Pulmonary hypoplasia
  Respiratory distress syndrome
  Pneumothorax
  Hemorrhage
  Pulmonary edema
  Pleural effusion

Inefficient alveolar–capillary gas transfer
  Diffusion defects
    Pulmonary edema
    Interstitial fibrosis
    Collagen disorders
    Pneumocystis carinii pneumonia
    Desquamative interstitial pneumonitis
    Adult respiratory distress syndrome secondary to shock, sepsis, and near-drowning

  Respiratory center depression
    Cerebral trauma
    Central nervous system infection
    Sedative overdoses
    Severe asphyxia
    Tetanus

2. **Securing a patent airway** may call for removal of bronchial secretions and use of bronchodilating agents, as well as intubation or mechanical ventilation.
   a. **Endotracheal or nasotracheal intubation** may be sufficient in upper airway obstruction. Placement of the tube should be verified promptly by auscultation and chest x-ray.
   b. **Humidifying the air** helps to reduce viscous bronchial secretions.

3. **Intubation and positive-pressure ventilation** may be required for an elevated arterial P_{CO_2} with respiratory acidosis.

III. ASTHMA

A. **Definition.** Asthma is a lung disease characterized by the following features.

1. **Airway obstruction** (or airway narrowing) that is reversible (but not completely so in some patients) either spontaneously or with treatment

TABLE 13-4. Clinical Signs of Respiratory Failure

Pulmonary Features	Cardiac Features	Neurologic Features
Tachypnea	Tachycardia	Headache
Altered depth and pattern of respiration	Hypertension	Restlessness
Chest retractions	Bradycardia	Irritability
Nasal flaring	Hypotension	Seizures
Cyanosis	Cardiac arrest	Coma
Diaphoresis		
Decreased air movement		
Grunting		

    2. Airway inflammation

    3. Airway hyperresponsiveness to a variety of stimuli

B. **Incidence.** Asthma is the most common chronic lung disease of children, affecting 5%–8% of all children.

    1. Before puberty, twice as many boys are affected, but at puberty the incidence of asthma in girls increases.

    2. Asthma is more severe in young children because they are more prone to viral infections (i.e., colds) and because the proportionately smaller airway size increases airway resistance.

    3. Asthma rarely is fatal, but causes 100 deaths in children each year.

C. **Triggering mechanisms** of increased airway hyperreactivity are many, and are listed in Table 13-5.

D. **Pathophysiology.** Every asthma attack has three **components;** bronchospasm, mucus production, and edema and inflammation of the airway mucosa. The components that predominate at any one time during an attack vary.

E. **Clinical features.** The reversible airway obstruction manifests as slowing of forced expiration. Resulting symptoms—which may occur singly or in any combination—include cough, chest tightness, wheezing, and dyspnea (tachypnea in young children). Symptoms may change in severity both spontaneously and as a result of therapy, making frequent clinical reassessment necessary. Hypoxemia results from airway obstruction, and arterial Po_2 continues to drop as the attack occurs. Initially, because of hyperventilation, arterial Pco_2 is low. During severe attacks, Pco_2 will subsequently rise as hypoventilation and respiratory failure ensue.

F. **Risk factors** for asthma are shown in Figure 13-1.

TABLE 13-5. Asthma Triggers in Children

Respiratory infections (viral, myco-plasma)	Changes in weather
Irritants (cigarette smoke, ozone, air pollution)	Emotional stress (crying, laughing)
	Medications (aspirin)
Exercise	Gastroesophageal reflux
Allergens	Chemicals (tartrazine, sulfites,
Inhaled	monosodium glutamate)
Ingested (rare)	

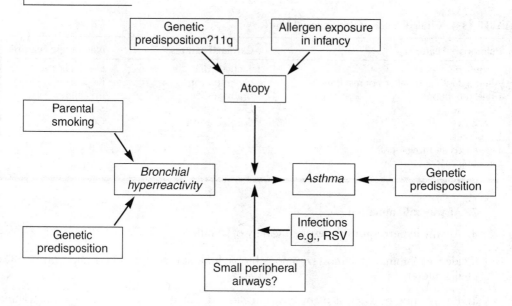

FIGURE 13-1. Possible risk factors for the development of asthma. *RSV* = respiratory syncytial virus. Reprinted from Loughlin GM, Eigen H: *Respiratory Disease in Children: Diagnosis and Management.* Baltimore, Williams & Wilkins, 1994, p 225.

G. **Diagnosis**

1. **Clinical diagnosis.** A description of the child's typical recurrent symptoms often is diagnostic. Diagnosis is more difficult when symptoms are atypical (e.g., chronic cough without wheezing or dyspnea) or when asthma begins in infancy.

2. **Differential diagnosis.** All that is needed to produce a wheeze is sufficient airflow through a sufficiently narrow orifice. Therefore, wheezing episodes can occur in many diseases. Those likely to be confused with asthma include bronchiolitis, cystic fibrosis, tracheomalacia, pertussis, bronchiectasis, tuberculosis with enlarged lymph nodes, foreign body aspiration, airway tumors (adenoma, carcinoid), congestive heart failure, and α_1-antitrypsin deficiency.

H. **Therapy**

1. **Management of the acute attack**
   a. **Emergency therapy** (Table 13-6)
      (1) Inhaled bronchodilators (e.g., isoetharine, albuterol) are rapidly effective and have minimal side effects in most patients. They are the drugs of choice in acute asthma management.
      (2) Subcutaneous epinephrine or terbutaline, 0.01 mg/kg (maximum 0.3 mg), should rarely be used except in the child with an altered level of consciousness as other measures are being undertaken. Although terbutaline has a longer duration of action than epinephrine, both drugs produce palpitations, pallor, and emesis.
      (3) In children older than 5 years of age, PEFR measurements can be obtained and used to follow effectiveness of therapy. PEFR less than 25% predicted is associated with elevated P_{CO_2}.
      (4) There is considerable debate about the use of intravenous aminophylline in the emergency department, with the weight of evidence not favoring its use.
      (5) Failure to respond to inhaled therapy is an indication for hospital admission. By definition, this is **status asthmaticus**.

TABLE 13-6. Emergency Management of Childhood Asthma

O_2 to keep O_2 saturation > 95%

Aerosolized albuterol (with O_2 6-liter flow)
0.15 mg/kg/dose (max. 5 mg/dose) q 20 min × 3

plus

Prednisone (1–2 mg/kg/dose bid) if steroid dependent or
no response after first aerosol

Good response: Discharge on additional medication

Inadequate response: Admit

b. In-hospital therapy (Table 13-7). Laboratory work on admission should include arterial blood gas analysis to check the patient's P_{CO_2} and P_{O_2} and electrolytes to look for albuterol-induced hypokalemia. A chest x-ray is advisable, if there are localized abnormalities on pulmonary auscultation.

2. **Maintenance therapy.** Three approaches are used in the management of asthma.
   a. **Avoidance** is the simplest, most direct treatment: If cats cause wheezing, they should be avoided. However, in many households this is easier said than done.
   b. **Desensitization** may be helpful when certain allergens (e.g., ragweed) cannot be avoided, but such immunotherapy is not a panacea.
   c. **Drugs** are the keystone of therapy. The key principle of therapy is to match therapy to symptom frequency and severity. In general, children with mild asthma require only as-needed therapy with β_2 agonists. Those with moderate asthma require regular, around-the-clock therapy with β_2 agonists and cromolyn or inhaled corticosteroids. Short bursts of oral prednisone may be required. Those with severe asthma require regular, around-the-clock therapy with β_2 agonists or cromolyn plus regular use of corticosteroids, either systemic alternate-day or inhaled agents, and should be evaluated by an asthma specialist.
   d. Drugs used include bronchodilators, corticosteroids, and cromolyn.
      (1) **Bronchodilators**
         (a) **Xanthine drugs** (theophylline and its derivatives) are effective bronchodilators but have significant side effects, and a narrow window of effectiveness. They have lost favor as primary bronchodilator therapy. Bronchodilation is directly related to the serum concentration, and blood levels are used to guide therapy and to monitor toxicity.
            (i) **Side effects** (irritability, hyperactivity, abdominal pain, tachycardia, hematemesis, seizures) can be minimized by beginning with a small dose and increasing it slowly.
            (ii) **Preparations.** There are numerous rapid-release and slow-release theophylline preparations. Fixed combinations and preparations containing alcohol or sugar should be avoided.
         (b) **β_2-Adrenergic agonists** include isoetharine, albuterol (salbutamol), terbutaline, epinephrine, isoproterenol, and metaproterenol (Table 13-8).

TABLE 13-7. In-Hospital Management of Childhood Asthma

O_2 to keep O_2 saturation > 90%

Aerosolized albuterol (0.15 mg/kg/dose q 1–2 h)

Methylprednisolone (1–2 mg/kg/dose IV or po q 6 h)

Aminophylline IV (or po theophylline) administered either
as a loading dose followed by continuous infusion or
bolus therapy q 6 h

TABLE 13-8. Bronchodilators in Asthma

β₂ Agonist	Oral Administration	Aerosol Administration	
		Formulations	Dose
Albuterol	2 mg/5 ml syrup 2 or 4 mg tablet 0.1–0.15 mg/kg/dose 3 times daily	0.5% solution	0.01–0.03 ml/kg (maximum 1 ml) diluted with 3 ml saline, up to 4 times daily
Metaproterenol	10 mg/5 ml syrup 20 mg tablets 0.3–0.5 mg/kg/dose 3–4 times daily	5% solution	0.01–0.02 ml/kg (maximum 1 ml) diluted with 3 ml saline, up to 4 times daily
Isoetharine		1% solution	0.5 ml diluted with 3 ml saline, up to 4 times daily
Terbutaline	2.5 or 5 mg tablets 0.075 mg/kg/dose 3 times daily	1% solution	0.03 ml/kg (maximum 1 ml) diluted with 3 ml saline up to 4 times daily
Salmeterol		Metered aerosol (21 µg/puff)	2 puffs 2 times daily
Bitolterol		Metered aerosol (370 µg/puff)	1–2 puffs 4 times daily
Anticholinergics Ipratropium bromide		Metered aerosol (20 µg/puff) 0.025% solution	2 puffs, 4 times daily 0.5–1.0 ml, 4 times daily

Modified and reprinted from Loughlin GM, Eigen H: *Respiratory Disease in Children: Diagnosis and Management.* Baltimore, Williams & Wilkins, 1994, p 234.

(i) **Side effects.** Albuterol and terbutaline are the most β₂-specific and, thus, cause less severe tachycardia and jitteriness than occur with epinephrine.

(ii) **Oral preparations.** As oral tablets or liquids, metaproterenol is short-acting; terbutaline and albuterol are medium-acting.

(iii) **Inhaled β₂-adrenergic agonist bronchodilators** can be administered by air compressor with nebulizer (for young children or patients in significant respiratory distress) or by a metered-dose inhaler (MDI). **Spacers** should be used in most children. These holding chambers allow children to use an MDI without needing to coordinate activation of the MDI with inhalation. Failure to respond to an MDI usually is the result of improper technique. Overuse can diminish the effectiveness of aerosolized bronchodilators (tachyphylaxis). Out of the hospital, they should not be used more often than six times per 24 hours. Salmeterol is a long-acting β₂ agonist that should not be used for acute asthma because it has an onset of action of approximately 20 minutes.

(c) **Anticholinergics** such as ipratroprium bromide, an atropine derivative, have a slower onset of action and provide less maximal bronchodilation than β₂ agonists. These compounds, however, have a longer duration of action, but are considered second-line therapy for acute asthma.

(2) **Corticosteroids** inhibit the late asthmatic response and the subsequent increase in airway reactivity induced by allergen challenge. They have significant side effects, when used orally for long periods. Oral preparations are extremely effective, however, as short-term therapy (usually 3–5 days) for status asthmaticus. Moreover, low-dose (preferably alternate day) steroid therapy can be very effective for patients whose asthma cannot be controlled with inhaled or oral

β_2-adrenergic agonists. Inhaled steroids because of high topical anti-inflammatory activity but low systemic absorption are highly effective and can be used safely for chronic asthma therapy. They are administered by MDI and are available in solution in some countries.

(3) Cromolyn is a mast cell stabilizer that inhibits pulmonary histamine release. It is given to prevent, not treat, asthma attacks. Cromolyn is administered three to four times per day by air compressor with nebulizer or by MDI. It has virtually no side effects but must be used daily to be effective.

(4) Nedocromil is chemically unrelated to cromolyn but has a very similar clinical profile. It is effective in long-term asthma management (4 mg by inhalation 2–4 times/day) but has no clear-cut advantage over cromolyn.

IV. **CYSTIC FIBROSIS.** The most common lethal inherited disease of whites, cystic fibrosis has an incidence of 1 in 1600 live births and an estimated carrier rate of 1 in 20. Covered in this chapter are the general aspects of cystic fibrosis and its pulmonary complications. Pancreatic insufficiency and other gastrointestinal manifestations of cystic fibrosis are covered in Chapter 11.

A. **Definition.** Cystic fibrosis is a disease of the exocrine glands that causes viscid secretions. The gastrointestinal and respiratory systems are most commonly and most severely affected.

B. **Underlying defect**

1. Cystic fibrosis is inherited as an **autosomal recessive trait**. The gene that causes cystic fibrosis is located on chromosome 7, and in 70% of patients in the United States there is an absence of a three-base pair that codes for the amino acid, phenylalanine (DF508). More than 400 different mutations have been discovered worldwide. The abnormal protein that the gene encodes for has been identified and named the **cystic fibrosis transmembrane regulator protein**.

2. The defect in cystic fibrosis is thought to be a **blocked or closed chloride channel** in the cell membrane of epithelial cells. This blockage traps chloride ions inside the cell and draws sodium ions and water into the cell. This process results in dehydration of mucus secretions.

C. **Clinical features** of cystic fibrosis vary considerably in nature and severity.

1. **Most common and most severe manifestations**
   a. **Respiratory insufficiency** occurs eventually in more than 95% of all patients and is caused by abnormal mucous gland secretion in the airways, producing airway obstruction and secondary infection, cough, dyspnea, bronchiectasis, and pulmonary fibrosis.
   b. **Malabsorption** of fats and protein due to pancreatic insufficiency and abnormal mucous gland secretions in the gastrointestinal tract occurs in 85% of patients (see Chapter 11), producing fatty stools, vitamin deficiencies, failure to gain weight, and retarded growth.

2. **Other manifestations and complications**
   a. **Electrolytes in sweat.** Concentrations of sodium and chloride in sweat are abnormally high in all patients. This can lead to heat intolerance and a hyponatremic, hypochloremic metabolic alkalosis.
   b. **Respiratory complications**
      (1) Hemoptysis is a common complication.
      (2) The incidence of pneumothorax is increased in adolescents and adults.
      (3) Cor pulmonale is a late complication.

    c. Other intestinal problems
      (1) Meconium ileus, in which abnormally viscid meconium completely obstructs the ileum, occurs in 10% of all infants born with cystic fibrosis.
      (2) A comparable fecal obstruction (meconium ileus equivalent, and recently called distal intestinal obstruction syndrome) can occur in older children as a result of dietary indiscretion or insufficient enzyme replacement therapy.
      (3) Rectal prolapse is a relatively common complication; less common is intussusception.
    d. Reproductive effects
      (1) Virtually all men with cystic fibrosis are sterile because of congenital obliteration of the vas deferens.
      (2) Women with cystic fibrosis produce thick, spermicidal cervical mucus and have reduced fertility.
    e. Hepatic effects. Focal biliary cirrhosis is present in 25% of all patients and is occasionally severe enough to produce portal hypertension and esophageal varices.
    f. Pancreatic effects
      (1) Abnormal glucose tolerance is present in 25%–75% of all patients.
      (2) Type II diabetes may develop in 1%–2% of all patients.
    g. Nasal effects
      (1) Chronic sinusitis with opacification of the sinuses occurs in all patients.
      (2) Nasal polyposis occurs in 5% of all patients.
    h. Musculoskeletal effects. Hypertrophic osteoarthropathy develops in some patients. This condition of unknown etiology consists of periostitis and arthritis, producing joint pain, edema, and decreased activity.

D. **Diagnosis.** The diagnosis of cystic fibrosis is made in 65% of patients in the first year of life, but in 10% of patients, the diagnosis is not made until after the age of 10 years. Diagnostic criteria for cystic fibrosis include a positive sweat test, typical pulmonary manifestations, typical gastrointestinal manifestations, and a positive family history.

  1. The **sweat test** is positive if the chloride concentration of sweat exceeds 60 mEq/L before age 20 years and 80 mEq/l in adults. Normal sweat chloride values are below 40 mEq/L.
    a. The test must be done correctly. The method of choice is quantitative pilocarpine iontophoresis by the Gibson and Cooke method or the Westcort method.
    b. False-positive results can occur in nephrogenic diabetes insipidus, hypothyroidism, mucopolysaccharidosis, adrenal insufficiency, ectodermal dysplasia, severe malnutrition, and anorexia nervosa.

  2. **DNA testing** is available for the 32 most common cystic fibrosis mutations and is indicated:
    a. if unable to collect adequate amounts of sweat for analysis
    b. if sweat test results are borderline or equivocal
    c. if sweat tests do not correlate with clinical symptoms
    d. in the in utero diagnosis such as a fetus with ultrasound evidence of ascites or dilated loops of bowel suggestive of meconium ileus, or in a fetus with a family history of cystic fibrosis

  3. Prenatal DNA testing should be offered to all families with a family history of cystic fibrosis.

  4. Evidence of meconium ileus is virtually diagnostic of cystic fibrosis. Failure to pass a stool in the first 24 hours of life, combined with small bowel obstruction (usually in the area of the ileocecal valve) and evidence of a microcolon, strongly suggests meconium ileus.

  5. Without evidence of meconium ileus, **a high index of suspicion** is required to make the diagnosis. The initial presentation may be subtle and often is missed. Any of the following initial signs and symptoms should suggest the possible need for a confirmatory sweat test.

    a. Respiratory signs and symptoms include a chronic cough; recurrent pneumonia and atelectasis; hyperinflation; digital clubbing; persistent crackles on lung auscultation; the presence of *Pseudomonas aeruginosa, Staphylococcus aureus,* and, in infants, *Klebsiella* or *Escherichia coli* in sputum; hemoptysis; and nasal polyposis.

    b. Gastrointestinal signs and symptoms include steatorrhea, chronic diarrhea, rectal prolapse, biliary cirrhosis, cholecystitis, and meconium ileus equivalent.

    c. Other signs and symptoms include failure to thrive, hyponatremic, hypochloremic metabolic alkalosis, and the symptom complex of hypoproteinemia, anemia, and edema in infants.

6. Neonatal screening using blood spots collected shortly after birth to detect elevated levels of immunoreactive trypsin (IRT) is available in some states. Preliminary studies suggest that early diagnosis may favorably affect outcome.

E. Therapy

1. Treatment of respiratory problems

    a. Antibiotics are given either continuously or intermittently to prevent or treat pulmonary bacterial infection.

        (1) Oral therapy usually consists of antistaphylococcal drugs (e.g., dicloxacillin), cephalosporins, trimethoprim-sulfamethoxazole, and chloramphenicol, and in older patients, oral quinolones.

        (2) Aerosolized aminoglycoside therapy is used to decrease chronic lung infection and reduce the need for hospitalization.

        (3) Intravenous therapy lasting 10–21 days may be needed for established infections. Usually, an aminoglycoside (e.g., tobramycin) and either a semisynthetic penicillin (e.g., piperacillin) or third-generation cephalosporin (e.g., ceftazidime) are given.

    b. Other drugs. Oral and inhaled **bronchodilators** are used frequently, and the **mucolytic** acetylcysteine sometimes is given. DNase, administered by aerosol, breaks down the DNA found as a by-product of bacterial breakdown and thins mucus, produces modest improvements in pulmonary function, and decreases hospitalization rates. Alternate-day **steroids** reduce inflammation and produce similar modest improvements in pulmonary function, but are associated with steroid side effects in some patients.

    c. Chest physiotherapy (breathing exercises, postural drainage with or without chest percussion, active cycle of breathing) is used to aid the clearance of viscid secretions. Some evidence suggests that regular vigorous exercise may produce the same benefit as chest physiotherapy.

    d. Lung transplantation is available to some patients with cystic fibrosis, with risks similar to those faced by other lung transplant recipients.

2. Treatment of digestive problems

    a. Pancreatic enzymes (freeze-dried extracts of animal pancreas) are given before each meal or snack. The dosage is adjusted on the basis of growth and stool pattern.

    b. A **high-calorie, high-protein diet** should be provided. For anorectic children, an oral or parenteral supplement may be needed to improve caloric consumption.

    c. Vitamin supplementation is given, especially the fat-soluble vitamins A, E, and K.

    d. Stool softeners are often helpful.

    e. Antacids and **H$_2$-receptor antagonists** are sometimes used to decrease gastric acidity and to improve the effectiveness of enzyme therapy.

3. Treatment of complications

    a. Meconium ileus usually requires surgery, although the obstruction sometimes can be cleared by instilling an enema composed of radiocontrast agent (meglumine diatrizoate) or acetylcysteine under fluoroscopic guidance.

    b. Meconium ileus equivalent usually can be relieved with enemas of soapsuds, acetylcysteine, or meglumine diatrizoate.

      c. Pneumothorax usually is treated by closed-tube thoracostomy if it is symptomatic or large. Persistent leaks require procedures such as sclerosis or pleural stripping and abrasion.

      d. Hemoptysis is treated with vitamin K and antibiotics. If bleeding is severe or life threatening, embolization of the bleeding vessel may be tried.

   4. Future therapy

      a. Gene replacement may prove to be promising; very early work suggests at least localized feasibility.

      b. Amiloride inhibits sodium and secondary water absorption, making secretions thinner; clinical trials are underway.

      c. Adenosine triphosphate-uridine triphosphate increases chloride secretion in cystic fibrosis airways, making secretions thinner; preliminary trials are underway.

F. **Prognosis.** The outlook for cystic fibrosis patients has improved significantly over the past 20 years, and mean life expectancy has reached 29 years of age. Most patients (95%) die of respiratory failure; others die of liver failure or other complications. Some individuals with cystic fibrosis live into the fifth or sixth decade of life.

V. BRONCHOPULMONARY DYSPLASIA

A. **Definition.** Bronchopulmonary dysplasia is a chronic pulmonary disease of infants that is characterized by the need for oxygen therapy beyond 28 days of life (more recently defined as an oxygen requirement at 36 weeks' corrected gestational age) and by a characteristic series of changes in the lung on x-ray. Bronchopulmonary dysplasia follows neonatal respiratory failure and is especially likely to occur after oxygen and mechanical ventilation therapy for hyaline membrane disease in a preterm infant. It also may occur in term infants after acute lung injury (e.g., pneumonia, meconium aspiration, diaphragmatic hernia).

B. **Pathogenesis**

   1. Important pathogenetic factors in bronchopulmonary dysplasia include:

      a. Oxygen toxicity from prior oxygen therapy at a concentration fraction of inspired oxygen (FIO_2) exceeding 0.8

      b. Barotrauma from mechanical ventilation with high airway pressure

   2. Other factors that may play a pathogenetic role include prematurity, fluid overload, damage caused by severe pulmonary disease, and a familial predisposition to asthma.

C. **Pathology.** The two most prominent features are:

   1. Diffuse alveolar injury with endothelial cell damage, resulting in interstitial pulmonary edema and fibrosis

   2. Necrotizing bronchiolitis with smooth muscle hypertrophy, resulting in areas of atelectasis and emphysema

D. **Clinical features** include retractions, tachypnea, wheezing, and cyanosis, especially with stress. Some infants show poor lung compliance, pulmonary edema, and pulmonary hypertension.

E. **Diagnosis**

   1. Pulmonary physical examination should emphasize the sleeping respiratory rate, the signs of the effort of breathing, and auscultation to determine the presence of crackles and wheezes.

2. A **baseline chest x-ray** should be taken, to delineate acute findings versus chronic changes.
   a. In the acute stage, there is near-total lung opacification on x-ray.
   b. In the chronic stage, x-rays show thickened fibrotic markings and cystic changes.

3. Blood gas analysis is important. However, the stress of obtaining an arterial specimen can produce significant hypoxemia in these infants, and oximetry plus capillary blood gas analysis may be preferable.

4. Electrocardiography and **echocardiography** help to identify the presence of cor pulmonale.

F. Therapy

1. Oxygen probably is the most important therapy in these infants. Oxygen is delivered by nasal cannula or feeding tube to maintain an oxygen saturation greater than 90% and to minimize the work of breathing. Some infants may require mechanical ventilation.

2. Diuretics. Infants with pulmonary edema or with respiratory crackles, marked elevations in P_{CO_2}, and persistent hypoxemia frequently benefit from diuretic therapy. Furosemide may cause nephrocalcinosis and should be avoided if possible for long-term therapy.

3. Bronchodilators. Inhaled β_2-adrenergic agents improve bronchospasm, decrease the work of breathing, and may improve oxygenation in some infants.

4. Dietary supplements. Infants with bronchopulmonary dysplasia require more calories than other infants, in part because of a higher basal metabolic rate and in part because of increased work of breathing. Increasing the caloric density of the formula or supplementing the diet with glucose polymers or medium-chain triglycerides often is sufficient, but some infants require nasogastric feedings or parenteral hyperalimentation for adequate growth.

G. Prognosis

1. Short-term prognosis
   a. Most infants, even those with severe bronchopulmonary dysplasia, will get better with time, and by age 5 years their pulmonary function may be similar to that of age-matched children. However, these patients may require oxygen for 6–12 months after hospital discharge, and in early childhood they may have some evidence of small airway obstruction.
   b. Many infants have hyperreactive airways and may require hospitalization for acute viral infections. During childhood these infants have a greater risk of asthma.

2. Long-term prognosis is not known because patients who were among the first reported cases are only now approaching adulthood. However, the marked pulmonary damage that occurs during the phase of rapid lung growth may predispose affected infants to chronic lung disease in adult life.

VI. APNEA OF INFANCY (see also Chapter 6)

A. Definition. In infants, apnea is the cessation of breathing for longer than 20 seconds or for any duration if it is associated with pallor, limpness, cyanosis, or bradycardia and if it requires vigorous stimulation for resuscitation. Apnea is a common symptom of disease in infants, not a disease itself.

1. SIDS (sudden infant death syndrome) is the sudden and unexpected death of an infant whose history or postmortem examination cannot demonstrate a specific cause of death.

SIDS is the leading cause of death in infants in the first year of life. Although probably not the major cause of SIDS, apnea may account for 5%–20% of SIDS deaths.

2. **ALTE** (apparent life-threatening event) is an episode of apnea associated with color change (pallor or cyanosis), marked change in muscle tone (usually limpness, rarely rigidity), or choking and gagging. Observers usually fear the child will die and intervene with vigorous stimulation or cardiopulmonary resuscitation.

B. **Types of apnea and their causes**

1. **Central apnea.** When there is no central neurologic drive to breathe, there is no chest wall or abdominal movement. There are several factors that lead to central apnea. It also may be idiopathic and may occur in infants with a positive family history of SIDS. Causes of central apnea are listed in Table 13-9.

2. **Obstructive apnea.** When airway obstruction results in apnea, chest wall and abdominal movements will be present in the absence of airflow at the nose and mouth. Causes of obstructive apnea are listed in Table 13-9.

3. **Mixed apnea.** A combination of central and obstructive apnea can occur. It usually begins with central apnea followed by airway obstruction.

C. **Evaluation of the infant with apnea**

1. **History.** In this important part of the evaluation, questions to be answered include the following.
   a. Was the child really apneic?
   b. Was the child asleep or awake?
   c. Were there rhythmic movements suggesting a seizure?
   d. What was the relationship to feeding?
   e. Was there mucus or vomitus in the mouth or nose?
   f. Was the child pale, limp, or cyanotic?
   g. How long was the child apneic?
   h. Did the apnea resolve on its own, and, if not, what intervention was needed?

2. **Physical examination.** Special attention should be paid to the neurologic and cardiac examinations as well as to the airway examination.

3. **Laboratory studies.** Depending on the suspected cause of the apnea and the findings on history and physical examination, the following tests may be useful:
   a. Arterial blood gas analysis
   b. Electroencephalography, both standard and during sleep
   c. Cranial ultrasonography

TABLE 13-9. Causes of Apnea in Infancy

Central Apnea	Obstructive Apnea
Prematurity (see Chapter 6)	Macroglossia (e.g., Down syndrome, hypothyroidism, or Pierre Robin syndrome)
Medications to mother or infant	
Infections, bacterial or viral	
Anemia	Enlarged tonsils and adenoids
Cardiac arrhythmias (especially Wolff-Parkinson-White syndrome)	Posterior pharyngeal muscle incoordination (e.g., from cerebral palsy or trauma)
Seizures	
Gastroesophageal reflux or aspiration (vagally mediated)	Laryngospasm
Hypoglycemia	Cleft lip repair
Central alveolar hypoventilation	Achondroplasia
Bronchopulmonary dysplasia	Obstructed tracheostomy

      d. Electrocardiography

      e. Chest x-ray

      f. X-ray of airway or bronchoscopy

      g. Barium swallow or gastrointestinal pH probe

      h. Various blood studies (e.g., complete blood count, electrolytes, calcium, blood sugar, blood cultures)

      i. Pneumography

D. Therapy

1. Treatment of hypoventilation and airway obstruction. Hypoventilation may require the use of a ventilator, and airway obstruction may call for tracheostomy.

2. Other treatments of apnea depend on its cause. Examples follow.

    a. Obstructing tonsils should be removed.

    b. Anemia or arrhythmias should be corrected.

    c. Seizures should be treated with anticonvulsants.

    d. Apnea due to bradycardia may be helped by the stimulant effects of theophylline or atropine.

    e. If the infant with gastroesophageal reflux is not helped sufficiently by an upright position and by adding cereal to thicken the formula, metoclopramide may be tried (see Chapter 11).

3. Home monitoring. Evaluation of the child with apnea may not identify a cause. Use of a home monitor may be recommended if the apneic episode is thought to be significant and if a recurrence could be potentially fatal (e.g., an ALTE).

    a. The home monitor sets off an alarm when apnea or bradycardia is detected. Families learn how to respond to an alarm and resuscitate their infant if necessary.

    b. Home monitoring has a significant negative impact on a family, however, and should not be recommended lightly.

VII. CONGENITAL MALFORMATIONS

that cause respiratory problems during the neonatal period are discussed in Chapter 6. The following discussion is focused on those congenital malformations that do not cause symptoms until after the neonatal period or that have late complications.

A. Laryngomalacia (infantile larynx).

This congenital disorder is the most common cause of stridor in infancy. The larynx appears disproportionately small and the supporting structures may be abnormally soft.

1. Clinical features

    a. Stridor begins within the first 4 weeks of life and is accentuated by increased ventilation (e.g., from crying or excitement) or by upper respiratory infections.

    b. Stridor usually resolves by age 12 months but may recur with respiratory infections until about 3 years of age.

2. Diagnosis is by fiberoptic bronchoscopy or direct laryngoscopy.

3. Therapy usually is not needed. Rarely, tracheostomy is required when stridor occurs in association with failure to thrive or in infants with life-threatening apnea or airway obstruction.

4. Other causes of stridor in children include bronchomalacia associated with primarily expiratory stridor, subglottic stenosis associated with inspiratory and expiratory stridor, and vocal cord paralysis associated with inspiratory stridor and hoarseness.

B. Vascular rings.

Congenital anomalies of the aortic arch or its branches can create a ring around the airway that compromises respiration.

   1. Types. Vascular anomalies most likely to compress the trachea are:

      a. A right aortic arch with a left ligamentum arteriosum or patent ductus arteriosus

      b. A double aortic arch

      c. An anomalous innominate or left carotid artery

      d. A pulmonary artery sling

   2. Clinical features

      a. Many of these infants present with stridor.

      b. Other respiratory symptoms can include raucous respirations, intercostal retractions, tachypnea, and dyspnea with prolonged exhalation; opisthotonos may make breathing easier.

      c. Respiratory symptoms may become worse with feeding.

   3. Therapy is surgical correction of the anomaly.

C. **Tracheoesophageal fistula** (see also Chapter 11). Children born with a tracheoesophageal fistula are prone to development of chronic pulmonary disease, particularly tracheomalacia, airway hyperreactivity, or bronchiectasis. Chronic aspiration is believed to be a major factor resulting from uncoordinated esophageal peristalsis.

D. **Bronchogenic cyst.** This congenital cyst lined with bronchial epithelium usually is found in the mediastinum.

   1. Clinical features. Symptoms result if the cyst compresses the airway or if the cyst becomes infected and suppurates through a tracheobronchial communication.

   2. Therapy is surgical removal of the cyst.

E. **Pulmonary sequestration.** A cystlike mass of nonfunctioning lung tissue, which lacks normal communication with the tracheobronchial tree, sometimes develops in the embryo, most often within the left lower lobe, but at times entirely outside the lungs. The nonfunctioning sequestration is nourished by systemic arteries.

   1. Clinical features

      a. Infection can result if a fistula develops between the sequestration and either the airway or the digestive tract.

      b. Children usually present with a history of recurrent, persistent, progressive pulmonary sepsis in the form of pneumonitis or lung abscess.

   2. Diagnosis

      a. Chest x-ray usually shows a density in the region of the sequestration, with displacement of the bronchovascular markings.

      b. Contrast bronchography shows the sequestration as an area that fails to fill, outlined by bronchi that are filled. Aortography will delineate the anomalous arterial supply from the aorta.

   3. Therapy is surgical removal of the sequestration.

F. **Pulmonary arteriovenous fistula.** A direct intrapulmonary connection between the pulmonary artery and vein, without an intervening capillary bed, produces an intrapulmonary right-to-left shunt. The fistula usually occurs in the lower lobes and is frequently small enough to be missed.

   1. Clinical features. When the shunt is severe enough to be symptomatic, children present with dyspnea, cyanosis, clubbing, hemoptysis, epistaxis, and exercise intolerance. Generalized telangiectasia is seen in 50% of these patients.

   2. Diagnosis

      a. Pulmonary arteriovenous fistula is suggested by laboratory tests showing polycythemia and oxygen desaturation at rest and during exercise, and by x-rays showing a homogeneous, noncalcified pulmonary density with irregular, sharp margins.

b. The diagnosis is confirmed by venous cineangiography with full chest x-rays, which not only may delineate the offending fistula but may uncover smaller fistulas that were not suspected.

3. Therapy. Symptomatic children with localized disease should undergo surgical correction.

VIII. **OTHER PULMONARY DISEASES.** Other pulmonary diseases not discussed in this chapter but found elsewhere in the book include aspiration of foreign bodies (see Chapter 2), aspiration of hydrocarbons (see Chapter 2), drowning (see Chapter 2), upper and lower respiratory tract infections (see Chapter 10), and pulmonary neoplasms (see Chapter 16).

A. **Pulmonary tuberculosis**

1. Incidence
a. Childhood tuberculosis accounts for about 4% of all new cases of tuberculosis each year, and the mortality rate is highest in infants and adolescents.
b. Susceptibility to infection is increased in children with chronic illness or malnutrition.

2. Etiology and pathogenesis
a. The etiologic agent is *Mycobacterium tuberculosis* and, in children, is frequently transmitted by an adult family member. Infrequently, the organism is transmitted transplacentally via seeded amniotic fluid.
b. The primary lesion occurs in the lung in 95% of cases of tuberculosis. After inhalation, tubercle bacilli spread to regional lymph nodes and then to other lymph nodes, with healing of the primary focus.

3. Clinical features and laboratory findings
a. Initial (primary) tuberculosis. A 2- to 10-week incubation period follows the initial infection.
   (1) Presenting symptoms usually are minimal and include a temperature that is slightly elevated (to 102°F) but persistent (lasting 2–3 weeks), weight loss, fatigue, irritability, and malaise. Initially, a chest x-ray may appear normal. Some patients are completely asymptomatic.
   (2) As the disease progresses, **x-ray findings** of pulmonary infiltration with hilar lymph node enlargement are evident. Mediastinal lymph node involvement is common and may result in bronchial obstruction, with labored breathing, a harsh cough, and tachypnea.
   (3) Tuberculous **pleurisy,** often a late complication, is marked by pleuritic pain, fluid in the chest, cough, and decreased breath sounds.
b. Reactivation (adult or chronic) tuberculosis. Many cases of pulmonary tuberculosis are caused by reactivation of *M. tuberculosis* after a long period of latency. Early lesions become encapsulated and then liquefy, spreading bacteria throughout the lungs.
   (1) Symptoms. A dry cough progresses to a productive cough that starts with mucoid sputum, changing to become mucopurulent and then blood-streaked. Other symptoms (e.g., low-grade fever, weight loss, night sweats) may be mild and overlooked initially; however, they progressively become more severe.
   (2) Chest x-ray reveals a well-defined, homogeneous shadow commonly located in the upper lobes.

4. Diagnosis. In childhood tuberculosis, important diagnostic points include:
a. A history of contact with the disease
b. A positive **tuberculin skin test,** with the amount of induration that constitutes a positive test varying with the clinical history and degree of suspicion

(1) A reaction with induration of 10 mm or more developing 48–72 hours after intracutaneous injection of purified protein derivative tuberculin is considered positive in young children and children at risk for exposure (homeless, immigrants from countries with high tuberculosis rates).

(2) A reaction of at least 5 mm is positive in a child with active or previously active tuberculosis household contacts, in an immunosuppressed child, or in a child with clinical evidence of tuberculosis or a chest x-ray compatible with active tuberculosis.

(3) A reaction 15 mm or larger is positive in a child older than 4 years of age without any risk factors.

c. Recovery of *M. tuberculosis* in sputum or gastric washings

5. **Therapy.** Because tubercle bacilli readily develop drug resistance, at least two drugs are given concomitantly in active tuberculosis. For pulmonary tuberculosis with hilar adenopathy, isoniazid (INH), rifampin, and pyrazinamide are used daily for 2 months, followed by 4 months of INH and rifampin. Dosing regimens and durations, however, are frequently changing.

6. **Prophylaxis.** Chemoprophylaxis with INH is recommended if the tuberculin test is positive and there is no evidence of disease. INH prophylaxis also is important for tuberculin-positive children undergoing prolonged therapy with corticosteroids or other immunosuppressants.

7. Prophylaxis with **bacille Calmette-Guérin** (BCG) vaccine is used in countries where the incidence of tuberculosis is high, and is never a contraindication to a tuberculin skin test.

B. **Desquamative interstitial pneumonitis (DIP).** In this disorder, macrophages, lymphocytes, and related cells accumulate in the interstitial tissue, followed by epithelial hyperplasia in alveoli and bronchioles. DIP is one of the restrictive lung diseases of children. The etiology is unknown but it most likely is immunologic.

1. **Clinical features.** Dyspnea is the most common feature. Other symptoms include fatigue, anorexia, weight loss, cyanosis, and digital clubbing. Copious crackles are audible on auscultation, particularly at lung bases.

2. **Laboratory findings**
   a. The chest x-ray shows a typical ground-glass appearance at the bases.
   b. Blood counts may show leukocytosis, eosinophilia, and low concentrations of immunoglobulins.
   c. Pulmonary function tests reflect the restrictive lung disease and decreased diffusing capacity.
   d. Blood gas analysis reveals arterial hypoxemia and hypocapnia (hypercapnia is a late finding).

3. **Therapy** is supportive. Once infectious pneumonitis has been ruled out, corticosteroids may be tried, but they are not always effective.

C. **Pulmonary hemosiderosis.** This uncommon disease is characterized by an abnormal accumulation of iron (as hemosiderin) in the lungs as a result of bleeding into the lungs. The etiology in most cases is unknown; in some cases, especially in young children, the disease is related to ingestion of cow's milk.

1. **Clinical features and diagnosis**
   a. Recurrent pulmonary symptoms include cough, hemoptysis, dyspnea, wheezing, and cyanosis.
   b. Blood counts show a hypochromic, microcytic, iron deficiency anemia.
   c. The chest x-ray is variable. Some patients show only transient infiltrates; others show massive parenchymal involvement with atelectasis, emphysema, and lymphadenopathy.

d. Gastric aspirates or bronchial washings show the presence of hemosiderin-laden macrophages.

e. Lung biopsy is necessary if the diagnosis is in doubt.

2. Therapy. Blood transfusions are given to correct the anemia. Corticosteroids may prove helpful. Milk-sensitive children benefit from a milk-free diet. If other measures fail, deferoxamine, a parenteral chelating agent, may be tried.

BIBLIOGRAPHY

Chernick V: *Kendig's Disorders of the Respiratory Tract in Children,* 5th ed. Philadelphia, WB Saunders, 1990.

Hillman BC: How to work up recurrent or persistent pediatric pneumonia. *J Respir Dis* 12:315–332, 1991.

Loughlin GM, Eigen H: *Respiratory Disease in Children: Diagnosis and Management.* Baltimore, Williams & Wilkins, 1994.

Starke JR: Childhood tuberculosis during the 1990's. *Pediatrics in Review* 13:343–353, 1992.

DIRECTIONS: Each of the numbered items or incomplete statements in this section is followed by answers or by completions of the statement. Select the ONE lettered answer or completion that is BEST in each case.

1. A 6-week-old infant presents with a history of noisy breathing. The noise was first noted shortly after birth, is inspiratory in nature, is worse now that the infant has a viral respiratory illness, and remits almost completely when the child is asleep. The most likely etiology of this child's noisy breathing is

(A) asthma
(B) bronchopulmonary dysplasia
(C) cystic fibrosis
(D) laryngomalacia
(E) tuberculosis

2. A 3-year-old girl presents with a history of recurrent pneumonia. On physical examination, wheezing and crackles are heard, and digital clubbing is evident. The most likely diagnosis is

(A) pulmonary sequestration
(B) bronchopulmonary dysplasia
(C) cystic fibrosis
(D) asthma
(E) laryngomalacia

3. A 4-year-old child presents with a history of chronic left lower lobe pneumonitis. On contrast bronchography, the area involved with the pneumonitis does not fill, whereas the area around it does fill. The most likely diagnosis is

(A) asthma
(B) pulmonary sequestration
(C) cystic fibrosis
(D) bronchopulmonary dysplasia
(E) bronchogenic cyst

DIRECTIONS: Each of the numbered items or incomplete statements in this section is negatively phrased, as indicated by a capitalized word such as NOT, LEAST, or EXCEPT. Select the ONE lettered answer or completion that is BEST in each case.

4. All of the following statements about asthma are correct EXCEPT

(A) its severity remits or exacerbates with or without therapy
(B) it is a disease of airway hyperreactivity
(C) it can be triggered by viral infections, exercise, or emotions
(D) the presence of wheezing is diagnostic
(E) inhaled sympathomimetics are effective therapy

5. A 15-year-old adolescent with asthma wakes up in the middle of the night with an acute asthma attack. He presents to the emergency room for therapy. On physical examination he is afebrile, with a normal respiratory rate, but is noted to be wheezing. His peak expiratory flow rate is 70% of predicted. Therapy for this adolescent should include all of the following EXCEPT

(A) aerosolized albuterol every 20 minutes
(B) measurement of oxygen saturation by oximetry
(C) peak flow measurements after albuterol aerosol
(D) prednisone if he fails to respond to aerosolized albuterol
(E) arterial blood gas

DIRECTIONS: Each set of matching questions in this section consists of a list of four to twenty-six lettered options (some of which may be in figures) followed by several numbered items. For each numbered item, select the ONE lettered option that is most closely associated with it. To avoid spending too much time on matching sets with large numbers of options, it is generally advisable to begin each set by reading the list of options. Then, for each item in the set, try to generate the correct answer and locate it in the option list, rather than evaluating each option individually. Each lettered option may be selected once, more than once, or not at all.

Questions 6–10

Match each pulmonary indication for imaging study with the appropriate procedure.

(A) Chest x-ray
(B) Chest computed tomography
(C) Barium swallow
(D) Chest ultrasonography

6. To evaluate an infant with apnea

7. To rule out diaphragmatic paralysis

8. To evaluate a child with chronic cough and wheezing

9. To differentiate a mediastinal mass lesion from a collapsed lung

10. To guide needle thoracentesis to sample a pleural effusion

ANSWERS AND EXPLANATIONS

1. The answer is D *[VII A]*. This infant's history and physical examination demonstrate stridor, which is inspiratory and is sensitive to changes in airflow. Of the causes of stridor in children, laryngomalacia is the most common.

2. The answer is C *[IV D 5 a]*. In children with a history of pulmonary disease, the presence of digital clubbing suggests cystic fibrosis until proven otherwise. Asthma, pulmonary sequestration, laryngomalacia, and bronchopulmonary dysplasia are not associated with clubbing.

3. The answer is B *[VII E 2 b]*. A pulmonary sequestration is a cystlike mass of nonfunctioning lung tissue, which most often is located in the left lower lobe. Children present with a history of chronic pneumonitis. Bronchography shows the sequestration as an area that does not fill with contrast, outlined by bronchi that are contrast-filled. Aortography demonstrates the anomalous arterial supply.

4. The answer is D *[III G 2]*. Although a clinical feature of asthma, wheezing also can occur in many other diseases, including cystic fibrosis, pertussis, foreign body aspiration, and bronchiolitis. Asthma is a disease characterized by airway hyperreactivity to a variety of stimuli, including upper respiratory infections, exercise, and emotions. The symptoms of asthma show remissions and exacerbations with or without therapy. β_2-Adrenergic agonists are effective bronchodilating therapy, and can be administered orally, by air compressor with nebulizer, or by a metered-dose inhaler.

5. The answer is E *[III H 1]*. This adolescent's history of waking up in the middle of the night with an acute asthma episode is very typical of asthma, which frequently exacerbates at night. His therapy should include oximetry, repeated peak flow measurements, aerosolized albuterol, and prednisone if he fails to respond to the aerosol therapy. An arterial blood gas analysis is not indicated at this point unless his peak flow drops below 25% of predicted, or if his asthma episode does not respond to therapy and admission to the hospital is planned.

6–10. The answers are: 6-C, 7-D, 8-A, 9-B, 10-D *[I C 3 a]*. A barium swallow or gastrointestinal pH probe may be useful in evaluating the possibility of gastrointestinal reflux as a cause of apnea in an infant. Chest ultrasonography is useful for evaluating diaphragmatic motility. It also can be used to distinguish pleural effusion from adjacent lung and to guide needle thoracentesis. With chest ultrasonography, the high levels of radiation exposure associated with chest fluoroscopy are avoided. Chest x-ray is indicated in the evaluation of a child with chronic cough and wheezing, to rule out chronic pneumonia, atelectasis, and hyperinflated lungs. In a child with asthma, increased peribronchial lung markings and air trapping are signs of chronic, poorly treated disease. Computed tomography (CT) scanning of the chest helps to differentiate among pulmonary lesions of differing radiographic densities that cannot be distinguished on chest x-ray (e.g., a collapsed lung versus a mediastinal tumor). CT scanning of the chest also is useful in determining the extent of pulmonary cysts and in detecting signs of bronchiectasis.

Chapter 14

Renal Diseases

Thomas L. Kennedy

I. GENERAL PRINCIPLES OF RENAL DISEASE IN CHILDREN

A. **Introduction.** Renal disease and dysfunction generally are considered in terms of the kidney's role in filtration, clearance, and excretion of nitrogenous waste. An equally important consideration, however, is the kidney's role in fluid and electrolyte balance, in blood pressure regulation, in acid–base homeostasis, and as an endocrine organ elaborating many hormones (e.g., erythropoietin, prostaglandins, renin, vitamin D, kinins). Other important aspects of renal disease in childhood are the limitations of normal function that exist at birth and the growth and maturational changes that occur through infancy and childhood.

B. **Evaluation of renal function**

1. **Urinalysis,** although not totally specific or sensitive, is a useful, noninvasive indicator of renal function and disease. Urine bags may be used to collect urine, or urine may be squeezed from a diaper for dipstick analysis.
   a. **Urine concentration and dilution** may be measured by specific gravity or osmolality. Specific gravity may be determined using a refractometer, which requires only a drop of urine. Dipsticks now are available that estimate specific gravity. Although in general it correlates well with urine osmolality, urine specific gravity measures the density of the solution and is disproportionately increased by high–molecular-weight substances, including protein, glucose, mannitol, and intravenous contrast agents.
      (1) Maximally diluted urine has a specific gravity of 1.002 (osmolality of 50 mOsm/kg).
      (2) Maximally concentrated urine has a specific gravity of 1.035 (osmolality of 1200 mOsm/kg).
      (3) Urine that is neither diluted nor concentrated (isosthenuria) has a specific gravity of 1.010 (osmolality of 300 mOsm/kg).
   b. **Urine dipsticks**
      (1) The dipstick technique provides a general estimate of **acidity** and indicates the presence or absence of **albumin, glucose, ketones, urobilinogen, bilirubin,** and **blood** (including free hemoglobin or myoglobin).
      (2) Other available dipsticks indicate **pyuria** (leukocyte esterase) or **gram-negative infection** (with organisms that convert urinary nitrates to nitrite) and estimate specific gravity.
   c. **Urine microscopy.** A freshly voided urine specimen is centrifuged, and the sediment is examined for **bacteria, cells,** and **crystals.**
      (1) **Bacteria.** It is difficult to distinguish infecting organisms from contaminants or amorphous material (e.g., phosphates, urates). A careful **Gram stain,** however, may help to identify bacteria. Also, pyuria is not a reliable indicator of infection because significant bacteriuria may occur in the absence of leukocytes, and pyuria may occur with acute illness in the absence of infection. Therefore, a **culture** must be obtained to confirm the diagnosis of a urinary tract infection and establish the antimicrobial sensitivities.
      (2) **Cells.** The **morphology** of red cells in urine may help to distinguish glomerular bleeding from blood loss elsewhere in the urinary tract. Crenated, dysmorphic red cells in fresh urine suggest a glomerular origin. These are best seen using **phase-contrast microscopy** or **Wright stain** of the urine.

(3) Casts of compacted red cells extracted from the tubular lumen (**RBC casts**) are the result of glomerular bleeding and usually are diagnostic of glomerulonephritis. **Leukocyte casts** occasionally are seen in pyelonephritis and interstitial nephritis. **Hyaline casts** and **granular casts** are not diagnostic of renal disease and may occur in sediment from children with oliguria of any cause.

(4) Crystals of many varieties may be present in the urine. They rarely are diagnostic of disease. In fact, they reflect factors such as the amount and concentration of solute and solubilizers and urinary pH and osmolarity. An exception is the hexagonal **cystine** crystal, which is diagnostic of cystinuria.

2. Tests of glomerular function use timed urine collections. Ideally, urine should be collected over 24 hours, but 8- to 12-hour collections are acceptable.

a. Glomerular filtration rate (GFR). Usually, endogenous **creatinine clearance** is used to measure GFR and is accurate unless the GFR is very low (< 20 ml/min), in which case it tends to overestimate GFR.

(1) The **normal GFR** in children 2 years of age or older is 120 ml/min/1.73 m².

(2) When timed urine collections are difficult to obtain (e.g., in a young child), GFR can be estimated as follows:

$$CC = \frac{K \ (\text{height in cm})}{\text{serum creatinine (mg/dl)}}$$

where CC = creatine clearance and K = 0.45 in infants younger than 1 year of age, 0.55 in infants older than 1 year of age, 0.33 in low–birth-weight infants, and 0.7 in adolescent boys.

(3) Because it is produced and excreted predictably, creatinine should be determined to check the accuracy of any timed urine collection. Young children should excrete at least 10 mg/kg/day and older, more muscular children 15–20 mg/kg/day.

b. Urinary protein excretion

(1) Total urinary protein should be less than 150 mg/24 hr, or less than 4 mg/m²/hr. Because timed collections may be difficult to obtain, a random urine specimen expressing the protein-to-creatinine ratio may be used to estimate proteinuria.

(2) Protein-to-creatinine ratio should be less than 0.2. A ratio exceeding 3.5 suggests nephrotic proteinuria.

3. Tests of renal tubular function

a. Concentrating, diluting, and acidifying capacity. Useful information is provided by tests that determine the kidney's capacity to concentrate, dilute, and acidify the urine. Renal concentrating capacity is easiest to assess. This is accomplished by a well-monitored overnight fluid deprivation test with determination of acute weight loss, urine output, and maximum urine specific gravity.

b. Reabsorptive capacity

(1) Tubular dysfunction is suggested by **detection of compounds in the urine that normally are reabsorbed completely by the renal tubules**. Such substances include glucose, amino acids, and β_2-microglobulin.

(2) The **tubular reabsorption of phosphate (TRP)** can be calculated using a small serum sample and random urine specimen. The TRP normally is greater than 85%. It is determined as:

$$TRP = 1 - \frac{\text{urine phosphate} \times \text{serum creatinine}}{\text{serum phosphate} \times \text{urine creatinine}} \times 100\%$$

4. Tests of bladder function and anatomy

a. Cystometry. Bladder function may be assessed using the urodynamic test, cystometry. Because it is an invasive procedure that uses catheters, rectal pressure balloons, and needle electrodes, and because it requires patient cooperation, cystometry is not used frequently. It is indicated in the evaluation of a child who has difficulty voiding (e.g., overflow incontinence, urine retention) or has urinary incontinence with a suspected neurologic cause. The test provides a profile of intravesical volume, pressure, and contractility.

b. Cystoscopy is the most direct method of visualizing the urethra and bladder. Because cystoscopy is invasive, requires general anesthesia, and adds little to other imaging techniques, it has little usefulness in children. Indications include preoperative evaluation of vesicoureteral reflux, investigation of congenital bladder anomalies, and suspicion of bladder neoplasia.

5. **Imaging procedures**
   a. **Ultrasonography** is the least invasive and most useful renal **anatomic imaging** technique for children. However, it cannot assess renal function and cannot demonstrate mild renal scarring.
      (1) Ultrasonography provides information on kidney location, size, shape, and consistency.
         (a) Serial studies are useful for evaluating renal growth.
         (b) Ultrasonography can be used to diagnose obstruction, malformations, cysts, calcifications, and tumors.
      (2) It is safe, and, because the equipment is portable, it can be performed on the most critically ill patients.
      (3) When combined with color Doppler imaging, blood flow velocity in the renal artery and renal vein can be evaluated.
   b. **Intravenous pyelography (IVP, excretory urography)** had been the standard anatomic renal imaging technique, but has limited usefulness compared to other imaging studies.
      (1) **Advantages**
         (a) IVP provides excellent, easily read anatomic images.
         (b) It reveals mild scarring and calyceal dilatation.
         (c) In a cooperative child, IVP may allow visualization of the bladder and bladder functioning.
      (2) **Disadvantages**
         (a) IVP requires intravenous injection of contrast material, which may produce an allergic reaction or nephrotoxicity.
         (b) Multiple radiographs cause relatively high radiation exposure.
         (c) IVP provides limited information regarding renal function.
         (d) Visualization is poor in patients with renal insufficiency, impaired concentrating capacity, or both.
   c. **Retrograde voiding cystourethrography (VCUG).** In this procedure, the contrast material is instilled by urethral catheter, and the bladder is visualized using fluoroscopy. The test defines the presence and magnitude of vesicoureteral reflux and provides information about the anatomy of the bladder and urethra.
   d. **Radionuclide scanning** is a useful test of renal function. Although it involves the intravenous injection of a radiolabeled tracer, radiation exposure is low—the gonadal dose is about 10% that of IVP.
      (1) **Evaluation of renal function.** Renal scanning can provide an estimate of total renal function, including GFR [with the use of technetium 99m (^{99m}Tc)-labeled diethylenetriamine pentaacetic acid] as well as tubular function [with the use of iodine 131 (^{131}I)-labeled o-iodohippurate]. It can also quantitate the contribution of each renal unit to total function. When images are obtained in the first seconds after the tracer is injected, information regarding renal blood flow may be obtained.
      (2) **Evaluation of vesicoureteral reflux.** Radionuclide scanning can be used to provide cystograms in the assessment of vesicoureteral reflux.
         (a) For cystography alone, the tracer is instilled directly into the bladder by catheter. For cystography in conjunction with a renal scan, it is given by intravenous injection of the nuclide ^{99m}Tc-mercaptoacetyltriglycine to a child able to cooperate by storing urine until instructed to void.
         (b) The major **advantage** of radionuclide cystography over standard radiographic cystography is the much lower gonadal radiation dose (less than 5% that of standard cystography). This is important because the child with reflux frequently needs serial cystograms.

(c) The major **disadvantages** of radionuclide cystography are its relatively poor structural delineation and its inability to evaluate the urethra. For these reasons, the VCUG is recommended initially, with follow-up studies done by radionuclide cystography.

(3) Evaluation of kidney infection. ^{99m}Tc-labeled dimercaptosuccinic acid, a tracer that localizes to tubular cells of functioning nephrons, is very valuable as an aid in the diagnosis of renal parenchymal infection and scarring by demonstrating focal areas of decreased uptake.

e. Other renal imaging techniques

(1) Computed tomography (CT) can be used to evaluate tumors or calcification of the renal tubules.

(2) Arteriography is useful for the evaluation of renovascular hypertension and vascular malformations.

(3) Magnetic resonance imaging (MRI) is used as an adjunct to tumor evaluation.

6. Renal biopsy is the definitive study for **histologic diagnosis** of renal disease. It provides tissue for examination by light, immunofluorescence, and electron microscopy.

a. Procedure. Renal biopsy usually is performed as a percutaneous closed procedure under fluoroscopic or ultrasonic guidance. In infants, renal biopsy is most safely carried out as an operative procedure under general anesthesia. For other patients, sedation and analgesia may be adequate.

b. Risks and contraindications. The risks of the procedure include obtaining insufficient tissue for diagnosis, causing bleeding or infection, and creating an arteriovenous fistula within the kidney. Contraindications to a percutaneous biopsy include bleeding disorders and the presence of a single kidney.

C. **Common presenting signs of renal disease**

1. Hematuria (blood in the urine) may be gross or microscopic.

a. Causes. Virtually any congenital anomaly, injury, or inflammatory disease of the kidney or urinary tract may cause hematuria.

(1) Isolated hematuria usually does not suggest a bleeding disorder or coagulopathy.

(2) Isolated microscopic hematuria is relatively common and usually is not indicative of serious renal disease. Most cases are idiopathic. However, when microscopic hematuria occurs in association with proteinuria, it is more likely to be a sign of significant disease.

(3) A common cause of microscopic hematuria in childhood is **idiopathic hypercalciuria,** which may be documented by a timed urine collection (normal urine calcium is less than 4 mg/kg/day) or a random urine sample for calcium-to-creatinine ratio (normally less than 0.2).

b. Evaluation

(1) Gross inspection of the urine and the **urine dipstick test** for blood may be useful in the diagnosis of hematuria, but **microscopic examination** of a fresh urine specimen is most important. Microscopic hematuria is considered significant if it is persistent and there are five or more red cells per high-power field. Urine that is brown or tea-colored suggests glomerular bleeding; a more specific indicator is the presence of crenated, dysmorphic red blood cells or red cell casts.

(2) Persistent, unexplained microscopic hematuria or a single episode of gross hematuria should be evaluated by **ultrasonography** to exclude abnormalities such as obstruction, renal cysts, or Wilms tumor.

2. Proteinuria refers to protein in the urine.

a. Causes

(1) Most commonly, asymptomatic proteinuria discovered in a random urine specimen is the protein excreted by some people when ambulatory and active. This **postural proteinuria** occurs in 5%–10% of children and young adults.

(a) Because it disappears when the patient is recumbent, it is identified by comparing the first morning urine with urine obtained later in the day.

(b) Although isolated postural proteinuria is a harmless finding, patients with significant renal disease may also show increased proteinuria in the upright position.

(2) Heavy proteinuria indicates **glomerulopathy**. Proteinuria that exceeds 960 mg/m^2/day defines the protein loss associated with **nephrotic syndrome**.

b. Evaluation. The **urine dipstick** is specific for albumin and does not detect tubular glycoproteins or globulins. **Sulfosalicylic acid precipitation** estimates total urinary protein.

3. **Oliguria** is defined as urine output less than 250 ml/m^2/day (urine volume insufficient to excrete even a minimal renal solute load in maximally concentrated urine).

   a. Causes. Oliguria is frequently a manifestation of **acute renal failure,** but it may also occur as an appropriate renal response to **hypovolemia** and **hypotension (prerenal oliguria).**

   b. Evaluation

   (1) Differentiation of oliguric renal failure from prerenal oliguria (appropriate renal salt and water retention) is often evident from the **history and physical examination.**

   (2) When volume depletion is suspected, differentiation is aided by response to an adequate **fluid challenge** with an intravascular volume expander, such as isotonic saline infusion (20 ml/kg given over 30–60 minutes).

   (3) Laboratory tests may also help to differentiate prerenal oliguria from renal failure.

   (a) The **blood urea nitrogen (BUN)-to-serum creatinine ratio** may be elevated (the normal ratio is 10:1 to 20:1; in prerenal oliguria the ratio exceeds 40:1) because urea is reabsorbed with water in prerenal states.

   (b) Also helpful is a **random urine sodium concentration,** which is very low (< 20 mEq/L) in prerenal oliguria but usually high (> 50 mEq/L) in renal failure.

   (c) Likewise, the **fractional excretion of sodium (FENa)** is low (< 1%) in prerenal oliguria and high (> 3%) in renal failure. The FENa is determined as follows:

$$\text{FENa} = \frac{\text{urine sodium} \times \text{serum creatinine}}{\text{urine creatinine} \times \text{serum sodium}} \times 100\%$$

4. **Polyuria** (excessive urine output) usually causes thirst and, therefore, is accompanied by **polydipsia** (excessive fluid intake). When free access to fluids is not possible, as with infants or the vomiting child, polyuria may contribute to dehydration and electrolyte disturbances.

   a. Causes (Table 14-1; see also Chapter 17). Polyuria most commonly is caused by disorders of renal concentrating ability or by diuretics, although it occasionally results from an abnormal desire for fluids (**psychogenic polydipsia**).

TABLE 14-1. Causes of Polyuria

Central diabetes insipidus (ADH deficiency)
Partial ADH deficiency
Complete ADH deficiency
Idiopathic diabetes insipidus
Acquired diabetes insipidus
Intracranial trauma or infection
Nephrogenic diabetes insipidus (ADH-resistant)
Inherited nephrogenic diabetes insipidus
Acquired nephrogenic diabetes insipidus
Interstitial nephritis, chronic renal insufficiency, papillary necrosis
Hypokalemia, sickle cell disease
Diuretic-induced polyuria
Osmotic agents (glucose, mannitol)
Volume expansion (intravenous fluids, resolution of acute renal failure)
Diuretic agents (furosemide)
Abnormal fluid ingestion (psychogenic polydipsia)

ADH = antidiuretic hormone (vasopressin).

b. Evaluation of polyuria involves a **fluid deprivation test** under close supervision in the hospital. Serum osmolarity, urine osmolarity, and body weight are monitored.

(1) Failure to achieve an adequate increase in urine osmolarity indicates a concentrating defect (e.g., maximum urinary concentration should occur with a serum osmolality exceeding 300 or with an acute 3% weight loss).

(2) The defect can be further categorized as vasopressin-deficient or vasopressin-resistant by the response to administration of vasopressin (also called antidiuretic hormone, or its analog, desmopressin).

II. THE KIDNEY IN THE NEWBORN

A. Developmental considerations

1. **Nephrogenesis** begins early in the first trimester of pregnancy and continues actively until 36 weeks' gestation. The very premature infant, therefore, is born with far fewer than the one million nephrons that exist in each kidney of the infant born at term.

2. The kidneys and genitourinary tract are the most common organ systems affected by **congenital anomalies,** although not all of these are significant.

3. The fetal kidney excretes urine into the amniotic fluid at a brisk rate—up to 10 ml/kg/hr. **Fetal oliguria or anuria** results in **oligohydramnios,** which is associated with pulmonary hypoplasia, other internal abnormalities, and a characteristic facial appearance with low-set ears (**Potter syndrome**). The pulmonary hypoplasia may be incompatible with life.

4. Significant intrauterine **urinary tract obstruction** may lead to abnormal and disorganized parenchymal development (**renal dysplasia**), and this may result in **renal insufficiency** even if the obstruction is relieved at birth.

B. Renal function at birth

1. Virtually every aspect of renal function has significant limitations at birth (Table 14-2). Because of these limitations, all **drug use** in the neonate must be evaluated in terms of renal excretion and potential toxicity. The more **premature** an infant is, the more severe and prolonged the limitations are.

2. **Serum creatinine.** In the first week of life, creatinine levels reflect maternal levels and do not accurately indicate infant renal function.

C. Renal diseases in the newborn

1. **Acute renal failure** in the newborn is uncommon, although transient rises in creatinine and oliguria in sick neonates are not.
   a. **Etiology**
      (1) **Perinatal insult** (e.g., asphyxia) is the most common cause of acute renal failure in newborns. Multisystem involvement worsens the prognosis.
      (2) **Congenital heart disease, congestive heart failure,** or **hypoperfusion.** Acute renal failure in this setting has a poor outcome.

TABLE 14-2. Renal Function in the Newborn

Function	Limitations
Glomerular filtration rate (GFR)	< 5 ml/min at birth; increases to 120 ml/min by 2 years
Sodium handling	Cannot maximally conserve or excrete sodium
Concentrating capacity	50%–60% of normal; achieves adult levels by 6 months
Diluting capacity	Low GFR impairs water excretion
Acidification	Bicarbonate reclamation and net acid excretion are impaired

(3) Congenital renal abnormalities (e.g., **dysplasia**) usually lead to renal failure after the neonatal period.

(4) Obstructive nephropathy must be bilateral (e.g., posterior urethral valves) to cause acute renal failure.

(5) Nephrotoxic agents (e.g., **aminoglycosides, contrast agents**) often cause non-oliguric renal failure.

b. **Diagnosis**

(1) Most newborns with **oliguria** (urine flow < 1 ml/kg/hr) do not have acute renal failure and respond to appropriate fluid challenge.

(2) Any infant with suspected renal failure should be evaluated for **obstruction** using ultrasonography. Obstruction should be promptly relieved.

c. **Therapy** for prolonged oliguric or anuric renal failure in the newborn may involve peritoneal dialysis to allow administration of the calories needed to prevent hypoglycemia and severe weight loss.

d. **Outcome** of acute renal failure in the newborn is usually good. Poor prognostic factors include multisystem organ failure, coexisting congenital heart disease, and need for dialysis.

2. **Congenital renal abnormalities,** including **hypoplasia** (too little normal parenchyma) and **dysplasia** (disorganized parenchyma), usually do not cause renal failure in the newborn, although they may progress to end-stage renal disease later in childhood.

3. **Renal venous thrombosis** may occur as a consequence of hyperviscosity (e.g., from polycythemia or severe volume depletion). The infant with this condition usually presents with a flank mass and hematuria. Severe hypertension or acute renal failure is uncommon. Treatment is supportive. Long-term sequelae include diminished GFR, tubular dysfunction, and hypertension.

4. **Renal artery occlusion** usually is caused by embolization from an umbilical artery catheter placed above the renal arteries. The infant presents with severe hypertension and signs of congestive heart failure. Therapy consists of antihypertensive medication to control the blood pressure.

III. NEPHROTIC SYNDROME

A. General considerations

1. **Definition.** Nephrotic syndrome is characterized by heavy proteinuria (urinary protein excretion exceeding 960 mg/m^2/day). This leads to hypoalbuminemia, edema, and hyperlipidemia. Nephrotic syndrome is not a single disease entity. It may accompany any glomerular disease.

2. **Pathogenesis.** Nephrotic syndrome develops when the glomerular basement membrane shows a marked, prolonged increase in permeability to plasma proteins. The underlying pathogenesis is unknown, but evidence suggests the importance of immune mechanisms.

B. Minimal change disease (also called **lipoid nephrosis** and **nil lesion**) is so named because the histologic changes visible on electron microscopy are limited to effacement of epithelial foot processes.

1. **Incidence and etiology.** Although uncommon, minimal change disease accounts for 80% of all cases of nephrotic syndrome in children. It occurs at all ages, but most commonly between 2 and 5 years of age. The cause is unknown.

2. **Clinical features and course**

a. The affected child usually presents with edema, which may be generalized and severe. Fatigue, anorexia, abdominal pain, diarrhea, infection, and intravascular volume depletion may be present.

b. Minimal change disease usually follows a relapsing course. Acute infections frequently trigger relapses, which may be detected promptly by urine testing with dipsticks.

3. **Diagnosis.** The typical patient with minimal change disease has normal renal function with no hematuria as well as normal blood pressure and serum complement levels, although exceptions are not uncommon.
   a. The best diagnostic indicator of minimal change disease, short of a renal biopsy, is the **response to steroid therapy**. A trial of steroid therapy should precede renal biopsy if minimal change disease is suspected.
   b. Table 14-3 lists other tests that are useful in establishing the diagnosis of nephrotic syndrome, in excluding other renal disease, and in monitoring for complications.

4. **Therapy**
   a. Steroids. Prednisone is administered daily, generally for 4 weeks. Alternate-day therapy is then given as a single, morning dose to mimic endogenous glucocorticoid release and to minimize steroid side effects. The dose is slowly tapered over many weeks to prevent a rapid recurrence of proteinuria as well as to prevent untoward steroid withdrawal effects.
   b. Alkylating agents. A child with minimal change disease who fails to respond to steroids or who manifests intolerable steroid toxicity may be treated successfully with either **cyclophosphamide** or **chlorambucil**. Because of their potentially serious side effects, these agents are used only when absolutely necessary.
   c. Diuretics. In the acute, edematous phase of minimal change disease, aggressive diuretic therapy may worsen the intravascular volume depletion. Diuretics do have a role in controlling the edema of chronic nephrotic states when intravascular volume depletion is not present.
   d. Cyclosporine. Cyclosporine is effective in inducing remission of nephrotic syndrome for children in whom steroid therapy is contraindicated. Its usefulness is limited by

TABLE 14-3. Tests Useful for Evaluating Nephrotic Syndrome

Purpose	Test
Establish the presence of nephrotic syndrome	Timed urinary protein excretion Total serum protein Serum protein electrophoresis Serum cholesterol and triglycerides

Exclude other renal disease*	Kidney function tests
	  Blood urea nitrogen
	  Serum creatinine
	  Creatinine clearance
	  Urinalysis (examine for cellular casts)
	Serologic tests
	  Complement component C3
	  Total hemolytic complement (CH_{50})
	  Antinuclear antibodies
	  Hepatitis B surface antigen
	  Circulating immune complexes
	Renal ultrasonography
	Renal biopsy

Monitor for complications (including those related to steroid therapy)	Complete blood count Appropriate cultures Serum electrolytes Bone densitometry (for steroid-induced demineralization) Eye examinations (for steroid-induced cataracts)

*Not all tests are necessary in all children.

its failure to maintain remission when it is discontinued, its expense, and potential nephrotoxicity.

    e. Supportive measures. Edema is managed by restricting sodium but not fluid intake. Dietary protein intake does not have to be increased above normal recommended levels. Pneumococcal vaccine should be given, ideally when the child is in remission and not taking steroids. Because nephrotic syndrome is a hypercoagulable state, deep venipuncture as well as intravascular volume depletion should be avoided.

  5. Prognosis. The long-term outlook is good because most cases of minimal change disease eventually remit permanently. The greatest concern is for steroid-related morbidity, especially growth retardation. Controversy surrounds the possibility that minimal change disease may rarely transform to another glomerulopathy, such as focal glomerulosclerosis.

C. **Other forms of nephrotic syndrome** (Table 14-4). The remaining 20% of cases of childhood nephrotic syndrome (i.e., those not associated with minimal change disease) occur with primary glomerulopathies, with systemic diseases, or secondary to toxic injuries. Accurate diagnosis is based on renal biopsy. Patients are less likely to be steroid-responsive and are more apt to progress to renal insufficiency than those with minimal change disease.

TABLE 14-4. Representative Causes of Childhood Nephrotic Syndrome

Primary nephrotic syndrome
  Without glomerulonephritis
    Minimal change disease
    Focal segmental glomerulosclerosis
    Congenital nephrotic syndrome

  With glomerulonephritis
    Mesangial proliferative glomerulonephritis
    Membranoproliferative glomerulonephritis
    Membranous nephropathy
    Acute postinfectious glomerulonephritis

Systemic diseases associated with nephrotic syndrome
  Infections
    Viral (e.g., AIDS, hepatitis B, cytomegalovirus, and Epstein-Barr virus infections)
    Bacterial (e.g., subacute bacterial endocarditis, shunt nephritis)
    Parasitic (e.g., malaria)

  Malignant diseases
    Lymphoma and leukemia
    Solid tumors (e.g., Wilms tumor, carcinomas)

  Metabolic diseases
    Diabetes mellitus
    Hypothyroidism

  Inflammatory diseases
    Systemic lupus erythematosus
    Systemic vasculitis
    Henoch-Schönlein purpura

  Other disorders
    Sickle cell disease
    Renal vein thrombosis
    Hemolytic–uremic syndrome

Exogenous agents associated with nephrotic syndrome
  Allergens (e.g., pollens, venoms)
  Vaccines (e.g., DTP)
  Toxic agents (e.g., heavy metals, heroin)
  Medications (e.g., captopril, penicillamine)

AIDS = acquired immune deficiency syndrome; DTP = diphtheria and tetanus toxoids with pertussis.

IV. GLOMERULOPATHIES are a heterogeneous group of diseases involving the glomerulus, which vary greatly in cause, presentation, course, and outcome. Most are immunologically mediated and are accompanied by varying degrees of hematuria, proteinuria, and azotemia. A large proportion of glomerulopathies are inflammatory, and thus are referred to as **glomerulonephritis**.

A. **Postinfectious glomerulonephritis** may follow many viral, bacterial, fungal, and parasitic infections.

    1. Acute poststreptococcal glomerulonephritis
      a. Pathogenesis. This prototype of postinfectious glomerulonephritis is mediated by the inflammatory response to immune complex deposition.
        (1) Glomerulonephritis usually **follows infection with several specific types of streptococci,** the so-called **nephritogenic strains**. There is a latent period of about 10 days (range, 1–4 weeks) between the streptococcal illness and the onset of glomerulonephritis.
        (2) Hypocomplementemia (decreased levels of complement component C3) develops transiently along with the nephritis in 90% of cases. (Other renal diseases associated with hypocomplementemia include membranoproliferative glomerulonephritis and glomerulonephritis that occurs in association with systemic lupus erythematosus, chronic infection, or inherited complement deficiencies.)
      b. Clinical features and course. The presentation may vary from mild, asymptomatic microscopic hematuria to gross hematuria, nephrotic syndrome, or severe renal failure. The typical affected child has a brief period of brownish urine, a sediment showing red blood cell casts, and mild renal insufficiency with volume-dependent hypertension and edema. The interval of azotemia (increased BUN) is short, and complete recovery of renal function is the rule. Microscopic hematuria, however, may persist for several years.

    2. Other infections that may lead to glomerulonephritis include:
      a. Bacterial (staphylococcal infection)
      b. Viral (hepatitis B, infectious mononucleosis)
      c. Fungal (histoplasmosis)
      d. Parasitic (toxoplasmosis, falciparum malaria)

B. Table 14-5 lists other forms of glomerulopathies that occur in childhood. None is commonly seen. All may be associated with the nephrotic syndrome.

V. TUBULOINTERSTITIAL NEPHRITIS (TIN)

A. **Definition and incidence.** Tubulointerstitial nephritis (TIN) refers to inflammation of the renal tubular cells and interstitium, the support structure between the tubules and vessels. Although more common in adults, TIN is frequently overlooked in children, in part because it often occurs in association with glomerular disease. It may also occur as a primary nephropathy.

B. **Etiology.** The most common causes of TIN in children are medication related, although infection-related TINs also occur frequently.

    1. Drug-related TIN may result from antibiotics (e.g., penicillin, cephalosporins), thiazide diuretics, and nonsteroidal anti-inflammatory drugs (e.g., ibuprofen).

    2. Infection-related TIN may be the direct result of pyelonephritis or an effect of the immune response. Bacterial, viral, fungal, and parasitic infections have been implicated (e.g., *Escherichia coli*, Epstein-Barr virus, *Candida*, *Toxoplasma gondii*).

TABLE 14-5. Uncommon Types of Childhood Glomerulonephritis

Types	Progression to Chronic Renal Failure	Therapy	Comments
Mesangial proliferative nephritis	Variable	Prednisone	Often steroid-dependent or steroid-resistant
Membranoproliferative nephritis	Common	Prednisone, every other day (ongoing)	At least three histologic types
Membranous nephritis	Variable	None	Spontaneous remission common; much more common condition in adults
IgA nephritis	Uncommon	None	Associated with upper respiratory infection
Henoch-Schönlein nephritis	Uncommon	None	Histologically identical to IgA nephropathy
Rapidly progressive nephritis (crescentic glomerulonephritis)	Common	Intravenous high-dose prednisone	May be associated with other forms of glomerulonephritis
Lupus nephritis	Variable	Prednisone, cyclophosphamide, or both	Several histologic types
Diabetic nephropathy	Rare in childhood	Preventive (e.g., good glycemic control)	Most common cause of end-stage renal disease in adults with antecedents in childhood
Sickle cell nephropathy	Unusual in childhood	None	Concentrating and acidifying defects most often seen

IgA = immunoglobulin A.

3. **Immune-mediated TIN** may be associated with membranoproliferative glomeru-lonephritis, systemic disease (e.g., systemic lupus erythematosus), renal allograft rejection, or uveitis.

C. **Clinical features and course.** TIN may present in several ways (Table 14-6). Manifestations vary from abnormalities of the urinalysis only, to anuric renal failure.

D. **Diagnosis.** Although the diagnosis of TIN may be suspected in a previously healthy child who, while taking a course of medication, suddenly manifests fever, constitutional symptoms, acute renal insufficiency, and proteinuria, hematuria, and sterile pyuria, definitive diagnosis must be made on **renal biopsy**. The presence of eosinophils in the urine, demonstrated on Wright stain, is virtually diagnostic of TIN, but in practice is detected uncommonly.

TABLE 14-6. Clinical Presentations of Tubulointerstitial Nephritis (TIN)

Abnormality	Comments
Acute renal failure	May be nonoliguric or oliguric
Tubular dysfunction	May involve proximal tubules (e.g., Fanconi syndrome), distal tubules (e.g., hyperkalemic renal acidosis), or general problems with concentrating ability (e.g., nephrogenic diabetes insipidus)
Nephrotic syndrome	Minimal change on biopsy

E. | **Treatment**

1. The underlying cause should be treated if possible.

2. Abnormalities of blood pressure and fluids and electrolytes should be treated.

3. **Prednisone** is thought to be efficacious in shortening the course of TIN.

F. | **Prognosis**

1. Most children with TIN have a full recovery.

2. Long-term follow-up studies show normal renal function.

VI. URINARY TRACT INFECTION

A. | **Incidence.** Urinary tract infection is common in infants and children. In newborns, it is twice as common in boys, but in childhood, it is 10 times more common in girls. About 5% of school-age girls will have a urinary tract infection, and 80% of these patients experience a recurrence.

B. | **Localization.** A urinary tract infection is frequently classified based on involvement of the renal parenchyma (**pyelonephritis**) or the bladder (**cystitis**). No laboratory study can accurately localize the infection, and localization usually is based on clinical findings (Table 14-7). Unfortunately, the symptoms of a urinary tract infection in infants and young children frequently are nonspecific and vague. Most infections do not involve the renal parenchyma.

C. | **Etiology and pathogenesis**

1. **Contamination by fecal flora.** In virtually all cases, a urinary tract infection results from fecal flora, especially coliform bacteria, ascending the urethra to the bladder (Table 14-8). Factors important to the development of urinary tract infection include the ability of organisms to adhere to the urinary epithelium, surface immunoglobulins, completeness of bladder emptying, and urine pH. Pyelonephritis implies that organisms have ascended the ureters, as can occur in vesicoureteral reflux (retrograde flow of urine up the ureters from the bladder).

2. **Vesicoureteral reflux** is present in 35% of children with a urinary tract infection; it is much less common in the general population. The relationship between vesicoureteral reflux and urinary tract infection is uncertain, but vesicoureteral reflux definitely increases the risk of pyelonephritis.

TABLE 14-7. Clues to the Localization of Urinary Tract Infections

Sign or Symptom	Pyelonephritis	Cystitis
Fever > 39°C	Common	Very unusual
Constitutional symptoms	Common	Very unusual
Leukocytosis	WBC frequently > 20,000	WBC usually normal
Elevated sedimentation rate	Virtually always	Unusual
Dysuria, frequency, urgency	Variable	Common
DMSA radionuclide scan	Areas of decreased uptake	Normal
Flank pain and costovertebral angle tenderness	Common (except in infants)	Absent

DMSA = dimercaptosuccinic acid.

TABLE 14-8. Organisms Causing Urinary Tract Infections in Infants and Children

Organism	Comments
Gram-negative organisms	
Escherichia coli	Accounts for 80% of urinary tract infections
Proteus	Urea splitters; urine often has a high pH
Haemophilus influenzae	Uncommon; does not grow well on usual media
Pseudomonas	Urinary tract anomalies (e.g., duplication, obstruction) are often a contributing factor
Gram-positive organisms	
Staphylococcus saprophyticus	Common cause in adolescents
Enterococcus	As with other gram-positive organisms, does not convert nitrates to nitrites
Group B *Streptococcus*	Unusual

    a. In most cases, vesicoureteral reflux is caused by a congenitally abnormal insertion of the ureter into the bladder wall. Mild vesicoureteral reflux may occur transiently with cystitis.

    b. Renal scarring is found in 50% of children with vesicoureteral reflux and infection. It is caused by reflux of urine into the renal parenchyma (**intrarenal reflux**). In most cases, such scarring occurs before age 2 years, indicating the need for prompt diagnosis and treatment of urinary tract infection in infants. It is not known if vesicoureteral reflux, in the absence of infection or obstruction, can injure the kidney.

D. **Clinical features.** Recognizing urinary tract infection in children, particularly infants, may be difficult. The classic symptoms of cystitis (i.e., dysuria, urgency, frequency) often are absent, as are the flank pains and shaking chills associated with pyelonephritis in adults. Children with urinary tract infection may present with unexplained fever, failure to thrive, vague gastrointestinal and abdominal complaints, and enuresis.

E. **Diagnosis**

  1. Urine culture. The diagnosis must be based on culture results, not on symptoms or urinalysis. Urine cultures should be obtained only in children in whom urinary tract infection is suspected, not in asymptomatic individuals. Reliable urine screening culture kits are available in outpatient settings.

    a. Definitive results. A count of 10^5 colony-forming units/ml for a single organism usually is accepted as proof of infection, although counts of 5×10^4 or less should not be discounted as contaminants.

    b. Methods of urine collection

      (1) Clean-catch samples can be 85% reliable.

      (2) Catheterization and suprapubic aspiration are more specific means of obtaining samples, but these methods may cause discomfort and involve some risk.

    c. Repeat culture is required if symptoms do not improve within 48 hours of initiating antimicrobial therapy.

    d. Follow-up culture should be obtained at least 72 hours after completion of antimicrobial therapy.

  2. Imaging is indicated for urinary tract infection in all children younger than 2 years of age, in all boys, in girls with parenchymal infection, and in all children in whom localization of the infection is in doubt. Uncomplicated cystitis in school-age girls does not require radiologic evaluation if follow-up is ensured.

    a. Ultrasonography should be performed to search for obstruction or urinary tract anomalies. It can be repeated serially to monitor renal growth.

    b. Voiding cystourethrography identifies vesicoureteral reflux and establishes the degree of reflux. The study is best performed after completion of therapy.

F. **Therapy**

1. **Uncomplicated cystitis.** Antimicrobial therapy is based on the results of urine culture and sensitivity testing. Usually, 10 days of therapy with amoxicillin or trimethoprim–sulfamethoxazole is effective and well tolerated. Although short-course therapy is established, effective therapy in adults, studies in children are equivocal, and therefore such therapy is not recommended.

2. **Pyelonephritis**
   a. The same drugs used for cystitis yield antimicrobial urinary levels that are adequate to treat renal parenchymal infections. Often, however, the child with pyelonephritis is vomiting and severely ill. Furthermore, until the organism is identified, parenteral broad-spectrum antibiotics may be desirable, and hospitalization for initial parenteral antibiotic and fluid therapy is then indicated.
   b. A single episode of pyelonephritis may be treated with 10–14 days of oral therapy. Recurrent episodes may require therapy for 4–6 weeks.

3. **Preventive therapy**
   a. **Risk factors** for urinary tract infections should be **investigated and eliminated**. These factors include:
      (1) **Congenital anomalies of the urinary tract** (e.g, diverticula of the bladder)
      (2) **Conditions associated with incomplete emptying of the bladder** (e.g., chronic constipation)
      (3) **Habits that lead to chronic infection or irritation of the perineal area** (e.g., bubble baths, wiping "back to front")
   b. The child with vesicoureteral reflux, other urinary tract anomalies, or a recurrent urinary tract infection requires **continuous antimicrobial therapy**. A single daily low dose of nitrofurantoin is effective and well tolerated. Bacterial resistance seldom develops.

G. **Complications and prognosis.** Although urinary tract infection is frequently recurrent, the risk of progression to chronic renal insufficiency, even with pyelonephritis, is very low.

1. **Hypertension** is the most common long-term sequela of recurrent pyelonephritis.

2. **Renal scarring** also can result from pyelonephritis.
   a. Renal scarring is seen in infants and young children; it rarely develops in older children and adults. The progression of renal scars is an immunologically mediated process that is not understood.
   b. Renal scarring is frequently focal, and hypertrophy of normal renal tissue maintains normal overall function. It may also result in a peculiar renal outline, referred to as **pseudotumor formation**.

3. **Severe vesicoureteral reflux.** Most vesicoureteral reflux in childhood resolves spontaneously, but severe reflux may require surgery. Serial cystograms, preferably with radionuclides, are obtained every 18–24 months to monitor the resolution of vesicoureteral reflux. Antimicrobial prophylaxis should be continued as long as reflux is present.

VII. HYPERTENSION

A. **Definition and incidence**

1. **Definition.** Hypertension in childhood is defined as a blood pressure reading greater than the ninety-fifth percentile for age obtained on three separate occasions. Approximately 1% of the pediatric population and 3% of adolescents are hypertensive by this definition.

2. **Blood pressure norms.** Figure 14-1 shows age-specific percentiles of blood pressure measurements in boys and girls, 1–13 years of age. Blood pressure values progressively increase from infancy to adolescence. A "normal value" does not imply freedom from the long-term risk of cardiovascular disease, and therefore is not necessarily a "healthy value."

A

B

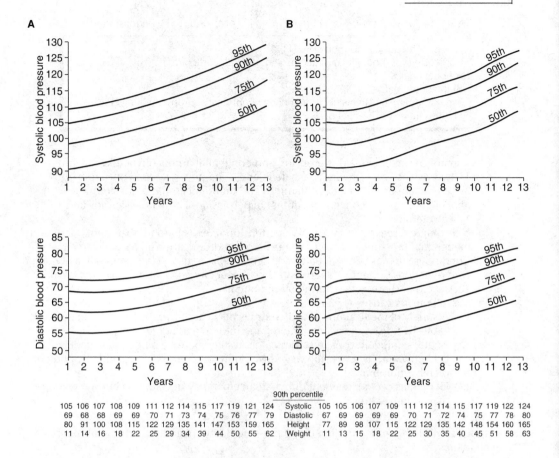

The 90th percentile data table:

105	106	107	108	109	111	112	114	115	117	119	121	124	**Systolic**	105	105	106	107	109	111	112	114	115	117	119	122	124
69	68	68	69	69	70	71	73	74	75	76	77	79	**Diastolic**	67	69	69	69	70	71	72	74	75	77	78	80
80	91	100	108	115	122	129	135	141	147	153	159	165	**Height**	77	89	98	107	115	122	129	135	142	148	154	160	165
11	14	16	18	22	25	29	34	39	44	50	55	62	**Weight**	11	13	15	18	22	25	30	35	40	45	51	58	63

FIGURE 14-1. Age-specific percentiles of blood pressure measurements in (A) boys and (B) girls, 1–13 years of age; Korotkoff phase IV (K4) used for diastolic blood pressure. Height is measured in centimeters and weight is measured in kilograms.

B. | **Etiology**

1. **Primary hypertension** (also called **idiopathic** or **essential hypertension**) is probably the most common form of hypertension (as defined earlier) in children. As in adults, primary hypertension is a heterogeneous group of disorders. The blood pressure elevation usually is mild to moderate and asymptomatic. If sustained for long periods, it becomes an important risk factor in the development of cardiovascular disease. Often, a strong family history of high blood pressure exists.

2. **Secondary hypertension**
   a. **Renal disease** is the most common cause of secondary hypertension. Virtually any renal disease, glomerular or interstitial, may be the cause. The hypertension may be transient or sustained and may be out of proportion in severity to the degree of renal insufficiency. Renal hypertension is caused by salt and water retention with volume expansion or by a renin-mediated increase in vascular resistance.
   b. **Vascular causes** of hypertension (e.g., coarctation of the aorta, renal artery stenosis, renal artery occlusion), although uncommon, are important to identify because they may lead to severe, symptomatic hypertension and they may be curable. Anatomic vascular abnormalities are identified by angiography.
   c. **Endocrine causes** of hypertension are very uncommon and are conditions associated with excess catecholamines or aldosterone. These include pheochromocytoma,

TABLE 14-9. Medications and Illicit Drugs That May Cause Hypertension

Adrenocorticotropic hormone (ACTH)
Corticosteroids (both glucocorticoids and mineralocorticoids)
Amphetamines
Birth control pills
Sympathomimetic agents (including phenylephrine eye drops in young children)
Phencyclidine (PCP, angel dust)

primary or secondary aldosteronism, and congenital adrenal hyperplasia with 11-hydroxylase or 17-hydroxylase deficiency. Diagnosis is based on serum and urine concentrations of catecholamines and their metabolites, aldosterone, and—in the case of congenital adrenal hyperplasia—17-hydroxysteroids and 17-ketosteroids.

   d. **Neurologic disease** as a cause of hypertension often is hard to document. Increased intracranial pressure and the Guillain-Barré syndrome are well recognized causes. Conditions such as cerebral palsy and seizure disorders are less definitely associated with hypertension. In the latter conditions, spasticity and hypertonicity may make accurate blood pressure determination difficult.

   e. **Miscellaneous causes**
      (1) A variety of **medications** and **illicit drugs** may cause hypertension in some people. Table 14-9 lists agents encountered in children and adolescents.
      (2) Acute, significant **rises in serum calcium** may increase blood pressure. Hypercalcemia and hypertension may develop in children who are suddenly and completely immobilized.
      (3) Hypertension independent of hypercalcemia may develop in children who are placed in **traction**.

C. **Diagnosis.** Most children with high blood pressure do not need an extensive or invasive evaluation.

   1. **Basic evaluation.** The evaluation of any child with elevated blood pressure should focus on three areas: (1) the likelihood of a secondary cause, (2) identifying risk factors for hypertension and cardiovascular disease (because hypertension is an important risk factor for the latter), and (3) recognizing the complications of hypertension already present.

      a. **History.** Significant items include previous growth and state of health, urinary tract symptoms or infections, medications, tobacco use, dietary intake, level of activity, and family history of hypertension, stroke, or premature cardiovascular disease.

      b. **Physical examination**
         (1) **Blood pressure readings** should be obtained when the heart rate is stable and repeated until values are consistent. Diastolic values are best expressed by both the phase 4 (muffling) and phase 5 (disappearance) Korotkoff sounds. Blood pressure readings should be obtained in all extremities, and pulses should be checked.
         (2) **Auscultation** for murmurs and bruits and **funduscopic examination** of retinal vessels are important.
         (3) Erroneous high blood pressure readings are frequently obtained because the **size of the cuff** is too small. An appropriate blood pressure cuff is the largest cuff that comfortably fits around the arm. The inflatable bladder should almost completely encircle the arm.

      c. **Laboratory studies** should include a urinalysis and measurement of serum electrolytes, BUN, and creatinine. A chest radiograph, an electrocardiogram, and occasionally an echocardiogram are indicated to exclude ventricular hypertrophy. Total cholesterol and high-density lipoprotein levels are important indicators of additional risk for cardiovascular disease.

2. Further evaluation for secondary hypertension may be indicated by findings on the initial evaluation or by any of the following:
   a. Very high blood pressure readings (e.g., above 120/80 mm Hg in infants, 140/90 mm Hg in children, 160/100 mm Hg in adolescents)
   b. Any level of blood pressure that causes **symptoms** (e.g., headache, vomiting, signs of congestive heart failure)
   c. Hypertension that is **progressive**
   d. Hypertension that is **refractory to therapy**

D. **Therapy**

1. **Initial therapy** in mild hypertension should be nonpharmacologic, namely, reduction in salt intake and, if indicated, weight reduction and increased physical activity.

2. **Drug therapy** is given when the preceding measures do not suffice.
   a. Approach. Drugs chosen should be those that can be taken infrequently and that will allow an active lifestyle, including competitive sports. The lowest possible effective dose is determined by starting a small, reasonable dose and increasing it until the desired control has been attained or until side effects intervene.
   b. Agents used most often to treat childhood hypertension are listed in Table 14-10. Many of the newer, more effective agents are not officially approved for use in pediatric patients, but nevertheless are commonly used by pediatricians who treat hypertension. One practical limitation to the use of these medications in small children is the fact that they are unavailable in liquid or appropriate low-dose pill form.

3. **Therapy for secondary hypertension** involves eliminating the cause when possible as well as administering antihypertensive medication to stabilize the blood pressure and the patient. Surgery or angioplasty is indicated for coarctation of the aorta and renal artery stenosis.

TABLE 14-10. Drugs Commonly Used to Treat Childhood Hypertension

Drug	Comments
Diuretics	
Hydrochlorothiazide	Seldom effective alone; ineffective in patients with a low GFR; may cause hypokalemia
Furosemide	Used to reduce intravascular volume; long-term effectiveness is limited
β-Blockers	
Propranolol	First and most commonly used of a large family of drugs; not selective; may cause bronchospasm
Atenolol	Cardioselective; once daily dosing
α-Blockers	
Prazosin	Commonly used with a β-blocker; well tolerated
Vasodilators	
Hydralazine	Causes salt and water retention; flushing; headache
Minoxidil	Very effective; severe hypertrichosis and fluid retention limit its use
Angiotensin-converting enzyme (ACE) inhibitors	
Captopril	Effective in children with high renin states; may decrease renal function in renovascular disease; may cause proteinuria and hyperkalemia
Enalapril	Once daily dosing
Calcium channel blockers	
Nifedipine	Effective; well tolerated; use with β-blockers should be avoided

GFR = glomerular filtration rate.

TABLE 14-11. Drugs Used to Treat Childhood Hypertensive Emergencies

Drugs	Comments	Side Effects
Vasodilators		
Diazoxide	Administered rapidly intravenously	Tachycardia
Nitroprusside	Immediate effect; continuous administration necessary	Hypotension, thiocyanate toxicity
Hydralazine	Administered slowly intravenously; not predictably effective	Headache, nausea
Calcium channel blockers*		
Nifedipine	Administered sublingually; safe and effective	Dizziness, headache
α-Adrenergic blockers		
Phentolamine	Used only when pheochromocytoma is suspected	Tachycardia, dysrhythmias
β- and α-Adrenergic blockers		
Labetalol	Administered intravenously	Bradycardia, bronchospasm

*Calcium channel blockers also act through vasodilation.

E. **Hypertensive emergencies.** When the blood pressure is severely elevated (e.g., 180/110 mm Hg), is producing symptoms, or is increasing rapidly, treatment must be given promptly (Table 14-11), and the child must be monitored continuously.

VIII. **FLUID AND ELECTROLYTE DISTURBANCES** in children commonly are the result of gastrointestinal illness (i.e., diarrhea, vomiting, or both) and involve some degree of dehydration. Most cases are mild and may be treated with oral fluids. When choosing among the several acceptable approaches to therapy, it is best to keep the approach as simple as possible.

A. **Maintenance water and electrolyte requirements** (Table 14-12) are the amounts required daily to maintain homeostasis in a person in a resting, basal state.

1. **Water.** Maintenance water requirements may be calculated as 1500 ml/m²/day for children weighing more than 1.5 kg. Surface area (SA) may be calculated as follows:

$$SA = (4W + 7)/(W + 90),$$

TABLE 14-12. Daily Maintenance Requirements for Water and Electrolytes

Substance	Requirement/24 hr
Water	1500 ml/m²*
Sodium	2–3 mEq/kg
Potassium	2–3 mEq/kg
Chloride	2–3 mEq/kg

*Amount of water is for patients weighing more than 1.5 kg.

TABLE 14-13. Approximate Composition of Gastrointestinal Fluids

Fluid	Sodium (mEq/L)	Potassium (mEq/L)	Chloride (mEq/L)	Bicarbonate (mEq/L)
Gastric	75	20	100	0
Small intestinal	135	15	100	30
Large intestinal	60	40	80	50
Diarrhea (in infants)	60	45	60	45

where W is the weight in kilograms. More commonly, maintenance water is estimated by body weight:

100 ml/kg for body weight kilograms 1–10

50 ml/kg for body weight kilograms 11–20

20 ml/kg for body weight kilograms > 20

Maintenance water balances the following **natural losses**.
   a. Insensible water loss. Approximately 40% of maintenance water replaces evaporative, electrolyte-free water lost from the skin and lungs.
   b. Fecal loss. About 5%–10% of maintenance water replaces fecal loss.
   c. Urinary loss. The remaining 50%–55% of maintenance water replaces urinary water loss. The amount of water lost in the urine is the amount necessary to excrete a basal renal solute load as urine that is neither concentrated nor diluted (i.e., with specific gravity of 1.010).

   2. **Electrolytes.** Maintenance electrolytes include sodium, potassium, and chloride; the daily requirements for these are shown in Table 14-12.

B. | **Dehydration states**

   1. **Etiologic considerations**
      a. Dehydration in the pediatric age group usually is the result of **acute gastrointestinal illness,** in which losses from diarrhea, vomiting, or both are combined with inadequate oral fluid intake. The serum electrolyte concentrations in a child with dehydration reflect the magnitude and electrolyte composition of the intake and losses. Table 14-13 lists the approximate composition of gastrointestinal fluids. Table 14-14 shows the composition of oral fluids used to treat mild or early cases of gastrointestinal illness.
      b. The increased water requirements induced by various disease states may be exacerbated by such factors as fever, hyperventilation, ambient humidity, sweating, and increased metabolic rate.

   2. **Diagnosis.** Table 14-15 lists the signs and symptoms of dehydration.

   3. **Types of dehydration.** Although the classification of dehydration states by plasma osmolality is based on serum sodium levels, it is simplest to consider the water deficit and sodium deficit separately.

TABLE 14-14. Composition of Oral Fluids Commonly Used to Treat Gastroenteritis

	Carbohydrate (g/dl)	Sodium (mEq/L)	Potassium (mEq/L)
Pedialyte*	2.5	45	20
Gatorade	4.6	23	3
Kool-Aid	10.5	3	0.1
Ginger ale	9.0	3.5	0.1
Rehydralyte*	2.5	75	20

*Oral rehydration solution.

TABLE 14-15. Signs and Symptoms of Dehydration

Signs	Symptoms
Sunken eyes (if subtle, may be noted only by parents)	Thirst
Dry mucous membranes	Lethargy, irritability
Decreased tears	Decreased urine output
Poor skin turgor	
Postural blood pressure change	
Sunken fontanelle (in quiet, sitting infants)	

    a. Isotonic dehydration. Net sodium and water losses are proportionate. This form of dehydration is found in approximately 75% of children hospitalized for dehydration.

      (1) Serum sodium values are within the broad range of normal (130–150 mEq/L).

      (2) Although extracellular fluid (ECF) tonicity remains normal, gastrointestinal losses are unevenly hypotonic, and there is a net loss of water from the intracellular fluid (ICF) as well.

    b. Hypertonic dehydration. Water is lost in excess of sodium.

      (1) Hypernatremia (serum sodium above 150 mEq/L) occurs in about 20% of cases of dehydration. Hypernatremia results when there is little oral intake, ongoing insensible water loss, and hypotonic diarrheal losses. Gastrointestinal water loss is increased with intake of relatively high carbohydrate-containing fluid. With hypernatremia, the water loss is primarily from the ICF, and the ECF is relatively well preserved.

      (2) Signs. The classic signs of dehydration frequently are absent. Instead, neurologic signs (e.g., irritability, lethargy, seizures) are prominent and the skin may feel doughy.

      (3) Associated abnormalities include hyperglycemia, metabolic acidosis, and hypocalcemia.

    c. Hypotonic dehydration. Sodium is lost in excess of water.

      (1) Hyponatremia (serum sodium below 130 mEq/L) occurs in about 5% of dehydrated children.

      (2) Signs

        (a) Because the losses are mainly from the ECF, the classic signs of dehydration and intravascular volume depletion (i.e., decreased skin turgor, decreased tearing, dry mucous membranes, sunken anterior fontanelle, tachycardia and orthostatic hypotension, low jugular venous pulsation) occur early.

        (b) Neurologic signs, including seizures, may occur and are directly related to both the serum sodium concentration and the rapidity with which hyponatremia develops.

      (3) Associated abnormalities. The various causes of hyponatremia (Table 14-16) must be considered.

TABLE 14-16. Causes of Hyponatremia

Pseudohyponatremia	Dilutional hyponatremia
Hyperlipidemia	Hyperglycemia
Hyperproteinemia	Congestive heart failure
Depletional hyponatremia	Nephrotic syndrome
Gastrointestinal loss	Liver disease
Sweat loss	Water intoxication
Renal loss (adrenal insufficiency, chronic	SIADH
renal insufficiency, diuretics)	Reset osmostat

SIADH = syndrome of inappropriate antidiuretic hormone secretion.

4. Degree of dehydration
   a. The extent of dehydration may be estimated from the change in body weight if the prior weight or growth charts are available. Acute weight loss may be assumed to equal water loss.
   b. Reasonable clinical estimates of dehydration can be made on the basis of history and physical assessment: A loss of 5% generally correlates with subtle evidence of dehydration, a loss of 10% with obvious evidence, and a loss of 15% with signs of shock.

5. Electrolyte deficits
   a. Sodium deficit occurs in all forms of dehydration, although the deficit is greatest in hyponatremic and smallest in hypernatremic states.
      (1) Isotonic dehydration. The losses include uneven hypotonic losses, so that the net water deficit from the ICF approximates the loss from the ECF. Therefore, a 1-L deficit in a child with a normal serum sodium concentration consists of 0.5 L of ECF (sodium 140 mEq/L) and 0.5 L of ICF (sodium 5–10 mEq/L).
      (2) Hypertonic dehydration. In hypernatremic states, the sodium deficit is smaller because losses from the ICF, where the sodium content is very low, comprise approximately three-fourths of the total loss.
      (3) Hypotonic dehydration. In hyponatremic states, ECF losses are accentuated, because the hypotonic ECF forces fluid to shift from the ECF into the ICF.
   b. Potassium deficit is difficult to estimate but in general approximates the sodium deficit found in isotonic states. The amount administered usually is limited by the concentration of potassium in intravenous fluids and should not exceed 40 mEq/L when infused into a peripheral vein.

6. Treatment of dehydration
   a. Shock. When signs of shock are present (e.g., weak, rapid pulse; mottled extremities; delayed capillary refill; hypotension), intravascular volume should be reexpanded promptly without regard to electrolyte status. An isotonic volume expander such as 0.9% (normal) saline is given at 20 ml/kg over 30 minutes. Further fluid resuscitation is often necessary and should be given as needed.
   b. Isotonic dehydration. Fluids that correct the deficit and provide daily maintenance requirements are given over 24 hours, with half of the total administered in the first 8 hours. Treatment of a 10% dehydrated child who weighs 10 kg (when well) and whose surface area is 0.6 m² is as follows.
      (1) The child should receive 1 L of water for maintenance (100 ml/kg) and 1 L of water for deficit replacement (10% of 10 kg). The child also should receive 20–30 mEq each of sodium and potassium for maintenance and 70 mEq each of these electrolytes for deficit replacement. (The sodium deficit represents the sodium concentration in the 0.5 L of deficit water estimated to come from the ECF. Again, the potassium deficit approximates the sodium deficit.)
      (2) Half of the total, or 1 L, of one-third normal saline in 5% dextrose should be given in the first 8 hours, and the remainder given over the next 16 hours.
      (3) The child must be reevaluated at regular intervals, watching for sources of ongoing losses (e.g., continued diarrhea).
   c. Hypertonic dehydration. To avoid too rapid a reduction in sodium concentration, the deficit amounts should be given slowly and evenly over 48 hours, along with maintenance fluids.
   d. Hypotonic dehydration
      (1) The sodium required to convert a hyponatremic dehydrated state to an isonatremic one may be calculated as follows:

required Na^+ (mEq) = 0.6 × body wt (kg) × [desired Na^+ (mEq/L) – observed Na^+ (mEq/L)]

      (2) The total sodium deficit should not be corrected completely because of the risk of neurologic damage, including **central pontine myelinolysis** (the osmotic demyelinization syndrome), which has been reported rarely in children.
         (a) In general, a corrected serum sodium concentration of 125 mEq/L is reasonable.

       (b) When the initial serum sodium is very low (e.g., < 110 mEq/L), the correction should be more modest (e.g., correct to 115–120 mEq/L).

       (c) The correction may be made with 3% saline (1 ml = 0.5 mEq of sodium) given at a rate to increase serum sodium 1–2 mEq/L/hr.

    (3) Further correction of the dehydration may then proceed as with isotonic dehydration.

IX. ACID–BASE DISTURBANCES

A. Normal acid–base homeostasis

1. Acid–base balance is maintained by the pulmonary excretion of carbon dioxide plus the renal excretion of excess hydrogen ions.

2. Acute changes in acid–base status are prevented by the body's buffer systems. The most important of these in the ECF is bicarbonate because it is plentiful, it can be conserved and generated by the kidney, and it links the lungs and kidneys by carbonic acid dissociation:

$$CO_2 + H_2O \rightleftharpoons H_2CO_3 \rightleftharpoons H^+ + HCO_3^-$$

3. The growing child excretes about 2–3 mEq of hydrogen ions per kilogram daily. Most of this net acid is derived from dietary protein. The kidney excretes net acid by acidifying the urine via the following mechanisms:
   a. Reclaiming all filtered bicarbonate
   b. Excreting urinary anions (e.g., phosphate), which combine with hydrogen ions to form titratable acid
   c. Producing ammonia in proximal renal tubular cells, which may bind hydrogen ions to form ammonium ions

B. Assessing acid–base status. Measuring a patient's serum electrolytes, blood pH, and blood gases provides the data for determining acid–base status.

1. **Serum electrolyte levels** provide the total carbon dioxide and permit calculation of the anion gap.
   a. The **total carbon dioxide** is almost identical to the serum bicarbonate plus small contributions of dissolved carbon dioxide and carbonic acid.
   b. The **anion gap** [serum sodium – (chloride + total carbon dioxide)] normally is less than 12 in older children and less than 17 in infants. A large anion gap means there is an excess of one or more unmeasured anions such as lactate or acetoacetate.

2. **Blood pH** indicates the net acid–base status and identifies **acidemia** (pH < 7.35) or **alkalemia** (pH > 7.45). The pH may be within the normal range in acid–base disorders if there is compensation for the primary disturbance or if there is a mixed disorder. Reasonable estimates of the pH change expected in an uncompensated, primary acid–base disturbance are as follows.
   a. For every change in the arterial partial pressure of carbon dioxide (Pa_{CO_2}) of 10 mm Hg, the pH will change inversely by 0.08.
   b. For every change in serum bicarbonate of 10 mmol/L, the pH will change 0.15.
   c. In situations in which the expected changes are not observed, there is either a mixed acid–base disturbance or compensation (or both).

3. **Arterial blood gas analysis** provides the carbon dioxide partial pressure (P_{CO_2}) that allows assessment of pulmonary ventilation. Analysis of blood gases also provides the amount of buffer base excess or deficit (negative excess), which is calculated by determining how much of a change in pH cannot be explained by a change in Pa_{CO_2}. The base excess (or deficit) equals 0.67 multiplied by the multiple of 0.01 pH unit unexplained. The base deficit can be used to estimate the total bicarbonate deficit using the formula (base deficit) × (body weight in kg) × (0.3).

C. **Acidosis** results from any process that reduces the body's pH.

1. **Respiratory acidosis**
   a. **Causes.** Respiratory acidosis is caused by the accumulation of carbon dioxide as the result of pulmonary hypoventilation. It may occur with any cause of respiratory failure, including pulmonary disease, neuromuscular disease, and central nervous system depression.
   b. **Compensation.** The body attempts to compensate for respiratory acidosis by the renal conservation of bicarbonate and by increased excretion of hydrogen ion.
   c. **Therapy** is directed at restoring adequate ventilation. Alkalinizing agents should not be used.

2. **Metabolic acidosis**
   a. **Causes.** Metabolic acidosis is caused by the accumulation of net acid or the excessive loss of bicarbonate.
      (1) **Accumulation of net acid** occurs with ingestion of acid (e.g., salicylate intoxication, which also causes respiratory alkalosis by stimulating central hyperventilation), excess production of acid (e.g., lactic acidosis, diabetic ketoacidosis), or decreased excretion of acid (e.g., in renal failure). These forms of acidosis usually have a **wide anion gap**.
      (2) **Excess loss of bicarbonate** commonly occurs with diarrhea. It may also occur in renal disease, although renal failure affects all phases of urine acidification. Metabolic acidosis resulting from bicarbonate loss usually has a **normal anion gap** and is called **hyperchloremic metabolic acidosis**.
   b. **Compensation.** The body's compensation for metabolic acidosis is increased respiratory minute ventilation (hyperventilation), leading to a reduction in P_{CO_2} and returning pH toward normal. Maximum hyperventilation can lower the P_{CO_2} to 12–15 mm Hg, which keeps the pH in the normal range with a bicarbonate concentration as low as 8 mmol/L.
   c. **Renal tubular acidosis** is the term given to a heterogeneous group of disorders, all of which are characterized by hyperchloremic metabolic acidosis and tubular dysfunction, but usually not by renal insufficiency. Renal tubular acidosis is classified broadly into three types. Table 14-17 lists representative causes for each type. Children with renal tubular acidosis may present with growth failure and with episodes of vomiting and dehydration.
      (1) **Distal renal tubular acidosis (type I)** is characterized by failure of the distal nephron to secrete the 2–3 mEq/kg/day of dietary acid (hydrogen ion) necessary to maintain acid–base homeostasis. The urine cannot be maximally acidified and new bicarbonate cannot be generated. Chronic positive hydrogen ion imbalance results in buffering by bone. This leads to increased skeletal calcium resorption, hypercalciuria, and increased risk of nephrocalcinosis and stones. In most children, there is also a urinary bicarbonate leak, which has implications in determining the amount of therapy needed to correct the acidosis.
      (2) **Proximal renal tubular acidosis (type II)** is characterized by decreased proximal tubular reabsorption of bicarbonate. A reduction in the normally variable renal threshold for bicarbonate causes a marked bicarbonate leak, which disappears when the serum bicarbonate falls below the threshold level (e.g., to 15 mmol/L). The defect may be isolated or may occur with other proximal tubular abnormalities, such as glycosuria, aminoaciduria, or depressed phosphate reabsorption. Diffuse proximal tubular dysfunction is termed the **Fanconi syndrome**.
      (3) **Type IV renal tubular acidosis** includes a group of disorders, all of which are characterized by defects in distal tubular hydrogen ion and potassium secretion, leading to hyperchloremic metabolic acidosis and hyperkalemia.
   d. **Therapy**
      (1) **Renal tubular acidosis** is treated with alkalinizing agents. Doses of either bicarbonate or citrate must be sufficient to correct the acidosis completely.

TABLE 14-17. Types of Renal Tubular Acidosis in Children and Representative Causes

Distal renal tubular acidosis (type I)	Proximal renal tubular acidosis (type II)

Isolated, primary
  Inherited
  Acquired
	Isolated, primary
	  Inherited
	  Acquired

Associated with heritable disorders
  Sickle cell disease
  Marfan syndrome
  Wilson disease
  Ehlers-Danlos syndrome
	Associated with carbonic anhydrase deficiency
	  Inherited
	  Acquired
	    Acetazolamide administration

Associated with renal disease
  Renal transplantation
  Obstructive uropathy
  Chronic pyelonephritis
  Acute tubular necrosis
	Associated with Fanconi syndrome
	  Inherited
	    Cystinosis
	    Lowe syndrome
	    Tyrosinemia
	    Galactosemia
	    Glycogen storage disease type I

Associated with other systemic disease
  Systemic lupus erythematosus
  Chronic active hepatitis
  Malnutrition
	Associated with renal disease
	  Renal transplantation
	  Nephrotic syndrome
	  Medullary cystic disease

Induced by drugs or poisons
  Amphotericin B
  Vitamin D
  Toluene
	Associated with other systemic disease
	  Rubella syndrome
	  Sjögren syndrome
	  Amyloidosis
	  Medullary cystic disease

	Induced by poisons
	  Heavy metals
	  Lindane

	Type IV renal tubular acidosis
	  Primary aldosterone deficiency
	  Hyporeninemic hypoaldosteronism
	  Mineralocorticoid-resistant hyperkalemia
	  Transient renal tubular acidosis in newborns

As much as 20 mEq/kg/day may be required to return the serum bicarbonate to a normal concentration. Adequate therapy restores normal growth in affected children.

    (2) **Metabolic acidosis other than renal tubular acidosis** sometimes is treated with alkalinizing agents, although such treatment is controversial.

        (a) In mild to moderate acidosis in which respiratory compensation has occurred and renal function is normal, therapy directed at the underlying cause of the acidosis is sufficient.

        (b) Although controversial, in severe acidosis (pH < 7.2), alkali therapy may be given to increase the serum bicarbonate concentration and to decrease the energy expended by compensatory respiratory effort. The amount of bicarbonate given should correct the pH to 7.2; it is essential to avoid fully correcting the base deficit, which places the patient at risk for **overshoot alkalosis**. Alkali should **never** be given unless adequate ventilation can be ensured.

D. **Alkalosis** results from any process that increases the body's pH through either a reduction in Pco_2 or an increase in bicarbonate buffer base.

    1. Respiratory alkalosis

        a. Causes. Respiratory alkalosis is caused by the excessive loss of carbon dioxide as the result of hyperventilation, which is usually centrally mediated (e.g., salicylate intoxication, head injury, hysteria).

b. Compensation. The body's attempt at renal compensation is through increased bicarbonate excretion.

c. Therapy is directed at the cause of the hyperventilation.

2. **Metabolic alkalosis**

a. **Causes and compensation.** Metabolic alkalosis is caused by a loss of hydrogen ions or an increase in base. Compensation is through a small and unpredictable decrease in minute volume to allow the $Paco_2$ to rise slightly.

(1) The **most common cause** of metabolic alkalosis in children is the use of diuretics, which leads to volume contraction and potassium and chloride depletion. These changes, in turn, lead to increased bicarbonate reabsorption and aldosteronism with increased hydrogen ion secretion. Volume contraction with significant chloride and potassium loss as a result of recurrent vomiting is another common cause. A gain of base can be the result of excessive alkali administration.

(2) **Less common causes** of metabolic alkalosis in children include Bartter syndrome, familial chloride diarrhea, chronic steroid administration, dietary chloride deficiency, chronic potassium depletion, and posthypercapneic states.

b. **Therapy.** Metabolic alkalosis is treated by restoring intravascular volume and replacing potassium and chloride deficits. Correction of the underlying cause of the alkalosis (e.g., surgery for pyloric stenosis, discontinuing diuretic therapy) is essential. The use of acid to correct alkalosis through the infusion of ammonium chloride or dilute hydrochloric acid rarely is indicated, and should be reserved for patients with severe alkalosis and those who cannot tolerate volume repletion.

X. RENAL FAILURE

A. **Definition.** Renal failure occurs when the kidneys no longer meet the body's need to maintain water, electrolyte, and acid–base balance and to eliminate the end products of protein metabolism.

1. Renal failure may be **acute or chronic.**
   a. Differentiation is important for prognosis and therapy.
   b. Differentiation is not always obvious because chronic renal insufficiency may present with acute signs and symptoms.

2. Renal failure may be **oliguric or nonoliguric.**
   a. Renal failure involves a fall in GFR but not necessarily a fall in urine output. For example, if the normal GFR of 120 ml/min fell to 1 ml/min and tubular reabsorption was 0, 1440 ml of urine would still be excreted per day.
   b. Just as renal failure is not always oliguric, oliguria does not always indicate renal failure. Differentiation is aided by history, physical examination, urine indices (see I C 3 b), and, if indicated, response to a fluid challenge.
   c. Nonoliguric and oliguric renal failure are equally significant, but nonoliguric failure is easier to manage because fluid restriction need not be so severe and the patient can be given drugs, electrolytes, and calories.

B. **Acute renal failure**

1. **Etiology and pathogenesis.** In childhood, acute renal failure frequently occurs as a component or complication of serious systemic illness (e.g., septic shock) or multiorgan injury (e.g., severe trauma). The pathogenesis is not completely understood but is multifactorial, involving hemodynamic, cellular, hormonal, and metabolic factors.
   a. **Categories.** Acute renal failure is divided into three categories, based on the nature of the insult or disease.

(1) Prenatal failure results from factors that decrease renal perfusion and impair the delivery of oxygen and energy substrate to the kidney. Prerenal factors include hypotension, severe hypertension, hypovolemia, hypoxemia, renal artery occlusion, decreased cardiac output, and hypoglycemia. Causes include dehydration, shock, septicemia, and heart failure.

(2) Renal parenchymal failure. Intrinsic renal parenchymal injury can affect glomerular function, tubular function, or both. Causes include all forms of glomerulonephritis, nephrotoxicity (e.g., from heavy metals, uric acid, myoglobin, or aminoglycoside antibiotics), and renal venous obstruction. Long-standing glomerular hyperperfusion, chronic hyperglycemia, and excessive protein loads may also cause renal parenchymal injury.

(3) Postrenal failure results from factors that injure the kidney by obstructing urine flow. Causes include stones, Wilms tumor, and congenital anomalies (e.g., obstructed ureteropelvic junction, posterior urethral valves).

b. Acute tubular necrosis. If prerenal, parenchymal, or postrenal insults are mild or promptly reversed, acute renal failure may not develop. If these factors are severe or prolonged, acute tubular necrosis will result.

(1) The renal failure that develops in acute tubular necrosis is usually self-limited and reversible, although chronic renal impairment and sequelae such as hypertension may result.

(2) If the insult is very severe, renal cortical necrosis may occur, with irreversible renal failure.

2. Complications

a. Water retention may lead to dilutional hyponatremia and possible neurologic effects ranging from lethargy to seizures or coma.

b. Sodium retention causes a compensatory expansion of the ECF, which can lead to edema, hypertension, or congestive heart failure.

c. Renal ischemia causes hyperreninemia, which can also lead to hypertension.

d. Hyperkalemia is a consequence of diminished filtration and failure of the distal nephron to secrete potassium. Hyperkalemia usually is not a serious problem unless there is a high potassium load (e.g., from tumor lysis syndrome) or until the GFR has fallen to less than 5 ml/min.

e. Metabolic acidosis develops from failure of renal acidification mechanisms and bicarbonate wasting.

f. Uremic syndrome, with anorexia, lethargy, and encephalopathy, results from the failure to excrete uremic toxins. These toxins remain poorly characterized.

3. Therapy

a. Initial treatment of acute renal failure is aimed at:

(1) Reversing or removing the underlying cause

(2) Minimizing the excretory work of the kidneys, especially reducing the nitrogen load by limiting protein intake and, if possible, drugs that are excreted by the kidneys

(3) Treating complications

(4) Providing adequate caloric intake

b. Dialysis is indicated when the preceding measures are inadequate. There is no specific BUN or creatinine level at which dialysis should be instituted.

4. Recovery from acute renal failure often involves a period of brisk urine output, the so-called **diuretic phase** or **recovery phase** of acute renal failure. Most often, this diuresis is appropriate and reflects excretion of water that accumulated in the earlier oliguric phase.

C. Hemolytic–uremic syndrome

1. Definition. Hemolytic–uremic syndrome is an unusual acute nephropathy characterized by the triad of microangiopathic hemolytic anemia, thrombocytopenia, and acute renal failure. Although the kidney often is the only organ affected, other organs also may be involved, including the central nervous system, gastrointestinal tract, lungs, and myocardium. With systemic involvement, it is impossible to differentiate hemolytic–uremic syndrome from thrombotic thrombocytopenic purpura.

2. **Incidence.** Hemolytic–uremic syndrome may occur at any age. It is the most common cause of acquired acute renal failure in infants and children. Although it usually is sporadic, clusters of cases occur.

3. **Etiology and pathogenesis**
   a. **Etiology.** Hemolytic–uremic syndrome usually is preceded by an infection, usually a gastrointestinal illness with diarrhea, although the syndrome has been reported as a sequela of virtually all types of viral and bacterial infections. The most common bacterial pathogen associated with hemolytic–uremic syndrome in the United States is the verocytotoxin-secreting *Escherichia coli* O157:H7.
   b. **Pathogenesis.** Endothelial injury leads to platelet aggregation and depletion. Platelet thrombi damage erythrocytes, causing hemolysis. The vascular injury leads to renal ischemia and acute renal failure.

4. **Clinical features and course**
   a. The anemia and thrombocytopenia may be mild or profound. Renal insufficiency varies from mild, nonoliguric renal failure to severe oliguria lasting several days to many weeks. Progression to end-stage renal failure is uncommon.
   b. Long-term sequelae may include hypertension and varying degrees of renal insufficiency. Recurrences are uncommon but are seen in some individuals, even after renal transplantation.

5. **Therapy**
   a. The acute renal failure and hematologic problems are the targets of therapy. Transfusions (red cell, platelet, or both) may be required.
   b. Supportive treatment includes careful attention to nutrition.
   c. Dialysis may be needed when prolonged acute renal failure occurs.

D. **Chronic renal failure** is a significant and irreversible reduction in GFR.

1. **Etiology.** Although any renal disorder, if severe enough, can lead to chronic renal failure, congenital nephropathies are the most common cause of chronic renal failure in childhood. Renal dysplasia, which may be a consequence of prenatal urinary tract obstruction, is the most common cause of progressive renal insufficiency in the first decade of life. Glomerulonephritis of all types is the second most common and the most frequent in adolescents.

2. **Course.** Although chronic renal failure progresses at different rates in different people, the course in a particular patient may often be predicted accurately by plotting the reciprocal of the serum creatinine versus time. The result is usually a linear relationship that predicts the approximate time when replacement therapy will be needed.

3. **Complications and their management.** Besides the complications seen with acute renal failure, several additional problems occur with chronic renal failure.
   a. **Problems with nutrition and growth** are the most significant complications seen in children.
      (1) **Nutrition.** The goal of dietary management is to maximize caloric intake, reduce excretory solute load, and preserve residual renal function. The diet should be high in carbohydrates and fat, with limited protein (1.0–1.2 g/kg/day) and phosphorus intake.
      (2) **Growth.** Most children with chronic renal failure grow poorly owing to a number of factors, including inadequate calories, acidosis, anemia, and renal osteodystrophy. Recent studies involving the use of **recombinant human growth hormone** have been very encouraging and demonstrate increased growth rates without significant side effects.
   b. **Renal osteodystrophy** results from several factors, including impaired vitamin D metabolism, decreased intestinal calcium absorption, phosphate retention (leading to

hyperphosphatemia), secondary hyperparathyroidism, and metabolic acidosis. The combination of skeletal demineralization and hyperparathyroidism retards growth and leads to rickets.

    (1) Therapy with vitamin D metabolites [e.g., calcitriol (1,25-dihydroxyvitamin D_3) or dihydrotachysterol] prevents or heals the skeletal abnormalities but does not dramatically improve growth.

    (2) Calcium carbonate is given to provide extra calcium for absorption and to act as a binder of dietary phosphate.

    (3) To prevent hyperphosphatemia, it often is necessary to limit phosphorus intake and to give phosphate binders. Either calcium carbonate or aluminum salts given with meals may be used.

  c. Hyperkalemia. Dietary potassium limitation usually is not needed until the GFR falls to very low levels (below 5 ml/min/1.73 m^2). Potassium balance is maintained in chronic renal failure by increased excretion from remaining nephrons and significant intestinal potassium loss. A potassium-binding resin (e.g., sodium polystyrene sulfonate) may be given orally or rectally to remove potassium.

  d. Anemia

    (1) Normochromic, normocytic anemia is common in chronic renal failure for several reasons.

      (a) Decreased erythropoiesis results from decreased erythropoietin levels and uremic inhibition of marrow.

      (b) Shortened erythrocyte survival results from uremic toxins and damage caused by hemodialysis.

      (c) Gastrointestinal blood loss results from the uremic bleeding diathesis.

      (d) Nutritional anemia may result from iron or folate deficiency, or both.

    (2) Until recently, effective therapy was not available except for the careful use of blood transfusions. The availability of **recombinant erythropoietin,** however, has provided an effective, although very expensive, treatment for the anemia. Erythropoietin injection therapy is well tolerated, although hypertension is a common side effect and hyperkalemia and hyperphosphatemia occasionally occur.

E. | **End-stage renal disease (ESRD).** When the progression of chronic renal failure is no longer adequately managed by medical means, replacement therapy is required, using hemodialysis, a peritoneal dialysis regimen, or transplantation.

  1. Incidence. The incidence of ESRD in the pediatric age-group (birth to 19 years) in the United States is approximately 11 per million population per year.

  2. Transplantation. Renal transplantation is the therapy of choice for children with end-stage renal disease because it provides the best opportunity for a normal, active lifestyle and for achieving good physical and cognitive growth. Approximately 600–800 renal transplants are done annually in children in the United States. Results are excellent, continue to improve, and remain slightly better with transplants from living, related donors than with cadaver transplants. Although renal transplantation may be carried out on a child of any size, infants, especially those weighing less than 10 kg, are at greater risk for surgical and infectious complications and have less favorable outcomes.

  a. Improvements in pretransplantation care include the use of erythropoietin, negating the need for transfusions and the risk of pretransplant sensitization to human leukocyte antigens (HLA).

  b. Advances in immunosuppressive therapy include better recognition and treatment of rejection, the routine use of cyclosporine, the more prudent use of corticosteroids, the selective administration of the monoclonal antibody OKT3, and the development of other potent immunosuppressives such as the maclide FK506.

  c. Problems. Posttransplantation growth acceleration ("catch-up growth") remains disappointing, particularly in older children and adolescents. Other problems that persist include:

    (1) The continued shortage of donor kidneys

(2) Complications of immunosuppressive drug use, such as drug toxicity, susceptibility to infection, and a small, but definite, risk of malignancy
(3) The absence of effective therapy to reverse chronic rejection
(4) Hypertension, which may persist or develop in more than half of transplant
recipients
(5) Persistent problems with preexisting urologic abnormalities
(6) Recurrence of disease in the transplanted kidney

3. **Dialysis**
   a. **Methods** (Table 14-18)
      (1) **Peritoneal dialysis** has been used for many years to treat acute renal failure, but
      only in the past 10–15 years has it gained wide acceptance as an effective ther-
      apy for ESRD.
         (a) **Continuous ambulatory peritoneal dialysis** involves the placement of a per-
         manent intraperitoneal (Tenckhoff) catheter that exits through a subcutaneous
         tunnel on the abdominal wall. Fluid is instilled into the peritoneal cavity,
         where solute diffuses from the extracellular fluid compartment to achieve
         dynamic equilibrium with the dialysate. The fluid is drained and the process
         repeated four to six times daily.
         (b) **Continuous cycling peritoneal dialysis** uses a mechanical cycler that controls
         exchanges through the night.
      (2) **Hemodialysis** has been used successfully to treat ESRD in children.
         (a) **Process.** In the pediatric age-group, hemodialysis is virtually always per-
         formed at a dialysis center and usually requires three sessions per week, last-
         ing 4–5 hours each.
         (b) **Major improvements in the success of pediatric hemodialysis** include the
         development of smaller and more efficient dialyzers, dialysis prescriptions
         better tolerated by children, and the use of chronically implanted, double-
         lumen Silastic catheters.
   b. **Disadvantages**
      (1) **Neither** peritoneal dialysis nor hemodialysis **addresses the problem of osteodys-
      trophy** or **is capable of reversing the poor growth** associated with chronic renal
      failure.
      (2) **Infections at the catheter site** are a problem with both procedures.
   c. **Factors that determine the success of dialysis**
      (1) **General**
         (a) Careful attention to use of medications and the effect of dialysis on pharma-
         cokinetics
         (b) Attention to and treatment of abnormalities and complications of chronic
         renal disease (e.g., hypertension, anemia)

TABLE 14-18. Comparative Advantages of Peritoneal Dialysis and Hemodialysis*

Peritoneal dialysis
  More easily carried out in infants
  May be done entirely at home; proximity to dialysis center not required
  Less expensive
  Peritoneal cavity access easier to achieve and maintain
  Less restriction of dietary intake and physical activity
  Less risk of disequilibrium (i.e., headache, nausea, cramps, and seizures resulting from
    osmolar shifts)
  Improved sense of well-being

Hemodialysis
  More efficient form of dialysis; less total time commitment
  Carried out by nursing staff; does not require participation of family
  Less chance of fatigue ("burn out") by child and family

---

*Both procedures carry an acceptably low long-term mortality rate and are well-established in the clinical setting.

        (c) Emphasis on normalizing the child's activity as much as possible

    (2) Peritoneal dialysis
        (a) Commitment and "stamina" of the child and family
        (b) Presence of an intact and well-perfused peritoneal lining
        (c) Prevention of infection at the catheter site and in the peritoneal cavity

    (3) Hemodialysis
        (a) Availability of skilled nurses and appropriate dialysis equipment
        (b) Adequate vascular access and good blood flow
        (c) Compliance with interdialysis fluid and caloric restrictions
        (d) Use of appropriate dialysis parameters to avoid disequilibrium

XI. **HEREDITARY RENAL DISEASES.** Most renal disease in childhood is not strictly heritable by dominant or recessive patterns. However, histocompatibility gene (HLA) associations occur with some conditions, including minimal change disease and membranoproliferative glomerulonephritis, making genetic predisposition likely. Some renal disorders are clearly heritable conditions. Several of the more common ones are considered in this section.

A. **Hereditary nephritis (Alport syndrome)** is a progressive disorder with variable severity. Although it appears to be autosomal dominant, it commonly affects boys more severely than girls.

    1. Clinical features
        a. The most common presentation in childhood is asymptomatic hematuria. Hypertension is also common. Renal insufficiency usually does not begin until the second decade.
        b. The nephropathy may occur alone or with auditory or visual problems. High-frequency sensorineural hearing loss occurs in one-third of the patients. Diverse eye problems, usually involving the lens, occur in 15% of patients.

    2. Diagnosis is made by renal biopsy showing characteristic abnormalities, notably lamellation and thinning of the glomerular basement membrane, which is visible on electron microscopy.

    3. Therapy. The only effective therapy is transplantation.

B. **Medullary cystic disease (nephronophthisis).** This serious and progressive disorder shows two distinct modes of inheritance that differ in age at presentation. Pathologically, both forms are characterized by small medullary cysts and tubular atrophy that progress to diffuse fibrosis and cystic enlargement.

    1. Clinical features
        a. The **juvenile form** (also called **familial juvenile nephronophthisis**) is an autosomal recessive disorder that presents in the first decade as growth failure, polyuria, salt wasting, anemia, hypertension, and progressive renal failure. Renal biopsy must include deep medullary tissue to be diagnostic.
        b. The **adult form** is an autosomal dominant disorder that presents in adolescence or adulthood as similar symptoms with a similar course.

    2. Therapy. There is no effective therapy. The disease does not recur in transplanted kidneys.

C. **Polycystic kidney disease.** Again, two types exist that differ in pattern of inheritance and age at onset.

    1. Infantile-type polycystic kidney disease is an autosomal recessive disorder usually detected at birth.
        a. Clinical features

        (1) The infant presents with large kidneys and oliguria. (If the oliguria is present during intrauterine life, severe pulmonary hypoplasia may result and the condition may be incompatible with life.) Renal insufficiency is slowly progressive, although it varies in severity.

        (2) The condition is virtually always associated with hepatomegaly due to **congenital hepatic fibrosis,** which causes portal hypertension and secondary varices.

    b. Therapy for infantile polycystic disease includes both renal transplantation and some form of portosystemic vascular shunt.

  2. Adult-type polycystic kidney disease is an autosomal dominant disorder that, despite its name, occasionally presents in childhood.

    a. Clinical features

        (1) Patients initially present with some combination of abdominal pain, flank mass, proteinuria, intermittent hematuria, hypertension, or urinary tract infection. Progressive renal failure develops later.

        (2) Adult polycystic disease is characterized by large cysts in both kidneys. Extrarenal cystic involvement of the liver, pancreas, or lungs is not unusual. Ten percent of patients have berry aneurysms.

    b. Therapy. Transplantation is the only effective treatment.

XII. UROLOGIC PROBLEMS

A. Renal trauma

  1. Etiology. Renal trauma in children is most commonly the result of a blunt blow to the abdomen or a deceleration injury (e.g., jumping from a height). Possible types of renal injury include contusions, cortical lacerations, calyceal lacerations, complete renal tears, and vascular pedicle injury.

  2. Clinical features. The injury need not be severe or dramatic to result in the most common manifestation, hematuria. Other common symptoms are abdominal pain and tenderness, which may mimic an acute abdomen or renal colic. A flank mass may be present.

  3. Diagnosis. Because the kidney with a cyst, tumor, or obstruction is more likely to bleed when injured, the kidneys should be imaged with ultrasonography and IVP. A nonfunctioning kidney suggests a vascular injury and should be investigated with arteriography.

  4. Therapy and prognosis

    a. Therapy should be conservative except in cases with vascular avulsion or with uncontrolled, massive bleeding. Surgery is required in severe cases.

    b. Preservation of renal function in the injured kidney is likely.

  5. Complications include delayed hemorrhage, urinoma, perinephric abscess, poor renal growth, obstruction due to clot or scar formation, and hypertension.

B. Urolithiasis during childhood is uncommon in the United States and consists mainly of renal stones. Although urolithiasis may be associated with chronic and recurrent urinary tract infection, most stones in children in the United States are related to metabolic causes and anomalies of the urinary tract. In some parts of the world, bladder stones are more common and appear to be related to dietary factors.

  1. Etiology (Table 14-19). The occurrence of a stone in a child should prompt evaluation to determine the cause.

  2. It is important to distinguish stones from **nephrocalcinosis,** although either condition may result from the same cause (e.g., hypercalciuria). Nephrocalcinosis is calcium

TABLE 14-19. Causes of Renal Calculi in Children

Increased excretion of solute	**Decreased excretion of solubilizing substances**
Calcium	Citrate
Idiopathic hypercalciuria	Distal renal tubular acidosis
Chronic furosemide therapy	Magnesium
Distal renal tubular acidosis	Pyrophosphate
Immobilization	
Vitamin D excess	**Urinary stasis or decreased flow rate**
Hyperparathyroidism	Poor fluid intake
Oxalate	Partial obstruction
Primary oxaluria	**Other disorders**
Small bowel disease (increased oxalate	Chronic urinary tract infection
absorption	Polycystic kidney disease
Ethylene glycol (antifreeze) intoxication	Medullary sponge kidney
Vitamin C excess	
Cystine	
Cystinuria	
Uric acid	
Cancer chemotherapy [e.g., for leukemia or	
lymphoma (tumor lysis syndrome)]	
Lesch-Nyhan syndrome	
Gout	

deposition within renal parenchyma. It may be diffuse when it results from a metabolic disorder, or patchy when it is the sequela of a renal insult (e.g., infection, trauma).

3. **Clinical features and diagnosis.** Signs and symptoms include hematuria and abdominal pain, which may be either vague or severe. The best diagnostic test is ultrasonography of the kidneys and pelvis.

4. **Therapy.** Maintenance therapy should be directed at prevention of further stones and close monitoring for their occurrence.
   a. High urinary flow rates are desirable in all causes of stones because they not only dilute solute, but avoid urinary stasis.
   b. In **hypercalciuria,** therapy is aimed at reducing urinary calcium with thiazide or dietary calcium restriction.
   c. Treatment of **cystinuria** (an autosomal recessive disorder with defective intestinal and renal transport of dibasic amino acids) involves urine dilution through round-the-clock intake of large amounts of water and alkalinization to keep the urine pH above 7.5. If these measures fail or cannot be maintained, D-penicillamine may be used to increase cystine excretion in a more soluble form.
   d. When a stone does not pass spontaneously, it generally should be removed. The treatment of choice is extracorporeal shock-wave lithotripsy (ESWL). If necessary, retrograde or antegrade ureteroscopy may be used to remove the stone or move it to the renal pelvis for ESWL. Open surgical removal is rarely indicated.

C. **Hypospadias** is the most common anomaly of the penis. There is a 10% risk of the defect in male siblings.

1. **Defect and associated anomalies**
   a. In hypospadias, the opening of the urethral meatus is on the ventral surface of the penis. Ventral curvature of the penis, known as **chordee,** usually is present.
   b. There is a 10%–15% risk of undescended testes with hypospadias. The risk of other anomalies of the urinary tract is not significant.

2. **Clinical features.** Hypospadias has a spectrum of severity. In its most common form, hypospadias is of no clinical significance. When severe, it can be associated with ambiguous genitalia and serious voiding difficulty.

3. **Therapy,** when necessary, is surgical. When severe, hypospadias may require serial procedures to construct a urethra. Because the foreskin is used in these procedures, the newborn with hypospadias should not be circumcised.

D. **Epispadias and exstrophy of the bladder.** This sporadic and uncommon spectrum of embryologic anomalies results from faulty disappearance of the cloacal membrane.

1. **Epispadias**
   a. **Defect.** Epispadias in boys is the opening of the urethra on the dorsal surface of the penis. In girls, the most common counterpart is a bifid clitoris; a shortened urethra and bladder neck involvement also may occur in girls.
   b. **Clinical features.** Epispadias in either sex may cause varying degrees of incontinence. When incontinence is present, a voiding cystourethrogram is indicated to evaluate reflux.
   c. **Therapy.** Surgery may be needed to reconstruct the urethra and bladder neck.

2. **Exstrophy**
   a. **Defect and associated clinical features.** Exstrophy is a serious anomaly in which the bladder extrudes through the abdominal wall. The kidneys and upper urinary tract usually are normal, but vesicoureteral reflux is common. When exstrophy is severe, there may be associated abnormalities of the pubic rami, the pelvic diaphragm, the vagina and uterus, the bowel and rectum, and the spinal cord.
   b. **Therapy.** Children with exstrophy require sophisticated care and extensive surgery. Immediate concerns include preventing infection and fluid and electrolyte disturbances.

E. **Cryptorchidism (undescended testes)** is present in 1% of 1-year-old boys.

1. **Defect and associated clinical features**
   a. Failure of the testis to descend into the scrotum may be unilateral or bilateral. The nonpalpable testis may be either undescended or absent. Ultrasound may sometimes be helpful, but a stimulation test with human chorionic gonadotropin (hCG) to demonstrate the production of testosterone is best to confirm the presence of testicular tissue.
   b. **An inguinal hernia** is often present. The true undescended testis must be differentiated from the **retractile testis** that results from an exaggerated cremasteric reflex. Careful and repeated physical examination will permit this distinction.
   c. The undescended testis is susceptible to testicular torsion and trauma, may be associated with infertility, and has an increased potential for malignant degeneration in adulthood. The risk of infertility is removed if the testicle descends before 2 years of age, but the risk of malignancy persists regardless of whether it is corrected or remains undescended.

2. **Therapy.** Treatment with hCG is sometimes successful in causing descent of the testis. If not, surgical treatment (**orchiopexy**) should be carried out before 2 years of age.

F. **Testicular torsion** (i.e., twisting of the testis and spermatic cord, causing ischemia) is uncommon in childhood. There are two incidence peaks, one in the perinatal period and the second at puberty.

1. **Clinical features.** Although the child usually complains of scrotal pain and swelling, severe abdominal pain may be the initial symptom.

2. **Differential diagnosis** includes epididymitis, mumps orchitis, incarcerated inguinal hernia, and testicular tumors. The diagnosis is made at surgery. Imaging studies (ultra-

sonography with Doppler) are not totally reliable and may cause significant delay in surgical correction.

3. **Therapy.** Testicular torsion is a true surgical emergency, because delay leads to infarction and testicular necrosis. A temporary measure to restore blood flow to the testicle before surgery is to twist the testis clockwise (facing the patient). At the time of surgical exploration, both testicles should undergo fixation in the scrotum.

G. Urethral stenosis. Stenosis of the urethral meatus in both sexes and urethral stenosis in girls are rare in children. True meatal stenosis occurs most commonly in the child with hypospadias.

1. **Clinical significance**
   a. These disorders are significant because they frequently are diagnosed incorrectly to explain a variety of urinary problems, such as recurrent urinary tract infections and enuresis.
   b. Because urethral stenosis is rare, girls with recurrent urinary tract infections and enuresis should not be subjected to cystoscopy and urethral dilation.

2. **Therapy** is meatotomy and dilation, but these are rarely indicated.

H. Neurogenic bladder

1. **Etiology.** Many neurologic conditions prevent adequate storage or elimination of urine from the bladder, but neurogenic bladder is most often the result of a spinal cord disorder, including meningomyelocele, trauma, and tumors.

2. **Clinical features.** Patients suffer from incontinence, regardless of whether the neurologic defect has caused spastic, flaccid, or uninhibited bladder emptying.

3. **Diagnosis.** Neurologic assessment must include attention to reflexes below the waist, including the anal and cremasteric reflexes. Cystometry and spinal cord imaging may be required.

4. **Therapy**
   a. Cholinergic agents may help to facilitate emptying the atonic bladder. Anticholinergic agents may help to inhibit uncontrolled or spastic bladder contractions.
   b. Repeated, regular bladder catheterization is the common approach in children with cord disorders who have sensory as well as motor deficits.
   c. Surgical procedures (urinary diversion, bladder enlargement, bladder neck reconstruction, antireflux surgery) are indicated in some children.

5. **Complications** of neurogenic bladder include recurrent or chronic urinary tract infection and obstruction. These, in turn, may lead to renal parenchymal damage.

BIBLIOGRAPHY

Engle W: Evaluation of renal function and acute renal failure in the neonate. *Pediatr Clin North Am* 33:129–151, 1986.

Fine RN: Recent advances in the management of the infant, child, and adolescent with chronic renal failure. *Pediatr Rev* 11:277–283, 1990.

Gaudio K, Siegel N: Pathogenesis and treatment of acute renal failure. *Pediatr Clin North Am* 34:771–787, 1987.

Hellerstein S: Fluids and electrolytes: clinical aspects. *Pediatr Rev* 14:103–115, 1993.

Hellerstein S: Fluids and electrolytes: physiology. *Pediatr Rev* 14:70–79, 1993.

Sherbotie J, Cornfeld D: Management of urinary tract infections in children. *Pediatr Clin North Am* 75:327–338, 1991.

STUDY QUESTIONS

DIRECTIONS: Each of the numbered items or incomplete statements in this section is followed by answers or by completions of the statement. Select the ONE lettered answer or completion that is BEST in each case.

1. A 10-year-old develops nephrotic syndrome. Several urinalyses reveal the presence of red blood cell casts. The creatinine is 2.8 mg/dl and the blood pressure is 145/95 mm Hg. The next best course of action is

(A) begin a course of oral prednisone
(B) follow the child and see if the nephrotic syndrome remits
(C) perform a diagnostic renal biopsy
(D) collect a 24-hour urine for creatinine clearance and protein excretion
(E) perform a renal scan

2. A 12-year-old girl has a physical examination so she can join the soccer team. A random urinalysis is normal except for 2+ protein on dipstick testing. The most reasonable next study would be

(A) blood urea nitrogen and serum creatinine measurements
(B) serum total protein and albumin measurements
(C) urine culture
(D) testing a 24-hour urine collection for total protein
(E) urinalysis of the first morning urine

3. A 14-year-old boy has a blood pressure of 140/88 mm Hg at a school physical examination. He is otherwise healthy. The next best step in his evaluation is

(A) obtain blood pressures on his parents
(B) perform an electrocardiogram, chest film, and echocardiogram
(C) obtain a urinalysis, renal ultrasound, and serum creatinine
(D) repeat his blood pressure on several different occasions
(E) refer to an ophthalmologist to examine for hypertensive retinopathy

4. A 12-year-old child with a history of posterior urethral valves and slowly progressive chronic renal insufficiency has a creatinine of 9.5 mg/dl (glomerular filtration rate 5 ml/min) and complains of fatigue, muscle cramps, and anorexia. The best course of therapy is

(A) proceed with transplantation from a matched, living, related donor
(B) institute a protein-restricted diet
(C) begin chronic peritoneal dialysis
(D) begin chronic hemodialysis
(E) begin erythropoietin therapy

DIRECTIONS: Each of the numbered items or incomplete statements in this section is negatively phrased, as indicated by a capitalized word such as NOT, LEAST, or EXCEPT. Select the ONE lettered answer or completion that is BEST in each case.

5. A 5-year-old, apparently healthy child has had three episodes of gross hematuria. All of the following laboratory procedures are indicated in the evaluation of this child EXCEPT

(A) examination of the urine for red cell morphology and casts
(B) renal and bladder ultrasonography
(C) prothrombin time, partial thromboplastin time, and platelet count
(D) urinary screening for hypercalciuria
(E) sulfosalicylic acid precipitation test for proteinuria

6. A 15-month-old girl has a history of poor oral fluid intake, occasional vomiting, rapid breathing, and decreased urine output. Physical examination reveals a pulse of 150/min, blood pressure of 120/80 mm Hg, and a respiratory rate of 60/min. There are bibasilar rales, and the liver is palpable 4 cm below the right costal margin. All of the following procedures might be helpful in evaluating the oliguria EXCEPT

(A) giving a fluid challenge with isotonic saline, 20 ml/kg
(B) determining the urine sodium concentration
(C) determining the blood urea nitrogen and serum creatinine levels
(D) giving a dose of intravenous furosemide
(E) calculating the fractional excretion of sodium

1. The answer is C *[III C]*. The nature of this child's nephrotic syndrome is unclear, but unlikely to be minimal change disease based on the child's age, the presence of red blood cell casts, the renal insufficiency, and the hypertension. To proceed in a reasonable way with therapy, biopsy for histopathologic diagnosis is indicated. Because the diagnosis of minimal change disease is unlikely, a course of prednisone therapy is not indicated. Because the child already has renal insufficiency, watchful waiting is not the best course. Given that the child has significant renal impairment and the nephrotic syndrome already is defined, another 24-hour collection would not prove helpful. A renal scan would indicate decreased function and would not add very much to an understanding of the clinical picture.

2. The answer is E *[I C 2 a (1)]*. The most common cause of proteinuria in an otherwise healthy child or adolescent is postural proteinuria. This possibility may be investigated by obtaining a urine specimen after prolonged recumbency (e.g., after a night's sleep) and repeating the urinalysis. Persistent proteinuria would suggest the need for further evaluation, including a timed urine collection for measuring protein excretion. The serum proteins should not be low unless the proteinuria is in the nephrotic range. Urinary tract infection does not cause significant proteinuria, and thus a urine culture would not be needed.

3. The answer is D *[VII C 1 b]*. Because blood pressure values are frequently labile and affected by such factors as anxiety, exercise, and relaxation, it is most important to repeat the blood pressure several times before any definite conclusions can be made on a child's true blood pressure. The other alternatives offered are all reasonable approaches in a child whose blood pressure is consistently elevated. Family history is an important risk factor for essential hypertension in children and adolescents. Cardiac evaluation is important to look for ventricular hypertrophy, although an echocardiogram is not usually necessary. Because renal disease is such an important cause of high blood pressure in children, evaluation with urinalysis, serum creatinine, and renal ultrasound is reasonable. Long-standing hypertension in children may result in retinal vascular changes that are not always obvious to a pediatrician.

4. The answer is A *[X E]*. The ideal course of therapy in a child or adolescent is renal replacement with a kidney transplant. If a matched, living, related donor, either a parent or older sibling, is available, the outcome of a renal allograft carried out at this time should be excellent. The institution of a protein-restricted diet, which can slow the progression of chronic renal insufficiency, is not adequate when end-stage renal failure is reached. Likewise, erythropoietin therapy, although effective in treating the anemia of renal disease, probably would have been instituted many months previously and will not correct the child's symptoms at this time. Beginning either peritoneal or hemodialysis at this time is a reasonable alternative, but not as good as transplantation if a donor is available.

5. The answer is C *[I C 1 a (1)]*. Prothrombin time, partial thromboplastin time, and platelet count are tests of the coagulation system. Hematuria rarely is the presenting sign of a bleeding diathesis, and so coagulation profiles are not necessary. Gross hematuria may occur in several forms of glomerulonephritis, including the mesangial proliferative form and immunoglobulin A nephropathy. It also may occur in disorders affecting genitourinary tract structure, such as tumors, cysts, and stones. Thus, urinary sediment examinations are important, and urinary tract imaging is essential. The common association of recurrent macroscopic and persistent microscopic hematuria with hypercalciuria makes it important to screen for this condition with the urine calcium-to-creatinine ratio. Testing for proteinuria is important, because the combination of proteinuria and hematuria is likely to signify a serious renal disease. Sulfosalicylic acid precipitation gives a measure of the total urinary protein.

6. The answer is A *[I C 3 b]*. Despite the history of poor intake of oral fluid, this infant presents with signs of congestive heart failure and fluid overload. In view of these findings, a fluid challenge could be dangerous, and it is unlikely that she would respond. If the oliguria is the result of congestive heart failure and poor renal perfusion, the urine sodium concentration and fractional excretion of sodium should be low, the blood urea nitrogen and serum creatinine should be normal or slightly elevated, and the child may respond well to furosemide.

Chapter 15

Hematologic Diseases

Arnold J. Altman

John J. Quinn

I. GENERAL PRINCIPLES

A. **Definition.** Hematologic disorders are those that produce either quantitative or qualitative defects in the cellular elements of the blood or in those soluble elements related to hemostasis. In evaluating hematologic data in the pediatric patient, it is important to recognize the normal developmental variations that are essential to proper interpretation of a particular blood response in infancy and childhood.

B. **Hematopoiesis**

1. **Prenatal hematopoiesis.** Hematopoietic tissue is derived from the mesenchymal layer of the embryo.
   a. The earliest evidence of hematopoiesis is seen in the blood islands of the **yolk sac** at about 2–3 weeks' gestation. After the yolk sac becomes connected to the systemic circulation, stem cells migrate to the embryo proper and seed future sites of hematopoiesis.
   b. At 5–6 weeks' gestation, hematopoiesis commences in the **liver,** which serves as the chief site of blood cell production until the sixth fetal month. The liver continues to produce hemic cells until 2 weeks after birth. The **spleen, lymph nodes,** and **thymus** are also sites of hematopoiesis during fetal life.
   c. Hematopoiesis commences in the **bone marrow** at about the fourth or fifth fetal month, and by the sixth month, the bone marrow becomes the chief focus of blood cell production.

2. **Postnatal hematopoiesis.** At birth, hematopoietic activity is present in most of the **bones,** especially the long bones. With progressive age, however, active marrow gradually recedes from the distal portions of the skeleton, so that by the age of 18 years, only the vertebrae, ribs, sternum, skull, and pelvis are active sites of blood production.

C. **Hematopoietic homeostasis.** Compared with most normal cells in the body, those in the peripheral blood have a relatively short life span—120 days for red blood cells, 10 days for platelets, and only 6–7 hours for neutrophils. Maintenance of adequate blood counts, therefore, requires continuous replenishment in massive quantities from the bone marrow. It has been estimated that the average adult must produce approximately 100–200 billion each of new red blood cells, neutrophils, and platelets daily to meet this demand.

1. **Requirements for hematopoiesis.** The following are major requirements for hematopoiesis:
   a. Pluripotential hematopoietic stem cells
   b. An inductive microenvironment
   c. Stimulatory factors for specific cell lines (e.g., erythropoietin, thrombopoietin)
   d. Nutrients (e.g., iron, vitamin B_{12}, folate, amino acids)

2. **Assessment of hematopoiesis.** In clinical practice, hematopoietic homeostasis is routinely assessed by **examination of the complete blood count and peripheral blood**

smear. When quantitative abnormalities of any of the cellular elements are encountered, it is useful to distinguish between disorders of production and disorders of destruction. Daily production of red blood cells can be estimated by means of the reticulocyte count, whereas neutrophil and platelet production usually are evaluated by **examination of the bone marrow**.

II. DISORDERS OF THE HEMATOPOIETIC STEM CELL

A. **Pancytopenia** is a reduction of red blood cells, white blood cells, and platelets. It is not a disease itself, but it may result from specific disease processes. The patient with pancytopenia may present with the pallor and lethargy of anemia, the infectious complications of neutropenia, or the hemorrhagic diathesis of thrombocytopenia. **Bone marrow examination** often is required to distinguish among bone marrow aplasia, bone marrow replacement (e.g., by leukemic cells), and peripheral autoimmune destruction (Evans syndrome).

B. **Bone marrow aplasia** severe enough to produce pancytopenia may be **congenital** or **acquired**. The distinction usually is not difficult because the congenital form is associated with characteristic phenotypic and cytogenetic abnormalities.

1. **Constitutional aplastic anemia (Fanconi anemia)**
   a. **Pathogenesis.** Fanconi anemia is an autosomal recessive disorder; it is associated with chromosome fragility, which results in excessive breaks and recombinations. This abnormality is not limited to hematopoietic cells but is found in all cells of the body.
   b. **Clinical features.** Although it is a congenital disorder, Fanconi anemia does not usually produce significant anemia or thrombocytopenia until the affected child is 3–8 years of age.
      (1) There are a variety of **associated phenotypic abnormalities** that are of diagnostic value. Among these are abnormal skin pigmentation, retarded growth, renal abnormalities, and skeletal deformities (e.g., absent or hypoplastic thumbs, aplasia of the radii, aplasia of the first metacarpals).
      (2) **Other abnormal findings** include macrocytic red blood cell indices and an elevated fetal hemoglobin (Hb F) level. The bone marrow is hypoplastic.
   c. **Therapy** involves appropriate supportive care with red blood cell and platelet transfusions. Some patients respond to androgen therapy, but the effect often is transient. Bone marrow transplantation is the treatment of choice if a human leukocyte antigen-matched donor is available.
   d. **Prognosis.** In the past, when the only treatment for Fanconi anemia patients with pancytopenia was blood transfusions, only rare patients survived more than 4 years. For patients who respond to androgens or bone marrow transplantation, the outlook is more favorable.

2. **Acquired aplastic anemia**
   a. **Etiology.** Acquired aplastic anemia may result from **exposure** to chemicals (e.g., benzene), drugs (e.g., chloramphenicol, sulfonamides), infectious agents (e.g., hepatitis virus), and ionizing radiation. In many instances, no clear-cut etiologic agent is identified, and the case is classified as **idiopathic**.
   b. **Clinical features.** The hypocellular marrow distinguishes acquired aplastic anemia from other forms of pancytopenia, such as leukemia and Evans syndrome, in which the marrow is not aplastic.
   c. **Therapy and prognosis.** Bone marrow transplantation is the treatment of choice. The prognosis of severe aplastic anemia is poor: 80% of patients die within 3 months of diagnosis unless a matched donor for a bone marrow transplant is available. Because exposure to sensitizing blood products compromises the success of the transplant, it is best to avoid transfusions (especially from family members) if transplantation is being considered.

III. ANEMIA

A. General considerations

1. **Definition.** Anemia is an abnormal decrease in the number of circulating red blood cells, in the hemoglobin concentration, and in the hematocrit. It is not a disease itself but is a symptom of another disorder.

2. **Normal red blood cell values** in the pediatric years are listed in Table 15-1. It is important to consider the following developmental variations when evaluating an infant or child for anemia.
   a. **Hemoglobin level** and **hematocrit** are relatively high in the newborn; these values subsequently decline, reaching a nadir at about 7 weeks of age for the premature infant and at 2–3 months of age for the term infant. (This condition is referred to as the physiologic "anemia" of infancy.) Total hemoglobin concentration and hematocrit rise gradually during childhood, reaching adult values after puberty.
   b. **Hb F** is the major hemoglobin of prenatal and early postnatal life. Hb F values decline postnatally; by 9–12 months of age, the Hb F values comprise less than 2% of the total hemoglobin concentration.
   c. **Mean corpuscular volume (MCV)** is relatively high during the neonatal period but declines during the latter part of infancy.

3. **Classification** (Table 15-2). In clinical practice, anemias are classified according to the morphologic appearance (i.e., color and size) of the red blood cells on the peripheral smear, and according to the MCV. The suffix "chromic" refers to color, and the suffix "cytic" refers to size. The primary classifications are:
   a. **Hypochromic, microcytic** (small, pale red blood cells; a low MCV)
   b. **Macrocytic** (large red blood cells; a high MCV)
   c. **Normochromic, normocytic** (cells of normal size and shape; a normal MCV)

B. Hypochromic, microcytic anemias

1. **General considerations**
   a. **Defect.** Hypochromic, microcytic red blood cells indicate impaired synthesis of the heme or globin components of hemoglobin.

TABLE 15-1. Red Blood Cell Values in the Pediatric Years

Age	Hemoglobin (g/dl)		Hematocrit (%)		Mean Corpuscular Volume (fl)		Mean Corpuscular Hemoglobin (pg/cell)	
	Mean*	Lower Limit*	Mean	Lower Limit	Mean	Lower Limit	Mean	Lower Limit
1–3 days (term infant)	18.5	14.5	56	45	108	95	34	31
1 month	14.0	10.0	43	31	104	85	34	28
2 months	11.5	9.0	35	28	96	77	30	26
3–6 months	11.5	9.5	35	29	91	74	30	25
½–2 years	12.0	11.0	36	33	78	70	27	23
2–6 years	12.5	11.5	37	34	81	75	27	24
6–12 years	13.5	11.5	40	35	86	77	29	25
12–18 years Female	14.0	12.0	41	36	90	78	30	25
Male	14.5	13.0	43	37	88	78	30	25

*Mean and lower limit of normal. Lower limit is 2 standard deviations below the mean. (Adapted from Dallman PR, Siimes MA: Percentile curves for hemoglobin and red cell volume in infancy and childhood. *J Pediatr* 94:26, 1979.)

TABLE 15-2. Anemias of Infancy and Childhood

Microcytic anemias
  Defects of heme synthesis
    Iron deficiency
      Nutritional
      Through blood loss (chronic)
    Chronic inflammation
    Sideroblastic anemia
      Due to lead poisoning
      Due to pyridoxine deficiency or dependency
  Defects of globin synthesis
    Classic thalassemias
    Thalassemic hemoglobinopathies
      Hemoglobin Lepore
      Hemoglobin E
      Hemoglobin Constant Spring
Macrocytic anemias
  With megaloblastic bone marrow
    Vitamin B_{12} deficiency
    Folic acid deficiency
    Hereditary oroticaciduria
  Without megaloblastic bone marrow
    Liver disease
    Hypothyroidism
    Bone marrow failure states
      Acquired aplastic anemia
      Fanconi anemia
      Diamond-Blackfan syndrome
      Myelodysplasia
	Normocytic anemias
	  Hemolytic disorders
	    Disorders of the external milieu
	      Antibody-mediated
	      Microangiopathic
	      Due to toxins
	      Due to infectious agents
	      Due to hypersplenism
	    Disorders of the red blood cell membrane
	      Hereditary spherocytosis
	      Hereditary elliptocytosis
	      Hereditary stomatocytosis
	      Paroxysmal nocturnal hemoglobinuria
	    Hemoglobinopathies
	      Hemoglobin S
	      Hemoglobin C
	      Unstable hemoglobins
	      Other hemoglobinopathies
	    Enzymopathies
	      Disorders of the hexose monophosphate shunt (e.g., G6PD deficiency)
	      Disorders of the Embden-Meyerhof pathway (e.g., PK deficiency)
	  Hemorrhage (acute or subacute)
	  Hypoproduction disorders
	    Pure red blood cell aplasia
	      Transient erythroblastopenia of childhood
	      Drug-induced aplasia
	      Chronic renal disease
	    Pancytopenia
	      Acquired aplastic anemia
	      Fanconi anemia
	      Bone marrow replacement (e.g., by leukemic cells)

G6PD = glucose-6-phosphate dehydrogenase; PK = pyruvate kinase.

      (1) Defective heme synthesis may be the result of iron deficiency, lead poisoning, chronic inflammatory disease, pyridoxine deficiency, or copper deficiency.
      (2) Defective globin synthesis is characteristic of the thalassemia syndromes.
    b. Evaluation. Laboratory studies that are useful in evaluating the hypochromic, microcytic anemias include determinations of serum iron levels, iron-binding capacity, and free erythrocyte protoporphyrin as well as quantitative measurements of the adult hemoglobin (Hb A_2) and Hb F levels.

  2. Iron deficiency anemia is by far the **most common cause of anemia in children**. Most cases result from inadequate intake of iron; however, loss of iron through hemorrhage must be considered in the differential diagnosis.
    a. Pathogenesis
      (1) Nutritional iron deficiency usually develops when rapid growth puts excessive demands on iron stores. This is seen mainly during:
        (a) Infancy, when iron stores at birth are inadequate owing to low birth weight or when the diet is composed exclusively of milk or cereals with low iron content
        (b) Adolescence, when a rapid growth spurt often coincides with a diet of suboptimal iron content (this is a particular problem in girls, who also lose iron with menses)

(2) Iron deficiency resulting from blood loss can occur prenatally, perinatally, or postnatally.
  (a) Prenatal iron loss can result from extrusion of fetal blood either into the maternal circulation (fetomaternal transfusion) or into the circulation of a twin (twin-to-twin transfusion).
  (b) Perinatal bleeding may result from obstetric complications such as placental abruption or placenta previa.
  (c) Postnatal blood loss may be of an obvious cause (e.g., after surgery or due to trauma) or may be occult, as occurs in idiopathic pulmonary hemosiderosis, parasitic infestations, or inflammatory bowel disease.
b. Clinical features. Iron deficiency is most commonly seen between 6 and 24 months of age. The typical patient is on a diet consisting almost exclusively of milk.
  (1) Symptoms. Although mild iron deficiency is relatively asymptomatic, as it becomes more severe, the infant manifests irritability, anorexia, lethargy, and easy fatigability.
  (2) Signs. On physical examination, the milk-fed infant is fat, pale, and sallow; other findings include tachycardia and a systolic murmur. If the anemia is very severe (i.e., hemoglobin < 3 g/dl) or if the patient has complications that put added stress on the cardiovascular system, there may be signs of congestive heart failure (i.e., a gallop rhythm, cardiomegaly, distended neck veins, hepatomegaly, and rales).
c. Diagnosis
  (1) Anemia may vary from very mild to very severe, depending on the degree and duration of iron deficiency. Small, pale red blood cells are evident on the peripheral smear, and this is reflected in the red blood cell indices; the reduction in MCV, mean corpuscular hemoglobin, and mean corpuscular hemoglobin concentration usually is proportional to the severity of the anemia.
  (2) The serum iron level is decreased, whereas the iron-binding capacity (the transferrin level) is increased and the percentage of saturation is low (usually less than 20%). The serum ferritin level is decreased (which is a reflection of low iron stores in the bone marrow), and the level of free erythrocyte protoporphyrin is increased.
  (3) Bone marrow examination usually is not clinically indicated to confirm the diagnosis. When performed, it demonstrates micronormoblastic hyperplasia of erythroid elements and decreased or absent stainable iron.
d. Therapy
  (1) Mild to moderate anemia (i.e., hemoglobin > 3 g/dl without signs of cardiac decompensation) can be managed by administration of iron. This can be provided by the oral route at a dosage of 6 mg/kg/day of elemental iron. Therapy is continued for a period of 2–3 months after the hemoglobin level has returned to normal; this allows replenishment of tissue iron stores. Dietary counseling must be given simultaneously to provide the patient with adequate amounts of dietary iron. Parenteral administration of iron sometimes is used when there is a gastrointestinal problem that would interfere with iron absorption or if there is concern about the reliability of administration.
  (2) Severe anemia. Although infants can tolerate remarkable degrees of anemia, particularly if the decline in the hemoglobin concentration is gradual, patients with extremely severe anemia in whom signs of cardiac decompensation have developed should be transfused slowly with packed red blood cells until the clinical condition has stabilized.

3. Anemia of chronic disease
  a. Pathogenesis
    (1) The anemia of chronic disease is associated with a variety of disorders, including:
      (a) Chronic inflammatory disease (e.g., Crohn disease, juvenile rheumatoid arthritis)
      (b) Chronic infection (e.g., tuberculosis)
      (c) Malignancy

(2) Iron is not released from its storage sites in the macrophages; thus, it is unavailable for hemoglobin synthesis in developing erythroblasts.

(3) A modest decrease in the survival of red blood cells and a relatively limited erythropoietin response to the anemia also contribute to the development of anemia.

b. Diagnosis

(1) The anemia is mild in degree (i.e., hemoglobin concentration is 7–10 g/dl) with hypochromic, microcytic indices.

(2) As in iron deficiency anemia, the serum iron level is reduced. However, in contrast with iron deficiency anemia, the iron-binding capacity is reduced and the serum ferritin level is increased.

(3) Bone marrow examination shows micronormoblastic hyperplasia. There is an increase in storage iron, but a decrease in the number of iron-containing erythroblasts (sideroblasts).

c. Therapy. The anemia resolves when the underlying disease process is treated adequately. Therapy with medicinal iron is unnecessary unless concomitant iron deficiency is present.

4. Sideroblastic anemia

a. Pathogenesis

(1) Among the conditions that produce sideroblastic anemia in childhood are:
  (a) Pyridoxine deficiency
  (b) Pyridoxine dependency
  (c) Lead poisoning

(2) Iron enters the erythroblast freely; however, because of a metabolic block, it cannot be incorporated into hemoglobin. Instead, it accumulates in the mitochondria, giving the cell a characteristic appearance (a ringed sideroblast) when stained for iron content.

b. Diagnosis

(1) All sideroblastic anemias are associated with hypochromic, microcytic indices. Stippled red blood cells may be found on the peripheral smear.

(2) The bone marrow shows micronormoblastic hyperplasia. Ringed sideroblasts and increased iron stores are evident when the cells are stained with Prussian blue.

c. Therapy

(1) A trial of pyridoxine (50–300 mg/day) should be instituted for several weeks.

(2) If the anemia is not responsive to the pyridoxine or related to a toxin that can be eliminated, treatment usually is not successful, and the patient may require support with red blood cell transfusions.

5. Thalassemias

a. Definition. Thalassemias are hereditary hemolytic anemias characterized by decreased or absent synthesis of one or more globin subunits of the hemoglobin molecule. **α Thalassemia** results from reduced synthesis of α-globin chains, and **β thalassemia** results from reduced synthesis of β-globin chains.

b. Pathogenesis

(1) Among the mechanisms responsible for producing thalassemias are:
  (a) Gene deletion, which is the most common cause of a thalassemia
  (b) An abnormality in the transcription or processing of messenger RNA, which occurs more frequently in β thalassemia
  (c) Thalassemic hemoglobinopathy, in which a structurally abnormal globin chain is produced in subnormal amounts (e.g., Hb Lepore, Hb E, Hb Constant Spring)

(2) Excess unpaired globin chains are a hazard to the red blood cell because they produce insoluble tetramers that precipitate, causing membrane damage. This makes red cells susceptible to destruction within the reticuloendothelial system of the bone marrow (resulting in ineffective erythropoiesis) and within the reticuloendothelial system of the liver and the spleen (resulting in hemolytic anemia).

TABLE 15-3. Clinical Manifestations of α Thalassemia Variants

Variant of Disease	Number of Genes Deleted	Characteristic Hb Pattern	Clinical Features
α Thalassemia major	Four	γ_4F (Hb Bart)	Hb Bart has high O_2 affinity—does not release it to tissues Hb Bart has poor solubility—forms inclusions in RBC Ineffective erythropoiesis Hemolytic anemia Hydrops fetalis/death in utero
Hemoglobin H disease	Three	γ_4F (Hb Bart)—fetus and early infancy	Sufficient α-globin chains produced in utero to allow fetus to come to term, albeit with severe anemia
		β_4A (Hb H)—beyond early infancy	Anemia persists throughout life
α Thalassemia minor	Two	Normal	Mild anemia No clinical symptoms
Silent carrier	One	Normal	No anemia Normal RBC indices

Hb = hemoglobin; RBC = red blood cell.

   c. α Thalassemias usually are the result of gene deletion.
     (1) α Thalassemia variants are found most often in populations of African or East Asian ancestry.
     (2) Normally there are four α-globin genes per cell; clinical manifestations of α thalassemia variants reflect the number of genes deleted (Table 15-3).
   d. β Thalassemias. Because normally there are only two β-globin genes per cell, only two general types of β thalassemia are possible.
     (1) Homozygous β thalassemia (β thalassemia major, Cooley anemia). Patients with this form of anemia usually are of Mediterranean background.
        (a) Defect. Molecular defects range from complete absence of β-globin synthesis (genotype β^0/β^0) to partial reduction in the gene product from the affected locus (genotype β^+/β^+).
        (b) Clinical features and course. Beginning in the middle of the first year of life, the infant manifests a progressively **severe hemolytic anemia** associated with marked **hepatosplenomegaly**. If untreated, the hepatosplenomegaly becomes progressive and anemia, failure to thrive, and **bone marrow hyperplasia** develop. The bone marrow hyperplasia produces characteristic features such as tower skull, frontal bossing, maxillary hypertrophy with prominent cheekbones, and overbite. Death due to congestive heart failure usually occurs within the first few years of life unless the patient is supported with blood transfusions.
        (c) Diagnosis
           (i) Despite the severity of anemia, there is reticulocytopenia, reflecting ineffective erythropoiesis. Peripheral blood smear shows marked hypochromia, microcytosis, anisocytosis, and poikilocytosis. The red blood cell indices are significantly reduced.
           (ii) On hemoglobin electrophoresis, Hb A is either markedly decreased or totally absent. Of the total hemoglobin concentration, 30%–90% is Hb F.
        (d) Therapy. The mainstay of treatment is **transfusion with packed red blood cells**. Splenectomy usually is considered when transfusional requirements exceed 250 ml/kg/year.
           (i) Even in the untransfused state, iron overload develops in thalassemic patients because of hyperabsorption of dietary iron. The iron load

becomes even greater with chronic transfusion therapy. When the bone marrow storage capacity for iron is exceeded, iron accumulates in parenchymal organs such as the liver, heart, pancreas, gonads, and skin, producing the complications of **hemochromatosis** ("bronzed diabetes"). Many patients succumb to congestive heart failure in their late teens and early twenties.

(ii) In an effort to prevent hemochromatosis, patients chronically on transfusion regimens are treated with chelating agents (e.g., deferoxamine), which promote iron removal from the body.

(2) Heterozygous β thalassemia (β thalassemia minor)

(a) **Clinical features.** The growth and development of patients with this disorder are normal. The only abnormality is mild anemia (a hemoglobin level that is approximately 10 g/dl).

(b) **Diagnosis**

(i) Hypochromia, microcytosis, and anisocytosis are found disproportionately severe to the degree of anemia.

(ii) Hemoglobin electrophoresis shows elevation of the Hb A_2 level and, sometimes, elevation of the Hb F level.

(c) **Therapy.** No treatment is necessary. It is important, however, that thalassemia minor is distinguished from iron deficiency to prevent inappropriate therapy with medicinal iron. Genetic counseling also is important.

C. **Macrocytic anemias**

1. General considerations

a. Defect. Macrocytic anemias are typified by large red blood cells (i.e., high MCV) in the peripheral blood. Some macrocytic anemias are associated with megaloblastic hematopoiesis, whereas others are not.

(1) Macrocytosis in association with megaloblastic hematopoiesis indicates a **defect in DNA synthesis,** usually caused by a deficiency of vitamin B_{12}, folate, or both. A much less common cause of megaloblastic anemia is **hereditary oroticaciduria,** a defect in nucleic acid processing.

(2) Macrocytosis in the absence of megaloblastic changes is seen in **liver disease, hypothyroidism,** and **dysmyelopoietic states** (e.g., Diamond-Blackfan syndrome, Fanconi anemia, preleukemia).

b. Evaluation

(1) Macrocytic anemia with megaloblastic marrow is characterized by the following hematologic and bone marrow findings.

(a) Macroelliptocytes and hypersegmented neutrophils are evident on the peripheral smear.

(b) The bone marrow is hypercellular with asynchrony between nuclear and cytoplasmic maturation. The nucleus remains relatively large with poor condensation of chromatin as the cytoplasm matures.

(2) Macrocytic anemia without megaloblastic marrow. Because young red blood cells generally are larger than mature cells, significant reticulocytosis due to any cause also produces macrocytes in the peripheral smear and elevates the MCV.

2. Folate deficiency

a. Etiology

(1) Dietary deficiency of folic acid is unusual in developed countries. However, folic acid deficiencies may develop in infants fed on boiled milk or goat's milk and in children with severe anorexia.

(2) Impaired absorption of folate is seen in malabsorptive states [e.g., regional enteritis (Crohn disease), celiac disease] that affect the small bowel (primarily the jejunum; see Chapter 11). Patients usually have a history of weight loss, poor weight gain, irritability, lethargy, and abnormal stools.

(3) Increased demand for folate is seen in conditions characterized by an increased cell turnover (e.g., pregnancy, chronic hemolysis, malignancy). Relative folate deficiency may develop if the diet does not provide adequate folate to meet these needs.

(4) Abnormal folate metabolism. Certain anticonvulsant drugs (e.g., phenytoin and phenobarbital) interfere with folate metabolism.

b. Diagnosis of folic acid deficiency is confirmed by the demonstration of a decreased folate level and by a hematologic response to a 50-g test dose of folic acid.

c. Therapy. The patient should receive 5–10 mg of folic acid orally daily until the anemia and megaloblastosis are corrected. Unless a true dietary deficiency exists, therapy should also be directed toward the underlying disease process.

3. **Vitamin B$_{12}$ deficiency**
   a. **Etiology.** Dietary vitamin B$_{12}$ deficiency is rare in developed countries; the one exception occurs in the infant who is breast-fed by a mother who is a strict vegetarian. The usual cause of vitamin B$_{12}$ deficiency is a selective or generalized **absorptive problem**.
      (1) Vitamin B$_{12}$ is absorbed primarily in the terminal ileum; combination with a factor produced by the gastric parietal cells (**intrinsic factor**) is necessary for absorption to occur. Once absorbed into the bloodstream, vitamin B$_{12}$ is transported in the plasma by means of a specific transport protein (**transcobalamin II**).
      (2) Any condition that alters intrinsic factor production, interferes with intestinal absorption in the terminal ileum, or reduces transcobalamin II levels reduces the availability of vitamin B$_{12}$.
   b. **Clinical features.** Vitamin B$_{12}$ deficiency affects multiple tissues, including the gastrointestinal mucosa (exemplified by diarrhea and weight loss) and the nervous system (seen in subacute combined degeneration of the spinal cord).
   c. **Diagnosis** is confirmed by the demonstration of a subnormal serum level of vitamin B$_{12}$. The mechanism of malabsorption can be demonstrated by the **Schilling test,** which measures the absorption and "flushing out" into the urine of a small dose of radioactive vitamin B$_{12}$.
   d. **Therapy** for most forms of vitamin B$_{12}$ deficiency requires intramuscular injection of a loading dose (1000 μg) of the vitamin followed by monthly maintenance of intramuscular doses (100 μg).

D. **Normochromic, normocytic anemias**

1. **General considerations.** Normochromic, normocytic anemias are a heterogeneous group of disorders. The distinction between those associated with shortened survival of red blood cells and those due to impaired production of red blood cells is facilitated by analysis of the reticulocyte count and analysis of the other cellular elements of the blood.
   a. A **low reticulocyte count** usually suggests bone marrow failure.
      (1) Anemia may be an isolated finding (pure red blood cell aplasia).
      (2) Anemia may occur in association with neutropenia and thrombocytopenia (pancytopenia).
   b. A **high reticulocyte count** with normal neutrophil and platelet counts is characteristic of a hemolytic or hemorrhagic disorder.

2. **Pure red blood cell aplasia**
   a. **Congenital anemia (Diamond-Blackfan syndrome)** is transmitted in an autosomal recessive fashion. Although usually associated with macrocytosis, Diamond-Blackfan syndrome is discussed in this section to simplify comparison with other forms of red blood cell aplasia.
      (1) Clinical features and diagnosis. In many patients, anemia becomes apparent within the first few months of life, and most patients manifest anemia within the first year. In addition to anemia, patients with this condition have reticulocytopenia, macrocytic red blood cell indices, and elevated Hb F levels.

      (2) Differential diagnosis. The early appearance of anemia, the presence of neu-
tropenia and thrombocytopenia, and a normal phenotypic expression differentiate Diamond-Blackfan syndrome from Fanconi anemia, the other congenital
anemia of childhood (see II B 1). The early presentation, macrocytosis, elevated
Hb F level, and chronic course distinguish Diamond-Blackfan syndrome from
transient erythroblastopenia of childhood.

      (3) Therapy. About 50% of patients with Diamond-Blackfan syndrome respond to
corticosteroids; in some of these patients, red blood cell production can be
maintained on remarkably low doses (e.g., 2.5–5.0 mg prednisone once or twice
weekly). Other patients may require red blood cell transfusions to maintain
hemoglobin at an adequate level.

   b. Acquired anemia (transient erythroblastopenia of childhood) is of unknown etiology
but probably results from the prolonged effects of viral suppression of erythropoiesis.

      (1) Clinical features and diagnosis. Transient erythroblastopenia of childhood is
seen somewhat later in infancy than is Diamond-Blackfan syndrome. The anemia, which sometimes can be very severe, is normochromic and normocytic.
Aside from reticulocytopenia, there are no other abnormalities in the peripheral
blood. The Hb F level is normal.

      (2) Therapy. Unless the anemia is severe enough to cause cardiac decompensation,
no therapy is required. Most patients recover spontaneously within 2–4 weeks.

   c. Other forms of acquired red blood cell aplasia

      (1) Disorders of the kidneys, liver, and **thyroid gland** may result in hypoprolifera-
tion of the bone marrow.

      (2) Hypoproliferative anemia may follow **bacterial** and **viral infections**. The etio-
logic agent that is documented most often is **parvovirus-B19**. Usually, the anemia is not severe unless the patient has an underlying hemolytic disorder; failure
of the bone marrow to meet the increased red blood cell turnover in this case
may lead to an **aplastic crisis**.

3. Hemolytic anemias are caused either by intrinsic defects of the red blood cell (**intracorpuscular**) or by factors extrinsic to the red blood cell (**extracorpuscular**). In general,
intracorpuscular defects are hereditary, and extracorpuscular defects are acquired.

   a. Hemolytic anemia associated with extracorpuscular defects. The external milieu of
the red blood cell consists of the plasma and the vascular endothelium. The presence
of autoantibodies or isoantibodies, toxic chemicals, or infectious agents in the
plasma may shorten red blood cell survival. Likewise, irregularities of the vascular
endothelium (microangiopathic changes) may be damaging to the red blood cell.

   b. Hemolytic anemia associated with intracorpuscular defects. Intracorpuscular
defects reflect abnormalities of the membrane, hemoglobin, or enzymes. With the
exception of paroxysmal nocturnal hemoglobinuria, these disorders are hereditary.

      (1) Membrane defects include hereditary spherocytosis, hereditary elliptocytosis,
hereditary stomatocytosis, and paroxysmal nocturnal hemoglobinuria.

      (2) Hemoglobinopathies result from a qualitative change in the structure of one of
the globin chains. This can result in one or more of the following consequences:

         (a) No functional change

         (b) Alteration in electrical charge, which allows identification by hemoglobin
electrophoresis

         (c) Alteration in solubility

            (i) Paracrystalline gel may form when hemoglobin is deoxygenated
(e.g., Hb S).

            (ii) The hemoglobin may precipitate as Heinz bodies (e.g., unstable hemo-
globins).

         (d) Alteration in oxygen affinity

            (i) High-affinity hemoglobins bind oxygen tightly and result in erythrocytosis.

            (ii) Low-affinity hemoglobins release oxygen easily and are associated with
a physiologic anemia.

      (e) Alteration in ability to maintain heme iron in a reduced (i.e., Fe^{2+}) state
         (i) Methemoglobin (i.e., Fe^{3+}) forms.
         (ii) The patient appears mildly cyanotic.
   (3) Enzymopathies generally involve either the glycolytic (Embden-Meyerhof) pathway or the hexose monophosphate shunt.
      (a) The most common glycolytic enzyme involved is **pyruvate kinase (PK)**.
      (b) The most common hexose monophosphate shunt enzyme involved is **glucose-6-phosphate dehydrogenase (G6PD)**.

4. Antibody-mediated hemolytic anemias
  a. General considerations
    (1) Major types
      (a) Autoimmune hemolytic anemias are the result of antibodies generated by an individual's immune system against his own red blood cells.
      (b) Isoimmune hemolytic anemias result from antibodies produced by one individual against the red blood cells of another individual of the same species.
    (2) Typical antibodies involved
      (a) Antibodies of the **immunoglobulin G (IgG)** class, for the most part, are **warm-reactive** (i.e., they have maximal activity at 37°C).
         (i) These are **incomplete antibodies** in that they do not agglutinate red blood cells, although they coat the surface of the red blood cells. These antibodies fix early complement components but cannot activate the complement cascade through the entire hemolytic sequence.
         (ii) Hemolysis occurs extravascularly owing to trapping of opsonized red blood cells by macrophages in the spleen and other reticuloendothelial organs.
         (iii) IgG antibodies are associated clinically with autoimmune diseases, lymphomas, and viral infections. Occasionally, no underlying etiology is demonstrable.
         (iv) They are identified by means of the direct Coombs test.
      (b) Antibodies of the **immunoglobulin M (IgM)** class usually are **cold-reactive** (i.e., most have maximal activity at low temperatures).
         (i) These are **complete antibodies** in that they agglutinate red blood cells and activate the complement sequence through C9, causing lysis of red blood cells.
         (ii) Hemolysis occurs intravascularly.
         (iii) IgM antibodies are associated clinically with mycoplasmal pneumonia, Epstein-Barr virus, and transfusion reactions.
      (c) Donath-Landsteiner antibody
         (i) Donath-Landsteiner antibody is of the **IgG** type, but it is exceptional in that it reacts best in the cold and can activate complement, causing hemolysis to occur intravascularly.
         (ii) Its clinical associations include syphilis and viral infections. It may also be idiopathic.
  b. Autoimmune hemolytic anemias
    (1) Etiology. Autoimmune hemolytic anemia may be idiopathic or the result of infectious agents, drugs, lymphoid neoplasms, or disorders of immune regulation (e.g., systemic lupus erythematosus, agammaglobulinemia).
    (2) Therapy depends on the etiology, clinical condition of the patient, and expected duration of the illness. Because most cases of childhood autoimmune hemolytic anemia are idiopathic or postinfectious and self-limited, supportive care and judicious use of transfusions and corticosteroids are the therapies most commonly used. Treatment modalities include:
      (a) Supportive care with bed rest and oxygen
      (b) Transfusion with packed red blood cells
      (c) Corticosteroids

(d) Splenectomy

(e) Immunosuppressive agents

c. Isoimmune hemolytic anemias can be seen in hemolytic disease of the newborn (see Chapter 6). Hemolytic transfusion reactions are associated with isoimmune hemolytic anemias (e.g., the transfusion of type A blood into an individual with type B blood).

5. Microangiopathic hemolytic anemias

a. Defect and pathogenesis. In these conditions, the red blood cells suffer mechanical damage due to irregularities in the vascular endothelium [e.g., in association with severe hypertension, chronic renal disease, artificial heart valves, hemolytic–uremic syndrome, giant hemangioma, or disseminated intravascular coagulation (DIC)]. The resulting hemolytic anemia occurs because of red blood cell fragmentation in the presence of small vessel disease.

b. Diagnosis is supported by demonstration of red blood cell fragmentation on the peripheral smear in the form of burr cells, helmet cells, and other irregularly shaped red blood cells.

c. Therapy involves supportive care and treatment of the underlying condition.

6. Hereditary spherocytosis

a. Defect. Hereditary spherocytosis is an autosomal dominant type of hemolytic anemia associated with a **defect in spectrin,** the major supporting protein of the red blood cell membrane. The defect leads to a loss of membrane fragments and the formation of small, spherical red blood cells with a high volume-to-surface ratio (**microspherocytes**).

(1) Microspherocytes have less deformability than normal red cells and, consequently, have difficulty in traversing small blood vessels.

(2) The microspherocyte membrane is excessively permeable to sodium. This puts a metabolic strain on the cell because energy in the form of adenosine triphosphate (ATP) is required to pump excess sodium out of the red cell.

b. Pathogenesis. The spleen plays a major role in the pathogenesis of hemolysis.

(1) The spleen has the smallest vessels in the body; thus, the rigid microspherocytes are trapped in its microvasculature.

(2) Glucose and oxygen levels are very low in the sluggish splenic sinusoids; thus, the excess metabolic demands of the microspherocyte for ATP cannot be met.

c. Clinical features

(1) Hereditary spherocytosis may present in the newborn as jaundice, which is sometimes severe enough to require exchange transfusions.

(2) Infants and children may present with pallor or splenomegaly.

(3) Occasionally, patients may present with severe hypoproliferative anemia due to an aplastic crisis after a viral infection [see III D 2 c (2)].

(4) Gallstones may develop in teenagers and adults, who present with the symptoms of **cholecystitis**.

d. Diagnosis

(1) Physical examination usually is positive for pallor, icterus, and mild to moderate splenomegaly.

(2) Laboratory findings

(a) Mild anemia and reticulocytosis usually are present. During aplastic episodes, the anemia may become severe and the reticulocyte count declines.

(b) Diagnosis is confirmed by the demonstration of increased osmotic fragility.

e. Therapy

(1) Supportive care involves folic acid supplementation (to meet needs imposed by increased red blood cell turnover) and red blood cell transfusion (during aplastic crises).

(2) Definitive therapy is splenectomy, which alleviates anemia, reticulocytosis, and icterus; however, characteristic microspherocytes persist after splenectomy.

(3) Because the asplenic patient is susceptible to overwhelming sepsis caused by encapsulated gram-positive cocci, special precautions should be taken (Table 15-4).

TABLE 15-4. Precautions Related to Splenectomy and the Hyposplenic State

1. Postpone splenectomy until older than 6 years of age
2. Immunize against pneumococci and *Haemophilus influenzae* before splenectomy
3. Administer daily oral penicillin prophylaxis postsplenectomy
4. Treat febrile illnesses as potential sepsis (blood cultures/intravenous antibiotics)

7. **Hereditary elliptocytosis**
   a. **Defect.** Hereditary elliptocytosis is an abnormality involving the shape of red blood cells. It is characterized by varying degrees of red blood cell destruction and hemolytic anemia.
   b. **Clinical features.** The clinical course is variable. Chronic hemolytic anemia develops in only 10%–15% of patients (these patients usually have red cells with increased osmotic fragility). The newborn may present with icterus; peripheral smear shows bizarre, fragmented forms of red blood cells as well as some characteristic oval-shaped cells. Later in life, the elliptocytes become more prominent.
   c. **Therapy.** Asymptomatic patients require no treatment. Patients with chronic hemolysis require splenectomy when they are older than 6 years of age.

8. **Hereditary stomatocytosis**
   a. **Defect.** Stomatocytosis is a rare hereditary disorder. Characteristically, red blood cells have a central slit, or stoma, when seen on dried smear. The physiologic defect is a red cell membrane that is unusually permeable to sodium.
   b. **Clinical features.** Most patients have mild symptoms associated with jaundice and occasional anemia.
   c. **Therapy.** If the anemia is of sufficient severity to warrant treatment, splenectomy has been found to be palliative but not curative.

9. **Paroxysmal nocturnal hemoglobinuria**
   a. **Defect.** Paroxysmal nocturnal hemoglobinuria is an uncommon, acquired membrane disorder characterized by red blood cells that are unusually sensitive to the action of hemolytic complement. Hemolysis is maximal during sleep, when carbon dioxide partial pressure (P_{CO_2}) rises and pH falls, thereby activating the alternative pathway of complement activation.
   b. **Clinical features.** The disorder is associated with attacks of hemoglobinuria, which usually—but not always—occur at night. The disorder often occurs in conjunction with hypoplastic anemia.
   c. **Diagnosis** is confirmed by demonstrating increased lysis in an acidified serum test (**Ham test**) or in isotonic, low–ionic-strength solutions (**sucrose-hemolysis test**).
   d. **Therapy** is symptomatic. When the anemia is severe, patients may be transfused with packed red cells (which should be washed to remove complement before transfusion).

10. **Hb S disorders**
    a. **Epidemiology.** This hemoglobinopathy is the most common cause of hemolytic anemia in the African-American population. It also is occasionally found in Greeks, Italians, Saudi Arabians, and Veddoids of southern India.
    b. **Defect and pathogenesis**
       (1) The molecular defect is the result of an abnormal autosomal gene that substitutes valine for glutamic acid in the sixth position of the β-globin chain. This substitution results in an unusual solubility problem in the deoxygenated state. Under conditions of hypoxia, the hemoglobin aggregates into long polymers that align themselves into rigid paracrystalline gels (tactoids), which distort the red cell into a sickle shape.

(2) The clinical consequences of the solubility anomaly are:
  (a) Shortened red blood cell survival (hemolytic anemia)
  (b) Microvascular obstruction, which leads to tissue ischemia and infarction
c. Heterozygous state (sickle cell trait). About 10% of African-Americans are heterozygous for the Hb S gene. Both Hb A and Hb S exist in individuals with sickle cell trait; there is more Hb A than Hb S.
  (1) Clinical features. Sickle cell trait usually is asymptomatic, unless the affected individual is subjected to hypoxemic stress. Otherwise, abnormalities may be limited to failure to concentrate urine, painless hematuria, or both.
  (2) Diagnosis. Patients with sickle cell trait do not routinely manifest sickle cells on peripheral smear. Sickle cell trait may be diagnosed by hemoglobin electrophoresis or by solubility tests (e.g., precipitation with dithionate and phosphate, sodium metabisulfite slide test). It is important to detect the trait for purposes of genetic counseling.
  (3) Therapy. No specific treatment is required; however, precautions to avoid hypoxemia associated with severe pneumonia, unpressurized flying, exercise at high altitudes, and general anesthesia are in order. Tourniquet surgery and deep hypothermia should be avoided.
d. Homozygous state (sickle cell anemia)
  (1) Clinical features
  (a) In the **asymptomatic period,** the high levels of Hb F during fetal life and during the first few months of postnatal life protect the patient.
  (b) The **earliest clinical manifestation** may occur at 4–6 months of age, when symmetrical, painful swelling of the dorsal surfaces of the hands and feet (hand–foot syndrome) develops. This is caused by avascular necrosis of the bone marrow of the metacarpal and metatarsal bones. During this same period, progressive anemia with jaundice and splenomegaly begins to develop.
  (c) Two major **life-threatening problems relating to the spleen** affect infants.
    (i) Splenic sequestration crises. The spleen may suddenly become engorged with red blood cells, trapping a significant portion of the blood volume. If not corrected rapidly, this can lead to hypovolemic shock and death.
    (ii) Overwhelming infection. Despite its large size, in the early childhood years, the spleen does not efficiently perform its filtering function with respect to blood-borne microorganisms. Patients are very susceptible to overwhelming infection, particularly with encapsulated bacteria such as pneumococci and *Haemophilus influenzae.*
  (d) Aplastic crises can occur at any age when there is suppression of erythropoiesis in response to a viral infection such as parvovirus-B19 [see III D 2 c (2)].
  (e) Vasoocclusive episodes can involve any tissue. Depending on the involved organ, a vasoocclusive episode can produce abdominal pain, bone pain, cerebrovascular accident (CVA), pulmonary infarction, hepatopathy, or hematuria. These episodes often are precipitated by infection, dehydration, chilling, vascular stasis, or acidosis.
    (i) The acute chest syndrome is characterized by fever, rales, pleuritic chest pain, and pulmonary infiltrates on chest radiography. Although frequently indistinguishable from an acute bacterial pneumonitis, it more often may result from pulmonary vascular occlusion and ischemia/infarction.
    (ii) Repeated vasoocclusive episodes in the spleen lead to infarction and fibrosis of this organ; it gradually regresses in size and usually is no longer palpable after the age of 5 years.
  (f) Late manifestations. By the time a patient reaches his late teens or early twenties, he is suffering the long-term consequences of chronic anemia, tissue hemosiderosis, and tissue infarction. Many succumb to progressive myocardial damage with congestive heart failure. Other long-term complications include gallstones, leg ulcers, renal damage, and aseptic necrosis of the long bones.

(2) Therapy
   (a) Infections. Because these patients suffer from functional asplenia, the same precautions to protect them from overwhelming gram-positive sepsis must be taken as for the patient whose spleen has been surgically removed (see Table 15-4).
   (b) Vasoocclusive episodes. Prevention involves the avoidance of dehydration, hypoxia, chilling, and acidosis. **Treatment** is as follows:
      (i) Analgesics should be given for pain.
      (ii) When a vital organ (the brain, liver, lung) is threatened, or when the episode does not respond to hydration, transfusion with packed red blood cells may be necessary.
      (iii) After a documented CVA, the patient remains at high risk for recurrent CVAs for an indefinite period of time; such patients should be maintained on a chronic transfusion program designed to keep the Hb S level at less than 30%. As is the case with chronic transfusion programs for thalassemias, iron overload may eventually necessitate chelation therapy [see III B 5 d (1) (d)].
   (c) Severe aplastic crises should be treated by transfusion with packed red blood cells.

11. Hemoglobin C disorder is mild and usually detected only during examination for an unrelated medical condition.
   a. Epidemiology. This β-globin variant is found primarily in African-Americans. Approximately 3% of African-Americans are heterozygous for the Hb A and Hb C genes, and 1 in 10,000 is homozygous for Hb C.
   b. Clinical features. An Hb AC trait is asymptomatic, but target cells are found in the blood smear. Hb CC homozygotes have mild to moderate hemolytic anemia with target cells on the peripheral smear.

12. Double heterozygous states. A combination of Hb S and another abnormal hemoglobin or a combination of Hb S with a thalassemia gene produces a variety of clinical syndromes of varying severity.
   a. The **Hb SC heterozygote** tends to have a milder disease than the Hb SS homozygote; splenomegaly may be more prominent and pulmonary infarction a more common problem.
   b. The **Hb S–β thalassemia heterozygote** may have a clinical picture that is as severe as Hb SS disease; Hb S–α thalassemia, on the other hand, may be mild.

13. Glucose-6-phosphate dehydrogenase (G6PD) deficiency is the most common red blood cell metabolic disorder. It usually is transmitted in an X-linked recessive fashion.
   a. Defects. There are about 150 G6PD variants. The two prototypic forms are the A- variant and the Mediterranean variant.
   (1) The **A- variant** is found mainly in the African-American population and is associated with an isoenzyme that deteriorates rapidly (it has a half-life of 13 days).
   (2) The **Mediterranean variant** is found mainly in individuals of Greek and Italian descent and is associated with almost complete absence of enzyme activity, even in young cells, due to extreme instability (it has a half-life of several hours).
   b. Pathogenesis
   (1) G6PD-deficient cells do not generate an amount of reduced glutathione that is sufficient to protect the red blood cells from oxidant agents. Exposed sulfhydryl groups of hemoglobin are oxidized, predisposing the molecule to denaturation.
   (2) The heme and globin moieties dissociate, with the globin precipitating as Heinz bodies, which form disulfide bridges to the red cell membrane. The damaged red cells are then removed by the reticuloendothelial system; severely damaged cells may lyse intravascularly.

c. Clinical features

(1) The classic picture of G6PD deficiency is an **episodic hemolytic anemia** that usually is drug induced. However, it may also present as hemolysis precipitated by infection, neonatal jaundice, chronic nonspherocytic hemolytic anemia, or favism.

(2) When patients with either the A- or the Mediterranean variant of G6PD deficiency are exposed to **oxidant drugs** (e.g., sulfonamides, salicylates, phenacetin), there is a lag period of 1–3 days, after which a brisk hemolytic process ensues. The subsequent course differs for the two variants, however.

    (a) Patients with the A- variant have self-limited hemolysis confined to the older red blood cell population. Recovery occurs as young red blood cells with enzyme activity sufficient to resist oxidant stress emerge from the bone marrow.

    (b) Patients with the Mediterranean variant have hemolysis that destroys most of their red blood cells and may require transfusions until the drug is eliminated from their bodies.

d. Therapy

(1) Patients with variants of G6PD deficiency that are associated with acute acquired hemolysis should avoid drugs that initiate hemolysis.

(2) Splenectomy does not benefit patients with G6PD deficiency.

14. Pyruvate kinase (PK) deficiency is clinically heterogeneous and is inherited in an autosomal recessive fashion.

a. Pathogenesis

(1) PK catalyzes the final step in the glycolytic pathway; the consequence of its deficiency is inadequate production of ATP. This puts metabolic stress on the red blood cells, because ATP is required to energize the pump that maintains intracellular sodium and potassium ions at the proper levels; thus, PK-deficient cells lose potassium and gain sodium.

(2) Reticulocytes, with their increased metabolic demands, are particularly vulnerable to destruction, especially in the sluggish splenic cords.

b. Clinical features

(1) The severity of hemolysis is variable; newborns may present with jaundice, chronic anemia, or splenomegaly.

(2) Although the signs and symptoms of PK deficiency are the same as those of other chronic hemolytic anemias, because of selective destruction of reticulocytes, there may be an inappropriately low reticulocyte count in response to the anemia.

c. Therapy.
Splenectomy has proven beneficial in individuals with severe enzyme deficiency. Paradoxically, the reticulocyte count rises after splenectomy because the reticulocytes are then able to survive longer.

IV. **POLYCYTHEMIA (ERYTHROCYTOSIS)** refers to a greater than normal number of red blood cells in the blood. The term sometimes also implies a greater than normal number of leukocytes and platelets. Erythrocytosis is, perhaps, a more accurate term because it implies an increase in total concentration of red corpuscles, not an increase of leukocytes and platelets.

A. **Etiology.** Erythrocytosis may be caused by an increase in red blood cell mass (**absolute erythrocytosis**) or by a decrease in plasma volume, in which case the total number of circulating red corpuscles is unaffected, although their concentration is increased (**relative erythrocytosis**).

B. **Pathophysiology.** Abnormal elevation of hematocrit usually is considered to be a hematocrit of 55% and above. Cardiac work is increased by an excessively elevated hematocrit, which can increase blood viscosity, leading to diminished blood flow and decreased oxygen delivery to tissues.

C. **Relative erythrocytosis** is commonly associated with **dehydration**. Because an elevated hematocrit may reflect either an expansion of total red blood cell mass (absolute erythrocytosis) or a decrease in plasma volume (relative erythrocytosis), it is necessary that dehydration be ruled out before the high hematocrit is considered significant.

D. **Absolute erythrocytosis** may be the result of a primary defect of the hematopoietic stem cell (**polycythemia vera**) or secondary to **elevated erythropoietin levels**.

1. **Polycythemia vera,** in which leukocytes and platelets also are increased in number, is extremely rare in childhood.

2. **Elevated erythropoietin levels,** leading to erythrocytosis, may be seen in the following clinical situations.
   a. **Hypoxia**
      (1) The most common cause of erythrocytosis in childhood is cyanotic cardiac disease. Pulmonary disease and high altitudes may also produce sufficient hypoxia to induce erythrocytosis.
      (2) Hemoglobins with a high affinity for oxygen do not release it readily to tissues. The consequent tissue hypoxia may be sufficient to induce an erythropoietin response, which can be diagnosed by demonstrating a P_{50} (the partial pressure of oxygen at which half of the hemoglobin has oxygen bound to it) that is lower than normal.
   b. **Inappropriate erythropoietin production** by renal cysts, renal tumors, and some other tumors (e.g., cerebellar hemangioblastoma)

V. **LEUKOCYTE DISORDERS.** In most clinical settings, the status of the leukocyte population is assessed by measuring the total white blood cell count and the differential count. In evaluating these parameters, it is important to remember that for the first 4 years of life, there is a relative preponderance of lymphocytes.

A. **Disorders of leukocyte morphology**

1. **Chediak-Higashi syndrome** is an autosomal recessive systemic disorder that is characterized by **giant cytoplasmic granular inclusions** in neutrophils.
   a. **Clinical features**
      (1) Recurrent, severe pyogenic infections
      (2) Partial albinism, photophobia, lymphadenopathy, and hepatosplenomegaly
      (3) A tendency to development of lymphoreticular malignancy
   b. **Diagnosis** is made by finding extremely large granules in peripheral blood neutrophils. Neutrophil movement also is impaired because of the large granules.
   c. **Therapy** involves antimicrobial treatment of the infections and blood or platelet transfusions for anemia.

2. **May-Hegglin anomaly** is a rare autosomal dominant disorder of leukocytes and platelets. **Döhle bodies** (large, pale blue inclusions) are found in the cytoplasm of neutrophils, eosinophils, basophils, and monocytes. The disorder is characterized also by thrombocytopenia, giant platelets, and large platelet granules. Neutrophil function remains intact, but there may be platelet function abnormalities.

3. **Pelger-Huët anomaly** is a common autosomal dominant trait that has no adverse effects on health. There is decreased nuclear segmentation of neutrophils, and neutrophil function is intact. Occasionally, Pelger-Hüet anomaly is seen as an acquired disorder (due to drugs, leukemia, infectious mononucleosis).

B. **Neutropenia**

1. **General considerations**
   a. **Definition.** Although the absolute neutrophil count (ANC) varies somewhat according to age and race, a value of 1500/mm^3 usually is considered the lower limit of normal. However, an increased propensity to infection is not seen until the ANC falls below 1000/mm^3. With an ANC of 500–1000/mm^3, patients are at higher risk for cutaneous and mucous membrane infections (e.g., furunculosis, gingivitis, mouth ulcers, perianal cellulitis). When the ANC is below 500/mm^3, the risk for severe visceral infections (including septicemia) increases proportionally to the lowering of the ANC.
   b. **Etiology and classification.** Neutropenia may occur in conjunction with anemia and thrombocytopenia as part of a generalized bone marrow dysfunction (e.g., aplastic anemia, malignancy) or as an isolated cytopenia. The discussion here is confined to isolated neutropenia. Isolated neutropenia may be the result of **either decreased production or increased destruction of neutrophils**. Determination of the etiology of neutropenia routinely requires bone marrow aspiration.

2. **Neutropenia due to decreased production of neutrophils**
   a. **Congenital or familial neutropenias.** A variety of chronic neutropenias, not all well defined, appear to be of congenital origin or to follow a familial pattern. These vary in severity from benign disorders detected accidentally by routine blood count to disorders associated with frequent life-threatening infections. It is not always possible to predict prognosis based on ANC or bone marrow examination; instead, a combination of family history and clinical follow-up often is the best guide to patient management.
      (1) **Cyclic neutropenia**
         (a) **Clinical features.** Cyclic neutropenia is characterized by regular development of marked neutropenia, usually at 21-day intervals. Coincident with the neutropenia, the patient has fever, oral ulcers, furunculosis, and other types of infection. Fatal infections are rare.
         (b) **Diagnosis.** Bone marrow changes are also cyclic, but are out of phase with changes in the peripheral blood (i.e., myeloid hyperplasia is present at the time of maximal neutropenia). The defect is most likely to occur at the pluripotential stem cell level, resulting from failure or inhibition of the bone marrow. Red blood cell and platelet production also are affected, but are not of clinical significance because of the longer half-lives of these cells.
         (c) **Management**
            (i) The patient with high fever in conjunction with ANC less than 500/mm^3 should be treated with broad-spectrum intravenous antibiotics.
            (ii) Patients with severe episodes of neutropenia may benefit from use of the growth factor known as G-CSF (granulocyte colony-stimulating factor) to stimulate neutrophil production.
      (2) **Chronic benign neutropenia**
         (a) **Clinical features.** This is a heterogeneous group of disorders, with variable inheritance patterns and morphologic features. Patients tend to have "nuisance" infections (i.e., mild furuncles, mouth ulcers) rather than life-threatening ones. The ANC usually is 300–1500/mm^3.
         (b) **Diagnosis.** The bone marrow often shows adequate numbers of myeloid precursors associated with an apparent arrest in development at any stage of maturation from promyelocyte to band form.

(3) Severe congenital agranulocytosis (congenital neutropenia; Kostmann disease) is inherited through an autosomal recessive gene. The bone marrow shows maturation arrest at the promyelocyte or early myelocyte stage. Severe and often lethal pyogenic infections of the skin and respiratory tract occur, often beginning in the first month of life. The outlook of these patients has improved markedly with the introduction of G-CSF to stimulate production of neutrophils.

(4) Neutropenia associated with metabolic or phenotypic abnormalities

    (a) Metabolic diseases associated with neutropenia include idiopathic hyperglycinemia, propionic acidemia, methylmalonic acidemia, and isovaleric acidemia. Patients with these diseases usually are quite ill with lethargy, vomiting, ketosis, and dehydration beginning in the neonatal period.

    (b) Cartilage–hair hypoplasia is a variety of short-limbed dwarfism that is characterized by fine, silky hair, moderate neutropenia, and variable immunologic abnormalities.

(5) Shwachman-Diamond syndrome is characterized by metaphyseal chondrodysplasia, dwarfism, pancreatic exocrine insufficiency, and neutropenia. Patients may present early in life with diarrhea, failure to thrive, and recurrent sinopulmonary infections. Neither the neutropenia nor the dwarfism is amenable to therapy.

(6) Neutropenia associated with immunologic disorders

    (a) Some cases of **congenital agammaglobulinemia** and **dysgammaglobulinemia** are associated with neutropenia, which may be transient, cyclic, or chronic.

    (b) Reticular dysgenesis is a lethal disorder characterized by a selective failure of stem cells committed to myeloid and lymphoid development. There is deficiency of granulocytic and lymphocytic development, although erythroid and megakaryocytic elements are spared. The bone marrow is devoid of myeloid elements, and the thymus and spleen are devoid of lymphocytes.

b. Neutropenia caused by infection. Various bacterial and viral agents are associated with neutropenia in children. The mechanisms responsible for the neutropenia are ill-defined and probably include myelosuppression as well as increased peripheral utilization, sequestration, and margination.

    (1) Viruses commonly causing neutropenia include influenza (A and B), hepatitis (A and B), respiratory syncytial, rubella, varicella, and Epstein-Barr viruses.

    (2) Bacterial infections that may produce neutropenia include typhoid, paratyphoid, brucellosis, and tularemia.

c. Drugs and toxic agents

    (1) Two patterns of drug-induced myelosuppression are recognized.

        (a) Cytotoxic drugs, such as methotrexate, cause regularly occurring, dose-dependent suppression of all marrow elements.

        (b) Idiosyncratic suppression of neutrophil production can be caused by drugs such as sulfonamides, synthetic penicillins, antithyroid agents, and phenothiazines.

    (2) Heavy metals and **benzene agents** also can suppress granulocytopoiesis.

3. Neutropenia due to increased destruction of neutrophils

a. Immune-mediated neutropenia. Antineutrophil antibodies may be self-produced (autoimmune) or transmitted to the patient from another individual (isoimmune).

    (1) Autoimmune neutropenia may be idiopathic or occur secondary to drug sensitization, systemic disease (e.g., lupus), a neoplasm (e.g., lymphoma), or viral infection. Some patients respond to corticosteroid therapy.

    (2) Isoimmune neutropenia results from the transfer of antineutrophil antibodies from the mother to the fetus. This may occur because the mother has been sensitized to an antigen on the fetal neutrophils or because the mother has an illness (e.g., lupus) that has induced an autoimmune process in her. When the neonatal neutropenia is severe, pyogenic infections of the skin, umbilical cord, respiratory tract, and bloodstream may develop. In most cases, the neutropenia resolves spontaneously when the maternal antibody is cleared from the infant's circulation.

      b. Drug-induced neutropenia. In addition to their myelosuppressive effects, drugs may produce neutropenia by acting as haptens in immune neutropenia or by directly damaging circulating neutrophils. Neutropenia may resolve after the withdrawal of the offending drug or through the use of steroids.

      c. Splenic sequestration (hypersplenism). Splenomegaly from any cause can lead to neutropenia due to trapping of the neutrophils. Red blood cells and platelets may be affected as well. Treatment of the underlying illness or splenectomy (if clinically indicated) usually resolves this form of neutropenia.

C. | **Disorders of neutrophil function** (see Chapter 9 II B 1)

VI. | **HEMOSTASIS.** Normal hemostasis requires the integrity of three elements: **blood vessels, platelets,** and **soluble clotting factors** (Figure 15-1). Hemorrhage may result from deficiency or disorders of any of these elements.

A. | **Hemorrhagic diathesis**

1. **Clinical features.** Indications of significant hemorrhagic diathesis include:
   a. Petechiae, purpura, or both
   b. Severe recurrent epistaxis (in the absence of an obvious local cause)
   c. Prolonged bleeding after dental extractions, surgical procedures, or major trauma
   d. Recurrent hemarthrosis

2. **Screening** the patient with a suspected hemorrhagic diathesis requires a battery of laboratory tests for assessing coagulation, including platelet count, bleeding time, partial thromboplastin time (PTT) [to measure intrinsic and common pathways], and prothrombin time (PT) [to measure extrinsic and common pathways].

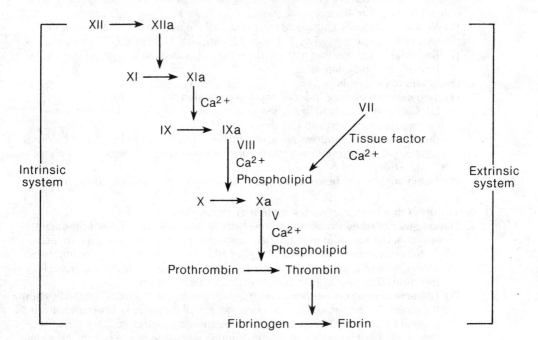

FIGURE 15-1. The coagulation cascade. The intrinsic pathway is initiated by activation of factor XII, whereas the extrinsic pathway is initiated by release of tissue factor and activation of factor VII. Both pathways converge with the activation of factor X. *a* = activated.

3. **General approach to management**
   a. **Drugs that compromise platelet function** (e.g., aspirin) must be avoided, as should deep venipunctures and intramuscular injections. The patient should be protected against trauma (especially to the head). Prolonged immobilization should be prevented.
   b. When the nature of the defect is identified, specific replacement measures should be employed.
   c. If the bleeding is life-threatening, fresh frozen plasma (10–20 ml/kg) can be used as a temporizing measure for defects in coagulation factors until a specific factor deficiency is identified.

B. **Disorders of blood vessels**

1. **Role of blood vessels in hemostasis.** Injury to a blood vessel elicits at least two responses that help to control bleeding.
   a. **Vasoconstriction** reduces blood flow through the injured vessel.
   b. **Subendothelial collagen** activates platelets and coagulation factors.

2. **Vascular abnormalities** leading to a bleeding diathesis include **vasculitis** as well as the following conditions.
   a. **Excessive capillary fragility** is seen in hereditary disorders of collagen synthesis (e.g., Ehlers-Danlos syndrome).
   b. **Hereditary hemorrhagic telangiectasia** is an autosomal dominant disorder. Vascular abnormalities occur throughout the body, especially on mucosal surfaces. Gastrointestinal bleeding may be severe. Iron deficiency anemia occurs invariably.
   c. **Vitamin C deficiency (scurvy)** results in impaired collagen synthesis. Walls of blood vessels are pliable owing to the poor collagen support. Bleeding may also be caused by qualitative platelet defects.
   d. **Henoch-Schönlein purpura** (see also Chapter 9 V D) is a disease of children and young adults that is associated with a variety of clinical features, including arthritis, nephritis, urticaria, a characteristic purpuric rash involving the buttocks and lower extremities, and gastrointestinal pain.

C. **Disorders of platelets.** Platelet defects can be quantitative or qualitative. **Quantitative disorders** are detected by platelet estimate on a peripheral blood smear or platelet count. **Qualitative disorders** are detected by bleeding time or platelet aggregation studies.

1. **Quantitative disorders. Thrombocytopenia** is a decreased number of platelets (the normal platelet count is 150,000–350,000/mm³); it is the most common cause of abnormal bleeding. The low platelet count may result from failure of production or from shortened survival. Platelet production is evaluated mainly by assessing the number of megakaryocytes in the bone marrow aspirate.
   a. **Thrombocytopenia due to decreased platelet production**
      (1) **Bone marrow failure** states associated with pancytopenia (see II and III C 1 a) are a cause of thrombocytopenia. Ineffective thrombopoiesis is associated with megaloblastic hematopoiesis.
      (2) **Amegakaryocytic thrombocytopenia** has a variable inheritance pattern, although when it is caused by the **thrombocytopenia–absent radius (TAR) syndrome,** it is inherited as an autosomal recessive trait. The thrombocytopenia in TAR syndrome may be associated with renal disorders and congenital heart disease.
      (3) **Wiskott-Aldrich syndrome** (see also Table 9-3) has an X-linked recessive inheritance. Clinically, it is characterized by eczema, recurrent infections due to deficiencies in T-cell and B-cell immunity, and thrombocytopenia. The thrombocytopenia may be severe, and the bleeding often is aggravated by sepsis. Small platelets (**microthrombocytes**) are seen on peripheral smear.
   b. **Thrombocytopenia due to shortened survival**
      (1) **Immune-mediated thrombocytopenia** may be associated with **viral infection** or **drugs,** but most cases in childhood are **idiopathic.** The term **idiopathic thrombocytopenic purpura (ITP)** refers to a thrombocytopenia for which exogenous

causes are not apparent. It seems that, in most patients, an autoimmune process increases platelet destruction. Opsonized platelets are trapped and destroyed in the reticuloendothelial system.

  (a) **Clinical features.** ITP may be seen after a mild viral illness or after an immunization. The onset usually is abrupt, with bleeding of the skin and mucous membranes. Bleeding is severe after trauma.

  (b) **Clinical course.** Severe internal hemorrhage is rare, despite a very low platelet count. In 80%–90% of cases, ITP resolves spontaneously within 1–6 months. However, some cases become relapsing or chronic. The mortality rate is less than 1%.

  (c) **Therapy.** Conservative management is advisable because the acute form of ITP observed in children resolves spontaneously in most cases. The use of corticosteroids is controversial, although some physicians advise a brief course early in acute, severe cases. Refractory cases may be treated with intravenous gamma globulin, splenectomy, or immunosuppressive agents.

  (2) Hypersplenism (see V B 3 c) is associated with thrombocytopenia, as well as anemia and neutropenia.

  (3) Disseminated intravascular coagulation (DIC) (see VI D 5) has also been associated with thrombocytopenia.

  c. **Thrombocytopenia in the newborn.** There are many causes of thrombocytopenia in the newborn. Among the most common are congenital infections (e.g., TORCH infections; see Chapter 8), bacterial sepsis, immune-mediated causes, and DIC. In **immune-mediated thrombocytopenia** in the newborn, antibody is formed by the mother against antigen on her own platelets (autoimmune antibodies) or on the fetus's platelets (isoimmune antibodies). IgG antibodies cross the placenta and opsonize the infant's platelets. Platelets are trapped and destroyed within the infant's reticuloendothelial system.

  (1) Autoimmune antibodies are produced by women with ITP, lupus, and drug-induced thrombocytopenia. The mother is usually thrombocytopenic.

  (2) Isoimmune antibodies are produced by the mother whose fetus's platelets possess an antigen that her platelets lack. The mother's platelet count is normal.

2. **Qualitative platelet disorders (thrombocytopathies)** may be congenital or acquired. Thrombocytopathies are associated with platelets that, although sufficient in number, are dysfunctional in hemostasis.

  a. **Congenital (inherited) thrombocytopathies** (Table 15-5)

  b. **Acquired thrombocytopathies**

  (1) Drug-induced (specifically aspirin-induced) **thrombocytopathia** is the most common cause of platelet dysfunction. Aspirin inhibits the platelet release reaction. Normal amounts of the dense granule contents (e.g., adenosine diphosphate) are not released by platelets. The second wave of platelet aggregation is deficient.

TABLE 15-5. Congenital Thrombocytopathies

Congenital Thrombocytopathy	Platelet Abnormality	Clinical Features
Bernard-Soulier syndrome	Glycoprotein 1_b membrane deficiency	Giant platelets Abnormal platelet adhesion to collagen Mild thrombocytopenia
Glanzmann thrombasthenia	Glycoprotein II_b–III_a membrane deficiency	Abnormal platelet aggregation
Gray platelet syndrome	Absent α-granules	Agranular platelets
Storage pool disease	Decreased dense granules	Normal aggregation reaction in response to exogenous ADP Poor release of endogenous ADP

ADP = adenosine diphosphate.

(2) Myeloproliferative disorders (disorders of bone marrow production) also are implicated in acquired platelet dysfunction.

D. **Disorders of soluble hemostatic factors**

1. **Hemophilia A and von Willebrand disease (factor VIII deficiency)**
   a. **General considerations.** Hemophilia A and von Willebrand disease are the most common hereditary coagulation disorders.
      (1) These two diseases involve different regions of the factor VIII molecule and are associated with different functions of the molecule. The factor VIII molecule is a complex of two proteins: the factor VIII procoagulant protein (antihemophilic factor; **VIII:C**) and the factor VIII-related protein (the von Willebrand factor; **VIII:R**).
      (2) Hemophilia A and von Willebrand disease can be distinguished from each other by a number of clinical and laboratory features (Table 15-6).
   b. **Hemophilia A**
      (1) **Pathogenesis.** Hemophilia A results from a deficiency of VIII:C, which is the small–molecular-weight unit of the molecule (the large–molecular-weight unit is present in normal amounts). VIII:C acts as cofactor of the intrinsic pathway of coagulation. The defective gene is located on the X chromosome.
      (2) **Clinical features.** The most characteristic features of hemophilia A are spontaneous or traumatic hemorrhages, which can be subcutaneous, intramuscular, or within joints (hemarthrosis).
         (a) In infants, excessive bleeding may occur after circumcision, but it is usually not evident in the first year of life.
         (b) Severely affected boys (i.e., those whose VIII:C activity is below 1%) show easy bruising and a propensity to hemarthrosis from the time they begin to walk.
         (c) In later life, soft tissue, muscle, and joint bleeding dominate the clinical course; life-threatening internal hemorrhage may follow trauma.
      (3) **Diagnosis.** The PTT is prolonged, indicating a deficiency in the intrinsic pathway. Factor VIII assay is required to confirm the diagnosis; a decrease in VIII:C activity with a normal level of VIII:R is diagnostic.
   c. **von Willebrand disease**
      (1) **Pathogenesis.** Transmission of the disease is variable. von Willebrand disease results from a deficiency of VIII:C as well as VIII:R, which plays a central role in platelet adhesion.
      (2) **Clinical features.** As is true with hemophilia A, the severity of von Willebrand disease varies with the degree of deficiency of factor VIII. Usually, the bleeding is mild, with mucosal and cutaneous (platelet-type) bleeding most dominant. However, severe hemorrhage may occur after trauma.
      (3) **Diagnosis.** There is prolonged bleeding time and prolonged PTT. Ristocetin-induced platelet aggregation is abnormal. VIII:R antigen measurement demonstrates deficiency.

TABLE 15-6. Clinical and Laboratory Features of Hemophilia A and von Willebrand Disease

	Hemophilia A	von Willebrand Disease
Molecular defect	VIII:C	VIII:C; VIII:R
Mode of inheritance	X-linked recessive	Autosomal dominant
PTT	Prolonged	Prolonged
Bleeding time	Normal	Prolonged
Ristocetin cofactor	Normal	Decreased
Bleeding diathesis	Deep muscle hematomas; hemarthroses	Mucous membranes

PTT = partial thromboplastin time.

d. Therapy. General supportive care is indicated for the hemorrhagic diathesis. Replacement therapy for severely affected patients is in the form of cryoprecipitate or factor VIII concentrate. Mildly or moderately affected patients may achieve adequate hemostatic levels of factor VIII after treatment with desmopressin, which releases the molecule from tissue stores.

    (1) Clotting factors derived from human blood products (fresh frozen plasma, cryoprecipitate, factor concentrates) all convey the risk of transmission of infectious agents, primarily hepatitis B and C and human immunodeficiency virus (HIV). Many hemophiliacs exposed to these products in the 1970s and early 1980s have been infected with these agents.

    (2) Current techniques for preparing factor concentrates (e.g., heat-inactivation, solvent/detergent exposure) inactivate HIV. However, there is always the possibility of a new viral agent, which is refractory to these techniques, contaminating the blood supply. Exploitation of molecular biology technology to generate recombinant factor VIII concentrates has provided a safe (albeit expensive) alternative to the use of blood-derived products.

2. Hemophilia B (factor IX deficiency; Christmas disease) is inherited as an X-linked recessive disorder.

    a. Clinical features. Hemophilia B has a bleeding diathesis similar to that of hemophilia A (i.e., deep-muscle hematomas, hemarthrosis, significant bleeding after trauma or surgery).

    b. Diagnosis. The PTT is prolonged. The activity of factor IX is decreased.

    c. Therapy. General supportive measures are indicated for the bleeding diathesis. Replacement therapy is with prothrombin complex concentrate (which is a mixture of coagulation factors II, VII, IX, and X).

3. Vitamin K deficiency. Coagulation factors II, VII, IX, and X (which are synthesized in the liver), as well as the antithrombotic factors protein C and protein S are dependent on vitamin K. When the vitamin is deficient, normal coagulation does not occur.

    a. Etiology

        (1) Vitamin K deficiency can occur in **malabsorption states** and other gastrointestinal disorders. **Drugs** (e.g., coumarin) that are vitamin K antagonists can interfere with metabolism of the vitamin.

        (2) Hemorrhagic disease of the newborn can occur in neonates if the now routine administration of vitamin K at birth is omitted.

    b. Therapy. Nutritional disorders and malabsorption states respond to parenteral administration of vitamin K. Fresh frozen plasma or the prothrombin complex concentrate is indicated for severe bleeding.

4. Liver disease. All of the coagulation factors, with the exception of factor VIII, may be deficient in liver disease. In addition, hepatic clearance of activated clotting factors may be impaired. Thus, both PTT and PT are prolonged. Fresh frozen plasma is indicated in therapy (prothrombin complex concentrates are to be avoided because activated factors may produce intravascular coagulation).

5. Disseminated intravascular coagulation

    a. Etiology. DIC occurs secondary to other disease processes.

    b. Pathogenesis. Intravascular activation of the coagulation cascade leads to fibrin deposition in the small blood vessels, tissue ischemia, release of tissue thromboplastin, consumption of labile clotting factors (i.e., platelets, factors II, V, and VIII, and fibrinogen), and activation of the fibrinolytic system.

        (1) Damage to the vascular endothelium occurs in renal disease, in sepsis, and in patients with giant hemangioma.

        (2) Introduction of thromboplastic substances into the circulation occurs in acute promyelocytic leukemia.

        (3) Impairment of clearance of activated clotting factors occurs in liver disease.

TABLE 15-7. Congenital Thrombotic Disorders

Classification	Function Compromised
Defective inhibitors of activated coagulation factors	
Antithrombin III deficiency	Heparin cofactor—inactivates thrombin, factors IX_a, X_a, XII_a
Protein C deficiency	Inactivates factors V_a, VIII_a
Protein S deficiency	Cofactor for protein C
Activated protein C resistance	Ability of activated protein C to inactivate V_a (due to mutation in factor V molecule)
Defects of fibrinolysis	
Dysfibrinogenemia	Forms fibrin polymers that can be lysed by plasmin
Defective plasminogen activator release	Converts plasminogen into plasmin
Excess inhibitors of fibrinolysis	
Cystathione β-synthase deficiency (homocystinuria)	Protects connective tissue (including vascular endothelium) from toxicity of homocysteine

    c. Clinical features
      (1) The bleeding diathesis is diffuse. There is oozing from venipuncture sites and around indwelling catheters; gastrointestinal and pulmonary bleeding as well as hematuria occur; bleeding occurs from traumatized sites.
      (2) Thrombotic lesions affect the extremities, skin, kidney, and brain.
    d. Diagnosis. The PTT and PT are prolonged. There is thrombocytopenia and hypofibrinogenemia. The levels of fibrin degradation products are elevated. Microangiopathic erythrocyte morphology is apparent on blood smear.
    e. Therapy. The primary disease process should be treated. Supportive measures are indicated for the bleeding diathesis. If bleeding persists or if thromboses are present, heparinization with replacement of platelets and clotting factors (i.e., fresh frozen plasma) should be considered.

E. | **Disorders predisposing to thrombosis.** Blood fluidity reflects the balance between activators and inhibitors of the coagulation and fibrinolytic pathways. Table 15-7 lists congenital disorders that may result in a propensity to thrombosis.

BIBLIOGRAPHY

Miller DG, Baehner RL: *Blood Diseases of Infancy and Childhood.* St. Louis, CV Mosby, 1993.

Nathan DG, Oski FA: *Hematology of Infancy and Childhood,* 4th ed. Philadelphia, WB Saunders, 1993.

STUDY QUESTIONS

DIRECTIONS: Each of the numbered items or incomplete statements in this section is followed by answers or by completions of the statement. Select the ONE lettered answer or completion that is BEST in each case.

1. Which one of the following statements regarding the anemia of chronic disease is true?

(A) Mean corpuscular volume (MCV) is elevated
(B) Serum iron level is elevated
(C) Serum iron-binding capacity is elevated
(D) Marrow iron stores are increased
(E) Iron therapy is required to raise hemoglobin level

2. Hemolytic–uremic syndrome is a disorder of which one of the following?

(A) The red cell membrane
(B) The vascular endothelium
(C) Hemoglobin
(D) The glycolytic pathway
(E) Immune regulation

3. Which of the following hemolytic anemias is associated with an extracorpuscular defect?

(A) Hereditary spherocytosis
(B) Sickle cell anemia
(C) Autoimmune hemolytic anemia
(D) Glucose-6-phosphate dehydrogenase (G6PD) deficiency

4. A 7-year-old patient with known hereditary spherocytosis presents with pallor, low-grade fever, and splenomegaly. Blood counts are as follows: hemoglobin 3 g/dl, reticulocyte count 2%, white blood cell count 8000/mm^3, and platelet count 200,000/mm^3. The most likely diagnosis is

(A) acute splenic sequestration crisis
(B) aplastic crisis
(C) hemolytic crisis
(D) acute leukemia
(E) superimposed iron deficiency

5. Proper management of a child with an absolute neutrophil count (ANC) of 100/mm^3 would be

(A) the start of broad-spectrum intravenous antibiotics
(B) careful physical examination and chest radiograph; close observation pending results of blood cultures
(C) granulocyte transfusion
(D) nutritional support with oral iron and intramuscular injection of vitamin B$_{12}$

6. A 6-month-old African-American boy in otherwise good health is found to be anemic. His red blood cell indices show an elevated mean corpuscular volume and his reticulocyte count is 0.1%. The most likely diagnosis is

(A) Fanconi anemia
(B) Diamond-Blackfan anemia
(C) aplastic anemia
(D) autoimmune hemolytic anemia
(E) sickle cell anemia

DIRECTIONS: Each of the numbered items or incomplete statements in this section is negatively phrased, as indicated by a capitalized word such as NOT, LEAST, or EXCEPT. Select the ONE lettered answer or completion that is BEST in each case.

7. All of the following conditions are characterized by hypochromic, microcytic red cells EXCEPT

(A) iron deficiency anemia
(B) thalassemia major
(C) thalassemia minor
(D) glucose-6-phosphate dehydrogenase (G6PD) deficiency
(E) anemia of chronic disease

8. All of the following disorders are associated with prolonged bleeding time EXCEPT

(A) hemophilia A
(B) von Willebrand disease
(C) aspirin-induced thrombocytopathia
(D) Bernard-Soulier syndrome
(E) idiopathic thrombocytopenic purpura (ITP)

9. Patients with disseminated intravascular coagulation (DIC) present with all of the following hematologic abnormalities EXCEPT

(A) thrombocytopenia
(B) microangiopathic blood smear
(C) hypofibrinogenemia
(D) prolonged partial thromboplastin time (PTT)
(E) low levels of fibrin degradation products

10. Which of the following is NOT a characteristic of Fanconi anemia?

(A) Hematologic abnormalities in infancy
(B) Pancytopenia
(C) Skeletal anomalies
(D) Chromosome fragility

ANSWERS AND EXPLANATIONS

1. The answer is D *[III B 3]*. The anemia of chronic disease is a hypochromic, microcytic anemia [i.e., anemia characterized by a low mean corpuscular volume (MCV)], which is associated with failure to release iron from marrow storage sites. Both serum iron and iron-binding capacity are low, but marrow iron stores are increased. The anemia improves when the underlying illness is treated, and usually does not respond to iron therapy.

2. The answer is B *[III D 5 a]*. Hemolytic–uremic syndrome is a microangiopathic hemolytic anemia that results from mechanical damage to the red cells due to irregularities in the renal vascular endothelium. This results in the characteristic red cell fragmentation on the peripheral smear, seen as burr cells, helmet cells, and other irregularly shaped red cells.

3. The answer is C *[III D 3 a, 4 b]*. Autoimmune hemolytic anemia results from an abnormality outside the red cell (i.e., the presence of antibody). Thus, it is an extracorpuscular defect. Hereditary spherocytosis is a disorder of the red cell membrane. Sickle cell anemia and glucose-6-phosphate dehydrogenase (G6PD) deficiency are disorders of hemoglobin and a constituent enzyme of the red cell, respectively.

4. The answer is B *[III D 6 c, d]*. Temporary suppression of erythropoiesis (as suggested in this patient by the inappropriately low reticulocyte count) can occur in conjunction with even a mild infectious process. In the patient with a hemolytic disorder, even a few days of reticulocytopenia can produce a profound decline in the hemoglobin level. The enlarged spleen represents the consequences of chronic hemolysis and possible early congestive heart failure; acute splenic sequestration crisis is characteristic of sickle cell anemia, not hereditary spherocytosis. Acute hemolytic crisis is characteristic of glucose-6-phosphate dehydrogenase (G6PD) deficiency. Acute leukemia is unlikely in view of the normal white blood cell and platelet counts. Superimposed iron deficiency is a possible diagnosis, but it is unlikely in a 7-year-old child unless there is a concomitant hemorrhage.

5. The answer is A *[V B 1 a]*. A child with an absolute neutrophil count (ANC) of 100/mm^3 is severely neutropenic and is at risk of death from overwhelming septicemia. Because most signs of infection (e.g., pneumonitis, pyuria) depend on the presence of neutrophils, serious infection may be present in such a patient without producing characteristic physical, radiologic, or laboratory findings. Thus, broad-spectrum antibiotics (to treat a variety of possible infections) must be initiated promptly after cultures are obtained. Deferring treatment until culture results are available may result in overwhelming septicemia and death. Granulocyte transfusions usually are not beneficial in these patients because of the short survival time of the cells in the bloodstream (plasma half-life is approximately 7 hours). Iron and vitamin B_{12} are treatments for nutritional anemias and are of no therapeutic value in neutropenia.

6. The answer is B *[III D 2 a]*. Diamond-Blackfan anemia is a hypoproliferative macrocytic anemia which manifests early in life. Fanconi anemia, which may also be hypoproliferative and macrocytic, usually does not become manifest until 4 years of age or older, and usually is associated with neutropenia, thrombocytopenia, or both. Autoimmune hemolytic anemia generally is associated with an elevated reticulocyte count. Sickle cell anemia is also associated with reticulocytosis and usually does not produce significant anemia until later in the first year of life.

7. The answer is D *[III D 3 b (3) (b)]*. In glucose-6-phosphate dehydrogenase (G6PD) deficiency, an enzymopathy, the red blood cell morphology is normochromic, normocytic. In other anemias listed in the question, failure of hemoglobin production due to lack of iron (iron deficiency), unavailability of iron (anemia of chronic disease), or defective globin chain production (thalassemia) leads to production of hypochromic, microcytic red blood cells.

8. The answer is A *[VI D 1 b (3); Table 15-6]*. Prolonged bleeding time usually reflects abnormalities of platelet number, platelet function, vessel wall, or von Willebrand factor (which mediates platelet adhesion and aggregation). In classic hemophilia (hemophilia A), the only abnormality is in the procoagulant component of the factor VIII molecule, which plays no role in platelet aggregation or adhesion. On the other hand, in von Willebrand disease, the entire factor VIII molecule is deficient, including the portion that interacts with platelets. Bernard-Soulier syndrome results from a defect in a platelet membrane receptor molecule that is associated with platelet adhesion. In idiopathic thrombocytopenic purpura (ITP), it appears that an autoimmune process causes increased platelet destruction. Aspirin inhibits platelet release.

9. The answer is E *[VI D 5 d].* In disseminated intravascular coagulation (DIC), activation of the coagulation system results in depletion of platelets as well as certain labile coagulation proteins (i.e., factors II, V, and VIII and fibrinogen). In addition, fibrin strands formed within the microvasculature can damage red blood cell membranes, resulting in microangiopathic morphologic abnormalities, such as helmet cells and burr cells on blood smear. The levels of fibrin degradation products are elevated in DIC.

10. The answer is A *[II B 1 b].* Although Fanconi anemia is a congenital disorder, the hematologic abnormalities associated with it usually do not appear until the patient is 3–8 years of age. Fanconi anemia is an autosomal recessive disorder of bone marrow, which may be severe enough to produce pancytopenia. The genetic defect is chromosome fragility, resulting in excessive breaks and recombinations. Among the many phenotypic abnormalities are skeletal anomalies and retarded growth.

Chapter 16
Oncologic Diseases
John J. Quinn
Arnold J. Altman

I. GENERAL PRINCIPLES OF ONCOLOGIC DISEASES IN CHILDREN

A. Incidence. Cancer develops in approximately 1 in 600 children between the ages of 1 and 15 years, making it the second most common cause of death, after injuries, in this age-group. Many of these children are cured, and, as a result, 1 in 1000 young adults is a survivor of childhood cancer.

B. Types

1. **Common types of cancer in children** (Table 16-1). **Leukemia and solid tumors** represent the majority of childhood neoplasms. The solid tumors are of diverse types and, in contrast to adult cancers, are **predominantly of nonepithelial origin** and are responsive to chemotherapeutic agents.

2. **Uncommon types of cancer in children.** Typical adult-type carcinomas (e.g., lung, colon, breast) are rare during childhood.

C. Oncogenesis

1. **Cells of origin.** In many childhood cancers, the malignant cells are immature precursor cells that fail to differentiate and accumulate because they proliferate more rapidly or die more slowly than normal cells. Under normal circumstances, these immature precursor cells would give rise to the more mature and functional cells of an organ or system. This is especially so for cancers that develop in younger children.
   a. In **acute lymphoblastic leukemia,** the malignant cells are precursors of the immune system's mature T or B lymphocytes.
   b. In **neuroblastoma,** the malignant cells are precursors of sympathetic ganglion cells.
   c. In **Wilms tumor,** the malignant cells are immature metanephric cells that give rise to the mature kidney.
   d. In **hepatoblastoma,** the malignant cells are precursors of mature liver cells.

2. **Mechanisms.** Malignant cells proliferate and develop abnormally because they have escaped normal control mechanisms. This escape is caused by genetic alterations within the malignant cells. Alterations are especially likely to **occur at periods of increased cell proliferation** such as gestation, infancy, and early childhood, when many systems and organs are developing. During these periods of rapid growth, innumerable cells are dividing, and this increases the chance that a normal cell will undergo one or more genetic alteration that will transform it into a malignant cell. Transformation provides the malignant cell with a proliferative advantage or blocks its programmed cell death (apoptosis), or both. **Two well-characterized causes of transformation are activation of oncogenes and loss of tumor suppressor genes.**
   a. **Oncogenes** are closely related to **proto-oncogenes,** which are normal regulatory genes that control cellular proliferation, differentiation, and development. Their products may be growth factors, growth factor receptors, cytoplasmic proteins that transmit messages from receptors to the nucleus, or nuclear regulatory proteins

TABLE 16-1. Types of Childhood Cancer

Cancer	Incidence	
	White Children (%)	African-American Children (%)
Leukemia	30.9	24.3
Central nervous system	18.3	21.6
Lymphoma including Hodgkin	13.8	11.3
Neuroblastoma	6.8	5.4
Soft tissue sarcoma	6.2	8.6
Wilms tumor	5.7	8.1
Bone	4.7	3.6
Eye	2.5	4.1
Germ cell	2.4	4.1
Liver	1.3	. . .
Other	7.4	8.9

(transcription factors) that control the expression of genes involved in cellular differentiation and proliferation. **An oncogene is an abnormally activated or an altered proto-oncogene** whose enhanced expression or altered product causes the cell to acquire and maintain malignant characteristics. Oncogenes behave in a dominant fashion, because their expression predominates over the unaltered gene on the other allele. **Oncogenes are produced in the following ways.**

(1) Translocation of proto-oncogenes to new locations in the genome where:

    (a) They may escape their usual regulatory mechanisms and instead come under the influence of new genes that inappropriately activate them.

        (i) In the B-cell malignancy Burkitt lymphoma, increased c-*myc* expression occurs by translocation of c-*myc* on chromosome 8 to an active genetic locus in B cells, such as the immunoglobulin heavy chain locus on chromosome 14 [t(8;14)] or the light chain loci on chromosomes 2 and 22 [t(2;8) or t(8;22)]. The c-*myc* oncogene is a member of the *myc* family of oncogenes. They encode for nuclear transcription factors that regulate expression of genes involved in cellular proliferation. When c-*myc* is inappropriately expressed in B cells with these translocations, increased cellular proliferation occurs.

        (ii) In T-cell acute lymphocytic leukemia (ALL), inappropriate activation of the SCL gene, a transcriptional regulator on chromosome 1, occurs by inversion that juxtaposes it to the active SIL locus on chromosome 1 or by translocation to the region of the T-cell receptor genes on chromosome 14. In either case, SCL, which normally is not expressed in T cells, becomes inappropriately activated by its close proximity to an active genetic locus in the developing T cell and causes increased proliferation of the genetically abnormal cells.

        (iii) In ALL associated with t(4;11), the MLL gene on chromosome 11 at q23 becomes activated when it is fused to the AF-4 gene on chromosome 4. MLL is a homeobox gene that encodes a transcription regulator that may be involved in early blood cell development. When MLL is appropriately activated in this and other translocations involving chromosome 11 at q23, primitive acute leukemias develop.

    (b) In whole or in part they form novel fusion products with other genes, which alter normal cellular function

        (i) In pre–B-cell ALL with t(1;19), a portion of E2A (a transcription factor gene on chromosome 19) fuses to PBX1 (a homeobox gene that codes for a developmentally important transcription factor) to produce a novel chimeric transcription factor, which transforms the cell into a malignant cell.

      (ii) In Philadelphia chromosome–positive chronic myelogenous leukemia (CML) and ALL, the t(9;22) produces a fusion gene consisting of a portion of the c-*abl* proto-oncogene from chromosome 9 and the *bcr* gene from chromosome 22 to produce a novel protein with tyrosine kinase activity that inhibits apoptosis.

      (iii) In acute promyelocytic leukemia, the t(15;17) produces a fusion gene containing a portion of the PML locus from chromosome 15 and the retinoic acid receptor alpha gene from chromosome 17 that codes for a novel fusion protein, which disrupts further differentiation of the cell by altering the retinoic acid receptor's function from inhibition to activation of transcription. As a consequence, the normal differentiation and apoptosis of the cell are blocked, and, therefore, promyelocytes accumulate rather than terminally differentiate and die.

  (2) Proto-oncogenes may undergo **point mutations** that alter their product. Point mutations of *ras* in acute nonlymphocytic leukemia (ANLL) result in increased *ras* activation and increased transmission of signals from the exterior to the interior of the cell.

  (3) Proto-oncogenes may undergo **gene amplification,** which enhances the output of their product. Amplification of the n-*myc* oncogene in neuroblastoma is associated with a more aggressive tumor and a poorer prognosis.

 b. Tumor suppressor genes inhibit cell growth and may do so by regulating oncogenes. They behave in a dominant fashion, because as long as one of two homologous suppressor genes remains, growth is inhibited. Uninhibited cell growth occurs only in the recessive state when both suppressor genes are lost. Loss of these genes can occur in either somatic or germ cells. When a gene is lost from germ cells, the condition can be inherited (see I D 1). Tumor suppressor genes are lost by:

  (1) Deletion

  (2) Recombination

  (3) Point mutation that inactivates them

D. **Predisposing factors.** Most childhood malignancies are of unknown cause and occur in otherwise healthy children. Certain children, however, are at an increased risk for cancer because of their constitutional makeup or because of exposure to cancer-causing agents.

1. Genetic factors

  a. Genetic mutations

    (1) Hereditary acquisition of these mutations may occur. Retinoblastoma and Wilms tumor are embryonal cancers of the eye and the kidney, respectively. Up to 40% of retinoblastomas and 20% of Wilms tumors are hereditary. These tumors have variable penetrance. They occur in young children and often are bilateral.

      (a) Retinoblastoma is postulated to evolve in two distinct steps, or **hits,** which produce genetic abnormalities that result in tumor formation:

        (i) Prezygotic (germline) inheritance of the first mutation

        (ii) Postzygotic (somatic) mutation, which induces malignancy in the tissue rendered susceptible by the first mutation

      (b) Each of the two mutations may inactivate or delete one of the two alleles of a regulatory gene carried on homologous chromosomes. If the affected alleles regulate or suppress an oncogene, their loss may result in uncontrolled expression of the oncogene and excessive growth of tissue under its influence.

      (c) Both alleles must be inactivated for tumors to develop. Tumors only form in individuals homozygous for defects at them; therefore, these sites of inactivation or mutation are termed recessive oncogenes. They may contain anti-oncogenes or tumor suppressor genes, which, if inactivated on both homologous chromosomes, permit expression of otherwise suppressed oncogenes (see I C 2 b).

      (d) Wilms tumor is postulated to develop in a manner similar to retinoblastoma. Abnormalities at a number of different genetic loci have been found in patients with Wilms tumor, suggesting that two hits at any of these loci may result in tumor formation, or, alternatively, that after the first two hits occur, additional genetic damage must be acquired for malignancy to develop.

    (2) Sporadic acquisition is more common than hereditary acquisition. Spontaneously occurring retinoblastoma and Wilms tumor comprise 60% and 80% of cases, respectively. Two steps (hits) also have been postulated for induction of retinoblastoma, and at least two steps are postulated for induction of Wilms tumor.

      (a) Occasionally, the first step occurs in the germ cells of the affected individual, and the mutation can be passed on to this person's progeny.

      (b) More frequently, both steps or mutations occur postzygotically. Their limitation to somatic tissue precludes their inheritance.

    (3) Germline and somatic mutations typically are not associated with detectable karyotypic abnormalities. When these abnormalities do occur, they can be detected in all of the patient's cells if one of the steps was germline, or in only the tumor cells if both steps were somatic.

    (4) Chromosome abnormalities

      (a) In both sporadic and hereditary cases of retinoblastoma, abnormalities localized to the long arm of chromosome 13 have been detected. This region is thought to contain the retinoblastoma gene, which is a tumor suppressor gene that blocks the uncontrolled proliferation of retinoblasts characteristic of retinoblastoma. Tumor formation occurs only in cells homozygous for abnormalities in this region of the chromosome. Cells susceptible to tumor formation have already received a first hit on one number 13 chromosome. They become tumor cells when they are rendered homozygous for the abnormality on chromosome 13 by development of a second hit on the other number 13 chromosome, a process that results in loss of constitutional heterozygosity for genetic information at this location.

      (b) In a few sporadic cases of Wilms tumor associated with aniridia, mental retardation, and genitourinary tract abnormalities, there has been deletion of genetic material from the short arm of chromosome 11, which is thought to contain a number of distinct genes that control the proliferation of cells of the developing kidney (metanephros).

  b. Defects in DNA repair cause increased chromosome fragility, which predisposes to malignancy. The following are examples.

    (1) Fanconi anemia. Patients with this constitutional aplastic anemia often have short stature, renal and skeletal abnormalities, and a propensity to development of leukemia (see Chapter 15).

    (2) Bloom syndrome. Leukemias, lymphomas, and carcinomas occur in high frequency in these individuals, with sun-sensitive facial telangiectasia, short stature, and immunodeficiency.

    (3) Ataxia–telangiectasia. Lymphoid malignancies are common in these patients, with widespread telangiectasia, cerebellar dysfunction, and immunodeficiency (see Chapter 18).

  c. Immunodeficiencies (see Chapter 9). Children born with congenital immunodeficiencies have a 100-fold increased risk of malignancy, particularly of the lymphoid system. In addition to Bloom syndrome and ataxia–telangiectasia, the congenital disorders include the following.

    (1) Wiskott-Aldrich syndrome is an X-linked disorder characterized by progressive T-cell dysfunction, eczema, thrombocytopenia, and a propensity to development of lymphomas.

    (2) Common variable immunodeficiency predisposes affected individuals to stomach cancer and lymphomas, both of which do not usually manifest until adulthood.

    (3) **X-linked lymphoproliferative syndrome** in males results in severe infections with the Epstein-Barr virus, which, if the acute infection does not end fatally, induces lymphoma formation.

  d. Abnormalities of chromosome number. Patients with trisomy 21 (Down syndrome) have an incidence of acute leukemia that is 15 times greater than that of the normal population.

  e. Neurocutaneous disorders

    (1) **Neurofibromatosis** is a dominantly inherited disorder characterized by neurofibromas, cutaneous pigmented lesions (café au lait spots), bony abnormalities, and a tendency for development of malignancy in the neurofibromas and in other tissues, which may result in leukemia, neuroblastoma, or soft tissue sarcoma (see also Chapter 18).

    (2) The NF1 gene produces a protein that inactivates *ras* and limits signal transduction from the exterior to the interior of the cell. In neurofibromatosis, one of the NF1 genes is inactivated by mutation. This serves as a first hit; if the second normal allele becomes inactivated by a second hit, *ras* remains active, and the cell is transformed. This sequence of events with NF1 serving as a tumor suppressor gene has been demonstrated to occur in some of the myeloid leukemias that develop in children with neurofibromatosis.

2. Infections. Two viruses that infect cells of the immune system have been associated with malignancy.

  a. Epstein-Barr virus has as its target the **human B cell**.

    (1) The virus renders the B cell capable of continuous cell division as well as inhibiting its apoptosis, so that it remains available to proliferate. If the patient is unable to mount an effective immune response that limits the B-cell proliferation, one of the continuously dividing B cells may undergo a specific chromosome change that transforms it into a malignant cell.

    (2) This sequence is seen with endemic **Burkitt lymphoma** and with similar lymphomas that develop in patients who have been immunosuppressed by chemotherapeutic agents or other factors.

    (3) The specific chromosome abnormality consists of translocation of a portion of the long arm of chromosome 8, which contains the c-*myc* oncogene, onto the area of another chromosome (14, 2, or 22), which controls immunoglobulin chain synthesis, a specific B-cell function.

  b. Human immunodeficiency virus (HIV), a retrovirus, has as its target the human helper T cell, which plays a critical role in modulating immune function.

    (1) Viral destruction of helper T cells may lead to **acquired immune deficiency syndrome (AIDS),** which is characterized by an increased susceptibility to opportunistic infections and malignancies (see Chapter 9). Children most often acquire AIDS perinatally from an HIV-infected mother or from transfusions.

    (2) Pediatric patients with AIDS are susceptible to lymphoid malignancies such as **Burkitt lymphoma,** but, to date, few children have had **Kaposi sarcoma**.

3. Environmental factors. Although many environmental carcinogens and toxic exposures are associated with the development of cancer in adults, childhood cancers caused by environmental factors and toxic exposures probably are rare.

  a. One known risk factor for childhood cancer is prior treatment of malignancy in a child (i.e., with chemotherapeutic agents, ionizing radiation, or both). For example, leukemias and lymphomas have developed in children who have been treated for Hodgkin disease with combined chemoradiotherapy, bone cancers have developed in children who have been heavily irradiated, and brain tumors have developed in children given cranial irradiation.

  b. Epidemiologic studies suggest possible links between in utero cannabis exposure and the development of ANLL. A link between exposure to electromagnetic radiation from power lines and the development of ALL has also been suggested.

TABLE 16-2. Malignant Abdominal Tumors in Children

Type	Origin	Age
Wilms tumor	Kidney	Infant and young child
Neuroblastoma	Adrenal medulla	Infant and young child
	Sympathetic ganglia	
Hepatoblastoma	Liver	Infant and young child
Non-Hodgkin lymphoma	Lymph node	Older child and adolescent
	Peyer patch	
Germ cell tumor	Ovary	Older child and adolescent
Rhabdomyosarcoma	Primitive mesenchyme	Older child and adolescent

E. | **Clinical features**

1. **Constitutional symptoms.** Fever, night sweats, and unintended weight loss of greater than 10% are nonspecific symptoms that are often associated with advanced cases of childhood cancer.

2. **Abdominal masses** (Table 16-2). The intra-abdominal tissues are the most common sites of solid tumor formation. Frequently, a visible or palpable mass is detected whose location is determined by the tissue from which it arises. Pain may be present, especially if the mass suddenly enlarges because of bleeding within it.
   a. **Common tumors** include **Wilms tumor** and **neuroblastoma.**
   b. **Rare tumors** include **rhabdomyosarcoma, Hodgkin disease** and **non-Hodgkin lymphoma, hepatoblastoma** and **hepatocellular carcinoma,** and **germ cell tumors. Leukemic infiltration** and **metastases** may cause enlargement of the liver, spleen, and intra-abdominal lymph nodes.

3. **Intrathoracic masses**
   a. **Mediastinal masses** are the most common type of intrathoracic mass. The type of tumor that causes the mediastinal enlargement determines the location of the mass within the mediastinum. Large masses may cause wheezing and hypoxia from severe airway compression, which is a medical emergency. Dysphagia and hoarseness can develop from compression of the esophagus and the recurrent laryngeal nerve, respectively.
      (1) **Anterior mediastinal masses** usually are the result of thymic involvement in non-Hodgkin lymphoma or ALL (see II B) but can also result from a malignant thymoma or a germ cell tumor.
      (2) **Middle mediastinal masses** suggest Hodgkin disease or metastatic involvement of leukemia, non-Hodgkin lymphoma, or neuroblastoma.
      (3) **Posterior mediastinal masses** usually are neural tumors, such as neuroblastoma or, in patients with neurofibromatosis, neurofibrosarcoma.
   b. **Intrapulmonary lesions** are less common than mediastinal masses and are metastatic in nature. Nodular pulmonary metastases develop in Wilms tumor, soft tissue sarcomas, bone cancers, germ cell tumors, hepatoblastomas, and Hodgkin disease. Neuroblastoma is the only solid tumor in which pulmonary metastases are rare.

4. **Lymph node enlargement** (lymphadenopathy) usually is the response to an infectious or inflammatory stimulus. However, it can also result from the proliferation of neoplastic cells within the lymph node.
   a. **Suppuration** strongly suggests an acute bacterial infection. Other findings, such as degree of hardness, matting, or tenderness, cannot reliably distinguish benign from neoplastic adenopathy.
   b. **Rapidly enlarging nodes** or nodes in the supraclavicular region should increase the suspicion of malignancy.
      (1) Leukemias, Hodgkin disease, non-Hodgkin lymphoma, and metastatic solid tumors can all cause nodal enlargement.
      (2) Metastases from abdominal tumors often enlarge the left supraclavicular nodes.
      (3) Metastases from thoracic tumors often enlarge the right supraclavicular nodes.

5. **Bone pain.** Expansion of the marrow cavity or destruction of cortical bone by leukemic cells or by a metastatic tumor can cause considerable pain.
   a. If the long bones of the lower extremities are involved, a limp or difficulty in walking may develop.
   b. If the skull is involved, proptosis or palpable nodules may develop.
   c. Neuroblastoma and the primary bone cancers (i.e., Ewing sarcoma, osteogenic sarcoma) are most likely to produce bone metastases. Primary bone cancers and histiocytosis X can also produce pain at their site of origin.

6. **Soft tissue masses.** Rhabdomyosarcomas often arise on the trunk or extremities and produce palpable tumors. Bone tumors that break through the cortex and infiltrate the soft tissues can also produce palpable tumors.

7. **Intracranial lesions.** Any space-occupying lesion can produce signs and symptoms of increased intracranial pressure (e.g., papilledema, ocular palsies, headaches, vomiting).
   a. Numerous primary intracranial malignancies usually arise below the tentorium.
   b. Discrete metastatic lesions from solid tumors also occur and are more often supratentorial.
   c. Central nervous system (CNS) involvement occurs in acute leukemia and takes the form of diffuse meningeal infiltration, which also causes increased intracranial pressure.

8. **Bone marrow failure**
   a. **Diffuse replacement** of the normal marrow elements characterizes the acute leukemias and results in anemia, thrombocytopenia, and a paucity of mature and functional leukocytes, especially neutrophils (see II A 3 a).
   b. **Less extensive infiltration** (e.g., as occurs with solid tumor metastases) may result in anemia and leukoerythroblastic changes on peripheral smear, consisting of teardrop-shaped, fragmented, and nucleated red blood cells and a shift in the granulocyte series to the left, down to and including the myeloblast stage. Tumor cells often are cohesive, and clumps of primitive cells in the marrow resulting from solid tumor metastases are termed **syncytia**.

F. **Staging.** Current classification systems employ numerical staging; advanced disease is indicated by high numbers and usually is associated with a poor prognosis. Staging systems apply only to solid tumors with a propensity to disseminate and do not apply to the leukemias, which always are disseminated at the time of diagnosis.

1. **Stage I** tumors are truly **localized** to their organ of origin and, if treated by surgery, must be totally resected with no microscopic or gross disease remaining.

2. **Stages II and III** refer to **more advanced localized** disease than stage I tumors, for which surgical resection does not result in complete tumor removal. Patients with stage II tumors generally have less residual disease after surgery than patients with stage III tumors. For malignancies primary to the lymph nodes, the meaning of stage II and III designations is somewhat different and indicates the degree of spread within the lymphoid system.

3. **Stage IV** is indicative of **disseminated** disease with hematogenous metastases or spread to distant nodes in tumors that are not primary to the lymph nodes.

G. **Therapeutic strategies.** Childhood cancers are among the most curable human malignancies. To achieve a cure, therapy often involves multiple disciplines working in concert.

1. **Surgery.** Total or partial removal (**debulking**) of solid tumors contributes greatly to the cure of disease. Very large tumors that cannot be removed at initial surgery sometimes can be rendered operable after their size has been decreased by radiotherapy, chemotherapy, or both.

2. **Radiotherapy.** The ionizing radiation beam can be directed at specific tumor locations. Radiotherapy plays an important role in the following situations:
   a. Destruction of localized residual tumor that cannot be surgically removed

b. Reduction in the size of large tumors to render them operable

c. Palliative and curative therapy of discrete metastatic foci

d. Eradication of leukemic cells in sanctuary sites (see II A 3 d)

e. Local control of selected malignancies of lymphoid, osseous, and mesenchymal origin for which surgery is not indicated

3. **Chemotherapy.** Many different antineoplastic drugs have been developed during the last 4 decades, and their use is based on the following principles.

a. Chemotherapy interferes with cell growth and division.

b. Chemotherapy produces adverse effects on normal as well as malignant cells.

(1) Normal cells that are most likely to be affected are rapidly dividing, particularly those of the bone marrow, gastrointestinal tract, and hair follicles. However, many types of cells and many diverse organs may be affected by the toxicity of a specific chemotherapeutic agent.

(2) The toxic effect of some agents is dose-related and may be avoided by not exceeding a certain dose.

(3) Drugs with dissimilar toxicities often can be used in combination to enhance a malignant cell kill without enhancing the toxicity to normal cells. Even when the toxicity of two or more agents is additive, they often can be used in combination if the toxicity is reversible and if the patient receives appropriate supportive care during the period of drug-induced toxicity.

c. Chemotherapy is most likely to effect a cure for any malignancy when the tumor cell burden is small. Chemotherapy, however, can be curative in any of the following situations.

(1) **Primary therapy for disseminated malignancy** (e.g., the leukemias). There is no opportunity to control the disseminated disease locally with either surgery or radiotherapy. The leukemias are the principal examples of systemic malignant diseases that are treated primarily with chemotherapy. Metastatic solid tumors also require chemotherapy for control but often are not as responsive as the leukemias.

(2) **Reduction in bulk disease.** Large solid tumors that cannot be managed initially with surgery, radiotherapy, or both can sometimes be successfully treated by these means if their size is first reduced by chemotherapy.

(3) **Destruction of micrometastases.** Patients with nonmetastatic solid tumors for which local surgery, radiotherapy, or both appear completely adequate often have recurrences at distant sites. They are thought to have clinically inapparent spread (**micrometastases**), which, in the absence of systemic therapy, produces gross metastatic disease. These patients—with their small tumor burdens—respond very well to adjuvant chemotherapeutic regimens designed to destroy micrometastases.

4. **Bone marrow transplantation.** Some disseminated malignancies that are not cured by standard doses of chemotherapy and radiotherapy, particularly leukemias, may be cured by high doses if the irreversible toxicity of the therapy can be avoided. Toxicity to bone marrow is the limiting factor in many treatment regimens. If marrow destruction by high therapeutic doses can be circumvented by transplantation of new marrow, then potentially curative doses of chemotherapy and radiotherapy can be administered.

a. Types of bone marrow transplantation

(1) In **syngeneic transplants,** the donor and recipient are identical twins and, thus, are genetically identical. This is a rare occurrence.

(2) In **allogeneic transplants,** the donor and recipient are not identical twins.

(a) Donors usually are related to the recipient. Most commonly they are siblings, but occasionally they can be other family members. Although there is no genetic identity between the donor and recipient, there must be histocompatibility [human leukocyte antigen (HLA) matching]. If there is not, either the new marrow will be rejected or, frequently, the T cells in the donated marrow will mount an immune response against the body of the recipient, which manifests as **graft-versus-host disease (GVHD)**. A related HLA-matched family member can be found for, at most, one in three individuals who require an allogeneic transplant. Less commonly, donors unrelated to the recipient can be identified. Because of the tremendous diversity of HLA antigens, it is more difficult to find an HLA match between two unrelated individuals. Searches for an unrelated donor require access to databases that have information on the HLA types of large numbers of potential donors.

(b) Even with histocompatibility between the donor and recipient of an allogeneic transplant, there is still a significant risk of GVHD. This can be particularly severe when the donor is not related to the recipient.

(3) In **autologous transplants,** the patient is the donor and the stem cells to reconstitute the marrow may be collected from **bone marrow** or from **peripheral blood** by leukapheresis.

(a) For these transplants, the patient's marrow or peripheral blood stem cells must be collected and stored before administering the marrow-ablative doses of therapy.

(b) There is no risk of GVHD with autologous transplants, but there is a risk of reinfusing malignant cells with the normal stem cells. Peripheral blood stem cells are less likely to be contaminated by malignant cells than marrow cells. When marrow is used for autologous transplants, techniques may be employed to "purge" the marrow in vitro of malignant cells before it is returned to the patient. Monoclonal antibodies directed against tumor-associated antigens or chemotherapeutic agents are most commonly used.

b. GVHD

(1) Clinical features

(a) GVHD produces mild to severe lesions in the skin, gastrointestinal tract, and liver.

(b) Profound immunodeficiency develops in patients with severe forms of GVHD, and they often die of complicating infections.

(2) Prevention

(a) Prevention of GVHD may be possible with posttransplant administration of immunosuppressive agents (e.g., methotrexate, corticosteroids, cyclosporine) and use of techniques that remove the T-cell mediators of GVHD from the marrow before its infusion into the recipient. These latter techniques often dramatically decrease the incidence and severity of GVHD, but may be associated with an increased risk of rejection of the transplanted marrow and with relapse of the malignancy.

(b) Intensive posttransplant immunosuppression or T-cell depletion could also extend the scope of bone marrow transplantation to include non–HLA-identical individuals as donors. This is an especially important consideration, because an HLA-identical family member donor cannot be identified for many patients in need of transplants.

II. THE LEUKEMIAS

A. **General considerations.** Collectively, these hematologic malignancies account for the greatest percentage of cases of childhood cancer (31% of all neoplastic disease in white children and 24% in African-American children).

1. **Classification.** Leukemias are classified on the basis of leukemic cell morphology into **lymphocytic leukemias,** which are proliferations of cells of lymphoid lineage, and **nonlymphocytic leukemias,** which are proliferations of cells of granulocyte, monocyte, erythrocyte, or platelet lineage. They are also classified on the basis of their natural history in the prechemotherapy era.

   a. Acute leukemias constitute 97% of all childhood leukemias. If untreated, they are rapidly fatal within weeks to a few months of the diagnosis; however, with treatment, they often are curable. The malignant cells, which are very immature in appearance and function, are termed **blasts**.

   (1) **Acute lymphocytic leukemia (ALL)** is also termed **acute lymphoblastic leukemia** owing to the distinguishing characteristic of the presence of large numbers of lymphoblasts in the bone marrow. ALL is the **most common pediatric neoplasm** and accounts for 80% of all childhood acute leukemia.

   (2) **Acute nonlymphocytic leukemia (ANLL)** accounts for the remaining 20% of cases of acute leukemia in children.

   b. **Chronic leukemias** comprise 3% of childhood leukemias; even without treatment, patients can survive for many months to years. Unfortunately, the chronic leukemias evolve into forms of acute leukemia that cannot be cured by available chemotherapy. All chronic leukemias in children are of **nonlymphocytic lineage**. The leukemic cells are more mature and functional than the blasts of acute leukemias.

2. **Epidemiology.** In addition to children with syndromes associated with abnormalities of chromosome number or stability or with immunodeficiency states (see I D 1 c–d), the following individuals are at increased risk for leukemia.

   a. **Identical twins** have a 20% risk of leukemia if it develops in one twin during the first 5 years of life.

   b. In **children with solid tumors** (e.g., Hodgkin disease, Wilms tumor) who have undergone intense treatment, leukemia may develop as a secondary malignancy.

   c. **Children with congenital marrow failure** states, such as **Shwachman-Diamond syndrome** (exocrine pancreatic insufficiency and neutropenia) and **Diamond-Blackfan syndrome** (congenital red cell aplasia), have an increased risk of leukemia.

   d. **African-American children** appear to have an increased incidence of ANLL and a decreased incidence of ALL.

3. **Clinical features**

   a. **Bone marrow failure.** Replacement of the normal hematopoietic elements by the leukemic cell population results in decreased production of red blood cells, normal white blood cells, and platelets. As a consequence, presenting clinical features of leukemia are similar to those of aplastic anemia. Signs and symptoms of marrow failure often predominate in the child with newly diagnosed leukemia, and most of these children will have one or more of the following symptoms.

   (1) **Anemia** that accompanies bone marrow failure is surprisingly well tolerated considering its degree of severity. It develops slowly, unless there is superimposed hemorrhage from thrombocytopenia. It does, however, produce:

   (a) Pallor

   (b) Irritability

   (c) Decreased activity

   (2) **Hemorrhagic diathesis**

   (a) Bleeding due to thrombocytopenia is common but usually superficial. It manifests as:

   (i) Petechiae and ecchymoses in the skin

   (ii) Mucosal bleeding, such as epistaxis or melena

   (b) If there is associated disseminated intravascular coagulation (DIC) or extreme leukocytosis [see II A 5 a (4)], occasionally there may be severe and life-threatening bleeding (e.g., in the CNS).

   (3) **Infection** due to a paucity of functional white blood cells, especially granulocytes, may be present.

   (a) Fever is the usual manifestation of infection.

   (b) Localized signs of infection, such as rales with pneumonia or pus formation in an abscess, may not be apparent in these granulocytopenic patients.

   (c) Infection often quickly disseminates and produces bacteremia and sepsis.

   b. **Reticuloendothelial system infiltration**

   (1) **Lymphadenopathy** is common, especially in ALL, and may be so massive as to resemble that in the lymphomas.

(2) Hepatosplenomegaly also may be present. Both the liver and the spleen can be minimally to massively enlarged.

c. **Bone pain** (see I E 5)

d. **Involvement of sanctuary sites.** Sanctuary sites are rarely involved at the time of diagnosis but may be involved with the recurrence of disease. These sites are the:

   (1) **CNS,** where involvement manifests as diffuse meningeal infiltration with signs of increased intracranial pressure (see I E 7 c)

   (2) **Testes,** one or both of which may be involved, with infiltration producing enlargement that is out of proportion to the child's sexual development

4. **Laboratory findings**

   a. **Peripheral blood.** A normal complete blood count does not preclude a diagnosis of leukemia, but abnormalities frequently are present.

   (1) **Anemia** is present in most patients and is normochromic and normocytic, with a low reticulocyte index indicative of decreased marrow production of red blood cells.

   (2) **Thrombocytopenia** also is very common. If the platelet count is less than 20,000/mm^3, as is often the case, there usually are hemorrhagic manifestations. Anemia, thrombocytopenia, or both are present in 90% of patients.

   (3) **Neutropenia** often is present. Even if the patient has a high total white blood cell count, few of the cells are mature neutrophils. The following distribution of white cells is seen:

   (a) Low (< 5000/mm^3) in one-third of patients

   (b) Normal (5000–20,000/mm^3) in one-third of patients

   (c) High (> 20,000/mm^3) in one-third of patients

   (4) **Blast cells** are commonly seen on peripheral smear, especially if the white blood cell count is normal or high.

   b. **Bone marrow** shows extensive replacement of the normal elements by leukemic cells. Even if there are blasts in peripheral blood, a diagnosis of leukemia should always be confirmed by bone marrow examination.

5. **Therapy**

   a. **Supportive care.** Treatment of any complications in the child with newly diagnosed leukemia is essential and lifesaving.

   (1) **Transfusional support** often is necessary. Blood products often are irradiated before transfusion to destroy any donor lymphocytes that could mount a graft-versus-host reaction in the immunocompromised leukemia patient.

   (a) Packed red blood cells are used to correct significant anemia.

   (b) Platelet concentrates are used for severe thrombocytopenia.

   (c) Granulocytes rarely are needed. Their use is controversial, but they may play a role in the management of granulocytopenic patients with infections that do not respond to antibiotics.

   (2) **Treatment of infection** is essential. Patients usually are granulocytopenic. If they become febrile, appropriate cultures (blood, urine, sites of local infection) should be obtained promptly and intravenous administration of broad-spectrum antibiotics begun immediately thereafter. A chest radiograph also should be obtained to look for infiltrates.

   (3) **Metabolic support** is necessary in patients with large malignant cell burdens as represented by a high white blood cell count or significant organ infiltration. These patients are likely to manifest a tumor lysis syndrome characterized by one or more of the following metabolic abnormalities.

   (a) **Hyperuricemia** may develop from a breakdown of purines released by dying leukemic cells. The uric acid can precipitate in the renal tubules and cause renal failure. This may be prevented by vigorous hydration to promote uric acid excretion, alkalinization of the urine to increase uric acid solubility, and administration of allopurinol, a xanthine oxidase inhibitor, to block uric acid formation.

    (b) Hyperkalemia also may develop and cause serious cardiac arrhythmias if not corrected.

    (c) Hyperphosphatemia also develops, which can cause a reciprocal fall in serum calcium, which may result in:

      (i) Tetany

      (ii) Potentiation of the effect of hyperkalemia on the heart

      (iii) Precipitation of calcium phosphate in the renal tubules

(4) Treatment of hyperviscosity. White blood cell counts greater than 100,000/mm³, especially in patients with ANLL, can cause significant hyperviscosity. The white blood cell count may be lowered by exchange transfusions or leukapheresis. Without treatment, the hyperviscosity may interfere with blood flow to the:

    (a) CNS, causing hemorrhagic infarction

    (b) Lungs, causing hypoxemia

(5) Treatment of compressive symptoms. Large collections of malignant cells in the anterior mediastinum may produce an obstructing mass, resulting in compressive symptoms such as hypoxemia from airway compromise and obstruction of the superior vena cava, producing a syndrome consisting of facial plethora, venous distention, and increased intracranial pressure. If the mass and the compressive symptoms do not decrease with the institution of chemotherapy, radiotherapy to the mass may be effective.

b. Antileukemic therapy is administered in distinct phases with distinct objectives.

(1) Remission induction. This initial phase lasts at least 4 weeks, during which maximal cytoreduction is achieved. If successful, at the conclusion of remission induction, bone marrow should demonstrate normal hematopoiesis and contain less than 5% blasts, complete blood count values should return to normal, and abnormal physical findings due to leukemia should be gone.

(2) Consolidation aims to:

    (a) Kill additional leukemic cells with further systemic therapy

    (b) Prevent leukemic relapse within the CNS by therapy specifically directed toward the CNS

(3) Maintenance is the longest phase of therapy. Its objectives are to:

    (a) Continue the remissions achieved in the previous phases

    (b) Produce whatever additional cytoreduction is necessary to cure the leukemia

(4) Discontinuation of antileukemic therapy is possible for patients who remain in remission throughout their prescribed course of maintenance therapy. During this phase, most patients continue in an indefinite remission and are cured of their leukemia. In a minority of patients, relapse (recurrence) occurs in either bone marrow or extramedullary sites, such as the CNS or testes.

B. **Acute lymphocytic leukemia (ALL)** is a malignant disease in which immature lymphoid cells (lymphoblasts) accumulate in the bone marrow and replace the normal hematopoietic elements. They are also released into peripheral blood, in which they spread throughout the body and infiltrate all organ systems.

1. Epidemiology. ALL is the most common type of childhood leukemia. It is more common in white children than in African-American children and more common in males than in females (1.2–1.3 times). ALL is associated with a peak incidence in the 3- to 5-year-old age-group for white children only.

2. Etiology. The immature lymphoid cells of ALL are derived from lymphoid precursor cells that reside in the bone marrow and normally give rise to mature B and T lymphocytes. B-cell development occurs within the bone marrow and T-cell development is completed within the thymus. Each distinct B or T cell synthesizes a unique antigen receptor molecule, a unique immunoglobulin molecule, or a unique T-cell receptor. There are billions of antigens for which immunoglobulins and T-cell receptors have specificity. As the immune system develops, the precursor cells give rise to billions of distinct B and T cells, each having a unique antigen receptor molecule. To accomplish this task, the limited amount of DNA devoted to the immunoglobulin chain genes and to the T-cell receptor genes undergoes innumerable rearrangements to produce each of the sequences specific for a given immunoglobulin molecule or T-cell receptor. Attempting to commit to a lineage, precursor cells commence to rearrange immunoglobulin chain genes and T-cell receptor genes into sequences that will direct the synthesis of a complete antigen receptor molecule. Cells that successfully rearrange their immunoglobulin chain genes develop into mature B cells, and cells that successfully rearrange their T-cell receptor genes become mature T cells. This process occurs predominantly during gestation, infancy, and early childhood, which is the period when the immune system rapidly develops. The numerous proliferating precursor cells undergo gene rearrangements and provide potential targets for development of additional genetic alterations that transform them into malignant cells.

a. Lymphoblasts of ALL patients usually demonstrate incomplete rearrangements of immunoglobulin and T-cell receptor genes. They were unsuccessful in completing a rearrangement that would have allowed them to mature fully. If they were normal precursor cells that failed successful gene rearrangement, they would have died; as malignant cells, they are thought to have developed genetic alterations that permit them to survive and proliferate. They remain frozen at an early stage of development, and their particular pattern of incomplete gene rearrangements and surface antigen expression reflects the point at which the block in their development occurred (see II B 3 b).

b. The malignant lymphoblasts of each patient with ALL are all thought to be descendants of a single abnormal precursor cell, and as such comprise a clone. They demonstrate a unique pattern of gene rearrangement that is identical in all the cells of the clone, and which distinguishes them from the clones of other ALL patients, and from the innumerable patterns in mature B and T cells.

3. Classification
a. Morphologic classification of ALL is based on the following features.
  (1) Appearance of the leukemic lymphoblasts. According to the French-American-British (FAB) classification, leukemic lymphoblasts subdivide into three categories.
    (a) COMPLETE lymphoblasts are small, with scant cytoplasm and absent or inconspicuous nucleoli. They are by far the most common type of cells in children with ALL.
    (b) L2 lymphoblasts are larger, with more abundant cytoplasm and one or more prominent nucleoli. They are much less common than L1 cells and are sometimes mistaken for myeloblasts.
    (c) L3 lymphoblasts are large, with deeply basophilic and vacuolated cytoplasm and prominent nucleoli. They are rare and usually indicative of the equally rare B-cell ALL.
  (2) Enzymatic evaluation. Terminal deoxynucleotidyl transferase (TdT) is a unique DNA polymerase that is found in almost all lymphoblasts but only rarely in ANLL blasts.
  (3) Histochemical evaluation shows:
    (a) Absence of enzymes characteristic of ANLL blasts
    (b) In many cases, block-like accumulations of glycogen on periodic acid-Schiff stain
b. Immunologic classification (Figure 16-1) considers ALL to be a heterogeneous group of malignancies comprising immature lymphoid cells arrested at various stages of development. On the basis of immunophenotype, ALL is divided into the following subtypes (Table 16-3).
  (1) Non-T, non–B-cell ALL accounts for 84% of all cases. Cells from patients with this type of ALL are lymphoid precursors that, under normal circumstances, would have differentiated into mature B cells capable of synthesizing a distinct immunoglobulin molecule or mature T cells capable of synthesizing a T-cell antigen receptor. Often, the malignant leukemic cells have begun to rearrange their antigen receptor genes, but not to the point that they can synthesize a functional gene product that indicates a commitment to a specific B-cell or T-cell

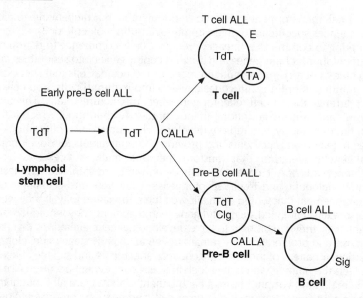

FIGURE 16-1. Scheme of B-cell and T-cell development and types of acute lymphocytic leukemia (*ALL*) that result from blocks at various stages of development. Current terminology considers both common acute lymphocytic leukemia antigen (*CALLA*)-negative and CALLA-positive early pre–B-cell ALL and pre–B-cell ALL as forms of non–T-, non–B-cell ALL. The exact precursor cell that gives rise to the T-cell lineage is not known definitively and may not be the cell depicted in this scheme. *TdT* = terminal deoxynucleotidyl transferase; *TA* = thymic antigen; *E* = sheep red cell receptor; *CIg* = cytoplasmic immunoglobulin; *SIg* = surface immunoglobulin.

lineage. Thus, these cells are blocked at very early stages of their development and referred to as non-T, non-B cells. In non-T, non–B-cell ALL, rearrangement of immunoglobulin chain genes is more common and more advanced than rearrangement of T-cell antigen receptor genes, and early B-cell differentiation antigens are expressed on the cell surface. Therefore, this type of ALL is considered to be a **malignancy of B-cell precursors**. Non-T, non–B-cell ALL is **subdivided based on reactivity with the common acute lymphocytic leukemia antigen (CALLA)** into the following subtypes.

(a) **CALLA-negative early pre–B-cell ALL** is much less common than CALLA-positive ALL and consists of early pre-B cells that are not yet able to synthesize CALLA or cytoplasmic immunoglobulin. It is most frequently seen in infants less than 1 year of age.

TABLE 16-3. Characteristics of the Different Types of Acute Lymphoblastic Leukemia

Immunophenotype	Age	White Blood Cell Count	Common Karyotype	Other
CALLA-negative early pre-B	Infant	High	Translocation	Worst prognosis
CALLA-positive early pre-B	Younger child	Low, normal	Hyperdiploidy	L1 morphology
Pre-B	Younger child	Low, normal	Translocation	Cytoplasmic immunoglobulin
T-cell	Older child Adolescent	High	Translocation	Mediastinal mass
B-cell	Older child Adolescent	Variable	Translocation	L3 morphology

CALLA = common acute lymphocytic leukemia antigen.

    (b) CALLA-positive ALL is much more common than CALLA-negative ALL and may be one of the following.

        (i) CALLA-positive early pre–B-cell ALL consists of cells that synthesize CALLA but not cytoplasmic immunoglobulin; this is the most common subtype in children with ALL.

        (ii) Pre–B-cell ALL consists of cells that usually continue to synthesize CALLA and have matured to the point where they synthesize cytoplasmic immunoglobulin consisting of only heavy chains, all of which are identical in the cells of any given patient.

  (2) B-cell ALL accounts for 1% of cases and is characterized by cells that lack TdT activity and often no longer express CALLA. These cells synthesize complete immunoglobulin molecules, which are expressed on their surface. The cells from any given patient all synthesize the same molecule, consisting of one specific light chain and one specific heavy chain. This is the most mature form of ALL of B-cell lineage and the only form of ALL in which the cells have a distinct appearance (L3) in the FAB classification. This form of ALL is closely related to Burkitt lymphoma, with which it shares clinical features (e.g., occurrence in older children and teenagers, predilection for males, intra-abdominal mass, and dissemination to the meninges) as well as karyotype features [see I C 2 a (1) (a) (i)].

  (3) T-cell ALL accounts for the remaining 15% of cases of ALL. The malignant cells show evidence of T-cell lineage by expression of various T-cell antigens, including the sheep red blood cell receptor, on their surface and by more advanced and definitive rearrangement of the genes for the T-cell antigen receptor. T-cell ALL has a characteristic clinical presentation that includes:

    (a) Occurrence in older children and teenagers

    (b) Predilection for males

    (c) High white blood cell count, often greater than 100,000/mm^3

    (d) Presence of anterior mediastinal mass

    (e) Early dissemination to meninges and testes

4. Prognosis. Presenting clinical and laboratory features for each patient with newly diagnosed ALL determine the probability that the child will remain in remission when treated with current antileukemic therapy. Certain factors (e.g., age, sex, leukemic cell burden as reflected by white blood cell count, immunophenotype, and karyotype) are used to determine prognosis. The Children's Cancer Group assigns patients to good or poor prognosis categories based on the following features (Table 16-4).

a. Good prognosis patients have an 80% or greater chance of cure.

b. Poor prognosis patients have less than a 60% chance of cure.

c. Other factors that may determine prognosis

  (1) Factors that **worsen the prognosis for any type of ALL** include **inadequate therapy, slow response to therapy, male sex, and CNS leukemia at diagnosis**.

  (2) For **non-T, non–B-cell ALL,** certain **karyotypic features** have a strong influence on outcome.

    (a) A **favorable prognosis** is associated with **hyperdiploidy,** especially if there are 53 or more chromosomes within the leukemic cells.

TABLE 16-4. Prognostic Groups in Acute Lymphoblastic Leukemia

	Good (All Required)	Poor (Any Sufficient)
Age	1 through 9 years	Less than 1 year, 10 years or older
White blood cell count	Less than 50,000	50,000 or higher
Lineage	Non-T, non–B-cell	T-cell or B-cell
t9;22	Absent	Present
t4;11	Absent	Present

          (b) Pseudodiploidy due to the presence of certain chromosomal translocations within the leukemic cells is strongly associated with a **poor prognosis**. These translocations include the Philadelphia chromosome t(9;22), which is seen in various types of non-T, non–B-cell ALL [see I C 2 a (1) (b) (ii)]; t(4;11), which is seen in some cases of early pre–B-cell ALL, especially in infants [see I C 2 a (1) (a) (iii)]; and possibly t(1;19), which is seen in some cases of pre–B-cell ALL [see I C 2 a (1) (b) (i)].

          (c) Hypodiploidy, due to less than 46 chromosomes in the leukemic cells, is also associated with a **poor prognosis**.

        (3) Pseudodiploidy is also characteristic of T-cell ALL and B-cell ALL [see I C a (1)].

     d. Morphology affects prognosis. Children whose blasts have a predominantly L1 morphology have a better prognosis than those with blasts with L2 morphology. L3 morphology, because of its association with the B-cell immunophenotype, carries a poor prognosis.

     e. Immunophenotype links certain prognostic features.

        (1) T-cell ALL carries a poor prognosis and is associated with such features as:

          (a) Age 10 years or older

          (b) A high white blood cell count

          (c) Pseudodiploidy

          (d) Predilection for CNS involvement

        (2) CALLA-positive non-T, non–B-cell ALL of the early pre–B-cell type (cytoplasmic immunoglobulin negative) carries a good prognosis and is associated with such features as:

          (a) Occurrence during the 3- to 5-year-old age peak

          (b) Association with a low or normal white blood cell count

          (c) Hyperdiploidy

5. Therapy

     a. Remission induction is successful in over 95% of children. At least three drugs—prednisone, vincristine, and L-asparaginase—are employed; other drugs are added to regimens for patients with a poor prognosis.

     b. Consolidation consists of continued systemic therapy, which may be very intense for poor prognosis patients. Intrathecal therapy with methotrexate, sometimes in conjunction with cranial irradiation, is given for CNS prophylaxis. Radiotherapy adds to the toxicity of CNS therapy and is reserved primarily for select poor prognosis patients. It may cause:

        (1) Learning disabilities, especially in young children

        (2) Transient somnolence syndrome

        (3) Fatal leukoencephalopathy (rare)

        (4) Brain tumors (rare)

     c. Maintenance therapy

        (1) Daily oral 6-mercaptopurine, weekly oral methotrexate, and periodic "reinduction" pulses of prednisone and vincristine is the recommended maintenance therapy for good prognosis patients. During early maintenance therapy, good prognosis patients often undergo a brief period of aggressive therapy termed **delayed intensification,** which is designed to eradicate any leukemic cells that escaped destruction during the initial induction and consolidation phases of therapy.

        (2) Poor prognosis patients should receive more intensive, multiagent therapy.

6. Outcome

     a. Continuous complete remission is the most common outcome for children with ALL and is especially likely in those with a good prognosis.

     b. Relapses still occur in 30%–40% of patients.

        (1) At least one half of relapses occur while initial chemotherapy is still being administered. Relapse can occur in the:

          (a) Bone marrow, which is the most common site of recurrence

          (b) CNS, which was the most common site of recurrence before CNS prophylaxis

          (c) Testes, which are becoming the most common site of extramedullary relapse

(2) Salvage chemotherapy sometimes can retrieve children with:
   (a) Isolated extramedullary relapses in the CNS or testes
   (b) Bone marrow relapses that occur later than 12 months after elective discontinuation of therapy
(3) Current chemotherapy regimens frequently produce additional remissions in children with bone marrow relapses on chemotherapy or within 12 months of its discontinuation, but they are rarely curative. Most of these patients will ultimately die of their ALL unless they can be retrieved by bone marrow transplantation. At least one-third of children with relapsed ALL who can undergo allogeneic transplantation from an HLA-matched relative are cured of their otherwise fatal disease. Results with other types of bone marrow transplants (unrelated HLA-matched, autologous) are not as good.

C. **Acute nonlymphocytic leukemia (ANLL).** ANLL is a malignant disease in which there is accumulation in the marrow of precursors of one or more of the following cell types: granulocytes, monocytes, erythrocytes, or platelets. These precursor cells also spread to the peripheral blood, in which they spread throughout the body and infiltrate all organ systems.

1. **Epidemiology.** ANLL accounts for 20% of all childhood leukemia. It is more common in males than in females and more common in African-American children than in white children. ANLL is not associated with an early childhood peak.

2. **Classification.** The FAB classification uses morphologic and histochemical information to subdivide ANLL into the following subtypes.
   a. **M1 (myeloblastic leukemia without maturation).** The cells have abundant cytoplasm and prominent nucleoli and resemble L2 lymphoblasts. However, they are TdT negative, and they are positive for one or more of the following histochemical stains:
      (1) Peroxidase
      (2) Sudan black B
      (3) Chloroacetate esterase
   b. **M2 (myeloblastic leukemia with differentiation).** The cells have the same histochemical features as M1 cells but also have readily discernible azurophilic granules, which may coalesce into Auer rods.
   c. **M3 (promyelocytic leukemia).** The abundant azurophilic granules in the cells may serve as a source of procoagulant material, which causes DIC and can greatly increase the severity of the bleeding tendency present at initial diagnosis. This form of ANLL is also associated with a distinct cytogenetic abnormality, t(15;17) [see I C 2 a (1) (b) (iii)].
   d. **M4 (myelomonocytic leukemia).** Some of the cells have myeloblastic features by morphology and histochemistry, others have monocytic features and stain for nonspecific esterase, and still others have features of both lineages. M4 with eosinophilia is a distinct subtype associated with:
      (1) Abnormalities of chromosome 16
      (2) Propensity for meningeal involvement
      (3) Good response to chemotherapy
   e. **M5 (monoblastic leukemia)** is characterized by nonspecific esterase-positive cells, propensity for gum and CNS involvement, and association with DIC.
   f. **M6 (erythroleukemia).** The malignant cells are predominantly megaloblastic erythroid precursors, but myeloblasts are also present.
   g. **M7 (megakaryoblastic leukemia),** unlike M1 through M6, cannot be defined by morphologic features alone. Its diagnosis requires one or both of the following:
      (1) Detection of platelet peroxidase by electron microscopy
      (2) Detection of platelet-specific proteins by immunologic techniques

3. **Therapy**
   a. **Remission induction** usually requires more intensive chemotherapy than that administered for ALL. Most regimens use at least an anthracycline and cytosine arabinoside. Myelosuppression is severe, and good supportive care is essential. Remission is achieved in 80% of children.

b. After remission induction, the following options are available:
  (1) Further chemotherapy consisting of:
    (a) Consolidation therapy with intensive systemic therapy and prophylactic therapy to the CNS
    (b) Maintenance therapy, which may not have the same benefit in ANLL that it has in ALL
  (2) Bone marrow transplantation (allogeneic if the patient has an HLA-matched donor, autologous if the patient does not)
c. For acute promyelocytic leukemia (M3), administration of large doses of *trans*-retinoic acid overcomes the block in differentiation and in apoptosis, and causes terminal differentiation and death of the leukemic cells. Retinoic acid alone can induce remission, but the remissions are not durable unless cytoreductive chemotherapy is also administered.

4. Prognosis
  a. The best chemotherapeutic regimens are curative for slightly less than half of the patients.
  b. The best allogeneic bone marrow transplantation regimens are curative for up to two-thirds of the patients.

D. | **Chronic myelogenous leukemia (CML)**

1. Classification. Two types of CML occur during childhood.
  a. Adult CML, which is twice as common as juvenile CML, is a clonal myeloproliferative disorder arising from a neoplastically transformed stem cell. The neoplastic cells almost invariably contain the Philadelphia chromosome t(9;22). This translocation results in fusion of the c-*abl* oncogene on chromosome 9 to the breakpoint cluster region (*bcr*) of chromosome 22. The hybrid c-*abl*/*bcr* region transcribes a novel tyrosine kinase that inhibits apoptosis.
  b. Juvenile CML is a form of myelomonocytic leukemia, which is characterized by a proliferation of cells of monocyte and granulocyte origin. It is not a variant of adult CML, and its cells do not contain the Philadelphia chromosome.

2. Clinical features
  a. Adult CML
    (1) Symptoms. Adult CML occurs in older children and teenagers who present with:
      (a) Lassitude and weight loss from hypermetabolism
      (b) Bone pain
      (c) Increasing abdominal girth from massive splenomegaly
    (2) Characteristic laboratory findings include:
      (a) Extreme hyperleukocytosis, which is characterized by a white cell count greater than 100,000/mm³, a predominance of more mature granulocytes on peripheral smear, and eosinophilia and basophilia
      (b) Normal to increased platelet count
      (c) Mild anemia
      (d) Extreme myeloid hyperplasia in the bone marrow
      (e) The Philadelphia chromosome
  b. Juvenile CML
    (1) Symptoms. Juvenile CML occurs predominantly in children younger than 5 years of age and in males, who present with:
      (a) Suppurative lymphadenopathy
      (b) Moderate hepatosplenomegaly
      (c) Desquamative, erythematous rash
      (d) Purpura
      (e) Pulmonary infiltrates
    (2) Characteristic laboratory findings include:
      (a) Anemia with characteristics of fetal erythropoiesis
      (b) Thrombocytopenia

(c) Moderate hyperleukocytosis, which is characterized by a mean white cell count of 60,000/mm^3 and an increase in monocytes and granulocytes in the peripheral blood

(d) An increase in monocytes and granulocytes and a decrease in megakaryocytes in the bone marrow

3. **Prognosis**
   a. **Adult CML** has a median survival of more than 2 years and can be subdivided into the following phases.
   (1) During **chronic CML,** the disease manifestations can be well controlled by chemotherapy.
   (2) During **accelerated CML,** clinical and laboratory findings show marked deterioration, and patient responsiveness to therapy diminishes.
   (3) During **blastic CML,** which is of short duration, the disease acquires the features of a fatal acute leukemia. Blast crisis can be:
      (a) **Myeloid,** which is more common than lymphoid and usually is unresponsive to further therapy
      (b) **Lymphoid,** which usually is briefly responsive to therapy
   b. **Juvenile CML** is more rapidly fatal, with a median survival of 9 months.

4. **Therapy**
   a. **Chemotherapy** is not curative of either type of childhood CML.
   b. **Bone marrow transplantation** has been curative of both adult and juvenile CML. For patients with adult CML, bone marrow transplantation is much more efficacious if it is done during the chronic phase.
   c. **Interferon** has been shown to decrease the proliferation of the Philadelphia chromosome–positive cells in adult CML. In some patients, there has been a transient decrease or disappearance of Philadelphia chromosome–positive cells from the bone marrow.

III. **NON-HODGKIN LYMPHOMAS** are a heterogeneous group of diseases characterized by neoplastic proliferations of immature lymphoid cells, which, unlike the malignant lymphoid cells of ALL, accumulate primarily outside the bone marrow.

A. **Epidemiology.** Non-Hodgkin lymphomas comprise approximately 6% of all childhood cancers. They occur predominantly in older children and teenagers and have a strong predilection for males.

1. **Childhood non-Hodgkin lymphomas** differ from many adult cases in that they are:
   a. Predominantly extranodal in presentation
   b. As likely to be T-cell lymphomas as B-cell lymphomas
   c. Highly aggressive
   d. Rarely of nodular histology

2. **Burkitt lymphoma** occurs in an endemic form in Africa, where it presents as a mass in the jaw or abdomen. Induction of the B-cell lymphoma in Africa has been linked to a prior Epstein-Barr virus infection occurring in a young child who has been immunosuppressed by malaria or another infection. Burkitt lymphoma and other closely related forms of B-cell lymphoma also develop in children immunosuppressed by HIV infection (see Chapter 9).

B. **Classification**

1. **Morphology.** Almost all cases are diffuse lymphomas and are classified as highly aggressive. The following types occur.
   a. In **lymphoblastic non-Hodgkin lymphoma,** the cells resemble the L1 and L2 cells seen in the usual cases of childhood ALL.

    b. In **nonlymphoblastic non-Hodgkin lymphoma,** the cells resemble transformed cells of the germinal center and may be:
      (1) Small noncleaved or Burkitt-type cells resembling L3 cells
      (2) Large transformed lymphoid cells, which, because of their size, have erroneously been called histiocytes

2. Immunology
    a. T-cell origin is demonstrated in almost half of the cases. The cells generally have a lymphoblastic morphology and contain TdT.
    b. B-cell origin is demonstrated in most other cases. The cells are nonlymphoblastic and lack TdT activity.
    c. Non-T, non–B-cell origin is uncommon.
    d. True histiocytic or nonlymphoid origin is rare.

C. | **Clinical features.** All childhood non-Hodgkin lymphomas are rapidly growing, and thus, symptom duration is short.

1. Anterior mediastinal masses, sometimes associated with pleural effusions, are the most common presentation of T-cell, or lymphoblastic, lymphomas. They can produce:
    a. Respiratory distress from airway compromise
    b. Superior vena cava syndrome [see II A 5 a (5)]

2. Abdominal masses are the most common presentation of B-cell, or nonlymphoblastic, lymphomas. They can cause:
    a. Abdominal enlargement from a rapidly growing tumor, sometimes producing pain, ascites, and urinary tract obstruction
    b. Intestinal obstruction, by serving as the lead point for an intussusception

3. Peripheral lymph node enlargement can be seen with any type of childhood non-Hodgkin lymphoma.

4. Less common presentations include:
    a. Obstructing nasopharyngeal tumor
    b. Bone tumor
    c. Skin tumor

D. | **Staging.** Various systems are employed for different types of childhood non-Hodgkin lymphoma. They all distinguish:

1. Local disease of limited bulk, often confined to one side of the diaphragm and carrying a good prognosis

2. Extensive disease within the mediastinum or abdomen

3. Hematogenous dissemination, especially to the bone marrow and meninges

E. | **Therapy**

1. Extensive surgical debulking (i.e., removal of at least 90% of the tumor) improves survival for individuals with abdominal lymphomas.

2. Systemic chemotherapy is needed in all cases to shrink the local tumor and to prevent dissemination to the bone marrow or to a leukemic phase. The intensity and duration of therapy depend on the type of lymphoma and on the stage of the disease.

3. CNS prophylaxis in some form is required in most patients.

4. Radiotherapy is indicated in treatment sites where there is:
    a. Life-threatening obstruction that does not respond to chemotherapy
    b. Bulk tumor for which chemotherapy alone is judged inadequate

F. Prognosis. With appropriate management of the metabolic consequences of rapid cell turnover [see II A 5 a (3)] and with the institution of therapy, a favorable outcome often is achieved. Without therapy, rapid and widespread dissemination occurs.

1. **T-cell lymphomas** spread to the bone marrow and meninges and then closely resemble T-cell ALL.

2. **B-cell lymphomas** of Burkitt type spread to the bone marrow and meninges and closely resemble B-cell (L3) ALL.

IV. HODGKIN DISEASE in children behaves similarly to the disease in adults.

A. Epidemiology. Hodgkin disease accounts for 4% of all childhood cancer. It occurs in older children and teenagers and has a slight female predominance.

B. Clinical features

1. **Localized adenopathy,** especially in the cervical region, is the most common presenting symptom.

2. **Systemic symptoms** occur in up to 30% of children and consist of:
   a. Temperature exceeding 38°C
   b. Drenching night sweats
   c. Weight loss in excess of 10% of body weight in 6 months

C. Classification based on histopathology divides Hodgkin disease into:

1. **Lymphocyte predominance,** with many lymphocytes and a few Reed-Sternberg cells

2. **Mixed cellularity,** in which there are more Reed-Sternberg cells admixed with a heterogeneous population of reactive cells

3. **Lymphocyte depletion,** with many Reed-Sternberg cells and a few reactive cells

4. **Nodular sclerosis,** in which dense fibrotic bands separate islands of reactive cells and Reed-Sternberg cell variants called **lacunar cells**

D. Staging. Approximate stage can be assigned by a combination of clinical and laboratory tests, but definitive staging often requires exploratory laparotomy with splenectomy, which is indicated if precise staging is needed to determine the type of therapy to be employed. Four stages are defined; however, for any given stage, patients are further subdivided into "A" or "B" depending on the absence (A) or presence (B) of systemic symptoms.

1. **Stage I.** Disease is confined to one group of nodes.

2. **Stage II.** Disease is present in more than one group of nodes but is limited to one side of the diaphragm. Approximately 60% of children have localized (stage I or II) disease.

3. **Stage III.** Disease involves nodes on both sides of the diaphragm, with the spleen considered a node.

4. **Stage IV.** There is hematogenous spread to the liver, bone marrow, lungs, or other nonnodal sites.

E. Therapy and prognosis. Prognosis is good and varies from a 90% cure of stage I disease to a 50% cure of stage IV disease.

1. **Radiotherapy** to involved nodes plus the next node group to which spread could occur is often used for localized disease. For patients treated with radiotherapy alone, chemotherapy can sometimes be used as successful salvage therapy for relapse.

2. Combination chemotherapy is indicated for all stage IV and many stage III patients and for patients with localized but bulky disease, such as a large mediastinal mass. Chemotherapy often is given in conjunction with radiotherapy.

3. Late effects of therapy are numerous. Most serious are:
   a. Secondary malignancies (e.g., ANLL, non-Hodgkin lymphoma) in patients treated with combined radiotherapy and procarbazine-containing chemotherapy regimens
   b. Thyroid gland dysfunction (hypothyroidism, benign and malignant tumors) after neck irradiation
   c. Growth disturbances after irradiation
   d. Sterility

V. **NEUROBLASTOMA** is a malignancy of neural crest cells, which, in the course of their normal development, give rise to the paraspinal sympathetic ganglia and the adrenal medulla.

A. **Epidemiology.** Its 7% incidence makes neuroblastoma the second most common solid tumor of childhood. Only brain tumors are more common. Neuroblastoma occurs predominantly in infants and preschool children, with over half of the patients younger than 2 years of age and one-third younger than 1 year. There is a slight male predominance.

B. **Clinical features** are extremely variable and reflect the widespread distribution of neural crest tissue.

1. Primary sites
   a. Abdominal tumors are the most common presentation, accounting for 70% of the cases; half arise from extra-adrenal tissue and half from the adrenal medulla. Presenting features are:
      (1) Abdominal mass, which often displaces the kidneys anterolaterally and inferiorly
      (2) Abdominal pain
      (3) Systemic hypertension, if there is compression of the renal vasculature
   b. Thoracic tumors are the next most common presentation and are located in the posterior mediastinum. Presenting features are:
      (1) Respiratory distress
      (2) Incidental finding on a chest radiograph that was obtained for unrelated symptoms
   c. Head and neck tumors present as palpable tumors sometimes with **Horner syndrome,** which consists of:
      (1) Miosis
      (2) Ptosis
      (3) Enophthalmos
      (4) Anhidrosis
      (5) Heterochromia of the iris on the affected side
   d. Epidural tumors arise from the posterior growth in dumbbell fashion of abdominal or thoracic tumors. They grow through the neural foramina into the epidural space, where they compress the spinal cord, producing back pain and symptoms of cord compression. Patients with this presentation require rapid evaluation with imaging studies to define the epidural component of the tumor and then therapy to prevent cord ischemia and its neurologic sequelae.

2. Metastases are common at diagnosis and often cause the symptoms that lead to the diagnosis of neuroblastoma.
   a. Nonspecific symptoms of metastatic disease include:
      (1) Weight loss
      (2) Fever
   b. Specific symptoms of metastatic disease include:
      (1) Bone marrow failure (see I E 8)

      (2) Cortical bone pain, resulting in a limp if present in the lower extremity

      (3) Orbit problems, resulting in:

          (a) Proptosis

          (b) Periorbital ecchymoses

      (4) Liver infiltration, causing hepatomegaly

      (5) Distant lymph node enlargement (see I E 4)

      (6) Skin infiltration, causing palpable subcutaneous nodules

  3. Remote effects occasionally are seen.

    a. Watery diarrhea may occur in patients with differentiated tumors, which secrete vasoactive intestinal peptide.

    b. Acute myoclonic encephalopathy is a rare manifestation associated with an excellent prognosis. Patients present with:

      (1) Opsoclonus (rapid eye movements)

      (2) Myoclonus

      (3) Truncal ataxia

C. **Staging** generally follows the pattern described in I F, with the following exceptions.

  1. Stage I and **stage II** tumors must not be large enough to cross the midline.

  2. Stage III tumors cross the midline.

  3. Stage IVS tumors are small primary tumors that occur in young infants with metastases limited to the skin, liver, and bone marrow but not to cortical bone.

D. **Tumor markers** are extremely useful in evaluating children with neuroblastoma.

  1. Urinary markers. Catecholamines are elaborated by most tumors and are useful for diagnosis, for following response to therapy, and for detection of recurrence. Particularly useful markers whose urinary excretion can be measured include:

    a. Vanillylmandelic acid

    b. Homovanillic acid

  2. Serum markers. Elevation of the following serum markers often is associated with a poor prognosis:

    a. Ferritin

    b. Lactic dehydrogenase

  3. Oncogene marker. Amplification of the n-*myc* oncogene within the tumor cells also is associated with a poor prognosis. This oncogene is a member of the *myc* family of oncogenes that encode transcription factors which regulate cell growth [see I C 2 a (1) (a) (i)]. The additional copies of this oncogene contribute to the rapid growth of the poor prognosis neuroblastomas with n-*myc* amplification [see I C 2 a (3)].

E. **Therapy**

  1. Surgery alone often suffices for stage I and stage II patients.

  2. Spontaneous regression without any therapy is common in stage IVS infants. Surgical removal of the small primary tumor is indicated to prevent late local recurrence.

  3. Chemotherapy often can produce dramatic tumor regression in stage III and IV disease, but it is infrequently curative, even when combined with radiotherapy and surgical debulking.

  4. Autologous and allogeneic bone marrow transplantation are being explored for stage III and stage IV patients who have a poor prognosis. Most transplants are autologous and use marrow that has been purged of contaminating neuroblasts by coating them with magnetic beads complexed to neural specific antibodies that attach the beads selectively to the neuroblasts. A magnetic field is used to separate the neuroblasts from the normal marrow cells, which are not coated with magnetic beads.

F. **Prognosis** depends on the following factors.

1. **Age.** Infants younger than 1 year of age have the best prognosis.

2. **Stage**
   a. Stage I and stage II patients and stage IVS infants have a good prognosis.
   b. Most stage III and stage IV patients have a poor prognosis.

3. **Histopathology** may be an important feature. The degree of differentiation of the tumor cells and the pattern of their growth may, in selected cases, influence prognosis.

4. **Tumor markers** (see V D)

VI. **WILMS TUMOR.** Neoplastic embryonal renal cells of the metanephros give rise to this kidney tumor, which is composed of an admixture of cells (blastemal, epithelial, and stromal) in varying proportions. The epithelial cells form tubules.

A. **Epidemiology.** Wilms tumor accounts for 6% of all childhood cancers. It is predominantly a tumor of the first 5 years of life, with an approximately equal incidence throughout each of those 5 years. There is an equal occurrence in males and females.

B. **Clinical features**

1. **Abdominal mass** is by far the most common presentation. On imaging studies, the mass characteristically occurs within the kidneys and displaces and distorts the renal collecting system.

2. **Abdominal pain,** especially with hemorrhage into the tumor, is characteristic. There may be associated fever and anemia.

3. **Hematuria** is not common but, when present, is more often microscopic than gross.

4. **Hypertension** occurs in approximately one-fourth of all patients and may be related to elaboration of renin by tumor cells or, less frequently, to compression of the renal vasculature by the tumor.

5. **Genetic factors** (see I D 1)

6. **Associated abnormalities** that occur in a few patients include:
   a. Hemihypertrophy
   b. Genitourinary tract abnormalities
   c. Mental retardation
   d. Aniridia
      (1) Children with sporadic (as opposed to hereditary) aniridia are at increased risk for development of Wilms tumor. In many of these children, a deletion of the short arm of chromosome 11 can be demonstrated.
      (2) Children with both sporadic aniridia and the chromosome deletion have an almost 50% chance for development of Wilms tumor.
      (3) Children with sporadic aniridia, chromosome deletion, and Wilms tumor may also have mental retardation and genitourinary tract abnormalities, including ambiguous genitalia in affected males.

C. **Staging** is similar to that for other solid tumors (see I F). An additional stage, **stage V,** designates those 5% of patients with tumor in both kidneys. Most patients have relatively localized disease; only 10%–15% of patients have distant metastases at diagnosis.

D. **Diagnosis**

1. **Appropriate imaging studies** are used to define the site of origin within the kidneys and to evaluate the contralateral kidney for tumor.

2. **Search for distant metastases** is undertaken. Sites may include:
   a. Lungs
   b. Liver
   c. Bone (in patients with an unfavorable histology)
   d. Brain (in patients with an unfavorable histology)

E. **Therapy.** Dramatic advances in survival have occurred with the use of combined modality therapy.

1. **Surgery** involves removal of the primary tumor, lymph nodes, and selected metastases.

2. **Radiotherapy** involves treatment of residual local disease and selected metastatic foci.

3. **Chemotherapy** varies in duration and intensity, depending on the patient's stage and histology.
   a. Actinomycin D and vincristine are used to treat all stages of disease.
   b. Additional agents, including doxorubicin, are used to treat patients with a poor prognosis.

F. **Prognosis.** Patients with localized disease and a favorable histology have a greater than 90% chance of survival. Poor prognosis patients have a less than 50% chance of survival.

1. **Stage**
   a. Patients with distant metastases (stage IV) do least well.
   b. Stage V patients often do well with individualized management of their bilateral tumors.

2. **Histopathology**
   a. Ninety percent of patients have a favorable histology, and most, in absence of distant metastases, do very well.
   b. Ten percent have unfavorable histologies and often do poorly, even if their disease is localized. They usually have:
      (1) Anaplastic Wilms tumor
      (2) Sarcomatous Wilms tumor

VII. **SOFT TISSUE SARCOMAS** are tumors of primitive mesenchyme.

A. **Rhabdomyosarcoma** arises from the embryonal mesenchyme from which skeletal muscle originates.

1. **Pathology.** Rhabdomyosarcoma can be divided into two pathologic categories.
   a. **Tumors of favorable histology** occur in 80% of affected children and are predominantly embryonal.
   b. **Tumors of unfavorable histology** occur in the remaining 20% of affected children and are of various subtypes.

2. **Clinical features.** Rhabdomyosarcoma is heterogeneous in presentation. The following are common sites of occurrence.
   a. **Head and neck** (38%)
      (1) **Orbit tumors** have a rapid onset of symptoms owing to their confinement by the bony orbit. They present as:
         (a) Exophthalmos
         (b) Ptosis
         (c) Eyelid swelling
      (2) **Nasopharyngeal and middle ear tumors** are associated with:
         (a) Discharge
         (b) Polypoid mass
         (c) Airway obstruction

       (d) Chronic otitis media

       (e) Spread to the adjacent meninges, causing increased intracranial pressure and cranial nerve palsies

    (3) Neck tumors cause:

       (a) Mass

       (b) Pain

       (c) Cervical and brachial plexus palsy

  b. Genitourinary tract (21%)

    (1) Bladder and prostate tumors cause:

       (a) Urinary obstruction

       (b) Hematuria

    (2) Vaginal and uterine tumors cause:

       (a) Vaginal bleeding

       (b) Polypoid tumor with glistening membrane (sarcoma botryoides, or "cluster of grapes") extruding from the vaginal orifice

  c. Extremity tumors (18%) present as solid masses on the upper or lower extremities.

  d. Miscellaneous presentations occur with a mass or obstructing lesion in the following locations:

    (1) Trunk

    (2) Retroperitoneum

    (3) Paratesticular region

    (4) Perianal region

    (5) Gastrointestinal and biliary tracts

3. Therapy

  a. Surgery

    (1) Complete excision is indicated for those locations where disfigurement will not result.

    (2) If disfigurement would result, chemotherapy, radiotherapy, or both are used as alternatives to surgery or to shrink the tumor to permit easier removal.

  b. Radiotherapy is used for local tumors and metastases.

  c. Chemotherapy is used as an adjuvant to other therapy and for local and metastatic tumors. The intensity of therapy depends on the location, stage, and histology of the tumor.

  d. Irradiation of adjacent meninges is indicated for patients with head and neck tumors that are close to the meninges ("parameningeal"). This prevents meningeal spread and greatly decreases the risk of recurrence in the CNS.

4. Prognosis has dramatically improved over the years by judicious use of all therapeutic modalities.

  a. Children with primary tumors of the orbit have an **excellent** (90%) survival rate without need for disfiguring surgery.

  b. Children with primary tumors of the genitourinary tract often are spared extensive pelvic surgery and still enjoy a good survival rate (as high as 75%).

  c. Poor prognosis is still seen with:

    (1) Extremity tumors

    (2) Retroperitoneal tumors

    (3) Metastatic disease

B. | **Rare soft tissue sarcomas**

1. Fibrosarcomas often arise in the distal portion of the extremities. They are more commonly seen in young children for whom the prognosis is excellent with surgical treatment alone.

2. Liposarcomas also are more common in young children and carry an excellent prognosis, provided that total surgical excision is possible.

3. Synovial sarcomas most commonly develop around the knee joint.

4. **Primitive neuroectodermal tumors** arise from peripheral nerves. These tumors have a characteristic translocation, t(11;22), which is also seen in Ewing sarcoma (see VIII A). Primitive neuroectodermal tumors often present as masses on the chest or extremities. Unlike other rare soft tissue sarcomas, those tumors have a greater metastatic potential and require aggressive systemic chemotherapy.

VIII. BONE TUMORS.
Primary malignant bone tumors account for 4% of childhood cancer. Two highly malignant tumors predominate: Ewing sarcoma and osteogenic sarcoma.

A. **Ewing sarcoma** is an undifferentiated sarcoma of uncertain histogenesis, which arises primarily in bone. A possible neurogenic origin has been suggested for the highly undifferentiated Ewing sarcoma cells because these cells have a t(11;22), which is the same translocation that is found in the cells from primitive neuroectodermal tumors of the peripheral nervous system (see VII B 4). This translocation fuses the transcription factor gene FLI-1 on chromosome 11 to the EWS gene on chromosome 22. A new fusion protein is produced, which leads to tumor formation. Occasionally, Ewing sarcoma arises in the soft tissues of the extremities and paravertebral region rather than in bone, and is referred to as **extraosseous** Ewing sarcoma.

1. **Epidemiology.** Ewing sarcoma is seen primarily in adolescents and is 1.5 times more common in males than females. It is rarely seen in African-Americans.

2. **Clinical features**
   a. Pain and localized swelling are the most common presenting complaints.
   b. Sometimes there are systemic manifestations, including:
      (1) Fever
      (2) Leukocytosis
      (3) Elevated erythrocyte sedimentation rate
   c. Any bone can be affected. Likely sites are:
      (1) Mid- to proximal femur and pelvic bones
      (2) Other long bones, the ribs, and the scapula

3. **Diagnosis**
   a. Radiographs characteristically show a destructive lesion possibly associated with periosteal elevation or a soft tissue mass.
   b. Metastases should be suspected, especially to the lungs and to other bones.

4. **Therapy**
   a. **Radiotherapy** is the usual mode of treatment of the primary tumor.
   b. **Chemotherapy,** which consists of cyclophosphamide and doxorubicin, as well as other agents such as ifosfamide and etoposide, plays an important role in:
      (1) Reduction of primary tumor bulk
      (2) Prevention of metastases
      (3) Treatment of patients with metastases at diagnosis

5. **Prognosis**
   a. The prognosis is very good for patients with distal extremity nonmetastatic tumors treated with chemotherapy and radiotherapy.
   b. The prognosis is poor for patients with:
      (1) Metastatic disease at diagnosis
      (2) Tumors of the pelvic bones
      (3) Tumors in the proximal femur

B. **Osteogenic sarcoma** is a malignant tumor of the bone-producing mesenchyme.

1. **Epidemiology.** Osteogenic sarcoma is the most common primary malignant bone tumor seen in pediatric patients. It is seen mainly in adolescents and is twice as common in males as in females.

2. Clinical features
  a. Pain and swelling are common.
  b. Systemic manifestations are rare.
  c. Half of all cases occur in the proximity of the knee joint.
  d. The most common tumor sites in decreasing order of frequency are:
    (1) Distal femur
    (2) Proximal tibia
    (3) Proximal humerus
    (4) Proximal femur
  e. Metastases are primarily to the lungs.
  f. Radiographic findings include:
    (1) Destructive lesions
    (2) Periosteal reaction, with a characteristic radial "sunburst" as the tumor breaks through the cortex and new bone spicules are produced

3. Therapy
  a. Surgery plays an important role.
    (1) Various limb salvage surgical procedures that limit resection to the tumor-bearing portion of the bone often are performed.
    (2) Amputation is performed when limb salvage is not possible.
  b. Chemotherapy also is of great importance and clearly improves disease-free survival. Particularly effective agents include:
    (1) High-dose methotrexate, which must be given with citrovorum factor rescue
    (2) Doxorubicin
    (3) Cisplatin

4. Prognosis. With aggressive adjuvant chemotherapy, survival is improved to greater than 50%. Aggressive treatment of metastatic disease is indicated because some patients can be salvaged with aggressive chemotherapy and surgical resection of pulmonary metastases.

IX. **BRAIN TUMORS.** Collectively, brain tumors are the **second most common form of childhood cancer,** accounting for 20% of the total. They are of diverse types, each with unique characteristics, locations, and growth rates.

A. **Special problems in management**

1. The blood–brain barrier limits the delivery of chemotherapy by the systemic route.

2. The developing brain of infants and young children is vulnerable to the toxicity of therapeutic modalities (e.g., radiotherapy).

3. The proximity of some tumors to important areas of brain function precludes their extensive surgical resection.

4. There is a tendency for the tumors to spread within rather than outside the neuraxis.

B. **Classification**

1. Location. Two-thirds of brain tumors arise below and one-third arise above the tentorium.

2. Histology. Most brain tumors fall into two distinct groups.
  a. Tumors of astrocytic origin
    (1) High-grade astrocytomas arise primarily above the tentorium and present as:
      (a) Focal neurologic deficits
      (b) Signs of increased intracranial pressure (see I E 7)
      (c) Focal seizures

    (2) Low-grade astrocytomas arise primarily below the tentorium in the cerebellum, where they present as:
      (a) Signs of increased intracranial pressure
      (b) Signs of cerebellar dysfunction (e.g., ataxia, nystagmus)
    (3) Brain stem gliomas present as:
      (a) Multiple cranial nerve palsies
      (b) Ataxia
      (c) Long tract signs

b. Tumors of neuroepithelial origin
    (1) Medulloblastoma is the most common malignant brain tumor in children and characteristically presents as a cerebellar tumor causing:
      (a) Signs of increased intracranial pressure
      (b) Cerebellar dysfunction
      (c) Propensity for rapid spread throughout the neuraxis by the cerebrospinal fluid (CSF) pathways, which is more common in young children and carries a poor prognosis
    (2) Primitive neuroectodermal tumors are much less common than medulloblastomas and are highly malignant. They present as cerebral masses with symptoms similar to those of cerebral astrocytomas.

C. Therapy

1. Surgery plays an important role in the management of tumors whose location permits resection.
  a. Resectable tumors include cerebellar and cerebral tumors.
  b. Brain stem gliomas usually are not resectable, and their location often makes even biopsy hazardous.

2. Radiotherapy plays a major role in the management of tumors in all locations and is indicated for most tumors except for completely resected low-grade astrocytomas.
  a. Unfortunately, the doses delivered often are associated with significant toxicity, which is especially severe in young children, and includes:
    (1) Learning disabilities
    (2) Growth failure
    (3) Primary hypothyroidism when the neck is in the radiation field
  b. For tumors that tend to spread throughout the neuraxis (e.g., medulloblastomas), the whole neuraxis (cranium and spine) must be irradiated.

3. Chemotherapy is a relatively recent addition to the armamentarium and has shown promise in:
  a. Prolonging survival of patients with high-grade astrocytomas
  b. Increasing the cure rate of select patients with medulloblastomas
  c. Controlling tumor growth in infants and young children so that radiation therapy may be postponed to a somewhat later age when it may be less toxic to the developing nervous system.

D. Prognosis

1. The prognosis is **excellent** for completely resected low-grade cerebellar astrocytomas.

2. The prognosis is **good** for many medulloblastomas, particularly if they:
  a. Occur in children older than 4 years of age
  b. Are relatively small in size
  c. Have not spread

3. The prognosis is **poor** for:
  a. Brain stem gliomas
  b. Medulloblastomas that occur in young children are large in size, and spread into the CSF and to distant sites in the neuraxis

X. LIVER TUMORS

A. **Epidemiology.** Liver tumors account for only 1% of childhood cancer. However, they are the most common epithelial malignancy of childhood.

B. **Clinical features.** Liver tumors present as a mass, primarily in the right upper quadrant. They often elaborate α-fetoprotein (AFP), which is a tumor marker useful for diagnosis, for following response to therapy, and for detection of recurrence. Two types of tumors occur.

   1. Hepatoblastoma, the most common type, occurs in infants and young children.
      a. It often is associated with thrombocytosis and metastasizes primarily to the lung.
      b. It has an outcome that depends on whether it can be completely resected.
      c. Hepatoblastoma that is not resectable sometimes may be sufficiently reduced in size by chemotherapeutic agents (e.g., doxorubicin and cisplatin) to permit curative resection.

   2. Hepatocellular carcinoma, which is less common than hepatoblastoma, is seen in older children and teenagers.
      a. It often is multifocal and is less curable than hepatoblastoma.
      b. Hepatocellular carcinoma may be related to a preceding hepatitis B infection, just as in adults.

XI. GERM CELL TUMORS arise from precursors of egg and sperm cells.

A. **Common sites of origin** include the **gonads** (testes, ovaries) and **ectopic sites** (sacrococcyx, anterior mediastinum).

B. **Histologies** represent the degree to which the cells remain pluripotent and undifferentiated.

   1. Multipotential cells form embryonal carcinoma.

   2. Cells with embryonic or somatic differentiation form teratomas, which may be benign or malignant.

   3. Cells with extraembryonic differentiation form:
      a. Yolk sac or endodermal sinus tumors
      b. Trophoblastic tumors or choriocarcinomas

   4. Cells with a commitment to pure germ cell differentiation form:
      a. Seminomas in males (rare in children)
      b. Dysgerminomas in females

C. **Diagnostic markers**

   1. AFP is produced by embryonal carcinomas and endodermal sinus tumors.

   2. Human chorionic gonadotropin is produced by embryonal carcinomas and choriocarcinomas.

D. **Clinical features**

   1. Testicular tumors present as painless intrascrotal swelling and always require radical orchiectomy with high ligation of the spermatic cord. Additional therapy and prognosis depend on:
      a. Age, with most infants younger than 2 years of age having an excellent prognosis with surgery alone
      b. Stage
      c. Histology
      d. Metastatic potential for spread to the retroperitoneal nodes and lungs via the lymphatics and blood, respectively

2. **Ovarian tumors** commonly present as abdominal or pelvic masses. They may sometimes produce severe pain of acute onset that results from torsion of the tumor. Uncommon presentations include precocious puberty or virilism. Therapy includes:
   a. **Complete surgical resection**
   b. **Chemotherapy** for patients with the most common histology, endodermal sinus tumor, and for selected other histologies

3. **Sacrococcygeal germ cell tumors** are the most common germ cell tumors and the most common solid tumor in newborns.
   a. These tumors usually are benign when diagnosed in the first 2 months of life.
   b. Such tumors in older infants and children often are malignant and associated with a poor prognosis.

4. **Mediastinal teratomas** are benign in 80% of cases. They are most likely to be malignant and carry a poor prognosis in older adolescents.

XII. **HISTIOCYTOSIS X** refers to a heterogeneous group of disorders that is characterized by proliferation of histiocytes. The wide range of clinical presentations has made classification confusing and suggests a spectrum of diseases—possibly associated with abnormalities of immune regulation—ranging from indolent to highly aggressive processes. Whether any of the forms of the disease are true malignancies remains disputed. Recent studies, however, indicate that in all types of histiocytosis X there is a monoclonal proliferation of Langerhans cells. This suggests that in its various forms histiocytosis X is a malignant disease with a wide spectrum of clinical behavior ranging from localized, indolent disease to disseminated, aggressive disease.

A. **Histology.** The proliferating histiocytes are dendritic cells. These weakly phagocytic cells are components of the bone marrow–derived mononuclear phagocytic system from which circulating monocytes and phagocytic tissue macrophages also arise. These dendritic cells are called **Langerhans cells**.

1. Langerhans cells primarily are located in the epidermis to which they migrated from the bone marrow.

2. These cells serve as antigen-presenting cells.

3. On electron microscopy, Langerhans cells contain an identifying structure called the **Birbeck granule**.

B. **Etiology.** Although the cause is unknown, an abnormality of immune regulation has been suggested because many cases are associated with dysmorphic changes in the thymus.

C. **Clinical features**

1. **Eosinophilic granuloma** is a benign and self-limited disease. It is uncommon in infants. Eosinophilic granuloma usually is limited to a single bone lesion that is painful and located in the femur or skull.

2. **Hand-Schüller-Christian disease** is a more chronic and extensive disease. It also is uncommon in infants. Hand-Schüller-Christian disease commonly involves the bone and skin. It occasionally presents as a classic triad of:
   a. Skeletal lesions
   b. Diabetes insipidus
   c. Exophthalmos

3. **Letterer-Siwe disease** is an acute disease that often terminates in fatal sepsis. It occurs in infants.
   a. Letterer-Siwe disease involves the skin, liver, spleen, lymph nodes, bone marrow, and lungs.

    b. Bone lesions are less striking than in the other forms of histiocytosis X.

    c. A poor outcome is heralded by dysfunction of one or more of the following: lungs, liver, and bone marrow.

XIII. **RETINOBLASTOMA** is a rare congenital malignancy that arises from neural tissue within the retina.

A. **Genetic factors** [see I D 1 a (1)]

B. **Clinical features**

1. Usually there is an abnormal white pupil, or **"cat's eye,"** and strabismus sometimes is present.

2. Most tumors are localized to the globe at diagnosis. Metastases occur late and spread to the:
   a. Meninges via the optic nerve
   b. Bone marrow and cortical bone via the blood

C. **Therapy** is highly specialized. The goal is to cure and to preserve useful vision whenever possible.

1. **Surgical enucleation** is indicated for:
   a. Most cases of unilateral disease
   b. The most severely involved eye in bilateral cases

2. **Radiotherapy** is indicated to:
   a. Treat any residual orbital disease
   b. Manage the remaining eye in bilateral cases along with other physical modalities (e.g., laser therapy, cryotherapy)

3. **Chemotherapy** is used in select cases as:
   a. An adjuvant
   b. Palliative treatment for the few patients with disseminated disease

D. **Prognosis**

1. The prognosis is **excellent** for those cases that are limited to the eyes.

2. There is a **poor** prognosis with dissemination.

BIBLIOGRAPHY

Cline MJ: The molecular basis of leukemia. *N Engl J Med* 330:328–336, 1994.

Crist WM, Kun LE: Common solid tumors of childhood. *N Engl J Med* 324:461–471, 1991.

Ferrara JLM, Deeg HJ: Graft-versus-host disease. *N Engl J Med* 324:667–674, 1991.

Pul CH, Behm FG, Crist WM: Clinical and biologic relevance of immunologic marker studies in childhood acute lymphoblastic leukemia. *Blood* 82:343–362, 1993.

Quinn JJ: Bone marrow transplantation in the management of childhood cancer. *Pediatr Clin North Am* 32:811–833, 1985.

Rivera GK, Pinkel D, Simone JV, et al: Treatment of acute lymphoblastic leukemia: 30 years' experience at St. Jude Children's Research Hospital. *N Engl J Med* 329:1289–1295, 1993.

Seeger RC, Reynolds CP: Treatment of high-risk solid tumors of childhood with intensive therapy and autologous bone marrow transplantation. *Pediatr Clin North Am* 38:393–424, 1991.

Tubergen DG, Gilchrist GS, O'Brien RT, et al: Improved outcome with delayed intensification for children with acute lymphoblastic leukemia and intermediate presenting features: a Children's Cancer Group phase III trial. *J Clin Oncol* 11:527–537, 1993.

DIRECTIONS: Each of the numbered items or incomplete statements in this section is followed by answers or by completions of the statement. Select the ONE lettered answer or completion that is BEST in each case.

1. An 11-year-old boy with hemophilia presents with a large left supraclavicular mass that has grown over a 3-week period. He has received many transfusions in the past but does not have a factor VIII inhibitor. The mass does not regress with factor VIII therapy. The most likely diagnosis is

(A) non-Hodgkin lymphoma
(B) metastatic neuroblastoma
(C) Kaposi sarcoma
(D) acute nonlymphocytic leukemia (ANLL)
(E) hemorrhage into the tissues of the supra-clavicular region

2. A 2-year-old boy presents with a large left-sided abdominal mass, which, on intravenous pyelogram, appears to arise within the left kidney and to distort and displace the collecting system. On chest radiography, multiple pulmonary nodules are present. The most likely diagnosis is

(A) neuroblastoma
(B) Wilms tumor
(C) non-Hodgkin lymphoma
(D) rhabdomyosarcoma
(E) hepatoblastoma

Questions 3–5

An 8-year-old girl presents with fever, numerous bruises over her entire body, and pain in both legs. Physical examination reveals pallor, a soft midsystolic murmur, the spleen at 2 cm below the left costal margin, and ecchymoses and petechiae on the face, trunk, and extremities. Findings on complete blood count (CBC) include a hemoglobin of 6.3 g/dl, white blood cell count (WBC) of 2800/mm^3 (10% neutrophils, 1% bands, 2% monocytes, 87% lymphocytes), and platelet count of 29,000/mm^3.

3. Which of the following would be the most appropriate initial diagnostic test?

(A) Heterophile antibody
(B) Bone marrow aspiration
(C) Sedimentation rate
(D) Skeletal survey
(E) Liver and spleen scan

4. If the patient's bone marrow were replaced by common acute lymphocytic leukemia antigen (CALLA)-positive lymphoblasts with L1 morphology, her risk of relapse would be

(A) high
(B) low
(C) undetermined
(D) zero

5. If the patient were to become febrile to 39.5°C, appropriate responses would include all of the following EXCEPT

(A) to administer aspirin for the fever
(B) to obtain a blood culture
(C) to obtain a chest radiograph
(D) to obtain a urine culture
(E) to start intravenous broad-spectrum antibiotics

6. A 7-year-old boy with T-cell acute lympho-blastic leukemia (ALL) in bone marrow remis-sion presents with headache, vomiting, stiff neck, and papilledema. He has no other abnormalities on physical examination. The most likely diagnosis is

(A) meningeal relapse
(B) adverse reaction to cranial irradiation
(C) bacterial meningitis
(D) superior vena cava syndrome
(E) intracranial hemorrhage

7. A 10-year-old girl presents with a 2-day his-tory of fever and a 4-cm warm, tender, and fluctuant left anterior cervical lymph node. The most likely diagnosis is

(A) Hodgkin disease
(B) acute lymphoblastic leukemia (ALL)
(C) histiocytosis X
(D) acute bacterial lymphadenitis
(E) metastatic neuroblastoma

Questions 8–10

A 2-year-old boy presents with bilateral prop-tosis and periorbital ecchymoses, a large right flank mass, and lower back and right arm pain. Evaluation demonstrates moderate ane-mia, a large right-sided mass that is distinct from the right kidney, clumps of primitive cells in the bone marrow, and bone scan showing increased activity in the right humerus, left and right orbits, and L1–L3 vertebrae.

8. The most likely diagnosis is

(A) histiocytosis X
(B) rhabdomyosarcoma
(C) neuroblastoma
(D) Wilms tumor
(E) lymphoblastic lymphoma

9. Laboratory features that may be associated with this disease include all of the following EXCEPT

(A) increased urinary vanillylmandelic acid excretion
(B) amplification of c-*myc* oncogene in the involved cells
(C) elevation of serum ferritin
(D) translocation (9;22) in the involved cells
(E) leukoerythroblastic peripheral blood smear

The patient experiences increased back pain and is unable to walk. Neurologic examina-tion reveals decreased strength in the lower extremities.

10. Management of this patient should begin with

(A) analgesic therapy for bone metastases with a nonsteroidal anti-inflammatory agent
(B) lumbar puncture
(C) imaging studies to evaluate the dorsolum-bar epidural space
(D) careful, serial neurologic examinations
(E) physical therapy to decrease lumbar mus-cle spasm and increase strength of lower extremity muscles

1. The answer is A *[I D 2 b; III A–C]*. The most likely diagnosis is non-Hodgkin lymphoma. The boy described in this case is at high risk for contracting a human immunodeficiency virus (HIV) infection and may, as a consequence, develop an acquired immune deficiency syndrome (AIDS)–associated, aggressive B-cell lymphoma. Kaposi sarcoma occurs less commonly than lymphoma in pediatric patients with AIDS. Metastatic neuroblastoma can present in this fashion, but the boy's age and hemophilia make this unlikely. Acute nonlymphocytic leukemia (ANLL) usually does not produce this degree of adenopathy, and would be unusual in a hemophiliac. Hemorrhage always is a possible diagnosis in a child with hemophilia, but failure of the mass to respond to appropriate treatment and absence of an inhibitor interfering with response to treatment make this very unlikely.

2. The answer is B *[VI B, D]*. The most likely diagnosis is Wilms tumor. The classic radiographic appearance of Wilms tumor is an abdominal mass that occurs within the kidney, distorting and replacing the renal collecting system; metastases to the lungs are noted on chest radiography. Neuroblastoma arises above the kidney and displaces it anterolaterally and inferiorly, and rarely metastasizes to the lungs. B-cell non-Hodgkin lymphomas often arise in the abdomen but not from the kidney, and they do not produce nodular pulmonary metastases. Rhabdomyosarcomas may arise in the retroperitoneum but are much rarer than Wilms tumor and are extrarenal. They do spread to the lungs. Hepatoblastomas most commonly arise in the right rather than left lobe of the liver and produce right-sided masses. They should not distort the intrarenal architecture. They do, however, metastasize to the lungs.

3–5. The answers are: 3-B *[I E 8 a; II A 3 a–c, 4 b]*, **4-B** *[II B 4 a; Table 16-4]*, **5-A** *[III A 3 a (2), (3), 5 a (2)]*. This child's presentation is typical of acute lymphoblastic leukemia (ALL). She has signs and symptoms of anemia and thrombocytopenia as well as bone pain and splenomegaly, and her complete blood count (CBC) values indicate pancytopenia. In this situation, bone marrow aspiration is the most appropriate test to see whether the bone marrow can produce adequate numbers of blood cells and, if not, whether the marrow is aplastic or replaced by malignant cells. A heterophile

antibody would be useful only if infectious mononucleosis were a strong possibility. Splenomegaly, immune thrombocytopenia, and hemolytic anemia can be seen with mononucleosis, but leukopenia and bone pain would not be expected to occur with a typical Epstein-Barr virus infection. The sedimentation rate is not a specific enough test to be useful in this patient, and would not provide a diagnosis. Skeletal survey may show leukemic lines, but their presence or absence cannot substitute for bone marrow examination, which is much more definitive and provides material for diagnosis of the specific type of leukemia. Liver and spleen scan would show splenic enlargement but would not provide a specific diagnosis.

A low white blood cell count (WBC), age of 8 years, and L1 morphology of lymphoblasts are typical of good-prognosis ALL. There are no high-risk features in this patient, such as a high WBC, age younger than 1 year or equal to or greater than 10 years, or T- or B-cell immunophenotype. Even with good-prognosis ALL, relapse occurs in 20% of cases and, therefore, risk is certainly greater than zero.

Aspirin should not be used as an antipyretic in a thrombocytopenic patient because salicylates interfere with platelet function and would worsen the bleeding tendency. Prompt institution of intravenous broad-spectrum antibiotics, however, is mandatory in the febrile, neutropenic patient. Blood and urine cultures should be obtained before initiating antibiotic therapy. A chest radiograph also should be performed to detect any infiltrates.

6. The answer is A *[I E 7; II B 3 b (3)]*. Meningeal leukemia is common in T-cell acute lymphoblastic leukemia (ALL). Meningeal relapse, which produces increased intracranial pressure, can occur in some patients with T-cell ALL even if they have received prophylactic therapy to the central nervous system (CNS). Cranial irradiation does not cause increased intracranial pressure. Acute bacterial meningitis can produce this symptom, but it would be rare in a leukemic child. Superior vena cava obstruction from a mediastinal mass is a possible but less common cause of increased intracranial pressure in a patient with T-cell ALL, and should be associated with facial plethora and signs of airway compromise. Intracranial hemorrhage may produce similar symptoms but would be uncommon, especially in a patient in remission who is unlikely to be severely thrombocytopenic and at risk for intracranial hemorrhage.

7. The answer is D *[I E 4 a].* Fever and signs of suppuration strongly suggest an acute bacterial infection. Hodgkin disease, acute lymphoblastic leukemia (ALL), histiocytosis X, and metastatic neuroblastoma may be associated with fever and adenopathy; however, their onset would not be as acute as that seen with acute bacterial lymphadenitis, and suppuration would be an unlikely presenting problem. Furthermore, histiocytosis X in this age-group is much more likely to involve the bones than the lymph nodes, and metastatic neuroblastoma is uncommon in children of this age.

8–10. The answers are: 8-C *[V B 1 a, 2 b],* **9-D** *[II D 1 a],* **10-C** *[V B 1 d].* This is a typical presentation of stage IV neuroblastoma, with the primary tumor arising from one of the paravertebral sympathetic ganglia and metastasizing to bone marrow, cortical bone, and the retroorbital tissues. Histiocytosis X may have a somewhat similar presentation and involve multiple bones, but it usually involves one rather than both orbits; the right flank mass and tumor clumps in the marrow of this patient also are not characteristic of histiocytosis X. Rhabdomyosarcoma may arise in the orbit but usually is unilateral; the tumor also rarely is associated with systemic metastases at initial diagnosis. Wilms tumor would produce a right renal rather than suprarenal mass and would metastasize to the lungs rather than to bone and bone marrow. Lymphoblastic lymphoma usually arises in the anterior mediastinum or peripheral nodes. Even if it were to present with widespread dissemination, abdominal rather than thoracic disease would be unusual and lymphoblasts rather than tumor clumps would be seen in the marrow.

The Philadelphia chromosome contains translocation (9;22) and is seen in adult chronic myelogenous leukemia (CML), not neuroblastoma. Increased urinary excretion of catecholamine metabolites (e.g., vanillylmandelic acid) is common in neuroblastoma. In many cases of neuroblastoma, the cells demonstrate amplification of the c-*myc* oncogene and elevated levels of ferritin are detected in serum. The presence of either or both of these findings often worsens the prognosis for neuroblastoma patients. Patients with marrow metastases from neuroblastoma often have leukoerythroblastic changes demonstrable on peripheral blood smear.

The development of back pain, inability to walk, and decreased lower extremity strength indicate a medically emergent situation in which the tumor has grown posteriorly through the intervertebral foramina into the epidural space. In this location, the tumor can compress the spinal cord and produce irreversible damage from ischemia to the cord. Prompt evaluation with a magnetic resonance imaging (MRI) or computed tomography (CT) scan is needed to detect the tumor in the epidural space. Lumbar puncture would not be useful unless it were combined with myelography to detect the encroachment on the cord. Institution of analgesic therapy or physical therapy would be inappropriate in this situation, as would serial neurologic examinations. Speed in establishing a diagnosis and in preventing permanent cord damage is critical.

Chapter 17

Endocrine and Metabolic Disorders
Susan K. Ratzan

I. DISORDERS OF CARBOHYDRATE METABOLISM

A. **Diabetes mellitus** is a heterogeneous group of disorders characterized by hyperglycemia and abnormal energy metabolism, caused by absent or diminished insulin secretion or action at the cellular level. **Insulin-dependent diabetes mellitus (IDDM), type I,** is the most common endocrine–metabolic disease in childhood, occurring in 1 in 500 children and adolescents. **Noninsulin-dependent diabetes mellitus (NIDDM), type II,** also occurs in childhood, but it is much less frequently diagnosed because of its milder or absent symptoms. Diabetes mellitus may be associated with other diseases or syndromes, such as cystic fibrosis (see Chapter 11), Prader-Willi syndrome (see Chapter 8), and Werner syndrome. A rare, usually transient form of IDDM may be seen in the newborn.

1. **IDDM**
   a. **Etiology.** Although the precise etiology of IDDM is unknown, the pathologic process that ultimately results in the loss of insulin secretion by the beta cells in the islets of Langerhans has been related to genetic, autoimmune, and environmental factors.
      (1) **Genetic factors**
         (a) There is an increased frequency of certain histocompatibility antigens [i.e., human leukocyte antigens (HLAs) DR3 and DR4] among individuals with IDDM. When both DR3 and DR4 are inherited, the relative risk for development of IDDM is additive.
         (b) There is an increased incidence of IDDM among first-degree relatives; IDDM will develop in 2%–5% of siblings and offspring. Concordance for identical twins is 30%.
      (2) **Autoimmune factors.** Evidence for an autoimmune basis for the disease consists of the presence of circulating islet cell antibodies in the serum of over 60%–80% of individuals with recent-onset IDDM and the increased appearance of the other autoimmune diseases (e.g., Hashimoto thyroiditis, Addison disease, celiac disease) in children with IDDM.
      (3) **Environmental factors.** The role of environmental factors in the pathogenesis of IDDM is less well understood. Although viruses have long been suspected to play a role, it is unlikely that a single virus is directly responsible for the development of the disease in all cases.
   b. **Pathophysiology** (Figure 17-1)
      (1) When 90% of the functioning beta cells have been destroyed, loss of insulin secretion becomes clinically significant. With the loss of insulin, the major anabolic hormone, a catabolic state develops, which is characterized by **decreased glucose utilization and increased glucose production** via gluconeogenesis and glycogenolysis, leading to **hyperglycemia**. In the state of insulin deficiency, levels of counterregulatory hormones (i.e., glucagon, epinephrine, growth hormone, and cortisol) are elevated. These hormones stimulate lipolysis, fatty acid release, and ketoacid production.
      (2) When the blood glucose concentration is persistently above the renal threshold for glucose reabsorption (i.e., 180 mg/dl), the resultant **glucosuria** causes an osmotic diuresis with increased urine output and increased fluid intake. Ketones

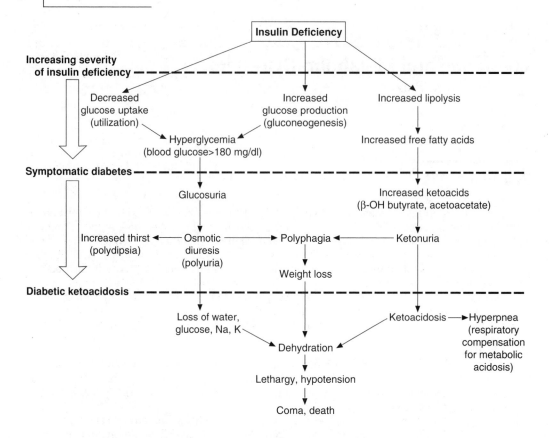

FIGURE 17-1. Pathophysiology of diabetic ketoacidosis.

are produced in abundant amounts when insulin deficiency is severe. If insulin treatment is not initiated, **diabetic ketoacidosis** ensues. This deranged metabolic state is characterized by hyperglycemia, metabolic acidosis (ketoacidosis), dehydration, and lethargy, which may progress to coma and death.

c. **Clinical features.** Although IDDM may present at any age, the most common time is in early adolescence. Typically, the child manifests frequent urination (**polyuria**) and increased thirst (**polydipsia**). Symptoms may wax and wane for a period of days or weeks but eventually become constant. Nocturia or enuresis may occur. If the disease is not discovered, significant **weight loss** may result, and with increasing insulin deficiency, the odor of ketones on the breath may be noted. Nausea, abdominal pain, and vomiting are symptoms of **diabetic ketoacidosis** and result in severe **dehydration**.

d. **Diagnosis** of IDDM in a child with polyuria, polydipsia, and glucosuria who is otherwise well rests on **documentation of hyperglycemia**.

(1) A **random blood glucose level** greater than 200 mg/dl, which is verified on a repeat test, is sufficient to make the diagnosis of IDDM.

(2) Early in the course of the disease, glucosuria and hyperglycemia may be transient. In this situation, a **fasting and 2-hour postmeal blood glucose** measurement may be helpful in making the diagnosis, if the fasting glucose level is higher than 140 mg/dl and the 2-hour glucose level is higher than 200 mg/dl. The presence of islet cell antibodies in the serum, increased levels of glycosylated hemoglobin, a family history of IDDM, or all three features may increase suspicion of developing IDDM. However, absence of these features does not rule out IDDM.

(3) A standard oral glucose tolerance test is not indicated if fasting hyperglycemia is present or if a random or 2-hour postmeal glucose level is greater than 200 mg/dl.

e. Therapy. The immediate goal of treatment is to **restore fluid and electrolyte losses,** either orally or intravenously, depending on the severity of the illness, and to **reverse the catabolic state** by replacing insulin.

(1) Insulin replacement

(a) Dosage. The usual insulin-dependent child or adolescent requires 0.75–1.0 U/kg of insulin daily when the diabetes is fully developed. However, early in the course of the disease, the requirement may be less than 0.5 U/kg/day, especially during the "honeymoon," or remission, phase of IDDM. For this reason, the initial dose should be tailored to the estimated degree of insulin deficiency and calculated for the child's weight (i.e., a ketonuric child or one who initially presented with ketoacidosis should be given 0.5 U/kg/day after the ketoacidosis is cleared).

(i) The total daily dose is divided between short-acting regular insulin and intermediate-acting [isophane insulin suspension (NPH) or Lente] insulin in a 1:3 proportion. It is conventional to give two-thirds of the daily dose before breakfast and one-third before the evening meal.

(ii) More intensive insulin replacement plans consist of multiple (three to four) doses of regular insulin before meals supplemented with intermediate-acting insulin once or twice daily.

(b) Source. Most children with IDDM now receive recombinant human insulin as opposed to insulin derived from animal sources (beef/pork or pork). Human insulin is less immunogenic than animal-source insulin.

(2) Diet. The principles of sound nutritional practices are the basis for diet and meal planning for children with IDDM.

(a) A meal plan that promotes normal growth and weight gain, that incorporates the prudent recommendations of the American Heart Association concerning fat intake, and that encourages high-fiber foods is appropriate. The American Diabetes Association Exchange Diet incorporates these healthful practices and provides consistency in type and distribution of calories throughout the day while allowing flexibility of food choices.

(b) Because food intake must match the time course of insulin absorption, meals and snacks must be roughly equivalent in calories from day to day and must be eaten on time. During and after periods of heavy exercise, increased food intake may be required to avoid hypoglycemia.

(3) Exercise. Children with IDDM should be encouraged to exercise regularly. Because strenuous exercise may result in hypoglycemia due to increased noninsulin-dependent uptake of glucose, physical education classes are best scheduled after meals, or extra food should be eaten before exercise. There should be no restrictions on individual or organized athletic programs because of IDDM.

(4) Patient education. Children with IDDM and their families should be taught the principles of home management by trained diabetes educators. This training should be individualized and include the pathophysiology of diabetes in lay language, the techniques of insulin injection and home blood glucose monitoring, the recognition and treatment of hypoglycemia and hyperglycemia, the significance of ketonuria, and the management of diabetes during intercurrent illness. Eventually, the child and family should learn how to make minor insulin dose changes. Education is an ongoing process, and periodic reinforcement is important as the child grows older and more independent of the family.

(5) Psychological support and counseling. The diagnosis of IDDM arouses strong emotional responses in the child and in family members, including grief, anger, guilt, resentment, and fear. Although these responses are normal, adjustment to the disease is facilitated by open discussion of these emotions.

(6) Medical follow-up. Regular follow-up visits every 3–4 months to a pediatrician with expertise in diabetes or to a regional pediatric diabetes program are indicated.

    (a) The glycosylated hemoglobin level should be measured as an objective index of blood glucose control over the preceding 2 months, and lipid levels should be measured periodically.

    (b) Because of the increased risk of autoimmune thyroid disease in children with IDDM, periodic assessment of thyroid function, including thyroxine level, T_3 resin uptake, thyroid-stimulating hormone (TSH) levels, and thyroid autoantibody determination should be carried out (see III A 2).

    (c) Although long-term complications of diabetes are rare during childhood, blood pressure measurement and funduscopic examination should be performed during each visit.

    (d) For adolescents who have had diabetes for more than 5 years, a more rigorous examination for retinopathy, nephropathy, and neuropathy should be carried out.

f. Complications of IDDM may be divided into **immediate complications,** which include hypoglycemia and diabetic ketoacidosis, and **late complications,** which are those generally associated with a long duration of IDDM.

  (1) Hypoglycemia (insulin reaction)

    (a) Symptoms of hypoglycemia may be related to sympathetic discharge (e.g., sweating, tremulousness, hunger) and should be readily recognizable by the child or family. More severe symptoms (e.g., lethargy, bizarre behavior, slurred speech, unconsciousness, seizures) are caused by glucose deprivation to the central nervous system (CNS). These may occur in combination with sympathetic symptoms or alone.

    (b) Therapy should be aimed at raising the blood glucose level above 100 mg/dl. The child should consume 4 oz of calorie-containing drink or food if he or she is able to swallow. When neuroglycopenic symptoms occur, the child needs assistance in treatment of the hypoglycemia episode. If the child is unconscious or having seizures, 1 mg of glucagon should be injected intramuscularly.

  (2) Diabetic ketoacidosis is caused by relative or absolute insulin deficiency, which results in **hyperglycemia** and **metabolic acidosis with respiratory compensation**. The most common cause of diabetic ketoacidosis in a known diabetic is **omission of insulin doses**. The condition may be triggered by intercurrent illness, which may be associated with some degree of insulin resistance.

    (a) Symptoms are polyuria, polydipsia, fatigue, headache, dry mouth, nausea, abdominal pain, and vomiting. Lethargy may progress to obtundation and coma.

    (b) Physical findings include tachycardia and hyperpnea (Kussmaul respirations), the respiratory compensation for metabolic acidosis; hypotension indicates marked dehydration and intravascular volume depletion. The child appears acutely ill, anxious, and dehydrated. The abdomen is mildly tender but without rebound or localized tenderness. Bowel sounds may be diminished. Physical examination must rule out intercurrent illness or infection.

    (c) Laboratory studies should include a complete blood count and determination of electrolyte, glucose, blood urea nitrogen (BUN), and creatinine levels, and, in more severe illness, arterial blood gas determination.

      (i) The hemoglobin and hematocrit usually are increased because of hemoconcentration. The white cell count may show marked leukocytosis (> 20,000), with a predominance of neutrophils and immature forms as a result of the metabolic stress.

      (ii) The serum sodium level usually is low or normal. A low serum sodium level may be caused by dilution from the osmotic effect of marked hyperglycemia (i.e., a glucose level > 700 mg/dl) or "pseudohyponatremia," an artifact of measurement if the patient's serum is lipemic.

      (iii) The serum potassium level usually is normal or high and does not reflect total body potassium depletion. A low serum potassium level (< 3.5 mEq/L) indicates profound potassium depletion and potential for life-threatening hypokalemia during the early course of treatment of diabetic ketoacidosis.

(iv) The bicarbonate level is low, ranging from 2–19 mEq/L, depending on the severity and duration of the illness.

(v) The BUN level may be considerably elevated on the basis of prerenal azotemia; the serum creatinine level is normal or minimally elevated.

(vi) Arterial blood gases indicate metabolic acidosis with respiratory compensation; pH typically is 6.9–7.3. Oxygen partial pressure (Po_2) is greater than 95 mm Hg (normal); carbon dioxide partial pressure (Pco_2) is less than 30 mm Hg (low) as the patient blows off carbon dioxide in an attempt to buffer the metabolic acid.

(d) **Therapy** should be carried out in an intensive care unit with frequent monitoring of the vital signs, neurologic status, and fluid input and output. If the patient is not alert, a nasogastric tube should be placed to empty stomach contents and prevent aspiration.

(i) The first aim of therapy is to replace fluids and electrolytes and to reexpand the vascular volume. The latter may be accomplished by an infusion of 10–20 ml/kg of normal saline over 2 hours.

(ii) The next consideration is insulin replacement. For all patients except those with mild diabetic ketoacidosis (i.e., a bicarbonate level > 15 mEq/L), continuous infusion of intravenous regular (crystalline) insulin is the most easily controlled and predictable. A priming intravenous dose of 0.1 U/kg of regular insulin is immediately followed by 0.1 U/kg/hour of regular insulin.

(iii) After the initial bolus of normal saline has been infused, half normal saline at a rate of one and one-half to twice the maintenance rate usually is adequate to begin to replace deficits. To this solution, 5%–10% dextrose should be added to maintain the blood glucose level between 200 and 300 mg/dl.

(iv) Vigorous replacement of potassium, using 40 mEq/L of potassium chloride, should begin as soon as urine output is established and the serum potassium level is less than 5 mEq/L.

(v) Correction of the acidosis with bicarbonate is controversial. Rapid infusion of bicarbonate is contraindicated because it may cause deterioration of neurologic function and depression of cerebrospinal fluid pH. In severe diabetic ketoacidosis (pH < 7.10), bicarbonate may be given over a period of 4 hours for partial correction of the acidosis.

(e) **Complications of diabetic ketoacidosis** include hypoglycemia, hypokalemia, and cerebral edema, which, although rare, is frequently fatal. A worsening mental status, confusion, unequal pupils, decerebrate posture, or seizures indicate cerebral edema. Early recognition and aggressive treatment to decrease intracranial pressure are associated with an improved outcome.

(3) **Late complications of IDDM.** There is evidence that long-term complications are related to chronic hyperglycemia, and improved glycemic control results in a decreased rate of development of complications. Efforts to maintain near-normal blood glucose must be balanced with the increased risk of hypoglycemia, especially in children and adolescents.

(a) Complications associated with a long duration (i.e., > 10 years) of IDDM include **microvascular disease** of the eye (**retinopathy**), the kidney (**nephropathy**), and the nerves (**neuropathy**). These problems may be seen in the older adolescent patient.

(b) The other major category of late complications is **large vessel atherosclerotic complications,** leading to premature myocardial infarction and stroke.

g. **Future directions of research in IDDM** include development of an implantable insulin pump, islet cell and whole pancreas transplantation, predicting diabetes risk and preventing diabetes in the high-risk person, and an improved understanding of the genetic and environmental factors in IDDM.

2. **NIDDM** occurs in children and adolescents, but because it is **usually asymptomatic,** it is infrequently diagnosed. In some families, NIDDM appears to be inherited as an autosomal dominant trait.

   a. **Etiology.** NIDDM is caused by insulin deficiency that is more modest than that in IDDM, and occasionally by resistance to insulin action, with normal or increased insulin secretion but decreased insulin receptors.

   b. **Therapy** consists of **maintenance of normal body weight.** Insulin treatment is indicated if there is fasting hyperglycemia (i.e., a glucose concentration > 140 mg/dl). Oral hypoglycemic agents usually are not used in children and adolescents.

B. **Hypoglycemia.** A variety of conditions and disease states may disrupt glucose homeostasis and result in hypoglycemia. Certain causes of hypoglycemia are more common at some ages than at others. This knowledge provides a useful way of approaching and understanding hypoglycemia in infancy and childhood.

1. **Glucose homeostasis.** Blood glucose is the major energy source for all tissues, and maintenance of normal glucose homeostasis is critical for efficient energy metabolism. Glucose homeostasis depends on the interplay of endocrine and metabolic or enzymatic processes that control glucose uptake and utilization, as well as on glucose production during periods of feeding and fasting to ensure a continuous supply.

   a. Blood glucose in the fetus depends on transplacental passage of maternal glucose and substrate reserves. At birth, the newborn is abruptly cut off from the maternal supply of glucose and depends on oral intake of calories and his or her own endocrine and metabolic function for maintenance of normal glucose levels.

   b. During the adjustment to extrauterine life, blood glucose levels are somewhat lower without apparent ill effects. Premature infants and infants with a low birth weight have slightly lower blood glucose levels than full-term infants.

   c. There is disagreement over the definition of hypoglycemia in infants and children and whether low blood glucose level is "normal" for premature infants. Thus, it is prudent to initiate therapy for any infant with a blood glucose below 40 mg/dl and to monitor closely any infant with a blood glucose of 40–50 mg/dl.

2. **Hypoglycemia in the newborn** has a varied presentation (see Chapter 6 V J).

3. **Hypoglycemia in infants and children.** Hypoglycemia beyond the neonatal period is quite rare. Hyperinsulinism, growth hormone (GH) deficiency, hypocortisolism secondary to **adrenocorticotropic hormone (ACTH) deficiency,** and primary adrenal insufficiency (**Addison disease**) may present as symptomatic hypoglycemia. Certain hepatic enzyme deficiencies, which result in impaired glycogenolysis or gluconeogenesis, may present during infancy as profound metabolic acidosis, ketonuria, and hypoglycemia. These deficiencies include glycogen storage disease types I, III, and IV; hereditary fructose intolerance; fructose 1,6-diphosphatase deficiency; and galactosemia. The presence of marked hepatomegaly with failure to thrive and hypotonia should suggest one of these defects; the actual diagnosis may require liver biopsy for assay of the specific enzyme.

   a. **Ketotic hypoglycemia.** In children 1–4 years of age, the most common cause of hypoglycemia is ketotic hypoglycemia. The typical child with this form of hypoglycemia is a toddler who has had one or more episodes of early morning lethargy, pallor, and sweating, with or without a seizure. The blood glucose level during an episode is lower than 40 mg/dl. Large amounts of ketones are present in the urine. The child is otherwise well. Episodes are associated with a decreased intake of food due to intercurrent illness.

      (1) **Etiology.** Ketotic hypoglycemia appears to be the result of a diminished tolerance for normal fasting. At the point of hypoglycemia, infusion of alanine (the major gluconeogenic substrate) results in prompt elevation of the blood glucose level, implying normal gluconeogenic mechanisms. GH and cortisol levels are high, and insulin levels are appropriately low. Glucose response to injected glucagon is minimal. This has been postulated to be an exaggeration of the limited ability of children to tolerate prolonged fasting compared to adults, perhaps related to smaller muscle mass, which limits substrate availability.

(2) Diagnosis is best made by monitoring blood glucose throughout a 24-hour fast. If the blood glucose level falls below 40 mg/dl, additional blood for insulin, glucose, cortisol, and GH measurement is obtained, as well as urine for ketones. The fast should be terminated when the blood glucose level is below 40 mg/dl with a glucagon tolerance test (i.e., glucagon is administered intramuscularly at 0.03 mg/kg, up to 1.0 mg, with the blood glucose level checked at 15 and 30 minutes).

(3) Therapy is avoidance of fasting by eating small meals frequently, up to six times daily. Monitoring urine for ketones during intercurrent illness may be helpful in alerting to symptoms of hypoglycemia. Symptoms usually disappear after the age of 6–8 years.

b. Hyperinsulinism. In the older child and adolescent, hyperinsulinism may present as erratic episodes of unpredictable or bizarre behavior, loss of consciousness, or seizures.

(1) Etiology. As opposed to the neonate or young infant with hyperinsulinism due to a diffuse functional process, in the older child, a functioning islet cell adenoma may be found.

(2) Diagnosis may be reached by monitoring the blood glucose level on a 24-hour fast. The child usually becomes hypoglycemic in 6–12 hours. Ketones are not present in the urine, and the glucose response to glucagon is brisk. Insulin levels are inappropriately and sometimes markedly elevated during hypoglycemia.

(3) Therapy. The tumor may be localized by arteriography. Surgical excision is curative.

c. "Reactive" hypoglycemia. Occasionally, parents relate concern about hypoglycemia as a cause of hyperactivity, inattentiveness at school, headache, and low energy. If clinical suspicion is low, documentation of the blood glucose level when symptoms are present may persuade parents that hypoglycemia is not present. If parental concern is great, a 24-hour fast documents normal fasting ability. There is little substantiation that reactive hypoglycemia is a defined entity in children. Oral glucose tolerance testing is not helpful in the evaluation of children for hypoglycemia.

II. **HYPERLIPIDEMIC DISORDERS.** Identification of hypercholesterolemia as a major risk factor for the development of coronary heart disease has focused attention on the diagnosis and treatment of lipid abnormalities. Recent evidence demonstrates that lowering the serum cholesterol level in adults reduces the risk for subsequent coronary morbidity. This information, as well as the recognition that atherosclerotic lesions can be identified in children and adolescents, has prompted a more aggressive approach to the diagnosis and treatment of hyperlipidemia in children.

A. **General considerations**

1. **Normal lipoprotein metabolism.** Cholesterol and triglyceride are transported in blood in particles called lipoproteins. There are **four major classes of lipoproteins,** which are classified according to density and electrophoretic mobility.

   a. Chylomicrons are large, triglyceride-rich particles produced in the intestine by dietary fat and cleared by the action of lipoprotein lipase.

   b. Very low-density lipoproteins (VLDLs) are rich in triglyceride and are synthesized in the liver and catabolized to low-density lipoproteins.

   c. Low-density lipoproteins (LDLs) are rich in cholesterol. LDLs must bind to specific LDL receptors to be taken into cells and degraded.

   d. High-density lipoproteins (HDLs) contain cholesterol and are synthesized from chylomicrons and VLDLs directly in the liver and intestine. A high HDL cholesterol level conveys low risk of coronary heart disease.

2. **Identification of individuals with hyperlipidemia** depends on the measurement of fasting total cholesterol, triglyceride, and HDL cholesterol levels. Elevated LDL cholesterol and low HDL cholesterol are associated with increased cardiovascular risk. LDL cholesterol may be calculated as

$$\text{LDL cholesterol} = \text{total cholesterol} - \left(\text{HDL cholesterol} + \frac{\text{triglyceride}}{5} \right).$$

   a. The definition of normal lipid levels depends on the reference population and the amount of saturated fat and cholesterol in the diet. In children in the United States, the ninety-fifth percentile for total cholesterol and LDL cholesterol are 200 mg/dl and 130 mg/dl, respectively, and the ninety-fifth percentile for triglyceride is 120 mg/dl.
   b. Although triglyceride levels rise slowly with age, cholesterol levels are relatively constant throughout childhood and adolescence, and the differences between the sexes are not of practical significance.

3. **Screening children for hyperlipidemia** (see Chapter 1 VII D 8). Because of increased interest in preventive medicine and proven cardiac benefit of reducing serum cholesterol in adults, there has been increasing interest in identifying children at risk. Although mass screening programs for hyperlipidemia in children have not been instituted, it is advisable at least to screen all children with a family history of hyperlipidemia or premature heart disease. For children with milder elevation of total cholesterol levels (200–250 mg/dl), a low-cholesterol, low-fat diet and identification of and counseling about reducing other risk factors (e.g., smoking, hypertension, obesity) are recommended.

B. **Primary hyperlipidemias.** Primary disorders of lipid metabolism are a heterogeneous group of genetically determined diseases. The expression of the diseases may be affected by diet, obesity, diabetes, or other environmental factors. Certain types of primary hyperlipidemias predispose affected people to premature atherosclerosis and others to pancreatitis or neurologic sequelae, usually in adulthood. Although five separate subtypes (i.e., subtypes I, II, III, IV, and V) were described in the past, it is more useful clinically to separate the hyperlipidemias by which fraction, or fractions, are elevated.

1. **Familial hypercholesterolemia** is characterized by marked elevation of total and LDL cholesterol levels with normal triglyceride levels. It is inherited as an autosomal codominant trait and occurs in about 1 in 500 people.
   a. **Pathogenesis**
      (1) The **heterozygous form** is associated with a total cholesterol level usually higher than 300 mg/dl (LDL cholesterol > 190 mg/dl) and a high risk of coronary heart disease by the age of 30–40 years. These people have approximately a 50% reduction in LDL receptor activity.
      (2) The **homozygous form** is associated with a total cholesterol level of 600–1000 mg/dl. In this rare condition, myocardial infarction in the first decade of life and death by the age of 20 years are common. This disorder is caused by a near total deficiency of LDL receptors, which prevents uptake and catabolism of LDL cholesterol.
   b. **Therapy**
      (1) Treatment of the **heterozygous form** of familial hypercholesterolemia in children consists of a **strict diet** low in cholesterol and total fat and an increased polyunsaturated-to-saturated fat ratio. Adherence to the diet may result in a 10%–15% reduction in the LDL cholesterol level. If the cholesterol remains above 300 mg/dl, the addition of cholestyramine or colestipol (bile acid–binding resins that remove cholesterol from the enterohepatic circulation) is safe and efficacious. Lovastatin, an inhibitor of cholesterol biosynthesis, has shown promising results in adults. There is little or no experience with other lipid-lowering drugs in children, and therefore they are not recommended.
      (2) The **homozygous form** of familial hypercholesterolemia is **very resistant to treatment** because there is virtually a total absence of LDL receptors in affected patients. Some lowering of the cholesterol level may be achieved by repeated exchange transfusion, portocaval shunting, or liver transplantation. Gene therapy (replacing the gene for LDL receptors) has shown promise in early clinical research trials.

2. **Familial combined hyperlipidemia (elevated cholesterol or triglycerides, or both).** This combination is more common than previously recognized in children and appears to be dominantly inherited. Adults have premature coronary artery disease and peripheral vascular disease. Treatment is the same as for familial hypercholesterolemia.

3. **Mild to moderate hypertriglyceridemia.** This pattern of hyperlipidemia also is rarely found in children. In adults, it has been associated with obesity, glucose intolerance, and hyperuricemia, and it may be aggravated by alcohol ingestion and some drugs.

4. **Severe hypertriglyceridemia.** In children and adolescents, elevation of fasting triglyceride levels over 1000 mg/dl may be caused by familial deficiency of lipoprotein lipase, which results in hyperchylomicronemia. This may result in recurrent pancreatitis, hepatosplenomegaly, and eruptive xanthomas. Treatment consists of severe restriction of dietary fat. Severe hypertriglyceridemia secondary to elevation of both chylomicron and VLDL levels is rare in children.

C. **Secondary hyperlipidemia.** Hypercholesterolemia may be secondary to hypothyroidism, nephrotic syndrome, diabetes, and liver disease, or it may be induced by a diet high in saturated fat and cholesterol. Elevated triglyceride levels may be present in poorly controlled diabetes, obesity, glycogen storage disease, and renal failure, or it may be secondary to use of certain drugs (e.g., oral contraceptives, thiazide diuretics, β blockers). In each of these instances, treatment is directed at the primary disease process, or the offending medication is removed.

III. DISORDERS OF THE THYROID GLAND

A. **General considerations.** A good understanding of thyroid physiology and the assessment of thyroid function in children is necessary to recognize, diagnose, and treat thyroid disorders.

1. **Thyroid function.** Thyroid hormone is critical for normal postnatal somatic growth and neurologic development in infants and children.
   a. Thyroid hormone is essential for normal maturation of the CNS in children. Deficiency of thyroid hormone in the first 2 years of life may result in severe psychomotor retardation.
   b. Thyroid hormone is also necessary for normal skeletal growth and maturation in growing children. In both children and adults, it plays a major role in oxidative metabolism and heat production.

2. **Thyroid metabolism**
   a. **Synthesis. Iodide** absorbed from the intestine is trapped in the thyroid gland and is organically bound to **tyrosine** residues of thyroglobulin. Iodination of tyrosine forms **monoiodotyrosine (MIT)** and **diiodotyrosine (DIT),** which condense to form **thyroxine (T_4)** and **triiodothyronine (T_3).**
   b. **Feedback control.** Thyroid hormone synthesis is controlled by a negative feedback loop involving the CNS at the level of the hypothalamus and pituitary gland.
      (1) Low levels of circulating thyroid hormones stimulate hypothalamic release of **thyrotropin-releasing hormone (TRH),** which then stimulates production of **thyroid-stimulating hormone (TSH)** in the pituitary gland. TSH stimulates increased production of T_4 and T_3 by the thyroid gland.
      (2) **Circulation.** T_4 and T_3 circulate in plasma bound to thyroid-binding proteins—thyroxine-binding globulin (TBG) and thyroxine-binding prealbumin. Protein-bound T_4 and T_3 account for over 99% of circulating thyroid hormones. The free (i.e., not protein-bound) T_4 and T_3 are the metabolically active forms of the hormone.

3. **Assessment of thyroid function** involves measurement of thyroid hormones and testing of thyroid responsiveness. The most commonly used tests are the following.
   a. **Radioimmunoassay** is used to measure the serum concentration of several hormones.
      (1) **T_4** as measured by radioimmunoassay may be affected by processes that increase either fraction of T_4. For example, estrogen treatment stimulates production of

TBG, thereby increasing the total T_4 by raising the T_4 bound to TBG. The free T_4 is normal, and the patient is therefore clinically euthyroid (i.e., the thyroid gland functions normally). Measurement of free T_4 is possible but usually not necessary for appropriate diagnosis.

(2) T_3 as measured by radioimmunoassay is particularly useful in diagnosing hyperthyroidism.

(3) TBG may be measured directly by radioimmunoassay.

(4) TSH measurement by radioimmunoassay is valuable in the diagnosis of primary hypothyroidism (elevated TSH). In newer, more sensitive assays, very low levels of circulating TSH can be distinguished from normal levels and may be supportive of a diagnosis of hyperthyroidism.

b. Thyroid gland imaging

(1) Technetium 99m (^{99m}Tc) scanning of the thyroid is the most commonly used thyroid imaging technique used in children.

(a) ^{99m}TC is most useful for identification of areas of **decreased uptake of the radionuclide ("cold" nodules)** and for localization of ectopic thyroid tissue or absence of thyroid tissue.

(b) ^{99m}Tc is trapped only by the thyroid and has a half-life of only 6 hours; thus, it is not a great risk to the child.

(2) Ultrasonography of the thyroid gland may be used for characterization of cystic lesions.

c. T_3 **resin uptake** is a widely used test that is an indirect measure of the patient's thyroid-binding protein, and, as such, is helpful in interpreting the effect of increased or decreased binding protein on the measurement of total T_4 (the test does not measure the patient's T_3). Radioactive T_3 is added to the patient's serum along with an insoluble binder of T_3, such as resin. Radioactive T_3 binds to unoccupied binding sites on the patient's binding proteins, and the remaining radioactive T_3 subsequently is bound to the resin added to the sample (Table 17-1).

(1) If the total T_4 is high because of an elevated protein-bound fraction (e.g., due to pregnancy or oral contraceptives), the T_3 resin uptake will be low.

(2) Conversely, if the T_4 is low because of a low protein-bound fraction (e.g., due to congenital deficiency of TBG), the T_3 resin uptake will be high.

(3) In hyperthyroidism, the T_4 (total T_4) and T_3 resin uptakes are high. In hypothyroidism, the T_4 and T_3 resin uptakes are low.

d. Free thyroxine index is an estimate of free T_4, taking into account the patient's level of thyroid hormone-binding protein as measured by T_3 resin uptake. This test is a calculation, not a direct measurement, based on the total T_4 and T_3 uptake.

e. TRH stimulation test measures the TSH response to an intravenous injection of TRH. Samples for TSH are measured before and every 15 minutes up to 1 hour after TRH injection.

(1) Because of negative-feedback suppression of T_4 on the pituitary thyrotroph, the TSH response to TRH is suppressed even in subtle hyperthyroidism.

TABLE 17-1. Differentiating Hyperthyroxinemia and Hypothyroxinemia from Thyroxine-Binding Globulin Excess or Deficiency

	T_4 RIA	T_3 RIA	T_3 Uptake	TSH
Hyperthyroidism	↑	↑	↑	↓
Hypothyroidism	↓	↓	↓	↑
TBG deficiency	↓	↓	↑	→
TBG excess (pregnancy, oral contraceptives)	↑	↑	↓	→

RIA = radioimmunoassay; T_3 = triiodothyronine; T_4 = thyroxine; TBG = thyroxine-binding globulin; TSH = thyroid-stimulating hormone.

(2) In hypothyroidism, the TSH response to TRH is increased. The test for hypothyroidism is more difficult to interpret than that for hyperthyroidism.

f. Thyroid receptor antibody tests measure a heterogeneous group of immunoglobulins that bind to the TSH receptor on thyroid cells and stimulate thyroid growth and function.

  (1) Two types of tests have been recently developed.

  (a) One measures **thyroid-stimulating immunoglobulins (TSI)**.

  (b) The other test measures **thyrotropin-binding inhibition immunoglobulin (TBII)**.

  (2) The presence of TBII and TSI correlates with disease activity in hyperthyroidism (Graves disease) in childhood, and their measurement may be useful in predicting the likelihood of clinical remission.

g. Radioactive iodine uptake rarely is performed in children as a diagnostic test owing to the high levels of radiation exposure. Iodine 123 (^{123}I) is preferred over ^{131}I because of its shorter half-life and lower radiation dose.

B. **Hypothyroidism** may occur at birth (**congenital hypothyroidism**) or at any time during childhood or adolescence (**juvenile hypothyroidism**). Because of the importance of thyroid hormone for normal brain growth and development in the first 2 years of life, the clinical considerations are different for infants than for older children and adolescents.

1. Congenital hypothyroidism, unlike acquired thyroid diseases, affects males and females equally.

  a. Etiology

  (1) Developmental thyroid defect (thyroid agenesis or dysgenesis) is the primary cause of congenital hypothyroidism.

  (2) Defective biosynthesis of thyroid hormone (frequently resulting in goiter) also may cause the disorder.

  (3) Transient congenital hypothyroidism may occur as a result of transplacental passage of maternally ingested goitrogens (e.g., iodide expectorants, antithyroid drugs, or maternal antithyroid antibodies).

  b. Clinical features. Because thyroid hormone does not appear to be necessary for fetal growth, infants with congenital hypothyroidism are normal in size. The severity of symptoms and physical findings correlates with the degree of hypothyroidism.

  (1) Symptoms. Although a newborn rarely may have some physical features of hypothyroidism in the first week of life, usually it is not apparent. Often the first symptom is **prolonged neonatal jaundice**. Other symptoms that develop in the first 1–2 months of life are feeding problems, lethargy, and constipation.

  (2) Physical findings are coarse facies with large, open fontanelles; large, protruding tongue; hoarse cry; umbilical hernia; cool, dry, mottled skin; hypotonia; and delayed development.

  (3) Severe manifestations. Severe congenital hypothyroidism is characterized by short limbs, epiphyseal dysgenesis, impaired physical growth and development, and mental retardation.

  c. Diagnosis

  (1) The diagnosis of congenital hypothyroidism is made by documenting decreased serum concentrations of total T_4, decreased T_3 resin uptake, and elevated serum concentrations of TSH.

  (2) Assessment of skeletal age (e.g., by knee radiography) may show retardation of skeletal maturation to less than 36 weeks' gestation, suggesting intrauterine hypothyroidism.

  (3) A ^{99m}Tc thyroid scan before initiating therapy may be helpful in ascertaining the etiology of congenital hypothyroidism, which may have prognostic and genetic implications.

  (a) Absence of ^{99m}Tc uptake indicates thyroid agenesis.

  (b) Increased ^{99m}Tc uptake in a normally positioned gland implies an enzymatic defect in thyroid hormone production.

  (c) An ectopic gland is demonstrated by abnormal localization of ^{99m}Tc uptake.

d. Therapy

(1) Thyroid hormone replacement, using synthetic L-thyroxine as a single daily oral dose, should be instituted after confirming blood tests are drawn. The dosage for infants is approximately 10 μg/kg. As the child grows, the dosage is adjusted to maintain the serum T_4 in the high-normal range (10–14 μg/dl).

(2) Follow-up. Growth and neurologic development are evaluated at regular follow-up visits every 2–3 months in the first 2 years, with somewhat less frequent follow-up visits after 2 years of age.

e. Prognosis. When the diagnosis of congenital hypothyroidism is delayed beyond 3 months of age, a high proportion of children suffer **permanent neurologic impairment**.

f. Screening. Because congenital hypothyroidism is a relatively common problem (occurring in 1 in 4000 births) and because it was expected that early recognition, before clinical suspicion was aroused, might prevent neurologic sequelae, techniques for mass screening for hypothyroidism were developed in the 1970s. Neonatal screening for hypothyroidism has become widely applied. The results from follow-up of children diagnosed through neonatal screening by 1 month of age indicate that neurologic function and intelligence are normal when compared to those of their siblings. Screening also enables genetic counseling for families of children with less common familial forms of congenital hypothyroidism (i.e., dyshormonogenesis).

2. Juvenile (acquired) hypothyroidism. When symptoms appear after the first year of life, hypothyroidism is presumed to be acquired. Juvenile hypothyroidism is more common in girls than in boys, as are most thyroid diseases.

a. Etiology

(1) The most common cause of juvenile hypothyroidism is **autoimmune destruction** of the thyroid secondary to chronic lymphocytic thyroiditis (Hashimoto thyroiditis).

(2) Other causes include ectopic thyroid dysgenesis, goitrogens (e.g., iodide cough syrup, antithyroid drugs), and surgical or radioactive iodine ablation for treatment of hyperthyroidism.

b. Clinical features

(1) Symptoms. Slow linear growth is the hallmark of hypothyroidism in childhood. Puberty usually is delayed although occasionally may be paradoxically precocious. Other symptoms include cold intolerance, small appetite, lethargy, and constipation. School performance usually is not impaired, and behavior problems are rare.

(2) Physical findings. Affected children may have coarse, puffy facies with a flattened nasal bridge; immature body proportions; stocky habitus; paucity of speech and spontaneous movement; dull, dry, thin hair; and rough, dry skin with a pale, waxy hue. Deep tendon reflexes show delayed relaxation time ("hung" reflexes).

c. Diagnosis

(1) The diagnosis is made on the basis of documentation of decreased serum concentrations of total T_4, decreased T_3 resin uptake, and elevated serum concentrations of TSH.

(2) Skeletal maturation may be markedly delayed and indicates the duration of hypothyroidism.

(3) The presence of circulating thyroid autoantibodies implies an autoimmune basis for the disease.

(4) A ^{99m}Tc thyroid scan is not indicated unless there are irregularities in thyroid consistency on palpation. In that case, a scan looking for a thyroid nodule would be appropriate.

d. Therapy

(1) Thyroid hormone replacement therapy is begun with synthetic L-thyroxine, approximately 3–5 μg/kg as a single daily oral dose. The adequacy of replacement can be judged by measurement of serum T_4 and TSH, which should be in the normal range.

(2) Transient deterioration of school performance and behavior as the child adjusts to newfound energy levels is common.

e. Prognosis
   (1) Unless hypothyroidism develops around the time of puberty when skeletal maturation is nearly complete, the prognosis for catch-up growth is good. However, there is some evidence that some children may not reach their genetic potential for growth. Other signs and symptoms resolve completely.
   (2) Children with autoimmune hypothyroidism are at increased risk for other associated autoimmune diseases, such as diabetes mellitus and adrenal insufficiency (Schmidt syndrome). Children with Down syndrome have an increased incidence of hypothyroidism and hyperthyroidism.

C. Hyperthyroidism

1. Etiology
   a. Graves disease (thyrotoxicosis), or hyperthyroidism secondary to diffuse thyroid hyperplasia (diffuse toxic goiter), is the most common cause of hyperthyroidism. It is an autoimmune thyroid disorder in which enlargement and hyperfunction of the thyroid gland may be stimulated by circulating immunoglobulins, particularly abnormal immunoglobulin G (IgG), a thyroid-stimulating immunoglobulin that binds to thyrotropin receptors on thyroid cells. The increased levels of free T_4 suppress TSH to undetectable levels. Thus, thyroid hyperfunction is not TSH dependent.
   b. Neonatal Graves disease. Neonatal hyperthyroidism is thought to be caused by transplacental passage of thyroid-stimulating immunoglobulins (i.e., IgG).
   c. Other etiologies for hyperthyroidism in children are rare but include hyperfunctioning "hot" thyroid nodule and acute suppurative thyroiditis.

2. Epidemiology. Girls are more commonly affected than boys (in a ratio of 4:1), and there often is a family history of Graves disease or Hashimoto thyroiditis. The usual age at presentation is adolescence; it is unusual before 5 years of age.

3. Clinical features
   a. Symptoms. The onset of symptoms is insidious, and emotional lability, increased appetite, heat intolerance, weight loss, frequent loose stools, deterioration of behavior and school performance, and poor sleeping are the most common symptoms. Weakness and inability to participate in sports sometimes are noted.
   b. Physical findings. On physical examination, the child appears fidgety, flushed, and warm. Marked tachycardia, fever, diaphoresis, nausea, and vomiting indicate **thyroid storm,** which is a sudden exacerbation of symptoms.
   (1) Proptosis and widened palpebral fissures may be present.
   (2) The thyroid gland usually is diffusely enlarged, smooth, firm but not hard, and nontender.
   (3) The precordium is hyperactive, and resting tachycardia and widened pulse pressure are present.
   (4) The skin is velvety smooth, warm, flushed, and moist.
   (5) A fine tremor of outstretched fingers may be seen. Proximal muscle weakness may be present.
   c. Graves ophthalmopathy is caused by lymphocytic infiltration of the conjunctiva, extraocular eye muscles, and retrobulbar soft tissue and may cause redness and edema of the conjunctiva, decreased mobility of the eye, and proptosis. Its course may not follow that of hyperthyroidism. Most of the 60% of children who have some evidence of ophthalmopathy experience mild symptoms; in only a few of the patients is the involvement severe or progressive.
   d. Neonatal Graves disease
   (1) Some infants born to women with Graves disease exhibit jitteriness, stare, hyperactivity, increased appetite, and poor weight gain.
   (2) Tachycardia is present, and thyromegaly may be detectable.
   (3) Thyroid hormone levels are elevated above the normal range for the newborn, and TSH is suppressed.

4. Diagnosis

    a. Hyperthyroidism is diagnosed by documentation of increased serum concentrations of total T_4 and total T_3, increased T_3 resin uptake, and low or suppressed levels of TSH. If T_4 levels are borderline, absence of the TSH response to TRH injection indicates autonomous thyroid hyperfunction.

    b. ^{131}I uptake is helpful if thyroid enlargement is not present. Increased T_4 with low ^{131}I uptake may point to surreptitious overdosing with thyroid hormone.

5. Therapy

    a. Medications

        (1) Initial treatment consists of antithyroid medication, either **propylthiouracil [PTU]** (300–600 mg/day) or **methimazole** (30–60 mg/day) in three divided doses. PTU offers the advantage of blocking the peripheral conversion of T_4 to T_3. The addition of propranolol (10–20 mg four times daily) may give symptomatic relief until preformed thyroid hormone is discharged from the thyroid and thyroid hormone levels begin to fall, usually in 2–4 weeks.

           (a) About 5% of patients experience side effects (e.g., skin rash, arthralgias, drug-induced hepatitis) while on antithyroid medication.

           (b) Less common, but more serious, is the occasional occurrence of **agranulocytosis**. If high fever, sore throat, or oral ulceration develops in the child, a white blood cell count should be obtained. Agranulocytosis usually is reversible, but alternative therapy for hyperthyroidism must be selected.

        (2) About 40%–50% of children with Graves disease go into a natural remission and may be taken off antithyroid medication after 12–24 months of treatment.

        (3) Recurrent hyperthyroidism, long-standing disease, and a large thyroid gland indicate continuing disease activity. More recently, the continuing presence of circulating TBII and TSI predicts continued disease activity.

    b. Surgery

        (1) **Subtotal thyroidectomy** usually is selected for recurrent hyperthyroidism after a course of medical treatment or if the patient is noncompliant with medical therapy.

        (2) **Complications** include postoperative hypoparathyroidism and recurrent laryngeal nerve damage in 1%–5% of patients. Most children require thyroid hormone replacement after surgery.

    c. Radioactive iodine. Although ablation of thyroid tissue by radioactive iodine has traditionally been reserved for adults, it has been used regularly in some centers as the preferred treatment for children with no untoward effects on subsequent fertility or fetal wastage.

        (1) The risk for immediate and long-term complications is low.

        (2) The choice of surgery versus radioactive iodine should probably be left to the patient and family after a thorough discussion of both forms of therapy.

        (3) As with surgery, most children eventually require thyroxine replacement for hypothyroidism after receiving radioactive iodine.

    d. Therapy for thyroid storm. The extremely hypermetabolic state of thyroid storm requires immediate hospitalization and treatment with iodide, PTU, β blockers, and supportive care as well as treatment of any other intercurrent illness that may have triggered the episode.

    e. Therapy for neonatal Graves disease. Therapy with PTU (5–10 mg/kg every 6 hours) is instituted. Propranolol and iodide solution may be added in very symptomatic infants. Initially, infants should be monitored closely for signs of congestive heart failure. Neonatal Graves disease usually resolves over the first several months of life.

D. **Thyroiditis** (i.e., inflammation of the thyroid gland) may be chronic, subacute, or acute. Each type has a distinct clinical presentation, course, and treatment.

1. **Chronic lymphocytic thyroiditis (CLT)** is commonly referred to as **Hashimoto thyroiditis** and is the most common thyroid condition in childhood and adolescence. Girls are affected more than twice as often as boys.
   a. **Clinical features**
      (1) **Asymptomatic thyroid enlargement (goiter)** is the most common presenting complaint or physical finding. The thyroid gland is diffusely enlarged, and the surface may feel pebbly. With long duration, the gland becomes hard and nodular.
      (2) Although most children are euthyroid, a few may be **hypothyroid** and very rarely some may have symptoms of **thyrotoxicosis (Hashitoxicosis)**. Occasionally, distinguishing Hashimoto thyroiditis from Graves disease may be difficult because elements of both diseases may coexist.
   b. **Diagnosis** is made on the basis of physical findings and laboratory data.
      (1) The most significant laboratory test supporting the diagnosis is the presence of high titers of thyroid autoantibodies in the serum. Antithyroglobulin and antimicrosomal antibodies are the most commonly found.
      (2) Measurement of serum concentrations of T_4 and TSH may be normal, or T_4 levels may be normal with elevated TSH (**"compensated" hypothyroidism**), or T_4 levels may be decreased with elevated TSH (hypothyroidism).
      (3) Thyroid scanning is not indicated unless a nodule is suspected.
   c. **Therapy** with L-thyroxine is reserved for those children with evidence of hypothyroidism, either decreased serum concentrations of T_4 or normal T_4 with elevated TSH. The disease may resolve completely with or without treatment in up to 50% of children with Hashimoto thyroiditis. In some children, thyroid function continues to deteriorate and permanent hypothyroidism results.

2. **Subacute thyroiditis** is a rare, nonsuppurative inflammatory disease of the thyroid, which is thought to have a viral etiology, although a specific virus is not identified in most cases.
   a. **Clinical features**
      (1) Typically, the child complains of sore throat and pain in the area of the thyroid gland. Pain may be referred to the angle of the jaw or the ear and is worse on movement of the neck.
      (2) Symptoms of systemic illness (e.g., fever, malaise) are frequent. Examination reveals a tender, swollen thyroid gland.
   b. **Diagnosis**
      (1) In the early stages of the disease, serum T_4 concentrations may be moderately elevated and TSH levels suppressed, presumably secondary to discharge of preformed thyroid hormone from the gland. Thyroid uptake of radionuclide is very low. Symptoms of hyperthyroidism usually are mild and do not require treatment.
      (2) Leukocytosis and elevated erythrocyte sedimentation rate are usual in the systemic phase of the illness.
      (3) In the later stages of the disease (2–6 months), hypothyroidism is common but ultimately resolves in almost all cases.
   c. **Therapy** is symptomatic. Aspirin and nonsteroidal antiinflammatory drugs to relieve pain and tenderness are sufficient in milder cases. Occasionally steroids are required for more severe cases.

3. **Acute thyroiditis** is a term usually reserved for acute bacterial infection of the thyroid, which may be suppurative or nonsuppurative. The most common causative organisms are *Staphylococcus aureus, Streptococcus hemolyticus,* and *Streptococcus pneumoniae.*
   a. **Clinical features.** The child presents with an acute, toxic febrile illness with marked tenderness in the area of the thyroid that is exacerbated by extension of the neck. The thyroid is extremely tender to palpation, and there may be increased warmth and erythema of the overlying skin.

b. Diagnosis
  (1) Laboratory studies show leukocytosis with a left shift and an elevated erythrocyte sedimentation rate. Unlike subacute thyroiditis, serum levels of T_4 and TSH are normal, as is the 24-hour uptake of radioactive iodine.
  (2) Ultrasonography may identify an abscess.
  (3) Needle aspiration for culture identifies the bacterial organism.
c. Therapy with high-dose parenteral antibiotics is begun immediately. An abscess requires surgical drainage.
d. Prognosis. Complete recovery with normal thyroid function is the rule.

E. **Thyroid nodules** are rare in children. Although the etiology is uncertain, there is a high incidence of palpable nodules found in young adults who received irradiation to the neck area during infancy or childhood.

1. Pathology. Thyroid nodules in children may be solitary nodules, which usually are benign (e.g., benign adenoma, cysts, lymphocytic thyroiditis) but may be malignant.
  a. The most common types of thyroid carcinoma are **well-differentiated papillary and follicular carcinomas**.
  b. An unusual and highly malignant, sometimes familial, form of thyroid cancer is **medullary thyroid carcinoma**. Medullary thyroid carcinoma is associated with **multiple endocrine adenomatosis type II (MEA II),** which includes pheochromocytoma and parathyroid hyperplasia or adenoma (see V B 1–2).

2. Diagnosis
  a. The patient history should seek to identify symptoms of hypothyroidism or hyperthyroidism, previous head or neck irradiation, and family history of thyroid or other endocrine disease.
  b. Laboratory evaluation includes measurement of T_4, T_3 resin uptake, TSH, and thyroid antibodies.
  c. The presence of a palpable mass in the thyroid is the major indication for performing a thyroid scan. As many as 30%–40% of isolated **"cold" nodules** (decreased radioisotope uptake) prove to be thyroid carcinoma in children. Most of the remaining nodules are benign adenomas or cystic lesions.
  d. Fine-needle aspiration by an experienced endocrinologist or pathologist is useful for differentiating benign from malignant lesions.
  e. Occult medullary thyroid carcinoma or precancerous C-cell hyperplasia of the thyroid can be detected by calcium or pentagastrin infusion. A positive calcitonin response to the stimulation test is an indication for total thyroidectomy.

3. Therapy
  a. Benign nodules. A nodule may be presumed to be benign if there is no predisposing condition or clinical characteristics of malignancy and the fine-needle biopsy is negative for malignant cells. In this case, observation of the patient while on thyroid hormone suppression is indicated.
  b. Malignant nodules require surgical removal. Hemithyroidectomy or subtotal thyroidectomy with lymph node excision is sufficient for well-differentiated unilateral carcinoma and usually affords an excellent prognosis. Total thyroidectomy is performed for medullary thyroid carcinoma. Postoperative drug therapy with L-thyroxine is used to suppress TSH.
  c. Metastatic thyroid cancer is treated with radioiodine ablation.

IV. **DISORDERS OF THE PITUITARY GLAND.** The pituitary gland is a complex structure that has two distinct portions—the anterior and posterior lobes—with different embryonic origins and separate hormonal functions.

A. **Disorders of the anterior lobe.** The anterior lobe of the pituitary gland (also called the **adenohypophysis**) is derived from a diverticulum of the primitive oral cavity. Hypothalamic polypeptides reach the anterior lobe through the median eminence and the portal vasculature of the pituitary gland. The hormones produced in the anterior lobe are **GH, TSH, ACTH,** gonadotropins [i.e., **luteinizing hormone (LH)** and **follicle-stimulating hormone (FSH)**], and **prolactin.** Children are more likely to have a deficiency than an excess of pituitary hormones. Hypersecretory pituitary adenomas, which are very rare in children, usually are prolactin- or GH-secreting adenomas.

1. GH disorders

    a. Normal GH function

        (1) GH is an anabolic polypeptide hormone that stimulates growth of all tissues. Its most striking effect is on the lengthening of long bones. Its action on long bone growth appears to be mediated through another polypeptide hormone, **insulin-like growth factor 1 (IGF-1),** which is generated in the liver and other tissues.

        (2) GH release from the anterior lobe is stimulated by the hypothalamic peptide, **growth hormone releasing factor (GRF),** and is inhibited by **somatostatin.**

        (3) Other substances and factors play a role in GH release, and many form the basis of testing for abnormalities of GH secretion, including sleep, exercise, hypoglycemia, amino acids (e.g., arginine), β blockers, sex hormones, and other drugs (e.g., L-dopa, clonidine).

    b. GH deficiency is associated with a variety of clinical conditions and syndromes, either as an isolated deficiency or in combination with other pituitary hormone deficiencies (**panhypopituitarism**).

        (1) Clinical features

            (a) Congenital hypopituitarism—a rare form of GH deficiency—may be familial and frequently is fatal if not diagnosed in the neonatal period. In these infants, profound hypoglycemia, prolonged jaundice, and low levels of cortisol, GH, and thyroid hormone require immediate treatment. When this syndrome is associated with optic nerve hypoplasia (blindness) and absence of the septum pellucidum, it is called **septooptic dysplasia.**

            (b) Secondary GH deficiency. GH deficiency may be secondary to **CNS tumors** (e.g., craniopharyngioma, glioma, pinealoma), **trauma, surgery** involving the hypothalamus or pituitary gland, **irradiation,** or malignant (histiocytosis) or infectious **infiltration.**

            (c) Idiopathic GH deficiency accounts for most cases of GH deficiency. Usually, the defect is in the hypothalamus, resulting in deficient GRF stimulation of pituitary somatotrophs.

                (i) Because GH does not appear to be necessary for fetal growth, affected newborns are of normal size. Growth velocity slows after 6–12 months of age, so that by 2 years of age, height is below the fifth percentile.

                (ii) Male infants may have microphallus secondary to intrauterine gonadotropin deficiency.

                (iii) Symptomatic hypoglycemia may occur in the newborn period.

                (iv) Older children with idiopathic GH deficiency have very short stature with growth velocities of less than 5 cm/year. They may have mild truncal adiposity, frontal bossing, a flat nasal bridge, and a high-pitched voice. Skeletal maturation is significantly delayed.

        (2) Diagnosis. Because GH is secreted in sporadic bursts, with the major surge coming after sleep onset (stages 3 and 4), GH levels are low throughout most of the day. To differentiate the normal low basal GH level from disease states associated with absent or diminished GH secretion, GH **provocative tests** have been developed.

            (a) GH levels greater than 10 ng/ml after exercise, insulin-induced hypoglycemia, and arginine infusion as well as L-dopa, glucagon, and clonidine administration are considered evidence of normal GH secretory capacity.

            (b) Peak levels of 7–10 ng/ml are intermediate and may indicate partial GH deficiency or a neurosecretory defect, and must be interpreted in the clinical context.

      (c) Levels less than 7 ng /ml on two separate provocative tests indicate classic GH deficiency. Children with normal or intermediate GH response to provocative testing may have a neurosecretory defect. In these children, a trial of GH therapy may be warranted.

    (3) Therapy. Before 1985, human GH extracted from human cadaver pituitary glands was used for treatment of GH-deficient children. In 1986, human recombinant GH became widely available and is currently the only GH approved for human use in the United States.

      (a) GH is given by subcutaneous injection daily or every other day. In young infants with hypoglycemia due to GH deficiency, daily injections are necessary.

      (b) With a theoretically unlimited supply of GH, new uses for GH in the treatment of short stature from other etiologies are being explored. GH has been shown to be effective treatment for growth failure in children with chronic renal insufficiency and Turner syndrome.

  c. GH-secreting adenomas cause acromegaly in the postadolescent child with fused epiphyses. In the younger child, it causes pituitary gigantism.

    (1) Clinical features include increased perspiration, headache, acral enlargement, and visual impairment. Carbohydrate intolerance, galactorrhea, joint pain, and delayed puberty also may be present.

    (2) Diagnosis

      (a) Elevation of GH levels may be variable, but integrated 24-hour GH secretion is increased as reflected in a significant increase in IGF-1 levels.

      (b) GH levels are not suppressible by glucose ingestion, as they are in healthy subjects.

    (3) Therapy. Neurosurgical excision of the adenoma relieves progression of symptoms. Drug therapy with bromocriptine may ameliorate symptoms of GH excess, but is not curative.

2. TSH deficiency. Isolated TSH deficiency is exceedingly rare. However, TSH deficiency in combination with other pituitary hormone deficiencies is common.

  a. Hypothyroidism secondary to TSH deficiency tends to be more subtle in its clinical manifestation than primary hypothyroidism. Therefore, all children who are being evaluated for GH deficiency should have evaluation of T_4, T_3 resin uptake, and TSH levels.

  b. GH therapy may induce or unmask TSH deficiency. Consequently, children on GH therapy should have yearly screening for secondary hypothyroidism. Treatment consists of thyroid hormone replacement.

3. ACTH deficiency as an isolated defect has been reported. More commonly, ACTH deficiency occurs along with deficiency of other pituitary hormones.

  a. Clinical features are secondary to hypocortisolism and include hypoglycemia, fatigue, and poor tolerance of intercurrent illness.

  b. Diagnosis is based on failure to increase cortisol levels after insulin-induced hypoglycemia (on an insulin tolerance test).

4. Gonadotropin deficiency

  a. Clinical features. Gonadotropin (LH and FSH) deficiency presents in infancy as microphallus in the boy. Hypogonadotropic hypogonadism becomes evident as the child's pubertal development falls significantly behind the expected age range for puberty (see VI B 1).

  b. Diagnosis

    (1) Gonadotropin deficiency may occur as an isolated defect, as part of a recognizable syndrome [e.g., Kallmann syndrome (anosmia and hypogonadism), Prader-Willi syndrome (characterized by hypotonia, obesity, short stature, mental retardation; see Chapter 8), and anorexia nervosa] or within the context of multiple pituitary hormone deficiencies.

    (2) There is no specific test that clearly separates hypogonadotropic hypogonadism from constitutional delay of puberty.

5. **Prolactin-secreting adenomas** may be very small (microadenoma) or large, creating primarily neurologic symptoms.
   a. **Clinical features** related to high prolactin levels include galactorrhea and delayed or arrested pubertal development.
   b. **Therapy.** Surgical excision is curative. If this is not possible, medical treatment with bromocriptine ameliorates symptoms and shrinks the size of the tumor with good long-term control of disease in many cases.

B. **Disorders of the posterior lobe.** The posterior lobe of the pituitary gland (also called the **neurohypophysis**) develops—along with the pituitary stalk—as a downgrowth of neural tissue from the area of the third ventricle. Neural fibers connect the neurohypophysis with hypothalamic nuclei, the site of synthesis of **arginine vasopressin** [antidiuretic hormone (ADH)] and **oxytocin,** which, together, comprise a neuroendocrine unit.

1. **ADH disorders**
   a. **Normal ADH function.** ADH is an octapeptide that has an antidiuretic effect on the collecting ducts in the kidney. This allows water to be reabsorbed and concentrated urine to be excreted, allowing the tonicity of body fluids to remain constant during periods of reduced water intake. ADH secretion is stimulated by hypovolemia through baroreceptors in the carotid sinus, by hyperosmolality through osmoreceptors in the hypothalamus, by the upright position, and by stress and anxiety.
      (1) Through an active process, sodium and chloride are removed from the glomerular filtrate in the ascending limb of the loop of Henle, which is impermeable to water. Therefore, urine delivered to the distal convoluted tubule is dilute.
      (2) In the presence of ADH, the collecting duct becomes permeable to water and water is passively reabsorbed into the hypertonic interstitium, concentrating urine to an osmolality greater than 1000 mOsm/L and reducing urine volume.
   b. **Diabetes insipidus** is a condition marked by the inability to concentrate urine appropriately despite a normal countercurrent osmotic gradient in the kidney. With loss of ADH secretion, 24-hour urine output may reach 5–10 L/day. Urine osmolality remains low (about 100 mOsm/L).
      (1) **Etiology.** Diabetes insipidus may occur as an isolated idiopathic defect, or it may be accompanied by anterior pituitary hormone deficiency (as in septooptic dysplasia). It may occur after head trauma, after surgical interruption of the pituitary stalk (e.g., for craniopharyngioma), and with tumors and infections of the CNS. There is a rare familial form of diabetes insipidus.
      (2) **Clinical features.** The patient has polyuria and polydipsia even when water-deprived. Frequently, the onset of symptoms of excessive thirst and urination is abrupt. The child prefers cold water to other fluids. Caloric intake diminishes, and growth and weight gain may fall off. Neurologic and visual complaints may be present if diabetes insipidus is secondary to a tumor.
      (3) **Diagnosis.** If the child's first morning urine is dilute (specific gravity of less than 1.015), a **water deprivation test** must be done. After a water load of 20 ml/kg is given in the morning, the child is not given anything by mouth until the test is ended. Meticulous hourly measurements of weight and urine output are recorded.
         (a) Urine specific gravity and osmolality are measured on each sample. Serum sodium and osmolality are measured hourly after 4 hours.
         (b) The test is terminated when 3%–5% of body weight is lost or when the serum osmolality rises to 300 mOsm/L or more and urine osmolality remains constant and dilute (< 250 mOsm/L) over a 2-hour period. Hemoconcentration may result in a high-normal serum sodium level.
         (c) At the end of the test, a long-acting analogue of ADH, dDAVP, 5–10 μg, is given intranasally, and the child may drink. A further rise in urine osmolality by 100 mOsm/L or more indicates ADH-deficient diabetes insipidus.
         (d) Documentation of responsiveness to ADH is important in differentiating ADH-deficient diabetes insipidus from nephrogenic diabetes insipidus and

other renal diseases associated with decreased concentrating ability (e.g., renal tubular acidosis, sickle cell disease, and other types of chronic renal disease) [see also Chapter 14].

(4) Therapy with dDAVP intranasally every 12–24 hours provides relief of symptoms of polyuria and polydipsia.

c. **Nephrogenic diabetes insipidus** is a rare X-linked recessive disease of renal unresponsiveness to ADH. Male infants are severely affected.

(1) Clinical features include polyuria, failure to thrive, and bouts of hyperpyrexia and vomiting, leading to severe hypernatremic dehydration in infancy.

(2) Diagnosis. Failure to respond to ADH at the end of the water deprivation test in the absence of other renal disease suggests the diagnosis of nephrogenic diabetes insipidus (see also Chapter 14).

(3) Therapy consists of provision of ample fluids at all times, including during the course of intercurrent illness. Thiazide diuretics, by promoting sodium diuresis and volume contraction, provide some relief of symptoms.

d. **Thirst and osmotic regulation abnormalities.** Children with these abnormalities usually have significant CNS disease.

(1) Clinical features and diagnosis. The serum sodium level is chronically elevated without symptoms of thirst, whereas urine remains dilute. With water deprivation and induction of more severe hyperosmolality, ADH may be secreted.

(2) Therapy with dDAVP allows urine concentration with normal serum sodium. Care must be taken by the patient to avoid excess fluids and hyponatremia while taking dDAVP.

e. **Psychogenic water drinking.** This disorder of compulsive water drinking is rare in children.

(1) The history of other neurotic behaviors, gradual onset of symptoms, failure to get up at night to drink and urinate, and the finding of low-normal serum sodium levels and osmolality with dilute urine may suggest this diagnosis.

(2) The ability to concentrate urine on a water deprivation test may be less than normal because of "washout" of the renal concentration gradient. However, urine osmolality eventually rises while serum osmolality and sodium remain in the normal range.

f. **Syndrome of inappropriate antidiuretic hormone (SIADH)**

(1) Clinical features. SIADH causes expansion of the vascular volume and hyponatremia, which may lead to lethargy, confusion, and seizures. In children, SIADH is occasionally associated with pulmonary and CNS disease (e.g., pneumonia, bacterial meningitis). It also is associated with some chemotherapeutic agents (e.g., vincristine, cyclophosphamide).

(2) Therapy involves fluid restriction. Symptomatic hyponatremia is treated with infusion of 3% sodium chloride solution.

2. **Oxytocin disorders.** Oxytocin is an octapeptide that differs from ADH by two amino acids, which results in marked reduction in antidiuretic properties. Its major function is in promoting uterine contraction and milk ejection. Deficiency of oxytocin is not associated with a recognized pediatric clinical problem.

V. DISORDERS OF THE ADRENAL GLAND

A. **Disorders of the adrenal cortex.** The products of adrenocortical steroidogenesis are glucocorticoids, mineralocorticoids, and sex steroids. **Cortisol,** the major glucocorticoid, is stimulated by pituitary ACTH under a negative-feedback loop. **Aldosterone,** the principal mineralocorticoid, is controlled by the renin–angiotensin system. The major sex steroids are **androgens**. Inherited deficiency of various enzymes involved in cortisol and aldosterone synthesis leads to a group of diseases called **congenital adrenal hyperplasia**. Autonomous hyperfunctioning of the adrenal cortex leads to **hypercortisolism** or

Cushing disease, and decreased adrenocortical secretion may be caused by primary adrenal insufficiency (**Addison disease**) or a lack of ACTH stimulation (**secondary adrenal insufficiency**).

1. **Congenital adrenal hyperplasia.** The clinical characteristics of congenital adrenal hyperplasia depend on which enzyme in the pathway of cortisol synthesis is deficient. Even for a specific enzyme, variability exists in the severity of disease expression and timing of onset of symptoms. It is helpful to review the pathways of adrenal steroido-genesis (Figure 17-2) to appreciate better the consequences of an enzyme defect on decreased synthesis of cortisol or aldosterone, increased ACTH production, and over-production of precursors that are shunted to androgens. The two most common defects are 21-hydroxylase deficiency and 11-hydroxylase deficiency.

   a. **21-Hydroxylase deficiency** accounts for 90% of cases of congenital adrenal hyper-plasia and occurs in several forms. These disorders are inherited as autosomal reces-sive traits. The gene is HLA-linked on the short arm of chromosome 6.

      (1) **Classic salt-wasting 21-hydroxylase deficiency** is a severe deficiency resulting in decreased cortisol and aldosterone secretion, increased ACTH, and increased precursor of the 21-hydroxylase step, **17-hydroxyprogesterone.** 17-Hydroxy-progesterone is metabolized to adrenal androgens, namely dihydroepiandro-sterone (DHEA) and androstenedione. There is a one in four recurrence rate in siblings of children with classic salt-wasting 21-hydroxylase deficiency.

         (a) **Clinical features**

            (i) Female infants are born with ambiguous genitalia. Clitoromegaly and labioscrotal fusion may lead to erroneous male sex assignment. Because there is normal ovarian development, internal genital structures are female. Male infants have no genital abnormalities.

            (ii) Symptoms of salt wasting, vomiting, dehydration, and shock develop in the first 2–4 weeks of life. Infants are hyponatremic, hyperkalemic, aci-dotic, and often hypoglycemic.

         (b) **Diagnosis** rests on measurement of markedly elevated levels of 17-hydroxy-progesterone in the serum. HLA family studies have shown that affected siblings share the same HLA type. Thus, after the birth of an affected infant,

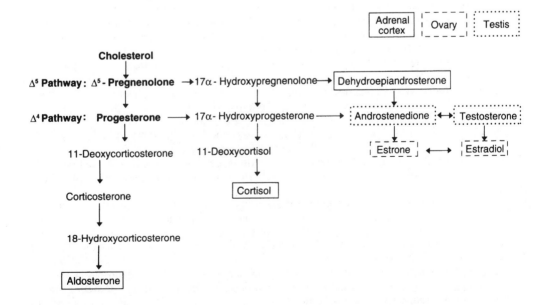

FIGURE 17-2. Summary of steroidogenesis in the adrenal cortex, ovary, and testis. (Reprinted from Bullock J, Boyle J, Wang M: *NMS Physiology,* 3rd ed. Baltimore, Williams & Wilkins, 1994, p 491.)

HLA typing of amniotic fluid cells, as well as measurement of elevated 17-hydroxyprogesterone in amniotic fluid, may permit prenatal diagnosis in subsequent pregnancies.

    (c) Therapy consists of:

        (i) Cortisol replacement (10–20 mg/m^2/day of oral hydrocortisone divided and given every 8 hours) to suppress ACTH and overproduction of androgens

        (ii) Mineralocorticoid (fludrocortisone 0.1 mg/day) adjusted to suppress the plasma renin level

        (iii) Surgical correction of female genital abnormalities

    (d) Follow-up. These children must be monitored closely for linear growth and sexual development.

        (i) Undertreatment, indicated by elevated 17-hydroxyprogesterone, androstenedione, and renin levels and by accelerated advancement of skeletal maturation, leads to excessive growth, premature sexual hair growth and virilization of male and female children, and ultimately to premature epiphyseal fusion and adult short stature.

        (ii) Overtreatment with cortisol suppresses growth and may cause symptoms of hypercortisolism.

(2) Simple virilizing 21-hydroxylase deficiency

    (a) Clinical features are caused solely by overproduction of adrenal androgens. Therefore, only female infants with ambiguous genitalia are diagnosed during the neonatal period. Boys and girls have excessive growth and premature appearance of pubic hair.

    (b) Diagnosis is based on the measurement of elevated 17-hydroxyprogesterone in serum.

    (c) Therapy. Principles of treatment with cortisol and follow-up are the same as for salt-wasters. Some children, even without clinical symptoms of salt wasting, have elevated levels of renin. The addition of a mineralocorticoid (fludrocortisone) facilitates suppression of adrenal androgens with smaller doses of cortisol.

(3) Nonclassic 21-hydroxylase deficiency (acquired or late-onset). This variant is most commonly diagnosed in female adolescents or adults.

    (a) Clinical features. Patients manifest signs and symptoms of androgen excess (i.e., menstrual irregularities, hirsutism, acne, advanced bone age).

    (b) Diagnosis. Basal levels of 17-hydroxyprogesterone may be only modestly elevated. However, the excessive rise of 17-hydroxyprogesterone after ACTH stimulation is diagnostic.

    (c) Therapy with a glucocorticoid suppresses adrenal androgens and ameliorates symptoms.

b. 11-Hydroxylase deficiency accounts for about 5% of cases of congenital adrenal hyperplasia. Lack of 11-hydroxylase results in decreased conversion of 11-deoxycortisol to cortisol, with precursors shunted toward overproduction of androgens, as in 21-hydroxylase deficiency. 11-Hydroxylase also is necessary for conversion of deoxycorticosterone to corticosterone in the aldosterone pathway.

    (1) Clinical features. Overproduction of deoxycorticosterone, which itself has mineralocorticoid activity, results in hypertension and hypokalemia in most of these patients.

    (2) Diagnosis is based on the measurement of increased 11-deoxycortisol and deoxycorticosterone in serum or their tetrahydrometabolites in the urine. Serum androstenedione and testosterone also are elevated, and renin and aldosterone are suppressed. In the milder nonclassic form, the biochemical abnormalities are expressed after ACTH stimulation.

c. Other defects. Other, extremely rare, forms of congenital adrenal hyperplasia may be caused by deficiencies of **cholesterol desmolase, 3β-hydroxysteroid dehydrogenase,** and **17-hydroxylase**. A nonclassic form of 3β-hydroxysteroid dehydrogenase may present clinically in prepubertal or pubertal girls as precocious adrenarche or excessive virilization. Treatment strategies are the same as for 21-hydroxylase deficiency.

2. **Primary adrenal insufficiency** may be congenital or acquired and results in decreased cortisol secretion alone or with diminished aldosterone.
   a. **Etiology**
      (1) Primary adrenal insufficiency in the newborn may be caused by adrenal hypoplasia, familial unresponsiveness to ACTH, adrenal hemorrhage, or overwhelming sepsis (**Waterhouse-Friderichsen syndrome**).
      (2) In older children and adolescents, **autoimmune adrenal insufficiency** may occur alone or in association with another autoimmune endocrinopathy (e.g., thyroiditis, IDDM). Tuberculosis and fungal destruction of the adrenal gland are rare.
      (3) **Adrenoleukodystrophy** is a group of X-linked recessive inherited disorders of long-chain fatty acid metabolism, resulting in progressive neurologic deterioration and adrenal insufficiency (see Chapter 18 XI D 2).
      (4) Adrenal insufficiency may occur after withdrawal of pharmacologic steroid therapy as a result of **suppression of pituitary ACTH**.
   b. **Clinical features**
      (1) **Symptoms** include weakness, nausea, vomiting, weight loss, and salt craving.
      (2) **Physical findings** include postural hypotension and increased pigmentation, especially over joints and on scar tissue, lips, nipples, and the buccal mucosa.
      (3) **Adrenal crisis** is characterized by fever, vomiting, dehydration, and shock that may be triggered by intercurrent illness, surgery, or trauma.
   c. **Diagnosis.** The characteristic electrolyte abnormalities are hyponatremia, hyperkalemia, and mild metabolic acidosis. The serum cortisol level is low (< 5 µg/dl) and fails to rise after acute injection of ACTH (cosyntropin at 250 µg intravenously). If the acute ACTH stimulation test results are abnormal, a prolonged ACTH stimulation test (3–5 days) is necessary to rule out an atrophic adrenal gland secondary to chronic ACTH deficiency (**secondary adrenal insufficiency**).
   d. **Therapy**
      (1) **Treatment of adrenal crisis.** Diagnostic studies should not delay treatment of this life-threatening illness. Rehydration and correction of electrolyte abnormalities are needed immediately.
         (a) Large quantities of 5% dextrose in normal saline are given, along with acute administration of intravenous glucocorticoid in stress doses (hydrocortisone at 100–200 mg/m^2/day divided and given every 4 hours).
         (b) Treatment with equivalent amounts of dexamethasone instead of hydrocortisone permits ACTH testing to be carried out while treatment is initiated, because dexamethasone does not interfere with measurement of cortisol after ACTH stimulation.
      (2) **Long-term treatment** of adrenal insufficiency consists of maintenance doses of oral glucocorticoid (hydrocortisone at 10–20 mg/m^2/day) and mineralocorticoid (fludrocortisone at 0.1 mg/day). The glucocorticoid dosage must be increased during significant intercurrent illness, trauma, or surgery to prevent acute adrenal insufficiency.

3. **Cushing syndrome** is a group of signs and symptoms that develop as a result of excessive cortisol, due to either endogenous overproduction of cortisol or exogenous treatment with pharmacologic doses of cortisol for other illnesses.
   a. **Etiology**
      (1) **Bilateral adrenal hyperplasia (Cushing disease)** is the most common etiology in children older than 7 years of age. This is now generally believed to be caused by chronic oversecretion of ACTH by a **pituitary tumor**. In many instances, the tumor is a microadenoma.
      (2) **Adrenal tumors** also may cause Cushing syndrome. Most adrenal tumors are adenomas, although in younger children and infants the possibility of malignant adrenal carcinoma is greater. Although most adrenal tumors are virilizing, rare feminizing adrenal tumors have been reported.
   b. **Clinical features.** The classic manifestations of Cushing syndrome in childhood are slow growth, truncal obesity, rounded "moon" facies, buffalo hump, purple striae, and acne. Hypertension and muscle weakness are common.

    c. Diagnosis. Initial laboratory studies document the presence of increased cortisol secretion. Elevated serum cortisol levels and absence of the normal diurnal variation are difficult to interpret in the stressed or hospitalized child.

        (1) A **24-hour urine test** for free cortisol is the most discriminating test. Failure to suppress the morning serum cortisol level to less than 5 µg/dl after receiving 0.3 mg/m^2 of dexamethasone at 11 P.M. the night before (the **overnight dexamethasone suppression test**) is supportive of possible Cushing syndrome.

        (2) A **prolonged dexamethasone suppression test** is needed to differentiate Cushing disease (bilateral adrenal hyperplasia due to pituitary adenoma) from Cushing syndrome due to adrenal tumor, if both the 24-hour urine free cortisol test and the overnight suppression test are positive. Low-dose oral dexamethasone (1.2 mg/m^2/day divided and given every 6 hours for 2 days) is followed by a high dose (4.8 mg/m^2/day for 2 days), with monitoring of serum cortisol and 24-hour urine free cortisol levels.

            (a) If serum and urine cortisol levels are suppressed to less than 50% of the baseline on the first 2 days, Cushing syndrome is not present.

            (b) Failure to suppress levels on the first 2 days (low-dose dexamethasone) but suppression on the last 2 days indicates bilateral adrenal hyperplasia due to pituitary adenoma.

            (c) Failure to suppress levels on high-dose dexamethasone indicates adrenal tumor.

        (3) **A computed tomography (CT) scan** of the pituitary and adrenal areas also is warranted.

    d. Therapy

        (1) Bilateral adrenal hyperplasia usually is treated by surgical excision of the pituitary adenoma. Transsphenoidal microsurgery is the treatment of choice for microadenomas. Some children have been treated with pituitary irradiation.

        (2) Adrenal tumors are treated by surgical excision. Chemotherapy for malignant metastatic disease may be palliative.

        (3) In all cases when surgery is performed, perioperative steroid coverage must be provided to prevent possible adrenal insufficiency.

B. **Disorders of the adrenal medulla.** The adrenal medulla is composed of chromaffin cells derived from neural crest tissue. The adrenal medulla produces catecholamines (**epinephrine** and **norepinephrine**) in response to sympathetic nervous system stimulation. Catecholamines exert widespread metabolic effects on glycogenolysis, lipolysis, and gluconeogenesis as well as effects on the cardiovascular system. The physiologic effects on vasodilation and cardiac muscle contractility are mediated through α- and β-adrenergic receptors on target cell surfaces. The major clinical problems arising from the adrenal medulla are tumors (see Chapter 16 for discussion of neuroblastoma).

    1. Pheochromocytoma is a rare tumor of chromaffin tissue. The most common site of occurrence is the adrenal medulla, but the tumor also may occur in extraadrenal sites in the chest and abdomen. Most tumors in childhood are benign. Morbidity and mortality result from the effects of overproduction of catecholamines. Pheochromocytoma may occur as an isolated tumor or in association with MEA types II and III (see V B 2 b–c).

    a. Clinical features. Hypertension usually is sustained but may be paroxysmal. Headache, vomiting, pallor, and sweating are prominent. Hypertensive encephalopathy may be life threatening.

    b. Diagnosis is based on finding elevated levels of epinephrine, norepinephrine, or their metabolites (e.g., metanephrine, normetanephrine) and 3-methoxy-4-hydroxymandelic acid in a 24-hour urine sample.

        (1) **Imaging studies.** An attempt to localize the tumor by noninvasive measures first should be made using abdominal ultrasonography and CT or magnetic resonance imaging (MRI) scanning. Tumors in the thorax may be identified on chest radiography or chest CT. ^{123}I-metaiodobenzylguanidine scintigraphy is helpful in imaging the adrenal medulla as well as extraadrenal chromaffin tissue.

    (2) Invasive procedures (e.g., venography for blood sampling for catecholamines, selective arteriography) may precipitate a hypertensive crisis and should be performed only after α-adrenergic blockade.

  c. Therapy for pheochromocytoma is surgical excision.

    (1) Careful attention must be given to perioperative control of hypertension and other symptoms. Preoperative medication consists of an α blocker, either the longer-acting phenoxybenzamine or prazosin, a shorter-acting α blocker, sometimes combined with a β blocker. During surgery, acute exacerbations of hypertension are treated with the short-acting α blocker phentolamine. The peripheral vasodilator nitroprusside may also be used.

    (2) Hypotension due to reduced vascular volume after the tumor is removed is managed with aggressive fluid replacement.

    (3) Glucocorticoids must be given if bilateral adrenalectomy is done.

  d. Follow-up. Postoperative levels of urinary catecholamines and metabolites should be normal. Persistent symptoms and elevated levels indicate residual tumor. Tumors may recur many years after initial successful treatment.

2. Multiple endocrine adenomatosis (MEA) syndromes are a group of familial disorders involving hyperplasia or neoplasia of a variety of endocrine tissues. Symptoms are related to the specific hormone that is secreted.

  a. MEA I. Tumors of the anterior lobe of the pituitary gland, the pancreatic islet cells, and the parathyroid glands may occur.

    (1) Nonfunctioning pituitary tumors may cause hypopituitarism. Hyperfunctioning pituitary tumors may cause acromegaly or gigantism, hyperprolactinemic syndromes, or Cushing disease.

    (2) Islet cell tumors may cause hypoglycemia (with secretion of insulin), intractable peptic ulcers (with secretion of gastrin), or hyperglycemia (with secretion of glucagon).

    (3) Hyperparathyroidism from hyperplasia or parathyroid tumor causes hypercalcemia.

  b. MEA II. This cluster includes pheochromocytoma, parathyroid hyperplasia, and medullary thyroid carcinoma (see III E 1 b).

  c. MEA III. This syndrome consists of multiple mucosal neuromas of the lips, eyelids, and tongue; marfanoid body habitus; and skeletal abnormalities, with medullary thyroid carcinoma and pheochromocytoma.

VI. DISORDERS OF THE GONADS

A. **Disorders of sexual differentiation of the newborn.** The diagnosis and management of clinical problems related to abnormal sexual differentiation of the newborn require an understanding of the process of normal sexual differentiation of male and female infants.

1. Normal sexual differentiation. The human embryonic gonad is undifferentiated before 45–50 days' gestation. The internal sexual ducts consist of both male (**wolffian**) and female (**müllerian**) structures at this early stage. Thereafter, sexual differentiation proceeds along distinctly different paths dictated by the genetic and hormonal factors in the male and female fetus.

  a. Male differentiation. The male genotype is 46,XY.

    (1) Determinants on the Y chromosome direct the synthesis of **testis-determining factor (TDF)**. In the presence of TDF, the undifferentiated gonad differentiates as a testis; in the absence of TDF, the undifferentiated gonad differentiates as an ovary.

    (2) The fetal testes secrete **testosterone** from Leydig cells under the direction of human chorionic gonadotropin (HCG) and fetal pituitary gonadotropin.

      (a) High local concentrations of fetal testosterone stabilize wolffian structures, which develop into the vas deferens, epididymis, and seminal vesicles.

    (b) Testosterone is converted to **dihydrotestosterone (DHT)** by the action of 5α-reductase. DHT is necessary for differentiation of the external genitalia into the scrotum, phallus, and phallic urethra, which is complete by 12–14 weeks' gestation.

    (c) The fetal testes also contain **Sertoli cells,** which secrete antimüllerian factor (AMF), causing regression of müllerian ducts in the male fetus by 8 weeks' gestation.

  b. Female differentiation. The female genotype is 46,XX. Female differentiation occurs in the absence of testicular determining factors (i.e., Y chromosome, TDF, testosterone, DHT, and AMF).

    (1) In the absence of a Y chromosome and TDF, the undifferentiated gonad develops as an ovary.

    (2) In the absence of AMF, müllerian ducts develop into the fallopian tubes, uterus, and upper one-third of the vagina.

    (3) In the absence of testosterone and DHT, the wolffian ducts degenerate and the external genitalia differentiate as the clitoris, labia majora and minora, and separate urethral and vaginal openings.

2. Abnormal sexual differentiation results in a newborn who appears sexually ambiguous.

  a. Male pseudohermaphroditism refers to infants who are 46,XY males (with testes) but who appear to have signs of incomplete masculinization, including hypospadias, a small phallus, and a poorly developed scrotum with or without descended testes. Male pseudohermaphroditism can be caused by a variety of endocrine disorders involving testosterone synthesis, metabolism, or action at the cellular level.

    (1) Defects in testosterone synthesis and metabolism are very rare and may be caused by one of five enzyme deficiencies inherited as autosomal recessive traits. The first three result in defects in cortisol synthesis as well, and therefore are classified as forms of **congenital adrenal hyperplasia** (see V A 1).

      (a) Cholesterol desmolase deficiency results in severe salt wasting. Profound deficiency in mineralocorticoid, glucocorticoid, and androgen results in death in infancy in spite of adrenal steroid replacement.

      (b) 3β-Hydroxysteroid dehydrogenase deficiency. Boys are incompletely virilized because of deficient testosterone synthesis. Girls may be mildly virilized. Diagnosis rests on measurement of elevated serum DHEA and 17-hydroxypregnenolone.

      (c) 17-Hydroxylase deficiency. Because this defect results in increased deoxycorticosterone, a weak mineralocorticoid, hypokalemia, and hypertension may be present. Boys have ambiguous genitalia because of the inability to produce sex steroids. Girls have normal sexual differentiation, but secondary sex characteristics fail to develop at puberty.

      (d) 17-Oxidoreductase deficiency prevents conversion of androstenedione to testosterone. Diagnosis may be made in infancy by finding an increased ratio of androstenedione to testosterone after stimulation with HCG.

      (e) 17,20-Desmolase deficiency is an extremely rare cause of male pseudohermaphroditism that results from the inability to convert progestogens to androgens. The defect can be demonstrated by an abnormal ratio of progestogens and androgens in the basal state and after HCG stimulation.

    (2) Defects in androgen action

      (a) 5α-Reductase deficiency impairs conversion of testosterone to DHT.

        (i) Boys are born with ambiguous genitalia because DHT is necessary for masculinization of the male external genitalia. Some of these infants are assigned a female sex because of the minimal virilization apparent at birth.

        (ii) At puberty, testosterone-dependent pubertal changes take place, such as clitoral enlargement and descent of inguinal testes into the rugated labioscrotal folds. Muscle mass increases, and the voice deepens. In one isolated community, a large number of affected children were raised as girls. Some of these individuals changed to a male gender role after puberty.

      (iii) The diagnosis of a 5α-reductase deficiency may be made in childhood by finding an increased ratio of testosterone to DHT after HCG stimulation.

  (b) **Androgen resistance syndromes (testicular feminization syndrome).** In the normal male newborn, testosterone levels are significantly elevated for the first several months. **Inappropriately elevated neonatal testosterone with high LH** might indicate androgen resistance due to a receptor defect or failure of normal negative-feedback suppression. The pattern of normal to high testosterone with high LH is well documented in postpubertal individuals with androgen resistance.

      (i) In **complete androgen resistance,** an XY male infant with testes appears unambiguously female because of complete resistance to androgen action at the cellular level. The first clue to this disorder may be the discovery of testes in inguinal hernia sacs in early childhood. Some children may present as female adolescents with primary amenorrhea. Because the undescended testes produce AMF in utero, the vagina is a shallow, blind-ending pouch. If the testes are not removed before the time of puberty, normal female breasts develop from the increased conversion of testosterone to estrogen by the testes.

      (ii) In **partial androgen resistance,** the affected XY individual has ambiguous genitalia. The diagnosis of partial androgen resistance is difficult to make in the newborn with an XY karyotype. Because it is inherited as an X-linked recessive trait, the infant's mother must be a carrier and half of her siblings would be expected to be female carriers or affected males. Therefore, a family history of infertile or cryptorchid relatives is suggestive.

b. **Female pseudohermaphroditism** refers to infants who are 46,XX females (with ovaries) but who appear masculinized at birth. Exposure of the female infant to increased androgen during the critical period of 8–12 weeks' gestation causes a variable degree of labioscrotal fusion, formation of a urogenital sinus, and clitoral enlargement. Exposure after the twelfth week cannot cause labioscrotal fusion, but it can induce clitoral enlargement. Some infants appear to be cryptorchid boys at birth.

  (1) **Congenital adrenal hyperplasia.** Defects that cause female pseudohermaphroditism are 21-hydroxylase deficiency, 11-hydroxylase deficiency, and 3β-hydroxysteroid dehydrogenase deficiency.

  (2) **Maternal androgen or progestin exposure.** With increasing awareness of the effects of medication and other drugs on the developing fetus, exogenous ingestion of androgenic substances is a rare cause of female pseudohermaphroditism. Occasionally, a virilizing tumor or disease during pregnancy in the mother may cause this syndrome. A detailed history of the pregnancy, including drugs taken and medical illness, should be obtained.

c. **Abnormal gonadal differentiation**

  (1) **True hermaphroditism** occurs when there is both ovarian and testicular tissue present in the gonads. In approximately 80% of cases, the karyotype is 46,XX, and in the remainder it is 46,XY or mosaicism. The exact etiology is unknown.

    (a) **Clinical features.** Usually there is significant masculinization, and consequently most true hermaphrodites are raised as boys. Gynecomastia and cyclic hematuria from uterine bleeding may occur.

    (b) **Diagnosis.** True hermaphroditism may be strongly suspected in an infant with ambiguous genitalia, an XX karyotype, and normal serum 17-hydroxyprogesterone levels, ruling out 21-hydroxylase deficiency. The final diagnosis rests with surgical exploration and demonstration of gonads containing both ovarian and testicular tissue.

  (2) **Mixed gonadal dysgenesis** involves a karyotype of 45X/46XY.

    (a) **Clinical features.** There is a spectrum of appearance of the external genitalia from completely male to completely female.

      (i) The gonads may appear as streak ovaries to dysgenetic testes and are often asymmetric. The more testicular tissue that is present, the greater is the likelihood of wolffian duct development on the side of that gonad.

      (ii) Because of the 45X cell line, some somatic features of Turner syndrome may be present (e.g., short stature, webbed neck, congenital heart disease) [see Chapter 8].

    (b) Diagnosis is made by karyotyping.

d. Other defects in external genital development include hypospadias and microphallus.

    (1) Hypospadias of varying degrees of severity may occur alone or with other birth defects, especially of the genitourinary system (see also Chapter 14).

    (2) Microphallus describes boys with abnormally small but well differentiated genitalia. Standards are available for assessing stretched penile length from infancy through adulthood. Male genital growth depends on fetal pituitary gonadotropin stimulation of the fetal testis.

        (a) Etiology. Microphallus may indicate postnatal hypogonadotropic hypogonadism, as in Kallmann syndrome, or may present as part of congenital hypopituitarism.

        (b) Therapy with testosterone (25 mg every 3 weeks for 3 months) may demonstrate responsiveness to testosterone and has a positive cosmetic effect, without significantly advancing skeletal maturation.

3. Management of the child with ambiguous genitalia

    a. Complete diagnostic evaluation should be undertaken as soon as possible after the birth of a child with ambiguous genitalia. Parents should be encouraged to delay naming and announcing the child's sex until diagnostic workup is complete. A careful family and pregnancy history and physical examination are the basis for further testing.

      (1) Physical examination. The size of the phallus, position of the urethra, palpable gonads (usually testes), and other dysmorphic or asymmetric features should be noted.

      (2) Laboratory studies initially include chromosome analysis and evaluation of electrolyte, testosterone, LH, FSH, and 17-hydroxyprogesterone levels. Radiographic dye study of the urogenital sinus often is helpful to delineate the presence of a vagina and cervix, and occasionally fallopian tubes may be seen. Pelvic ultrasonography may demonstrate the presence of ovaries and a uterus.

        (a) If the karyotype is 46,XX and the 17-hydroxyprogesterone level is elevated, the most likely diagnosis is 21-hydroxylase deficiency. If the 17-hydroxyprogesterone level is normal, true hermaphroditism is likely. Measurement of 11-deoxycortisol and DHEA levels rules out the remote possibility of 11-hydroxylase deficiency or 3β-hydroxysteroid dehydrogenase deficiency.

        (b) If the karyotype is 46,XY, measurement of gonadal and adrenal steroids before and after ACTH and HCG stimulation identifies rare forms of congenital adrenal hyperplasia and defects in testosterone synthesis and metabolism.

          (i) Infants must be monitored closely for evidence of salt wasting and glucocorticoid deficiency while awaiting diagnostic test results.

          (ii) Diagnosis of partial androgen resistance depends on a family history compatible with X-linked recessive inheritance. High neonatal testosterone levels with elevated LH levels are suggestive of androgen resistance.

    b. Gender assignment. It is important to arrive at the most specific diagnosis possible for a variety of therapeutic and management considerations.

      (1) Even markedly **masculinized girls with 21-hydroxylase deficiency** should be raised as female because they have reproductive potential with adequate medical management of their disease and cosmetic repair of the external genitalia.

      (2) For **46,XY boys with ambiguous genitalia,** gender assignment should be based on consideration of the possibility of normal adult male sexual function. This generally depends on the size of the phallus and the surgeon's estimation of surgical correctability of the hypospadias.

        (a) Dysgenetic testes and ovotestes should be removed because of their potential for malignant transformation.

      (b) Gonads that do not agree with gender assignment should be removed to avoid the possibility of undesirable hormonal influences at puberty.

  c. Therapy

      (1) Appropriate hormonal replacement at the usual age of puberty should be provided.

      (2) Genetic and sexual counseling for families and for children is an important aspect of medical care.

      (3) In general, full but sensitive disclosure of all test results in an age-appropriate manner leads to successful psychosexual adjustment in adulthood.

B. **Disorders of puberty.** Normal pubertal development occurs as the period of transition from sexual immaturity to the sexually mature adult state (see Chapter 5; Tables 5-1–5-3; Figures 5-2, 5-3). During this time, secondary sex characteristics are acquired and reproductive capacity is attained as a result of the secretion of gonadal steroids under the direction of gonadotropin-releasing hormone (GnRH) and pituitary gonadotropins (i.e., FSH and LH). Deficiencies or defects in the functioning of these secretions may result in abnormal pubertal development.

  1. Delayed puberty

    a. Female delayed puberty. By definition, the absence of secondary sex characteristics at 13 years of age is considered delayed. Normal secondary sex characteristics but absence of menarche by 16 years of age also is considered delayed (**primary amenorrhea**).

      (1) Constitutional delay of puberty is less commonly diagnosed in girls than in boys.

        (a) Etiology. Constitutional delay of puberty is a designation reserved for otherwise healthy children (see VIII B 1). Delayed puberty may also be secondary to a variety of endocrine and systemic diseases, such as hypothyroidism, sickle cell anemia, rheumatoid arthritis, inflammatory bowel disease, chronic renal failure, and others.

        (b) Clinical features. Girls with constitutional delay of puberty frequently are short but growing at normal prepubertal growth velocities. Bone age often is significantly delayed; however, there is no evidence of other endocrine or systemic disease. There is frequently a strong history of delayed puberty or menarche in adult family members. Late but otherwise normal puberty occurs.

      (2) Primary ovarian failure. Girls with primary ovarian failure have castrate levels of gonadotropins by the usual age of puberty (10–12 years) because of lack of feedback of gonadal steroids on the pituitary gland.

        (a) Turner syndrome is the most common cause of primary ovarian failure (see Chapter 8).

        (b) Prepubertal surgical removal or irradiation of the ovaries for treatment of cancer also may cause primary ovarian failure.

        (c) Autoimmune ovarian failure may occur in association with other autoimmune diseases, adrenal insufficiency, thyroiditis, hypoparathyroidism, and IDDM.

      (3) Hypogonadotropic hypogonadism may be difficult to distinguish from delayed puberty because, in each situation, gonadotropin levels are low and the response to GnRH stimulation is also minimal. This disorder often is part of other recognizable syndromes.

        (a) Kallmann syndrome involves anosmia with hypogonadotropic hypogonadism.

        (b) Hypopituitarism may include gonadotropin deficiency as one of several deficient pituitary hormones.

        (c) Hypothalamic and pituitary tumors such as adenoma, microadenoma (especially one secreting prolactin), craniopharyngioma, and pinealoma may be associated with hypogonadotropic hypogonadism.

        (d) Anorexia nervosa may cause delayed puberty or, in older adolescents, secondary amenorrhea due to gonadotropin deficiency.

        (e) Prader-Willi syndrome is characterized by short stature, obesity, mental retardation, and hypogonadotropic hypogonadism (see Chapter 8).

b. Male delayed puberty. The earliest sign of puberty in boys is testicular enlargement. Absence of any evidence of puberty by 14 years of age is considered delayed.

  (1) Constitutional delay of puberty is the most common cause of delayed puberty in boys. Frequently these boys are short (at or below the fifth percentile) but growing at a low to normal prepubertal growth velocity. The bone age is significantly delayed. The physical examination is negative except for sexual immaturity. There usually is a family history of delayed pubertal development.

  (2) Primary testicular failure. In boys with primary testicular failure, gonadotropin levels are elevated in the castrate range by the usual age of puberty because of the lack of testosterone feedback on the pituitary gland.

  (a) Congenital bilateral anorchia ("vanishing testes" syndrome). Boys with this syndrome have normal male sexual differentiation with apparent cryptorchidism. However, no testes are found on surgical exploration, and there is no testosterone response to HCG stimulation. Because there are normal male external genitalia and there are no müllerian remnants internally, it is presumed that testes must have been present in early fetal life and subsequently "vanished."

  (b) Chemotherapy, irradiation, surgical excision, trauma, and infection in the prepubertal boy may result in testicular failure.

  (c) Primary testicular failure also may be associated with the normal onset of puberty. In **Klinefelter syndrome** (see also Chapter 8), a common cause of testicular failure, puberty begins at the usual age and secondary sex characteristics are acquired. However, these boys have small, firm testes and often have gynecomastia.

  (3) Hypogonadotropic hypogonadism. As in girls, isolated hypogonadotropic hypogonadism in boys may occur alone or as part of a recognizable disease (e.g., Kallmann syndrome, hypopituitarism, CNS tumors, Prader-Willi syndrome).

c. Diagnosis

  (1) A careful **history** and **physical examination** should be taken, including height and weight, Tanner staging of pubertal development (see Tables 5-1–5-3), smell testing, and presence of dysmorphic features or signs of other endocrine or systemic disease.

  (2) Laboratory studies include an evaluation of skeletal maturation (bone age) as well as FSH, LH, prolactin, T_4, TSH, and testosterone or estrogen levels. To rule out systemic disease, complete blood count, erythrocyte sedimentation rate, electrolyte, and BUN levels may be helpful. Depending on the clinical situation, CT or MRI scan of the head and testing of other pituitary hormones may be indicated.

d. Therapy

  (1) Treatment with appropriate sex steroid replacement for adolescents with a permanent cause of delayed puberty (either primary gonadal failure or hypogonadotropic hypogonadism) should be instituted at the usual age of puberty. Because sex steroids promote epiphyseal fusion while stimulating linear growth, this effect must be taken into consideration when treating children with short stature, especially that caused by GH deficiency.

  (2) For adolescents with constitutional delay of puberty, smaller doses of the appropriate sex steroid may be used for a short course of treatment (3–6 months). This will initiate some development of secondary sex characteristics and be psychologically beneficial while not promoting premature epiphyseal fusion and loss of adult height.

2. Precocious puberty. Sexual development is considered to be precocious if there are any secondary sex characteristics present in girls before 7 years of age and in boys before 9 years of age. True **central (gonadotropin-dependent) precocious puberty** appears to be more common in girls than in boys. In girls, there rarely is underlying CNS disease, and it is therefore considered "idiopathic." There is a significant incidence of CNS pathology, especially tumors, in boys with central precocious puberty.

a. Premature thelarche refers to the frequent finding of **isolated breast development** in very young girls. The usual age of onset is 12–24 months.
 (1) Etiology. It has been postulated that premature thelarche is caused by transient bursts of estrogen from the prepubertal ovary or from increased sensitivity to low levels of estrogen in some prepubertal girls.
 (2) Clinical features. Gonadotropins and serum estrogen levels are in the prepubertal range. Linear growth acceleration and advanced skeletal maturation are not present. Breast development does not progress, and no other signs of puberty develop.
 (3) Diagnosis. This nonprogressive, benign condition can be distinguished from true precocious puberty by the normal growth rate and bone age associated with premature thelarche.
b. Premature adrenarche describes the **early appearance of sexual hair** (i.e., before 8 years of age in girls and 9 years of age in boys).
 (1) Etiology. This benign condition is believed to be caused by early maturation of adrenal androgen secretion (adrenarche) in some children.
 (2) Clinical features. Levels of adrenal androgens are normal for pubertal stage but elevated for chronologic age. Bone age may be slightly, but not usually significantly, advanced.
 (3) Diagnosis. Children with premature adrenarche must be evaluated for other causes of increased androgen production, such as congenital adrenal hyperplasia due to 21-hydroxylase, 11-hydroxylase, or 3β-hydroxysteroid dehydrogenase deficiency or adrenal tumor. In children with clinical evidence of significant androgen effect (e.g., advanced bone age, growth acceleration, acne), measurement of adrenal steroids and androgens before and after ACTH will identify those with congenital adrenal hyperplasia.
c. Precocious isosexual puberty may be divided into two types—gonadotropin-dependent and gonadotropin-independent. This distinction has etiologic and therapeutic considerations.
 (1) Gonadotropin-dependent precocious puberty (GDPP) may be considered normal puberty beginning at an abnormally early age.
  (a) Etiology. GDPP may be idiopathic (as it is in most girls) or secondary to structural or functional disturbance in the CNS where the onset of puberty originates. However, a variety of diseases of the CNS have been associated with GDPP, including tumors (e.g., glioma, pinealoma, hamartoma), hydrocephalus, head injury, congenital malformation, and infection.
  (b) Clinical features are progressive development of secondary sex characteristics, beginning in girls before 7 years of age and in boys before 9 years of age, accompanied by a growth spurt, causing the child's height to cross isobars on the growth curve. If the GDPP is secondary to a CNS problem, a history of neurologic disease or abnormal neurologic findings on physical examination may be present. Because sex steroids stimulate growth while promoting epiphyseal fusion, precocious puberty causes tall stature in childhood, premature closure of the epiphyses, and adult short stature. Behavior problems related to early sexual development are relatively common.
  (c) Diagnosis is based on evidence of growth acceleration, significantly advanced bone age, and pubertal levels of gonadotropins and estrogen or testosterone. Because of the episodic secretion of gonadotropins and sex steroids early in GDPP, random daytime measurements may be low. A pubertal pattern of elevated gonadotropins after an intravenous infusion of GnRH is indicative of GDPP.
  (d) Therapy. Goals are to diminish secondary sexual characteristics, inhibit menses in girls, and slow growth velocity and skeletal maturation to a normal prepubertal rate. The recent development of long-acting analogues of GnRH that inhibit gonadotropin release has provided effective treatment in GDPP for the first time.

(2) Gonadotropin-independent precocious puberty (GIPP) is a rare cause of precocious sexual development. Examples of GIPP are McCune-Albright syndrome (polyostotic fibrous dysplasia of bone), some cases of familial male precocious puberty (testitoxicosis), and Leydig cell tumors and hyperplasia. Gonadotropins are low, and there is no increase in gonadotropins after GnRH infusion. GIPP does not respond to treatment with analogues of GnRH.

(3) Ectopic HCG production by neoplasms may stimulate Leydig cell growth and hypersecretion of testosterone with the clinical presentation of precocious puberty in boys. Tumors include hepatoblastoma, pinealoma, and retroperitoneal carcinoma. High LH levels (due to cross-reaction with HCG in radioimmunoassay) and low FSH levels are a clue to ectopic HCG production.

(4) Hypothyroidism paradoxically may be associated with sexual precocity. Both gonadotropins and prolactin are elevated. Galactorrhea may be present. Unlike the case in other forms of precocious puberty, growth is arrested in hypothyroidism and bone age is delayed. Treatment of hypothyroidism may stop progression of sexual development.

VII. DISORDERS OF CALCIUM METABOLISM. Calcium and phosphorus homeostasis is maintained by having adequate nutritional intake of calcium, phosphorus, and vitamin D and a normally mineralized skeleton, the major reservoir of these minerals. The serum calcium and phosphorus are finely regulated by the action of **parathyroid hormone (PTH),** which acts on the bone and kidneys to raise the serum levels of calcium and lower the levels of phosphorus. Abnormalities of vitamin D and PTH may have profound effects on the serum levels of calcium and phosphorus and on the skeleton.

A. Disorders of the parathyroid glands

1. **Primary hyperparathyroidism** is rare in childhood. The disorder may be isolated or occur as part of MEA I or II (see V B 2). Increased PTH levels cause increased mobilization of calcium and phosphorus from bone. The effect of increased PTH on the kidneys is decreased tubular reabsorption of phosphorus. Thus, the serum levels of calcium are elevated (**hypercalcemia**) and the phosphorus levels are low.
   a. Clinical features
      (1) Symptoms are related to hypercalcemia and include nausea, vomiting, constipation, lethargy, confusion, and weakness.
      (2) Hypertension and renal colic secondary to kidney stones are common.
   b. Diagnosis
      (1) Laboratory studies show elevated serum levels of calcium (total and ionized), low levels of phosphorus, increased alkaline phosphatase, and low tubular reabsorption of phosphorus (less than 80%). PTH levels are elevated relative to the elevated serum calcium. PTH secretion is autonomous.
      (2) Radiographs of bone show subperiosteal bone resorption that is especially evident in the clavicles.
   c. Therapy involves excision of the tumor if an adenoma is found and subtotal parathyroidectomy for hyperplasia.

2. **Secondary hyperparathyroidism.** Diseases that cause **hypocalcemia** stimulate PTH to be released. The elevated PTH then restores the serum calcium to normal, but not elevated, levels, but at the expense of having low phosphorus levels.
   a. Etiology. Conditions that are associated with secondary hyperparathyroidism are chronic renal disease, liver disease, and lack of vitamin D. In each of these situations, the initiating event is related to lack of intake, absorption, or metabolism of vitamin D, which leads to the hypocalcemic stimulus for PTH secretion.
   b. Diagnosis and therapy. The radiographic manifestation is rickets, and treatment is provision of adequate vitamin D.

3. **Hypoparathyroidism**
   a. **Idiopathic hypoparathyroidism** may present in the neonatal period or at any time during childhood. The etiology may be autoimmune.
      (1) **Clinical features.** Symptoms are caused by low serum levels of calcium and include seizures, tetany, numbness of the face and extremities, and carpopedal spasm. Associated diseases may be thyroiditis, diabetes, adrenal insufficiency, and mucocutaneous candidiasis.
      (2) **Diagnosis.** At the time when serum calcium levels are low and phosphorus levels are high, the PTH levels are inappropriately low, indicating lack of PTH response to the hypocalcemia signal.
   b. **Pseudohypoparathyroidism** also presents as symptomatic hypocalcemia, but PTH levels are very high, indicating PTH unresponsiveness due to a receptor or post-receptor defect. Patients with pseudohypoparathyroidism may have distinctive skeletal and facial characteristics, including short stature, round facies, a short, thick neck, and short metacarpals. Mental retardation is common.
   c. **Therapy**
      (1) **Vitamin D** is the treatment for idiopathic hypoparathyroidism and pseudohypo-parathyroidism.
         (a) Because low levels of PTH inhibit 1,25-hydroxylation of vitamin D in the kidneys, PTH deficiency is associated with a deficit of 1,25-dihydroxyvitamin D_3 (calcitriol), the most active metabolite of vitamin D. Treatment with 1,25-dihydroxyvitamin D_3 overcomes the deficit and also stimulates increased calcium absorption in the intestine.
         (b) Other forms of vitamin D, such as 25-hydroxyvitamin D_3 (calcidiol) and vita-min D_3 (cholecalciferol), also are effective but are required in larger doses. Because of the longer half-life of vitamin D_3, however, toxicity (hypercal-cemia) is more serious.
      (2) **Oral calcium supplementation** may speed the restoration of normal calcium levels. These children should have serum calcium and phosphorus levels moni-tored frequently to avoid hypercalcemia and potential nephrocalcinosis and renal damage.

4. **Neonatal hypocalcemia**
   a. **Early hypocalcemia** (serum calcium levels < 7 mg/dl) in the first 24–48 hours of life usually is associated with prematurity.
      (1) Immaturity of the parathyroid response to the normal fall in serum calcium levels after birth is believed to be the cause.
      (2) Clinical conditions associated with hypocalcemia in the first 2 days of life are birth asphyxia and maternal diabetes.
      (3) Hypocalcemia may be treated with oral calcium supplementation or intravenous calcium infusion for seizures.
   b. **Late hypocalcemic tetany** may occur in the first few weeks of life in infants receiving high-phosphate diets (i.e., cow's milk). Increased phosphate intake precipitates hypocalcemia, and therefore is not recommended.
   c. **Idiopathic hypoparathyroidism** may present in the neonatal period with hypocal-cemic seizures.

B. | **Rickets**

1. **General features of rickets**
   a. **Defect.** Rickets is characterized by bone lesions that are caused by **failure of osteoid,** the growing cellular matrix of bone, **to become mineralized**. The undermineralized bone is less rigid and the growing, remodeling bone bends and twists abnormally.
   b. **Clinical features**
      (1) Characteristic physical findings are bowing of the legs, thickening of the costo-chondral junction (rachitic rosary), knobby prominence of the wrists and knees, and growth failure. In infants, craniotabes (thinning of the skull bones) and frac-tures are common.

(2) The radiographic manifestations are readily visible in views of the wrists and knees, with widening of the space between the end of the metaphysis and the epiphysis. The ends of the metaphysis are cupped, widened, and irregular or frayed.

2. **Variants of rickets** may be caused by vitamin D deficiency secondary to decreased intake, decreased absorption or decreased metabolism of vitamin D, or by lack of adequate calcium and phosphorus for normal bone mineralization caused by either deficient mineral intake or increased losses by the kidneys.

   a. **Nutritional rickets.** Lack of vitamin D in the diet results in decreased calcium absorption in the intestine. Hypocalcemia stimulates PTH secretion, which then causes increased reabsorption of calcium from bone and decreased renal reabsorption of phosphorus.

   (1) Etiology. Despite fortification of many foods with vitamin D to provide the minimum requirement of 400 IU daily, nutritional rickets still occurs in people with low vitamin D intake, such as food faddists. Often other aggravating factors are present besides decreased vitamin D intake, such as decreased exposure to the sun due to dark skin pigmentation, urban living conditions, and the winter season.

   (2) Clinical features. In classic nutritional rickets, the serum calcium level is low (or it may be normalized by the secondarily high PTH), the phosphorus level is low, and the alkaline phosphatase level is high because of active bone resorption from secondary hyperparathyroidism.

   (3) Therapy with 5000–10,000 IU/day of vitamin D_3 (cholecalciferol) for several weeks, followed by provision of 400 IU/day in the diet, is curative.

   b. **Rickets associated with abnormal metabolism of vitamin D**

   (1) Vitamin D-dependent rickets, an autosomal recessive disease, is caused by absence of the renal enzyme 1α-hydroxylase, which converts 25-hydroxyvitamin D_3 to the active metabolite 1,25-dihydroxyvitamin D_3.

   (a) Clinical features. Vitamin D-dependent rickets presents in the same way as nutritional rickets. The serum calcium level is low (or normal), the phosphorus level is low, and PTH is elevated. Usually 25-hydroxyvitamin D_3 levels are normal, whereas 1,25-dihydroxyvitamin D_3 levels are low.

   (b) Therapy with physiologic doses of 1,25-dihydroxyvitamin D_3 is curative.

   (2) Chronic renal disease. One of the factors leading to **renal osteodystrophy**—the complex of osteopenia, osteitis fibrosis, and rickets associated with chronic renal failure—is decreased activity of 1α-hydroxylase in the kidneys. Therefore, treatment of renal osteodystrophy includes 1,25-dihydroxyvitamin D_3.

   (3) Chronic liver disease, such as biliary atresia and other cholestatic diseases, may result in rickets from decreased intestinal absorption of vitamin D, a fat-soluble vitamin, or from decreased 25-hydroxylation in the liver itself. The treatment of choice is 25-hydroxyvitamin D_3 or 1,25-dihydroxyvitamin D_3.

   (4) Chronic anticonvulsant therapy. Phenobarbital and phenytoin cause increased metabolism of calcidiol and may be associated with rickets. Usually other nutritional and environmental factors also are present in children with seizure disorders who present with clinical rickets. Increased demand for vitamin D can be satisfied by increasing the daily intake to 1000–2000 IU/day for children on chronic anticonvulsant therapy whose exposure to sunlight and nutritional intake is marginal.

   c. **Rickets due to mineral deficiency**

   (1) X-linked hypophosphatemia (familial hypophosphatemia). The primary defect in this inheritable form of rickets is a renal tubular defect resulting in phosphate "wasting." The serum calcium level is normal, the phosphorus level is low, and the alkaline phosphatase level is elevated. The 25-hydroxyvitamin D_3 level is normal, but the 1,25-dihydroxyvitamin D_3 level is low or normal, which is inappropriate given the hypophosphatemic stimulus for increasing 1α-hydroxylase activity. This may imply a defect in vitamin D metabolism as an additional etiologic factor.

(a) **Clinical features.** Biochemical abnormalities and radiographic signs of rickets are evident in the first few months of life. Subsequently, these children have severe rickets and short stature.

(b) **Therapy** consists of oral phosphate to replace renal losses and 1,25-dihydroxy-vitamin D_3. Care must be taken to avoid vitamin D intoxication with hypercalciuria, nephrocalcinosis, and hypercalcemia.

(2) **Rickets of prematurity (metabolic bone disease of the premature infant).** Infants born prematurely have decreased bone mineralization compared to full-term infants because they do not benefit from the major skeletal accretion of calcium and phosphorus occurring in utero during the last trimester.

(a) **Clinical features.** Human milk and standard infant formulas that provide adequate calcium and phosphorus for the full-term infant are not adequate for the needs of the premature infant, as evidenced by the occurrence of severe osteopenia and rickets, resulting in fractures, in some premature infants. In these infants, serum calcium level is normal, and phosphorus level is low. 1,25-Dihydroxyvitamin D_3 levels are elevated, probably because of the hypophosphatemic stimulus.

(b) **Therapy.** Fortifying human milk or formulas with additional calcium and phosphorus results in improvement in bone mineralization and healing of fractures and rickets.

VIII. APPROACH TO THE PEDIATRIC PATIENT WITH SHORT STATURE. This section discusses the general approach to the evaluation of the child or adolescent with short stature. Many of the specific endocrine disorders that may result in short stature are described in detail elsewhere in this chapter.

A. Growth assessment

1. **Growth charts.** Assessment of growth in childhood begins with accurate and serial measurements that are plotted on the appropriate growth chart. The most widely accepted charts for children in the United States are those compiled by the United States National Center for Health Statistics.

2. **History.** Information that may have a bearing on the child's growth is gathered from talking with the child and his or her caregivers, usually the parents.
   a. Birth history, review of past growth and medical records, and a careful review of symptoms referable to each organ system must be obtained.
   b. Behavior problems and school performance should be noted.
   c. Growth records kept by the parents, school, and doctors' offices are helpful. If such records are not available, indirect information about growth may be ascertained by asking about frequency of shoe and clothing size changes and height relative to siblings and peers.
   d. Information about genetic potential for height may be gathered by recording the heights of parents, siblings, and other relatives. A family history of other medical problems also is relevant.
   e. The child should be questioned sensitively about the impact of short stature on his or her relationships with peers, participation in sports, and other social activities. Parents' perceptions also should be noted in these matters.

3. **Physical examination.** The following aspects should receive special attention during a physical examination.
   a. **Height**
      (1) **Recumbent length** is plotted for children from birth to 24 months of age. **Standing heights** are plotted for children 2–18 years of age. A **stadiometer** or other measuring device fixed to the wall measures height most accurately.
      (2) In addition to height, **arm span** and **upper-to-lower body segment ratio** should be measured.

   b. **General appearance and activity.** Dysmorphic features in a pattern suggestive of a specific syndrome, obesity, and general appropriateness of behavior to the examiner and family members should be noted.
   c. **Skin** is examined for abnormal pigmentation or cyanosis, and the skin and hair texture are noted for possible clues to hypothyroidism.
   d. **Head, ears, and eyes** are examined for midline defects (e.g., clefts) and for ocular or dental anomalies. Visual field examination is performed. Funduscopy is performed to look for optic nerve abnormalities, which might indicate increased intracranial pressure or an underlying CNS disease causing GH deficiency.
   e. **Neck.** The thyroid is palpated to determine its size, consistency, and the presence of nodules.
   f. **Chest and heart** are examined for evidence of chronic cardiopulmonary disease or heart murmur.
   g. **Abdomen.** Tenderness or bloating may indicate chronic gastrointestinal disease, such as celiac disease or inflammatory bowel disease.
   h. **Genitalia.** Anomalies of the genitalia, such as undescended testes and hypospadias in boys and clitoromegaly and labial fusion in girls, should be noted. Stretched penile length and testicular size should be recorded. Tanner staging for breast and pubic hair development in girls and genital and pubic hair development in boys should be documented.
   i. **Extremities.** Abnormalities of digits, joints, and body proportions should be noted and compared to published norms for age and sex.
   j. **Neurologic examination** is performed to rule out underlying CNS disease, especially any tumor that might cause GH deficiency.

B. **Short stature** generally can be ascribed to several broad categories of medical problems. On the basis of previous growth and medical records and the current medical, family, and social history and physical examination, the laboratory evaluation focuses on a relatively small number of tests of both diagnostic and prognostic significance. Broad diagnostic categories are discussed in the order of those most frequently found among children presenting to an endocrinologist with the complaint of short stature.

   1. **Constitutional delay of growth and development** is a more common diagnosis among boys referred for short stature than among girls, perhaps because of greater social value placed on height for boys than for girls.
      a. **Growth assessment**
         (1) These children grow at or below the fifth percentile at normal growth velocities, which results in a curve that is parallel to the fifth percentile.
         (2) Puberty is delayed and usually reflects significantly delayed skeletal maturation. Because these children fail to enter puberty at the usual age, their short stature and sexual immaturity are accentuated at this time compared to those of normally developing peers.
         (3) Family members usually are of average height, but there often is a family history of short stature in childhood and delayed puberty in other family members.
      b. **Diagnosis.** Minimal diagnostic tests are indicated, including thyroid studies, complete blood count, erythrocyte sedimentation rate, electrolytes, BUN, and bone age assessment. These children have no findings suggestive of other endocrine or chronic systemic disease, and the normal growth velocity argues against such diagnoses.
      c. **Counseling.** These children and their families should be counseled about this pattern of growth and development as a variant of normal conditions and reassured about their potential for normal height, usually in the range expected for their families.
      d. **Therapy.** In many instances, reassurance that no significant endocrine disease exists and that normal growth and puberty with reasonable adult stature are expected is all that is required. Treatment with the anabolic steroid oxandrolone is controversial but appears to be helpful in some boys, mostly for the psychological benefit

of modestly increasing muscle mass and growth velocity. There is no convincing evidence that final adult stature is either augmented or reduced by this treatment. Because of the illicit use of anabolic steroids by many athletes, oxandrolone is no longer available in the United States for treatment of short stature. For boys and girls with no signs of puberty by 14 years of age and with a diagnosis of constitutional delay of growth and development, a short course (4–6 months) of the appropriate sex steroid may be helpful.

2. Familial (genetic) short stature
   a. Growth assessment
      (1) These children establish growth curves at or below the fifth percentile by 2–3 of age years. They are otherwise completely healthy, with a normal physical examination. Bone age in these children is normal. Therefore, puberty occurs at the usual age, and thus limits potential for growth late into adolescence.
      (2) Short stature usually is found in at least one parent. However, because the inheritance of height is complex, occasionally short stature may be present only in more distant relatives.
   b. Diagnosis. The same minimal diagnostic evaluation may be performed in these children as for those with apparent constitutional delay of growth to rule out subtle thyroid dysfunction or chronic disease.
   c. Counseling. Because puberty occurs at the expected time, these children seem to be at less of a disadvantage socially and emotionally compared to those with constitutional delay, despite the fact that their potential for adult height in the normal range is less.

3. GH deficiency (see also IV A 1 b). Fewer than 5% of children referred to endocrinologists for short stature have GH deficiency.
   a. Growth assessment. Children with classic GH deficiency grow at subnormal growth velocities (< 5 cm/year) and have significant retardation of skeletal maturation. Therefore, evaluation with GH testing should be reserved for children who satisfy those criteria.
      (1) A history of birth asphyxia or neonatal hypoglycemia, or physical findings of microphallus or midline defects, is strongly suggestive of idiopathic GH deficiency.
      (2) GH deficiency secondary to a hypothalamic or pituitary tumor usually is associated with other neurologic or visual complaints and findings. In an older child with more recent onset of subnormal growth, the index of suspicion for tumor should be high.
   b. Diagnosis. After establishing that current growth velocity is less than 5 cm/year and that thyroid function is normal and other systemic disease is unlikely, GH testing should be carried out. Evaluation for other pituitary hormone deficiencies also should be performed.
   c. Therapy
      (1) For children deemed GH-deficient, recombinant human GH (0.03–0.05 mg/kg) is given by subcutaneous injection every day. Accelerated growth velocity on GH treatment results in some catch-up growth in most children.
      (2) If puberty is delayed beyond 14 years of age, the addition of sex steroids may be considered, both to augment the growth response to GH and to stimulate secondary sexual development. In children who have permanent gonadotropin deficiency, sex steroids may need to be replaced indefinitely, as physiologically as possible.
      (3) Treatment with cortisol, thyroid hormone, and vasopressin (ADH) may be needed, depending on the degree of hypopituitarism.
      (4) Although some GH-deficient children release GH when stimulated by GRF, treatment with GRF currently is not an available alternative to GH therapy except in the research setting.

4. **Primary hypothyroidism** (see also III B) causes marked growth failure, with growth velocity less than 5 cm/year, and marked retardation of skeletal maturation. Because primary hypothyroidism is easily treatable, almost all children with short stature should have T_4, T_3 resin uptake, and TSH levels measured, even in the absence of obvious symptoms, to rule out any degree of hypothyroidism.

5. **Cushing disease** [see also V A 3 a (1)] is a very rare cause of short stature in children. However, **hypercortisolism** (from either exogenous treatment with pharmacologic doses of steroids or endogenous oversecretion) may have a profound growth-suppressing effect. Usually other features of Cushing syndrome are evident.

6. **Primordial growth failure** has been used to describe a large, diverse group of children who have normal endocrine function but who have inherent limitations on skeletal growth.
   a. **Etiology.** The cause of short stature in these children usually is easily identified on the basis of abnormal body proportions (skeletal dysplasias), dysmorphic features (chromosome abnormalities), and other characteristics of the history or physical examination (e.g., Prader-Willi syndrome, Noonan syndrome, intrauterine growth retardation) [see Chapter 8 VI C 6].
   b. **Diagnosis.** Special attention should be given to the evaluation of **girls with short stature**. Although a short girl with all of the physical stigmata of Turner syndrome may be easily identified, the features may be quite subtle in some girls. Therefore, girls with short stature and delayed puberty should have gonadotropins and chromosomes measured. Elevated gonadotropins indicating primary ovarian failure and chromosome abnormalities are diagnostic of Turner syndrome (see Chapter 8).
   c. **Therapy.** Although children with primordial growth failure are not thought to have classic GH deficiency, the response to GH treatment in these children is being explored.

7. **Chronic systemic disease.** The impact of chronic systemic disease on growth is well known.
   a. **Types of diseases**
      (1) Cyanotic congenital heart disease, poorly controlled diabetes mellitus, and severe rheumatoid arthritis have a deleterious effect on growth, probably related to a combination of nutritional deficits and increased metabolic demands created by the disease process.
      (2) Some chronic diseases may have minimal symptoms and yet have a significant effect on growth. The two best known categories of chronic diseases that may present first as short stature are gastrointestinal diseases, specifically inflammatory bowel disease (Crohn disease) and celiac disease, and renal disease associated with renal tubular acidosis or uremia.
   b. **Diagnosis.** Screening studies that may be helpful are complete blood count, erythrocyte sedimentation rate, serum electrolytes, and BUN. In some children where there is no explanation for growth failure, additional diagnostic tests for gastrointestinal disease are performed.

8. **Psychosocial deprivation.** In some children, a hostile, abusive, or neglectful environment appears to result in functional GH deficiency.
   a. **Clinical features.** Children with psychosocial deprivation characteristically show bizarre behavior, including hoarding food, gorging, drinking from puddles and toilet bowls, immature speech, disturbed sleep–wake cycles, and diminished perception of pain. Clinically, they resemble children with GH deficiency, with marked retardation of bone age and delayed puberty.
   b. **Diagnosis.** If GH testing is done while the children remain in the hostile environment, it usually shows a blunted response. When taken out of that environment, the children show catch-up growth, and testing reverts to normal.

C. **Tall stature.** Occasionally children appear to be growing too rapidly. Children who are growing above the ninety-fifth percentile should be examined carefully for signs of precocious puberty or adrenal androgen excess.

1. Most children have **familial tall stature**. Occasionally, early adolescent girls with familial tall stature may request treatment to reduce adult stature. High-dose estrogen may induce premature epiphyseal fusion and reduction of final height.

2. Other, more unusual causes of tall stature are GH excess (causing **acromegaly** and **gigantism**), hyperthyroidism, Marfan syndrome, and homocystinuria.

BIBLIOGRAPHY

Kappy MS, Blizzard RM, Migeon CJ: *Wilkins Diagnosis and Treatment of Endocrine Disorders in Childhood and Adolescence,* 4th ed. Springfield, IL, Charles C Thomas, 1994.

STUDY QUESTIONS

DIRECTIONS: Each of the numbered items or incomplete statements in this section is followed by answers or by completions of the statement. Select the ONE lettered answer or completion that is BEST in each case.

1. Autoimmunity is thought to play a pathogenetic role in which of the following conditions?

(A) Hypophosphatemic rickets
(B) Familial hypercholesterolemia
(C) Congenital hypothyroidism
(D) Insulin-dependent (type I) diabetes mellitus (IDDM)

2. A 12-year-old boy is referred to his pediatrician by his teacher for poor attention span, deteriorating school performance, and frequent trips to the bathroom. By the pediatrician's records, the boy has lost 5 lb since his previous visit 6 months earlier. On physical examination, the boy's resting pulse is 110 beats/minute, his blood pressure is 130/50, and his thyroid gland is about twice the normal size. The most likely diagnosis is

(A) Hashimoto thyroiditis
(B) medullary carcinoma of the thyroid
(C) insulin-dependent diabetes mellitus
(D) juvenile hypothyroidism
(E) thyrotoxicosis

3. A 15-month-old girl is brought to the emergency room because she is lethargic and may have had a "seizure." Her appetite has been decreased for 24 hours because of an intercurrent viral illness. Urinalysis reveals 3+ ketones, and blood chemistry evaluation reveals:

$[Na^+] = 140$ mEq/L
$[K^+] = 5.0$ mEq/L
$[Cl^-] = 100$ mEq/L
$[CO_2] = 19$ mEq/L
[glucose] = 31 mg/dl

Based on the history and initial laboratory evaluation of this child, what is the most appropriate course of action?

(A) Treat with intravenous glucose and admit to hospital for (diagnostic) 24-hour fast
(B) Treat with intravenous glucagon
(C) Perform oral glucose tolerance test
(D) Let the child eat and discharge from emergency room
(E) Obtain an electroencephalogram and begin treatment with phenobarbital

DIRECTIONS: Each of the numbered items or incomplete statements in this section is negatively phrased, as indicated by a capitalized word such as NOT, LEAST, or EXCEPT. Select the ONE lettered answer or completion that is BEST in each case.

4. Factors most likely to contribute to the development of diabetic ketoacidosis include all of the following EXCEPT

(A) overeating
(B) vomiting
(C) omission of insulin doses
(D) infection
(E) lack of patient education

5. All of the following conditions may lead to elevated total serum cholesterol levels EXCEPT

(A) low-density lipoprotein (LDL) receptor deficiency
(B) pancreatitis
(C) acquired hypothyroidism
(D) high-fat diet
(E) diabetes

6. A 14-year-old child who presents with delayed skeletal maturation (bone age) may have any of the following disorders EXCEPT

(A) growth hormone (GH) deficiency
(B) psychosocial deprivation
(C) hypothyroidism
(D) nonclassic (late-onset) 21-hydroxylase deficiency
(E) constitutional delay of puberty

7. All of the following may be manifestations of an insulin reaction (hypoglycemia) in an insulin-dependent diabetic patient EXCEPT

(A) loss of appetite
(B) sweating
(C) lethargy
(D) bizarre behavior
(E) slurred speech

8. All of the following are goals of newborn screening for congenital hypothyroidism EXCEPT

(A) to ensure normal linear growth
(B) to ensure normal intellectual function
(C) to facilitate genetic counseling
(D) to prevent sudden infant death syndrome

9. A newborn infant with ambiguous genitalia is found to have a 46,XX karyotype. All of the following are diagnostic possibilities EXCEPT

(A) 21-hydroxylase deficiency
(B) partial androgen resistance syndrome
(C) true hermaphroditism
(D) maternal virilizing tumor

10. A child with pheochromocytoma may present with all of the following signs and symptoms EXCEPT

(A) headache
(B) weight loss
(C) seizures
(D) sweating
(E) flushing

11. A 5-year-old boy is discovered to have pubic hair during his prekindergarten physical examination. His mother says that recently he has been complaining of headaches. Additional findings on physical examination include height on the ninetieth percentile and acne. All of the following diagnostic studies are appropriate in this case EXCEPT

(A) serum testosterone measurement
(B) computed tomography scanning of head
(C) serum human chorionic gonadotropin measurement
(D) smell testing to detect anosmia
(E) serum 17-hydroxyprogesterone measurement

DIRECTIONS: The set of matching questions in this section consists of a list of four to twenty-six lettered options (some of which may be in figures) followed by several numbered items. For each numbered item, select the ONE lettered option that is most closely associated with it. To avoid spending too much time on matching sets with large numbers of options, it is generally advisable to begin each set by reading the list of options. Then, for each item in the set, try to generate the correct answer and locate it in the option list, rather than evaluating each option individually. Each lettered option may be selected once, more than once, or not at all.

Questions 12–16

For each disorder, select the characteristic serum electrolyte pattern.

	$[Na^+]$ (mEq/L)	$[K^+]$ (mEq/L)	$[Cl^-]$ (mEq/L)	$[CO_2]$ (mEq/L)
(A)	131	3.4	100	24
(B)	128	5.8	103	16
(C)	135	6.0	106	10
(D)	138	4.2	102	27
(E)	144	5.0	105	26

12. Diabetic ketoacidosis

13. Acute adrenal crisis

14. Diabetes insipidus

15. Psychogenic water drinking

16. Insulin shock

ANSWERS AND EXPLANATIONS

1. The answer is D *[I A 1 a (2)]*. Insulin-dependent (type I) diabetes mellitus (IDDM) is thought to have an autoimmune basis. Evidence for this is the presence of circulating islet cell antibodies in most newly diagnosed patients and the association of IDDM with other autoimmune disorders, such as Hashimoto thyroiditis, Graves disease, and Addison disease. The other disorders listed in the question are not thought to be autoimmune in nature. Hypophosphatemic rickets is caused by an inherited defect in renal phosphate handling, familial hypercholesterolemia is caused by an inherited deficiency of low-density lipoprotein receptors, and congenital hypothyroidism is caused by thyroid dysgenesis or defective thyroid hormone synthesis.

2. The answer is E *[III C 3]*. The 12-year-old boy described in the question has symptoms of thyrotoxicosis (Graves disease), particularly weight loss, deterioration of behavior and school performance, and tachycardia. Medullary thyroid carcinoma presents as an asymptomatic nodule or mass in the neck. In children with juvenile hypothyroidism, school performance usually is not impaired, and clinical symptoms include lethargy and constipation. Hashimoto thyroiditis usually presents as an asymptomatic goiter. Transient symptoms of thyrotoxicosis very rarely are present in Hashimoto thyroiditis. Insulin-dependent diabetes mellitus would not account for thyromegaly, widened pulse pressure, and tachycardia.

3. The answer is A *[I B 3 a]*. This child is hypoglycemic and ketonuric. The differential diagnosis includes idiopathic ketotic hypoglycemia, growth hormone (GH) deficiency, and cortisol deficiency as well as some rare inborn errors of metabolism. After the acute episode is treated with intravenous glucose, the child should be fed and observed as she recovers from her intercurrent illness. She should then be admitted to the hospital for a 24-hour fast with frequent monitoring of blood glucose and urinary ketones. If she becomes hypoglycemic (blood glucose level < 40 mg/dl), blood should be obtained for measurement of electrolytes, cortisol, GH, and organic acids (blood and urine). If the patient's GH and cortisol levels are elevated (as they should be during the hypoglycemic stress) and she is not acidotic, the most likely diagnosis is idiopathic ketotic

hypoglycemia. An oral glucose tolerance test is not an appropriate test for a child with hypoglycemia and ketonuria. In the presence of ketonuria, intravenous glucagon is unlikely to raise the blood sugar; therefore, it is not an appropriate treatment.

4. The answer is A *[I A 1 f (2)]*. Central to the development of diabetic ketoacidosis is absolute or relative lack of insulin, most commonly due to omitted insulin doses. Inappropriate actions, such as withholding insulin during intercurrent illness—especially when vomiting—may play a role in an uninformed patient. Infection also is frequently associated with insulin resistance, which necessitates a compensatory increase in insulin dose to prevent ketoacidosis. Overeating may cause excessive hyperglycemia, but as long as the patient continues his or her usual insulin dose, there should be enough insulin present to suppress ketogenesis and subsequent ketoacidosis.

5. The answer is B *[II B]*. Pancreatitis may be a complication of severe hypertriglyceridemia but, by itself, is not associated with hypercholesterolemia. Familial hypercholesterolemia is caused by a deficiency of low-density lipoprotein (LDL) receptors. Individuals with familial hypercholesterolemia may be heterozygous (one defective gene for LDL receptor activity, and thus half the normal number of LDL receptors) or homozygous (two defective genes for LDL receptor activity, and thus an absence of LDL receptors). Hypothyroidism, diabetes, nephrotic syndrome, and liver disease are causes of secondary hypercholesterolemia. In some people, a high-fat diet induces hypercholesterolemia.

6. The answer is D *[V A 1 a (3)]*. Children with nonclassic 21-hydroxylase deficiency have advanced skeletal maturation (i.e., bone age) in childhood owing to the effect of adrenal androgen on bone maturation. Growth hormone (GH) deficiency and hypothyroidism cause marked retardation of skeletal maturation. Psychosocial deprivation may cause "functional" GH deficiency, which is reversible when the child is moved to a more nurturing environment. Children with constitutional delay of puberty have mild to moderate retardation of bone age secondary to prepubertal levels of gonadal steroids.

7. The answer is A *[I A 1 f (1) (a)]*. Insulin-dependent diabetes mellitus (IDDM) is characterized by a loss of insulin secretion by pancreatic beta cells. With the loss of insulin—the major anabolic hormone—a catabolic state develops. When treating IDDM with insulin, there is a risk of relative insulin excess, with resultant hypoglycemia. Symptoms of hypoglycemia may be related to a sympathetic discharge and include sweating, tremulousness, and hunger (not loss of appetite). More severe symptoms (e.g., lethargy, bizarre behavior, slurred speech, seizures) are caused by glucose deprivation to the central nervous system.

8. The answer is D *[III B 1 f]*. There is no known association of congenital hypothyroidism and sudden infant death syndrome. Children with congenital hypothyroidism diagnosed on clinical grounds usually manifest poor linear growth and weight gain and are developmentally delayed. With institution of thyroid hormone replacement, growth and weight gain improve, but there often is permanent neurodevelopmental impairment. With early diagnosis (usually by 4 weeks of age) through newborn screening, children with congenital hypothyroidism have neurologic function and intelligence comparable to their nonaffected siblings. Most affected children have a sporadic form of congenital hypothyroidism with no increased risk to subsequent offspring. Children with an enzymatic defect in thyroid hormone synthesis (dyshormonogenesis) usually have milder disease; however, there is a 25% chance of other siblings being similarly affected.

9. The answer is B *[VI A 2 a (2) (b)]*. Infants with partial androgen resistance may have ambiguous genitalia, but the karyotype is 46,XY. These infants have testes and high levels of testosterone, which are incompletely effective in virilizing the external genitalia in a normal male pattern. The defect is at the level of the androgen receptor. Female infants with congenital adrenal hyperplasia due to 21-hydroxylase deficiency may exhibit a variable degree of masculinization of the external genitalia because of prenatal exposure to high levels of circulating adrenal androgens. Most infants with true hermaphroditism have a 46,XX karyotype. However, gonadal tissue includes both ovarian and testicular elements. The testicular androgens cause external virilization, leading to ambiguous genitalia. In a similar fashion, a maternal virilizing tumor may expose a female fetus to high levels of androgen.

10. The answer is E *[V B 1 a]*. The excessive production of catecholamines by a pheochromocytoma results in episodic or sustained hypertension, which usually is severe. Headache and seizures are symptoms typically related to hypertension and hypertensive encephalopathy. Sweating and weight loss are a result of a true hypermetabolic state caused by catecholamine excess. The usual appearance during a paroxysm is pallor; catecholamines do not cause flushing.

11. The answer is D *[VI B 2]*. This 5-year-old boy presents with signs of precocious sexual development. The cause of his disorder could be congenital adrenal hyperplasia, gonadotropin-dependent precocious puberty, or, possibly, a central nervous system tumor secreting human chorionic gonadotropin (HCG). Smell testing for anosmia might be indicated for the evaluation of delayed puberty—because of the association of hypogonadotropic hypogonadism and anosmia (Kallmann syndrome)—but not in the evaluation of precocious puberty.

12–16. The answers are: 12-C *[I A 1 f (2) (c)]*, **13-B** *[V A 2 b, c]*, **14-E** *[IV B 1 b]*, **15-A** *[IV B 1 e]*, **16-D** *[I A 1 f (1)]*. Diabetic ketoacidosis results in an anion gap metabolic acidosis because of overproduction of strong organic ketoacids, thus lowering the serum bicarbonate (HCO_3^-) level. In the face of metabolic acidosis, potassium (K^+) is drawn out of cells, elevating the serum K^+ level, whereas total body K^+ actually is low because of urinary losses. In acute adrenal crisis, lack of mineralocorticoid causes hyperkalemia due to urinary sodium (Na^+) wasting and K^+ retention. With increased renal excretion of HCO_3^-, the patient also becomes acidotic. The patient with diabetes insipidus loses water because of inability to produce a concentrated urine. This may result in hemoconcentration and a high-normal serum Na^+ level. The effect of psychogenic water drinking is to cause dilutional hyponatremia. In insulin-induced hypoglycemia (insulin shock), serum electrolyte levels are normal. This is helpful in distinguishing insulin shock from diabetic ketoacidosis in an unresponsive patient with insulin-dependent diabetes mellitus.

Chapter 18

Neurologic Diseases
Carol R. Leicher
Barry S. Russman

I. GENERAL PRINCIPLES OF PEDIATRIC NEUROLOGIC DIAGNOSIS

A. History

1. A well-performed history should emphasize whether the neurologic problem being analyzed is:
   a. Focal or diffuse
   b. Acute or insidious
   c. Static or progressive

2. An attempt should be made to obtain eyewitness accounts of "spells" or suspect behaviors. Special attention should be given to the developmental history and school function.

B. Physical examination. Special aspects of the pediatric neurologic examination include evaluation of the developmental reflexes (Table 18-1), measurement of head circumference, assessment of developmental milestones, and a search for birthmarks, which can signal a neurologic defect.

C. Diagnostic studies. Useful procedures, depending on the clinical problem, can include:

1. **Lumbar puncture and cerebrospinal fluid (CSF) examination** (e.g., for infectious, metabolic, and degenerative diseases)

2. **Electroencephalography (EEG)** [for epilepsy]

3. **Electromyography (EMG)** and nerve conduction studies (for motor unit diseases)

4. **Measurement of cortical evoked potentials** [for assessment of central nervous system (CNS) function]

5. **Neuroimaging studies**
   a. **Skull radiography** (e.g., for depressed skull fracture)
   b. **Computed tomography (CT) scan** (useful in emergencies and detection of calcification and blood or bony abnormalities)
   c. **Magnetic resonance imaging (MRI) scan** [for anatomic abnormalities, especially in the midline structures; optimal for assessing gliosis or other abnormalities of gray and white matter. New techniques (magnetic resonance angiography) also permit assessment of the cerebral vasculature]
   d. **Arteriography** (for vascular disease)
   e. **Positron emission tomography (PET) scan** (research tool for assessment of brain metabolism)

6. **Biopsies** of muscle, peripheral nerve, skin, liver, bone marrow, rectal mucosa, and, rarely, brain (for evaluation of a degenerative disease)

TABLE 18-1. Developmental Reflexes

Reflex	Test Position	Stimulus	Response	Age at Onset	Age at Disappearance	Significance
Moro	Support head and shoulders 30° above horizontal	Allow head to drop to horizontal	Extension of upper extremities at shoulders and elbows	28 weeks' gestational age	6 months	**Absence** suggests severe myopathy or severe CNS abnormality **Persistence** suggests CNS abnormality
Asymmetric tonic neck	Supine with head in midline	Passive or active neck rotation to left or right	Extension of arm and leg on face side, with flexion of arm and leg on occiput side	37 weeks' gestational age	6 months—never obligatory*	**If obligatory or persistent** suggests CNS pathology
Parachute	Support infant in vertical position	Sudden tip of upper body downward	Arms extend to break fall	6–8 months	Persists	**Should be symmetric** **If not developed at appropriate time** suggests CNS abnormality
Suck	Any	Finger or pacifier placed in mouth	Sucking	37 weeks' gestational age		**Absence** suggests either CNS or muscle dysfunction
Rooting	Any	Touching side of mouth with cheek	Head turns	37 weeks' gestational age		**Absence** suggests CNS depression
Grasp (palmar)	. . .	Finger in palm	Grasp of finger	20 weeks' gestational age	4–5 months	**Absence** suggests CNS dysfunction
Placing	Held upright	Touching dorsum of foot	Places foot onto surface	37 weeks' gestational age	Covered by voluntary action	**Absence** suggests CNS dysfunction

CNS = central nervous system.
*An obligatory reflex is defined as a tonic neck posture that is maintained beyond 30 seconds after the head is turned.

TABLE 18-2. Glasgow Coma Scale—Finding Score*

Best verbal response:	**Eyes open:**
Oriented 5	Spontaneously 4
Confused 4	To speech 3
Inappropriate words 3	To pain 2
Incomprehensible	None 1
sounds 2	
None 1	
Motor response:	
Obeys commands 5	
Able to localize pain 4	
Flexion to pain 3	
Extension to pain 2	
None 1	

*Scoring is as follows: 3–7, severe head injury; 8–11, moderate head injury; 12–14, mild head injury.

II. ALTERED STATES OF CONSCIOUSNESS.

When assessing a child's altered state of behavior or decreased responsiveness, the child's developmental age and how the child typically responds to various stimuli must be considered (determined by history).

A. Definitions

1. **Delirium** is an altered state of behavior in which the patient appears alert, but is confused, irritable, and has inappropriate reactions to stimuli.

2. **Coma** is a state of unarousable unresponsiveness. This is a consequence of bilateral cerebral dysfunction or involvement of the periventricular gray matter in the brain stem. Assessment of a patient in coma should include a description of the stimulus used and the response observed. Inexact terms (e.g., "stupor," "lethargy," "semi-coma") are best avoided. The Glasgow Coma Scale is reliable (Table 18-2).

B. Etiology.

There are many possible etiologies of delerium and coma (Table 18-3).

TABLE 18-3. Etiology and Clues to Delirium and Coma

Etiologies	Diagnostic Clues
Infection—meningitis, encephalitis	Fever, nuchal rigidity, history of preceding illness, exanthem
Cerebrovascular disease—arteriovenous malformation, stroke	Focal neurologic signs, nuchal rigidity, papilledema
Trauma	Scalp or facial bruises, hemotympanum (blood behind the eardrum)
Metabolic disorders—abnormalities of electrolytes, glucose, oxygen content	Signs of dehydration, acetone on breath, cyanosis; laboratory evaluation is necessary to establish the etiology
Toxic (poisoning)—one of the most common causes of altered consciousness in toddlers and adolescents	Breath may smell of the ingested agent, such as cleaning fluids, alcohol; parents should be questioned on medications available in the home
Postictal state—depressed level of consciousness secondary to an unwitnessed seizure	Prior history of seizures, abnormal electro-encephalogram may be helpful

C. **Diagnosis**

1. **History.** The patient history must be obtained rapidly, usually while the child is being stabilized. Particular attention should be paid to the events leading to altered consciousness, past medical conditions, and availability of toxins.

2. **Physical examination.** In addition to establishing the patient's standing on the Glasgow Coma Scale, special attention should be given to the following areas.
   a. **Eyes.** Pupil size and reaction to light may suggest the presence of a toxic substance or a brain stem injury. Abnormal extraocular movements, as elicited by the "doll's eye" maneuver or caloric testing, will suggest brain stem damage. Papilledema suggests elevated intracranial pressure.
   b. **Motor status.** Spontaneous movements should be observed and carefully recorded. The presence of decorticate or decerebrate posturing or seizures should be specifically noted.
   c. **Respiratory pattern.** The rate of respiration as well as breathing abnormalities (e.g., Cheyne-Stokes respiration, central neurogenic hyperventilation, Biot breathing) should be noted.

3. **Laboratory studies.** Tests to be ordered are determined by the history and physical examination.
   a. **Blood** should be analyzed for metabolic abnormalities (e.g., hypoglycemia).
   b. **Urine** can be analyzed for the presence of toxic substances, heavy metals, sugar, and acetone.
   c. **CT scan** screens for most emergency conditions (i.e, hemorrhage, mass lesions, blunt trauma); MRI scan provides more detailed information about other intracranial lesions.
   d. **EEG** can help to diagnose seizures as the cause of the coma (see V C).
   e. **Lumbar puncture** should be performed if an infection is suspected.

D. **Therapy**

1. **Supportive treatment** includes establishing an airway, maintaining hydration, and decreasing intracranial pressure. Hyperventilating the patients is the quickest way to lower intracranial pressure. Medications (e.g., mannitol, steroids) also are helpful.

2. **Specific treatment** depends on the etiology of the delirium or coma.

III. MALFORMATIONS OF THE CNS

A. **Epidemiology**

1. Approximately 3% of all infants have at least one minor CNS malformation.

2. About 40% of infants who die in the first year of life have one or more developmental abnormalities of the nervous system.

3. Fully 75% of fetal deaths are associated with a major CNS malformation.

B. **Disorders of embryogenesis** (induction disorders) occur during the first 4 weeks of fetal development.

1. **Posterior midline lesions** (also called **neural tube defects** or **dysraphia**) can range from complete failure of the brain to develop (**anencephaly**) to a clinically insignificant posterior defect of the vertebral bodies (**spina bifida occulta**). Neural tube defects occur because the neural groove fails to fuse completely during formation of the neural tube. These defects usually show a multifactorial inheritance pattern (see Chapter 8).

a. Spina bifida cystica is a herniation of the meninges (**meningocele**) or the meninges plus the spinal cord (**meningomyelocele**) through a vertebral defect, usually in the lumbar area.

   (1) Clinical features depend on the level and severity of the lesion. Bladder and bowel sphincters may be affected. Distal orthopedic problems (e.g., clubfoot) are common. Cerebral deficits and seizures can develop as a result of secondary meningitis, hydrocephalus, or associated CNS anomalies.

   (2) When the **diagnosis** is suspected before birth, the α-fetoprotein level in maternal serum and in amniotic fluid should be tested. Fetal ultrasonography also may establish an early diagnosis.

   (3) Therapy begins with surgical closure of the defect to prevent infection. A multi-disciplinary approach provides the best management of a patient with a severe lesion, because ongoing neurosurgical, orthopedic, urologic, and psychological care will be necessary.

   (4) Prognosis for ambulation correlates with the level and severity of the defect.

b. Arnold-Chiari malformation is an elongation and protrusion of medullary and cerebellar tissue through the foramen magnum and into the cervical spinal cord. The condition often accompanies meningomyelocele.

   (1) Several variations of this malformation are described. **Chiari type 1** is an isolated protrusion of the cerebellar tissue. **Chiari type 2** combines type 1 plus hydrocephalus, and **Chiari type 3** is a combination of these defects plus a cranium bifidum, with or without protrusion of cerebral tissue (encephalocele). In patients with hydrocephalus, the presenting symptoms are those of increased intracranial pressure. Respiratory distress because of lower cranial nerve abnormalities is a common clinical sign of this abnormality.

   (2) Surgery to prevent compression of the neural tissue at the foramen magnum may be necessary. Shunting procedures may be necessary if the hydrocephalus is symptomatic.

c. Other dysraphic states can occur when embryonic nervous tissue comes in contact with the dermis.

   (1) Tethered cord results when the filum terminale becomes entangled with fibrous and fatty tissue, preventing the normal upward migration of the spinal cord that occurs with age.

      (a) Symptoms develop as the child grows. Typically, a gait disturbance, caused by spasticity and weakness, develops during the third to sixth year of life.

      (b) Therapy consists of surgical release of the cord.

   (2) Diplomyelia and diastematomyelia are, respectively, a duplication and a cleft in the spinal cord.

      (a) Clinical features of these lesions usually appear as the child grows.

      (b) Therapy. Prompt surgical treatment prevents further loss of function.

   (3) Syringomyelia is a fluid-filled cavity or cyst (syrinx) in the cord. A decompression laminectomy or decompression of the syrinx itself can alter the otherwise relentless progression that causes loss of sensation and weakness below the level of the cyst.

   (4) Sacral dysgenesis may be seen in offspring of diabetic mothers. The major neurologic disabilities are urinary incontinence and weakness of the lower extremities. Treatment is symptomatic.

   (5) Neurodermal sinus usually does not cause a neurologic problem. However, exploration and closure are important because the tract may extend from the skin into the spinal cord, leading to recurrent meningitis.

2. Anterior midline defects (holoprosencephaly) can cause hypoplasia of the hypothalamus and a single ventricle.

   a. Symptoms include poor body temperature control, apnea, seizures, and severe psychomotor retardation. Midline facial defects suggest the underlying brain abnormality.

   b. Diagnosis is made by CT or MRI scan or ultrasonography.

3. **Developmental anomalies of the base of the skull**
   a. **Platybasia** is an upward displacement of the base of the skull, leading to narrowing of the foramen magnum.
      (1) **Clinical features** result from compression of the cervical cord and include spasticity in the lower extremities, shooting pain in the arms, and weakness of the proximal arm muscles.
      (2) **Therapy** consists of surgical decompression.
   b. **Klippel-Feil syndrome** results from the absence or fusion of several cervicovertebral bodies. The symptoms are similar to those noted for platybasia. Commonly associated abnormalities include spina bifida, syringomyelia, sensorineural hearing loss, and congenital heart disease.

C. **Disorders of cellular migration and proliferation** usually occur for unknown reasons, although they have been associated with maternal ingestion of toxic substances (e.g., alcohol, phenytoin) during pregnancy as well as with chromosomal and other genetic abnormalities.

1. **Agenesis of the corpus callosum** can be diagnosed best by MRI scan. The corpus callosum is absent and there are often abnormalities in the cerebral hemispheres. Clinical manifestations depend on the extent of associated anomalies and range from severe psychomotor retardation and seizures to minimal or no symptoms.

2. **Microcephaly** (see also Chapter 8) is, by definition, a head circumference more than two standard deviations below the norm; it most often occurs as a result of a small brain (**micrencephaly**), because the skull generally grows in response to brain growth.
   a. **Etiology.** Microcephaly occurs idiopathically, as a chromosomal anomaly, and as an autosomal recessive disorder. It has also been noted in patients with hypothyroidism, Hurler syndrome, or rickets, and secondary to maternal irradiation during early pregnancy.
   b. **Differential diagnosis.** Skull radiographs help determine whether **craniosynostosis** (i.e., premature closure of the sutures) is the cause of the microcephaly.
      (1) **Craniosynostosis** may occur alone or in association with other syndromes (e.g., Crouzon, Apert, Carpenter).
      (2) **Therapy.** Surgical intervention rarely is necessary to relieve pressure caused by craniosynostosis. Most often, surgery is performed for cosmetic reasons.

3. **Macrocephaly** (see also Chapter 8) is a large head circumference. Either the brain is too large (**macrencephaly**) or a space-occupying lesion (including enlarged ventricles) is the cause.
   a. The most common cause of macrocephaly in infants is **hydrocephalus**.
   b. Macrocephaly can also be caused by several **inherited metabolic or chromosomal anomalies** and several leukodystrophies (e.g., Canavan disease, Alexander disease; see XI D 3). **Arachnoid cysts** can also cause an enlarging head circumference; they are best diagnosed by MRI scan.

4. **Hydranencephaly** is a severe necrosis of the cerebral cortex that occurs in utero, with subsequent accumulation of CSF. The etiology is still uncertain; a migration disorder and bilateral internal carotid artery occlusion are popular theories.

D. **Hydrocephalus** is enlargement of the cerebral ventricles due to excessive accumulation of CSF. This relatively common condition is the most frequent cause of an enlarged head in neonates.

1. **Noncommunicating (obstructive) hydrocephalus** is caused by an obstruction of CSF flow within the ventricular system. **Communicating hydrocephalus** results from a dysfunction in the absorption of CSF.

2. **Etiology.** Causes of hydrocephalus can be related to time of onset.
   a. Prenatally or during the first month of life, the common causes are intraventricular hemorrhage, infection, or congenital malformations (e.g., aqueductal stenosis).
   b. During the first few years of life, a brain tumor must be suspected if the patient presents with hydrocephalus. Also, an asymptomatic partial obstruction might manifest itself at this age.

3. Abnormal rate of head growth, irritability, lethargy, vomiting, and headache (in the older child) suggest this diagnosis. Obtaining head circumference measurements over time is more important than a one-time measurement.

4. A CT or MRI scan can reliably diagnose hydrocephalus, as can ultrasonography if the anterior fontanelle is still open.

5. **Therapy** includes the use of dehydrating agents (e.g., mannitol, acetazolamide, furosemide), serial spinal taps, and shunting procedures.

6. **Prognosis**
   a. Arrested hydrocephalus designates the termination of the hydrocephalic condition, with subsequent return to normal intracranial pressure. However, the ventricles commonly remain enlarged.
   b. The child's future cognitive and motor functions are related to several factors, including the cause of the hydrocephalus, how rapidly it developed, the duration of asymptomatic hydrocephalus, the frequency of shunt infections, and the presence and type of associated malformations.

E. Congenital defects of cranial nerves and related structures

1. **Möbius syndrome** is characterized by facial diplegia and ophthalmoplegia. Lack of development of the cranial nerve nuclei in the brain stem is the main pathologic finding. No treatment is indicated other than possible cosmetic surgery.

2. **Sensorineural hearing loss** in many cases is the result of a congenital defect (see Chapter 4).

F. **Cerebellar malformations** include **total agenesis of the vermis** and the **Dandy-Walker malformation** (i.e., cystic dilation of the fourth ventricle, with obstructive hydrocephalus secondary to a blockage or atresia of the foramen of Magendie and foramen of Luschka). Shunt procedures invariably are required.

IV. CEREBRAL PALSY

A. **Definition.** "Cerebral palsy" is a descriptive term that refers to abnormal control of motor movements due to a nonprogressive (static) lesion of the immature brain. The lesion or lesions may occur prenatally, perinatally, or postnatally.

B. **Etiology and risk factors.** The cause of cerebral palsy is unknown in approximately 70% of patients. Approximately 20% of cases can be correlated with risk factors, including prematurity, cerebral anoxia, and trauma. Specific causes include embryologic malformations and infection.

C. **Clinical features**

1. **Typical clinical patterns.** The classification system for cerebral palsy considers the number of limbs involved and the type of motor abnormality (Table 18-4).

2. **Injuries to the brain** that result in motor problems may have other, more widespread effects. Problems associated with cerebral palsy include epilepsy in approximately 30% of patients, mental retardation or learning disabilities in approximately 40%–50%, behavior problems in 20%, and strabismus in approximately 40% of patients.

TABLE 18-4. Anatomic and Physiologic Classifications of Cerebral Palsy

Anatomic classification
    Diplegia: the lower limbs are more affected than the upper limbs
    Hemiplegia: one side of the body is involved more than the other, and the arm usually is affected
        more than the leg
    Quadriplegia: all four limbs are similarly affected
    Double hemiplegia: both sides of the body are affected, the arms more than the legs
    Paraplegia: both legs are affected; the arms are spared

Physiologic classification
    Spasticity: an increase in muscle tone
    Dyskinesia: a collective term for several movement disorders:
        Chorea: abrupt, jerky movements
        Athetosis: slow, writhing, continuous movements in the extremities
        Dystonia: writhing movements leading to sustained, bizarre postures
            of the trunk and extremities
    Ataxia: an incoordination of movement; commonly associated with hypotonia, at least during the
        first few years of life

D. **Diagnosis**

   1. **History.** The patient presents with a history of a motor delay, but is not losing skills that
   have been attained.

   2. **Physical examination.** Findings on physical examination place the lesion in the CNS
   and commonly include any or all of the following:
      a. Hyperactive reflexes
      b. Abnormal movements of chorea, athetosis, or dystonia
      c. Abnormal absence or persistence of infantile reflexes (see Table 18-1)

   3. **Differential diagnosis.** Distinguishing cerebral palsy from a progressive neurologic disorder may be difficult early on because the infant is in the initial stages of developing
   skills, and a loss of minimal skills may be impossible to determine. If a progressive disease is of concern, screening tests are available for a number of the inherited metabolic
   disorders.

E. **Therapy.** Early on, physical therapy programs are usually indicated. When the patient
   reaches the toddler or school-age stage, orthopedic intervention (e.g., special shoes,
   braces, surgery) often is necessary. The treatment of associated problems (e.g., learning disabilities, seizures) is no different for cerebral palsy patients than for children who are
   impaired in other ways.

V. SEIZURES AND EPILEPSY

A. **Definitions**

   1. **Seizures** represent abnormal neural discharges in the cerebral cortex that result in
   abnormal function. The nature of the clinical manifestation depends on the region(s) of
   the brain affected by the discharge. Seizures may be the result of a known cerebral
   insult or may arise without detectable cerebral disturbance.

   2. **Epilepsy** is a condition in which the patient is subject to recurrent, unprovoked
   seizures.

   3. **Status epilepticus** is a prolonged seizure lasting more than 30 minutes or a series of
   seizures without return to consciousness for more than 30 minutes.

4. An **epileptic or seizure syndrome** describes a seizure type(s) that occurs in association with characteristic EEG findings, demographic characteristics, and prognosis. There are several epileptic or seizure syndromes in childhood.

B. | **Classification.** There are several ways to classify seizures. By classifying seizures by type or by etiology, it is possible to recognize certain clinical patterns and determine appropriate diagnostic testing and treatment.

1. Classification by seizure type

a. Partial seizures arise from a localized portion of the cerebral cortex. Because of the limited cortical involvement, consciousness may not be affected by the seizure activity.

  (1) A **simple partial seizure** may have motor manifestations or sensory manifestations, depending on the location of the seizure discharge, without loss of consciousness.

  (2) In **complex partial seizures,** there is a greater degree of cortical involvement. In addition to the motor and sensory phenomena, consciousness is clouded or lost. The motor manifestations of this seizure type are often complex and semipurposeful [i.e, picking at clothing, walking in circles (automatisms)]. There is usually a period of confusion or exhaustion after the seizure, called the "postictal" state.

  (3) When a partial seizure spreads to involve both sides of the brain, a full convulsion may result, a **partial seizure with secondary generalization**. This seizure is distinguished from a generalized seizure by the aura, or focal onset, which consists of localized abnormal movements or abnormal sensations preceding the generalized convulsive activity.

b. Generalized seizures arise simultaneously from both cerebral hemispheres. The manifestations may involve motor function, consciousness, or both.

  (1) The **absence** seizure (or petit mal) is characterized by staring and loss of awareness of the environment. There is no warning to the patient that the seizure is about to happen. Absence seizures are brief, rarely longer than 30 seconds, and terminate as abruptly as they began, with no postictal state. There may be minor motor movements, such as eyeblinking or finger twitching.

  (2) Myoclonic seizures are brief, generalized motor seizures consisting of symmetric jerks of the trunk or upper extremities. These seizures may occur in flurries. There is no apparent loss of consciousness or postictal state.

  (3) Atonic and **akinetic** seizures are brief generalized seizures characterized by either sudden, momentary loss of truncal tone ("head drop seizures") or sudden freezing of activity.

  (4) The **grand mal** or **major motor** seizure begins abruptly with no warning. There may be sustained tonic or clonic movement of both sides of the body. The patient may have labored breathing, cyanosis, or excessive salivation. Urinary or fecal incontinence may occur. After the seizure, the patient may experience a period of confusion, headache, and lethargy. This seizure type can be distinguished from the partial seizure with secondary generalization by the lack of an aura and focal motor signs.

2. Classification by etiology. Seizures that occur without a discernable cerebral abnormality are considered idiopathic or cryptogenic. A seizure that is the consequence of a discernable cerebral abnormality is considered a symptomatic seizure. This category is further divided into those disorders that acutely produce seizures, and chronic disorders associated with recurrent seizures (Table 18-5).

C. | **Epileptic/seizure syndromes.** An epileptic syndrome describes a particular type or types of seizure associated with typical EEG findings and patient characteristics. The concept of the epileptic syndrome is useful diagnostically and in treatment because it allows for accurate prognostic statements to be made and also helps in choosing appropriate anticonvulsant therapy.

TABLE 18-5. Etiology of Seizures

Acute Symptomatic Seizures	Chronic Symptomatic Seizures
Metabolic disturbances (hypoglycemia, hypoxia, electrolyte disturbances)	Cerebral malformations Acquired cerebral injuries Neurocutaneous syndromes Tumors Inborn errors of metabolism
Intoxications (cocaine, tricyclic antidepressants, antipsychotics) Fever Head injury CNS infections (meningitis, encephalitis) Vascular accidents (CVA, AVM)	

AVM = arteriovenous malformation; CNS = central nervous system; CVA = cerebrovascular accident.

1. **Febrile seizures** are not typically considered to be epileptic because they are provoked events, not spontaneous. This seizure type is typically seen in infants from 6 months to 3 years of age, but may occur until 6 years. This is a frequent syndrome, affecting between 3–8/1000 children. The seizures occur in the context of a febrile illness, often an upper respiratory infection or otitis media.
   a. **Seizure type.** The classic seizure type is a brief generalized seizure lasting less than 5 minutes.
   b. **EEG findings.** The interictal EEG is usually normal. If an EEG is done shortly after the seizure, background slowing may be present.
   c. **Prognosis.** The risk of recurrent febrile seizures is 30%. In a small number of children, afebrile seizures and, ultimately, epilepsy will subsequently develop. Abnormal neurologic examination results and the presence of atypical seizure features (focal involvement, prolonged seizure, or multiple seizures in 24 hours) are risk factors for the development of epilepsy.
   d. **Treatment.** Because most of the seizures are brief and nonrecurrent, fever control is the only warranted therapy. In the event of multiple febrile seizures, phenobarbital and valproate are effective. Oral diazepam administered during febrile illnesses has also been effective. Phenytoin and carbamazepine are not useful.

2. **Absence seizures (petit mal) of childhood.** This idiopathic syndrome is thought to be inherited as an autosomal recessive trait in children who are otherwise normal. The onset is between 4–10 years of age.
   a. **Seizure type.** The seizures are generalized, 10–20 seconds in duration, and characterized by staring, with minimal clonic activity [see V B 1 b (1)].
   b. **EEG findings.** The characteristic findings are bursts of 3–cycle-per-second spike waves. These may be precipitated by hyperventilation or use of a strobe. During the episodes, the patient often will not hear or be able to answer a question.
   c. **Prognosis.** Sixty percent of children with this syndrome will have remission of seizures by late adolescence. Children with concurrent grand mal seizures are more likely to have lifelong epilepsy.
   d. **Treatment.** Ethosuximide or valproate are the drugs of choice for this type of epilepsy. Clonazepam may be useful as a second-line medication. Phenobarbital, phenytoin, and carbamazepine are not effective.

3. **Benign focal epilepsy of childhood.** This is one of the most common idiopathic epileptic syndromes of childhood. The age of onset is 4–10 years. This syndrome is not associated with underlying cerebral disorders.
   a. **Seizure type.** If the patient is awake, the typical seizure is a focal seizure, involving the face, pharynx, and possibly the arm. The patient is conscious, but is unable to speak and may drool. Nocturnal seizures may be generalized convulsive seizures, but may also have focal motor involvement, or involvement of the pharyngeal muscles. Gagging is a common symptom of the nocturnal seizures in this syndrome.

    b. EEG findings. The interictal EEG shows discharges in either one or both central and midtemporal electrodes, corresponding to the rolandic gyrus. These may be limited to the sleep portion of the recording.

    c. Prognosis. This syndrome has a high remission rate, with 99% resolution by 16 years of age.

    d. Treatment. Carbamazepine and phenytoin are the most commonly used anticonvulsants in this disorder.

4. Infantile spasms. This syndrome may be symptomatic (e.g., tuberous sclerosis) or idiopathic. The onset is typically from 4–18 months of age.

    a. Seizure type. Infantile spasms are massive myoclonic seizures, with either forceful flexion or extension of the trunk. The spasms occur in clusters at short intervals for periods of 30 minutes or more. The child may cry or be extremely irritable during these periods.

    b. EEG findings. The EEG pattern, called "hypsarrhythmia," shows extreme disorganization of the background activity with very high-voltage and frequent, multifocal spike wave discharges.

    c. Prognosis. If not treated, the outcome of this syndrome is poor, with lifelong epilepsy and severe neurodevelopmental disability. Idiopathic infantile spasms are more likely to respond to aggressive treatment, and 40% of the patients may have excellent outcome. Outcome of treatment of the symptomatic form of infantile spasms is less successful and may reflect the severity of the underlying disorder. The spasms may progress to akinetic or atonic seizures later in life.

    d. Treatment. Intramuscular adrenocorticotropic hormone (ACTH) is the most effective treatment for infantile spasms. This is administered for a 4–8-week period of time. Valproate and clonazepam may also be useful as secondary agents.

5. Juvenile myoclonic epilepsy is an idiopathic form of seizure disorder that typically begins in adolescence.

    a. Seizure type. There are three types of seizures present in this syndrome, grand mal or major motor, absence, and myoclonic.

    b. EEG findings. The interictal abnormality is generalized spike and wave (4.5–5 Hz).

    c. Prognosis. Although the seizures usually are readily controlled with medication, the rate of relapse is high. Treatment usually is lifelong.

    d. Treatment. Valproate is the drug of choice. Phenytoin or carbamazepine can also be used in combination with clonazepam.

D. | **Diagnosis.** The diagnosis of seizures or epilepsy is usually made on the basis of the description of the event. This is usually obtained from an observer, but in the case of the partial seizure, the patient may be able to relate some of her own symptoms. The physical and neurologic examination may provide clues to the diagnosis in patients with symptomatic epilepsy, but is usually negative in patients with idiopathic epilepsy. Provocative maneuvers, such as hyperventilation, may allow the physician to observe an event. This is particularly useful in absence seizures. **Ancillary tests** include the following.

    1. An **EEG** is the most commonly ordered test in the evaluation of epilepsy. An EEG is the recording of the electrical activity at the surface of the cortex. The resting patterns of the brain change according to location of the electrodes on the scalp and the state of the brain. During a seizure, the brain generates high-voltage, chaotic activity that peaks rapidly, giving the appearance of a "spike" or "sharp wave." The cells giving rise to the clinical seizure may produce a sustained abnormal discharge, the "ictal" pattern, which accompanies the clinical seizure. Between clinical seizures, shorter discharges may be recorded; this is called the interictal pattern. It is much more common to record interictal abnormalities than ictal abnormalities. The chances of recording an abnormality can be increased by recording during sleep, or with hyperventilation or stimulation with a strobe light.

    2. In the event that a routine EEG captures no abnormality, or fails to define the nature of the clinical event, **videotelemetry** may be helpful. This consists of simultaneous recording of EEG and videotaping of behavior for a prolonged period of time. This increases the likelihood of capturing an event and defining the nature of the abnormality.

3. Neuroimaging procedures such as **CT** or **MRI** are useful in the evaluation of symptomatic seizures. An imaging study should be performed in the case of a partial seizure, or when the neurologic examination is positive. When the clinical history and EEG findings are consistent with an idiopathic epileptic syndrome, such as absence seizures of childhood, an imaging study is not required. CT is often more readily available in emergencies, and is adequate for evaluating the presence of most mass lesions, hemorrhage, or gross cerebral abnormalities. MRI is superior in the evaluation of subtle cerebral abnormalities and white matter changes.

E. **Treatment.** Once the presence of seizures and epilepsy has been established, treatment usually consists of the use of anticonvulsant medication. Not every child who has a seizure will be started on anticonvulsants. The decision will be based on the circumstances of the seizure and the prognosis for further seizures.

1. **Counseling.** The child with epilepsy should lead as normal a life as possible. Physical and social activities should be encouraged. Family and teachers may need counseling to provide the needed psychological support.

2. **Anticonvulsant medication.** The choice of drug is based on the seizure type and EEG findings. Blood levels are guidelines only: some patients need lower drug doses, whereas others need and can tolerate higher doses. Medication must be increased slowly to avoid side effects (e.g., lethargy) and withdrawn slowly to avoid precipitating seizures.

3. **Diet.** A ketogenic diet is used for grand mal or absence seizures that are difficult to control with medication, and is most effective in children 2–5 years of age.

4. **Surgery.** When drug treatment is unsuccessful, surgical excision of the epileptic focus or corpuscallosotomy (i.e., surgical splitting of the corpus callosum) can be considered. Most patients who undergo surgery still require anticonvulsant medication.

F. **Prognosis.** Anticonvulsant medication can control seizures in 35%–50% of patients. Adequate control is less likely when seizures begin early in life, occur frequently, are mixed in type, and are associated with mental retardation or abnormal results on neurologic examination. If a patient is seizure-free for at least 2 years, discontinuing medication should be considered.

VI. NONEPILEPTIFORM PAROXYSMAL DISORDERS

A. **Migraine** is characterized by recurrent attacks of headache, pulsatile in character, sometimes unilateral, and often accompanied by neurologic disturbances as well as nausea, vomiting, and photophobia. Migraine attacks may be precipitated by stress or by ingestion of certain foods or substances, such as chocolate, peanuts, tyramine (found in aged cheese, chicken liver, and beer), nitrites, and quinine.

1. **Clinical features and diagnosis.** There are many variants of migraine.
   a. In **classic migraine,** the patient has an **aura** preceding the attack (visual scotoma, flashing lights.) The headache is unilateral, pulsatile, and associated with gastrointestinal upset and photophobia. The patient will frequently report relief with sleep. The physical examination typically is negative. In approximately 75% of cases, a positive family history exists.
   b. In **common migraine,** the headache tends to be diffuse rather than unilateral, and no aura is present. Nausea and vomiting are variably present.
   c. There are several forms of **complicated migraine**.
      (1) Patients with **hemiplegic migraine** manifest a transient neurologic deficit just before, or in association with, the headache. The neurologic deficit may consist of aphasia, hemiparesis, hemianopsia, or third-nerve palsy.

    (2) Patients with **basilar artery migraine** have attacks resembling basilar artery occlusion, with confusion, vomiting, vertigo, and loss of vision. A positive family history of migraine helps to distinguish this form from vascular malformation, although the latter must always be considered.

    (3) Cyclic vomiting—recurrent attacks of pernicious vomiting without systemic illness—is thought to be a childhood variant of migraine. This can present in infants and toddlers and can result in hospitalization for dehydration. Metabolic evaluation of these patients is unrewarding, and as they grow older, more typical migraine attacks with prominent headache may occur.

2. Therapy. Many drugs have been tried in the management of migraine, including vaso-constrictors (ergotamine), serotonin antagonists (cyproheptadine), serotonin agonists (sumatriptan), drugs that prevent reuptake of norepinephrine (amitriptyline), prostaglandin inhibitors (aspirin, ibuprofen), membrane stabilizers (phenytoin), calcium channel blockers, and other agents (e.g., propranolol).

3. Prognosis is extremely variable, and no helpful predictive factors have been found. The patient can go into remission for years, only to have the migraine return decades later.

B. **Sleep disorders**

1. Sleepwalking (somnambulism), sleeptalking, and **night terrors** are common in children younger than 5 years of age. These disorders occur in stage 4 (deep) sleep. There is no recollection of the event the following day. An EEG sometimes is necessary to rule out a seizure disorder. Diazepam may be helpful if the sleepwalking is a danger to the patient.

2. Narcolepsy is characterized by paroxysmal attacks of irrepressible sleep. Hypnagogic hallucinations, cataplexy (sudden loss of body tone precipitated by strong emotion), and sleep paralysis are also seen in these patients. This disorder most commonly presents in the second decade, although it has been reported in younger children. The characteristic abnormality on EEG consists of a shortened latency from full alertness to onset of rapid eye movement sleep. Narcolepsy is treated by regulating nighttime sleep schedules and allowing for brief daytime naps, if possible. When the symptoms are severe, stimulants may be helpful.

C. **Other paroxysmal disorders**

1. Syncope (fainting, with loss of consciousness) occurs because of decreased blood flow in the posterior circulation of the brain secondary to vagal stimulation. It is essentially a benign disorder and is treated by reassurance. Cardiac arrhythmias must be considered as a possible etiology.

2. Breath-holding spells occur between 3 months and 6 years of age. The child initially cries and then holds his breath, turns cyanotic, and becomes limp. Occasionally, the patient has a short-lived tonic seizure. This is a benign disorder; reassurance is the treatment.

VII. **MOVEMENT DISORDERS**

A. There are several disorders that present in childhood with involuntary movements (see Table 18-4). These are usually associated with abnormalities of the basal ganglia. **Chorea** is a quick involuntary movement affecting any part of the body. These movements are variable, as opposed to tics, which also are usually brief muscle movements, but have a stereotyped quality. **Dystonia** is a more prolonged abnormal movement, resulting from simultaneous contracture of agonist and antagonist muscles. **Myoclonus** is characterized by rapid muscle jerks. Movement disorders may be transient and symptomatic, or chronic and progressive.

TABLE 18-6. Abnormal Movements Due to Medications

Movement	Medication Type
Chorea	Anticonvulsants
	Stimulants
	Phenothiazines
Tics	Stimulants
Dystonia	Phenothiazines
	Haloperidol
	Metoclopramide

B. Symptomatic movement disorders

1. **Drug-induced movements.** Medications can produce multiple types of abnormal movements (Table 18-6).

2. **Systemic disorders**
   a. **Sydenham chorea (rheumatic chorea).** Chorea is one of the cardinal symptoms of rheumatic fever (see Chapter 9). The child presents with choreic movements of the extremities and face. Hypotonia and emotional lability may also be seen. Recovery is gradual and usually complete. The patients must be treated for rheumatic fever, and the chorea may respond to diazepam, haloperidol, or phenobarbital.
   b. **Lupus erythematosus** may occasionally present with chorea. The symptoms are indistinguishable from Sydenham chorea and the diagnosis is established by serologic testing. Treatment with corticosteroids is indicated.

C. Idiopathic or genetic movement disorders (see also XI B)

1. **Tourette syndrome** is characterized by multiple and vocal **tics,** persistent for at least 12 months. It is an autosomal dominant disease with variable expression.
   a. **Etiology.** The biochemical basis for the disorder has not been determined. Stimulant medications may precipitate tics or worsen tics in susceptible individuals. There is a high frequency of coexistent conditions such as attention deficit hyperactivity disorder (50%–70%), learning disability (40%–50%), and obsessive-compulsive disorder.
   b. **Clinical features.** The motor tics—involuntary, rapid movements—may appear first in the head or neck. Complex tics consisting of gestures or complete utterances may occur. **Coprolalia** refers to complex verbal tics with obscene or inappropriate content. This occurs in approximately 30% of patients. The tics commonly are exacerbated by anxiety or excitement. The onset is between 5 and 10 years of age, a time when many children display tics. The diagnosis requires multiple tics, both motor and vocal, that are persistent for at least 1 year.
   c. **Therapy.** Dopamine antagonists such as haloperidol and pimozide are the most effective medications for tic suppression, but produce significant side effects. Clonidine and clonazepam have also been used for tic control, but are less effective.
   d. **Prognosis.** Approximately 30% of children will have lifelong symptoms. Thirty percent experience complete remission of symptoms, and the rest have milder symptoms as they enter adulthood. Prognosis depends on the severity of tics and associated disorders.

2. **Benign hereditary (essential) tremor** is an autosomal dominant disorder with variable expression.
   a. **Clinical features.** The tremor consists of a rhythmic, oscillating movement of the distal muscles of the extremities. It does not worsen as the patient approaches a target. The major effect of the tremor is on performance of fine motor skills. The disorder is mildly progressive.

    b. Diagnosis. Essential tremor can be associated with many toxic, metabolic, and infectious disorders as well as hereditary CNS diseases. It is important to establish that a tremor is not a symptom of an underlying disorder.

    c. Therapy is indicated only if the tremor adversely affects functions such as handwriting. Propranolol has been successful in alleviating the tremor in some patients.

3. Dystonia musculorum deformans is a disorder that manifests as slow, twisting movements causing what appears to be a fixed deformity, only to disappear with relaxation. The movements involve the trunk, extremities, and head. The disorder may be dominant, recessive, or sporadic. The genetic dystonias tend to be progressive; the sporadic types are static as a rule.

    a. Clinical features. Intermittent or continuous muscle spasms are noted when the patient tries to move the muscles purposefully. The truncal muscles are affected initially in the dominant form and the extremity muscles in the recessive form. Sporadic dystonia may occur secondary to birth trauma or other trauma, exposure to toxic substances (e.g., lead), or vascular disease.

    b. Diagnosis is established by physical examination and, in the hereditary forms, by a positive family history. A CT or MRI scan is not helpful because no anatomic site has been identified.

    c. Therapy. Thalamotomy has been reported to alleviate the symptoms, possibly for up to 2 years. Clonazepam, trihexyphenidyl, and carbamazepine have provided moderate, but temporary, improvement in some patients.

4. Segawa syndrome is a rare movement disorder characterized by diurnal episodes of dystonic posturing; the patient has an underlying motor deficit (cerebral palsy). This movement abnormality usually responds to dopamine.

VIII. TRAUMA

A. Head trauma (see also Chapters 2 and 7)

1. Clinical features

    a. Concussion produces a transient loss of consciousness, with amnesia for the event but with no obvious pathologic cerebral changes.

        (1) Diagnosis. Neurologic examination is unremarkable except for the change in mental status. Nystagmus and a positive Babinski reflex may be present for several hours.

        (2) Therapy is symptomatic. Headache, dizziness, and poor attention span may persist for up to 1 year after the injury.

    b. Contusion and **laceration** of the brain can be the result of a depressed skull fracture, a penetrating injury, or a closed injury.

        (1) Control of intracranial pressure is essential because cerebral edema commonly occurs. The level of coma usually is greatest by the third to fifth day, when cerebral swelling is at its maximum level.

        (2) Depressed skull fractures and penetrating injuries require surgery as soon as the patient is stable, or at least within 24 hours of the injury, to minimize the possibility of meningitis.

2. Complications

    a. Epidural hematoma occurs within hours of the injury in an adult but may not develop for 1–2 days in a child. Tearing of the dural veins or the middle meningeal artery is responsible for this complication, which should be suspected when a patient's condition deteriorates. The diagnosis is established by CT scan. Surgical evacuation is necessary.

    b. Subdural hematoma can develop even more slowly than epidural hematoma. Especially in an infant younger than 6–9 months of age, this problem might not develop for several weeks after the head injury. A common presenting sign is an enlarging head circumference; this, plus a change in feeding habits or in personality, heralds the onset of the problem. In the infant who still has an open anterior fontanelle, a subdural tap might be the only treatment necessary. If this is unsuccessful, surgical intervention is indicated.

c. **Parenchymal hematoma** (blood clot within the brain) rarely requires surgical intervention. However, if swelling cannot be controlled by medical means, evacuation might be necessary.

d. **Transtentorial herniation** may occur as a result of generalized cerebral edema or a space-occupying lesion. This complication is suspected with the observation of dilated pupils that are nonresponsive to light and the development of sixth nerve palsy. Rapid treatment with a dehydrating agent (e.g., mannitol) and hyperventilation often are necessary.

e. **Recurrent meningitis** is a risk when the injury provides an entrance for bacteria. The cause is not always obvious. CSF rhinorrhea or otorrhea should be sought. The former may occur as a result of a cribriform plate fracture.

f. **Arachnoid (leptomeningeal) cyst** typically occurs in a linear fracture. It can develop in children of any age but is more likely to occur in those younger than 3 years of age. Onset usually is several months after the injury. The patient's presenting feature is an enlarging head circumference. Excision of the cyst may be necessary.

3. **Prognosis**
a. The duration of coma after head injury correlates with the extent of the future disability. Normal cognitive and motor function is unlikely if the coma lasts more than 1 week in an adolescent or adult, or 2–4 weeks in an infant or young child.

b. A seizure at the time of the impact does not correlate with future epilepsy. On the other hand, coma lasting more than 24 hours does correlate with future epilepsy. A depressed skull fracture or a penetrating injury leads to a seizure disorder in 70%–80% of cases. (Prophylactic use of anticonvulsants does not appear to prevent future seizure development.)

c. Posttraumatic personality and learning problems are common after significant injury and may be an exacerbation of the pretraumatic personality and cognitive skills.

B. **Spinal cord injuries** (see also Chapter 7 VI D 4)

1. **Clinical features.** The level of injury is determined by the lack of sensation below the level of the lesion. The absence of a normal wheal-and-flare response also may help to identify the level of the lesion.

2. **Diagnosis.** MRI scan is the most helpful procedure in determining whether a lesion is amenable to surgery.

3. **Therapy.** Once the patient's vital signs are stabilized and appropriate surgery is performed, the most immediate concern is the prevention of urinary retention. Catheterization of the bladder often is necessary.

4. **Prognosis.** The patient may be areflexic distal to the injury for several weeks, after which spasticity commonly appears. Complete paralysis 5–10 days after the injury suggests permanence.

C. **Peripheral nerve injuries**

1. **Clinical features** include sensory loss as well as weakness and wasting of the muscles innervated by the affected nerves.

2. **Therapy** includes removal of the compressing force and reanastomosis of severed nerves, if possible, as well as minimizing complications, including contractures (with a physical therapy program) and causalgia (with medication).

3. **Prognosis** can be determined by EMG. The presence of reinnervation potentials augurs well for recovery.

IX. **CEREBROVASCULAR DISORDERS.** Stroke is an uncommon cause of acute neurologic dysfunction in children.

A. Vascular occlusion

1. **Thrombosis.** Arterial thrombosis can occur as a result of cerebral arteritis, trauma, or a congenital vascular abnormality (e.g., carotid artery stenosis).
   a. **Moyamoya disease** is an idiopathic disorder characterized by progressive occlusion of the carotid arteries and sometimes the basilar arteries. Collateral circulation in the form of small vessels occurs, resulting in a typical "puff of smoke" appearance on angiography. Patients typically present with alternating focal symptoms secondary to vascular insufficiency. Seizures may also be a symptom of this disorder.
   b. **Acute hemiplegia of childhood** usually occurs before 3 years of age, often as a result of an internal carotid artery thrombosis. Associated focal or generalized seizures occur in 60% of patients.
      (1) **Differential diagnoses** include systemic vascular disorders such as periarteritis nodosa, sickle cell anemia, and systemic lupus erythematosus. Vascular occlusion must also be differentiated from Todd paralysis (which occurs up to 24 hours after a focal seizure), and hemiplegic migraine. Todd paralysis and hemiplegic migraine are distinguished by the patient's recovery without sequelae.
      (2) **Therapy** combines physical therapy for the motor deficit with the use of appropriate anticonvulsants for the seizures, which often are difficult to control.

2. **Embolism.** Cerebral embolism is seen in patients with congenital heart disease (see Chapter 12). These patients may experience embolism through right-to-left shunting, or as a result of cardiac catheterization or open heart surgery.

B. **Hemorrhage.** Intraventricular hemorrhage in the neonate is discussed in Chapter 6. Angiomas and other malformations of blood vessels are uncommon as causes of intracranial hemorrhage in children.

C. **Arteriovenous malformation (AVM)** is the most common of the brain angiomas. AVM rarely is hereditary.

1. **Clinical features**
   a. **Seizure** is the most common presentation. Rupture of an AVM causes sudden symptoms, which may include coma, nuchal rigidity, and paresis.
   b. **Malformation of the vein of Galen** usually does not present as a CNS hemorrhage. Rather, congestive heart failure may be the presenting problem in the newborn period, hydrocephalus at 6 months of age, and seizures at 18 months of age.

2. **Diagnosis** of AVM is established by a contrast CT scan or MRI scan. Arteriography is necessary to determine the extent of the malformation.

3. **Therapy.** Surgery is considered if the AVM is accessible. Embolization techniques are used for surgically inaccessible lesions. Even without operative intervention, 85% of the patients are alive 5 years later.

X. **DISEASES AFFECTING BOTH THE SKIN AND THE CNS.** Neurocutaneous disorders (**phakomatoses**) are disorders that have in common lesions of the skin, brain, and eyes. Most of these disorders are inherited.

A. **Neurofibromatosis** is an autosomal dominant disease with variable expression. There are two distinct forms of neurofibromatosis, although variant forms also exist. It is estimated that 1 in 3000 people have at least a very mild variety of this disease.

1. Clinical features and diagnosis

a. Neurofibromatosis-1 (NF-1; von Recklinghausen disease). The diagnosis of NF-1 is established by the presence of two or more of the following:

(1) Six or more café-au-lait spots larger than 5 mm in greatest diameter in prepubertal individuals and larger than 15 mm in postpubertal individuals

(2) Two or more neurofibromas of any type or one plexiform neurofibroma

(3) Freckling in the axillary or inguinal region

(4) Optic glioma

(5) Two or more Lisch nodules (pigmented hamartomas of the iris)

(6) A distinctive osseous lesion (e.g., sphenoid dysplasia or thinning of long bone cortex with or without pseudoarthrosis)

(7) A first-degree relative with NF-1 according to above criteria

b. Neurofibromatosis-2 (NF-2). Diagnosis of NF-2 is established by the presence of:

(1) Bilateral eighth nerve masses seen with appropriate imaging techniques, or

(2) A first-degree relative with NF-2 and either unilateral eighth nerve mass or two of the following: neurofibroma, meningioma, glioma, schwannoma, or juvenile posterior subcapsular lenticular opacity.

c. Important considerations. Screening for visual change, hearing loss, and learning disabilities should be routine. A CT scan should be ordered if there is any clinical indication that a tumor may be present.

2. Therapy and prognosis. If tumors are confined to peripheral nerves only, a normal life span without deficits is very likely. Genetic counseling is indicated.

B. **Tuberous sclerosis (Bourneville disease)** is an autosomal dominant disease of variable expression, which affects approximately 1 person in 30,000.

1. Clinical features. Tuberous sclerosis is characterized by the triad of skin lesions, seizures, and mental retardation.

a. Skin lesions are seen by 3 years of age in 40% of patients. The lesions include flat, hypopigmented "ash-leaf" spots (visible under a Wood lamp), shagreen patches (unevenly thickened skin areas), and café-au-lait spots. During the second decade, angiokeratomas appear on the face. Retinal hamartomas are noted in 50% of patients.

b. Epilepsy may begin early in life and may be difficult to control.

c. Periventricular tumors may occur, leading to hydrocephalus and, if large enough, causing the patient's death. Autistic features are noted in about 10%–15% of patients.

d. Cysts and **malignant tumors** may develop in the heart, kidneys, pancreas, and peritoneal cavity.

2. Therapy and prognosis. The various clinical problems are treated as they are in patients without tuberous sclerosis. Prognosis is related to the severity of the seizure disorder and the cognitive dysfunction.

C. **Sturge-Weber syndrome** is most likely a sporadic disease, although familial cases have been described.

1. Clinical features. A port-wine stain (capillary hemangioma) occurs unilaterally in a trigeminal distribution (over the forehead and, often, the maxillary area); occasionally it is bilateral. Glaucoma develops later in 50% of patients. A seizure disorder is likely.

2. Therapy and prognosis. Anticonvulsant therapy often is unsuccessful, and surgical removal of the damaged cortex is necessary. Prognosis is related to the ease of seizure control.

D. **von Hippel-Lindau disease** is an autosomal dominant disorder characterized by vascular tumors in the cerebellum and spinal cord. Associated retinal hemangiomas are seen in 50% of patients, and renal carcinoma is seen in 45%. The skin is not involved in this syndrome.

E. **Ataxia–telangiectasia (Louis-Bar syndrome)** is an autosomal recessive disease affecting the cerebellum, skin, and immune system.

  1. **Clinical features.** The ataxia typically develops during the first 5 years of life; it is distinguished from cerebral palsy because the ataxia is progressive; it is distinguished from Friedreich ataxia by the neurologic examination. The telangiectasias, most apparent on the conjunctiva and the ears, become prominent during the second 5 years of life. Lung infections, secondary to immunoglobulin A deficiency, develop by about 10 years of age, and malignant lymphomas begin to develop at approximately 15–20 years of age.

  2. **Therapy and prognosis.** Treatment is symptomatic. The disease is progressive, and death usually results from infection or malignancy.

XI. DEGENERATIVE CNS DISEASES

A. **General approach to the patient with a degenerative CNS disease**

  1. **Clinical features.** Degenerative CNS diseases are characterized clinically by a deterioration of function over an extended period of time. Most of the diseases are genetic, and many have a metabolic basis. The clinical condition may start with seizures or with losses in motor, cognitive, or language skills. These losses may be subtle and difficult to recognize in the very young child.

  2. **Diagnosis**
     a. **History.** In evaluating the patient with a suspected neurodegenerative disease, a careful and probing history is necessary. An infant may show a lack of normal motor and social development and may have recurrent episodes of altered consciousness or unexplained vomiting. A toddler may show a loss of motor, cognitive, or social milestones. An older child may have problems with schoolwork.
     b. **Laboratory studies** may aid in the diagnosis of degenerative CNS diseases.
        (1) **Urine screening** should include:
           (a) Quantitative determination of amino acids (for phenylketonuria, maple syrup urine disease, and other aminoacidopathies)
           (b) Quantitative determination of organic acids for disorders of fatty acid metabolism
           (c) Bile acids for disorders of peroxisomal function such as Refsum disease or neonatal adrenoleukodystrophy
        (2) **Blood screening** should include tests for fasting blood sugar, ammonium, lactate, and pyruvate levels; pH and carbon dioxide partial pressure (Pco_2); and lysosomal enzymes.
        (3) **Radiography** of the skull and vertebral bodies may be helpful.
        (4) **Fibroblast evaluation.** Fibroblasts in skin and other tissues should be evaluated for microscopic abnormalities and missing enzymes.

B. **Degenerative diseases of the basal ganglia.** The major abnormalities noted in these diseases are movement disorders (e.g., tremor, chorea, athetosis, dystonia).

  1. **Wilson disease (hepatolenticular degeneration;** see also Chapter 11 IX F 2) is an autosomal recessive disorder that causes copper to accumulate progressively in the liver, brain, cornea, kidney, and other tissues. The patient who presents in the second decade of life may show choreoathetoid movements. A grayish hue surrounding the iris (**Kayser-Fleischer ring**) is seen on slit-lamp examination in 75% of children who present in the first decade of life and in all children with this disorder who have a neurologic defect.

  2. **Other pediatric basal ganglia disorders** include:
     a. **Hallervorden-Spatz syndrome** (progressive spasticity, dystonia, rigidity, and choreoathetosis, with iron deposits in the basal ganglia)
     b. The childhood form of **Huntington chorea**

      c. Lesch-Nyhan syndrome (choreoathetosis, mental retardation, and self-mutilation, due to a defect in purine metabolism)

      d. Fahr disease (calcification of the basal ganglia and cerebellum)

C. | **Degenerative diseases of the cerebellum, brain stem, and spinal cord.** These diseases often present as **gait ataxia**. Other signs and symptoms include disorders of eye movements, hearing loss, facial palsy, and swallowing difficulties. These and other features, including the pace at which the disease progresses, lead to a specific diagnosis.

1. **Friedreich ataxia,** an autosomal recessive disease, is the best understood of the genetic ataxias. The disease presents during the latter half of the first decade of life.
   a. **Clinical features.** Progressive ataxia is the presenting sign, with associated weakness and wasting of the distal muscles and, occasionally, spasticity. In addition, most patients have skeletal deformities (pes cavus, kyphoscoliosis), and a few show nystagmus or deafness. The electrocardiogram becomes abnormal by 20 years of age. Cardiomyopathy leading to congestive heart failure is the usual cause of death. Patients seldom live past 30 years of age.
   b. **Diagnosis.** The combination of ataxia, a positive Babinski sign (cortical spinal dysfunction), a loss of vibration and position sense with minimal loss of sensation of sharp pain (posterior column dysfunction), and depressed or absent reflexes (peripheral neuropathy) is virtually diagnostic. Nerve conduction velocities are mildly slowed and sensory conduction velocities are unobtainable.
   c. **Therapy.** A physical therapy program and appropriate orthopedic intervention can help patients with Friedreich ataxia.

2. **Other pediatric disorders of the cerebellum, brain stem, and spinal cord** include a varied group of hereditary cerebellar ataxias, dentate cerebellar ataxia (Ramsay Hunt syndrome), familial spastic paraplegia, abetalipoproteinemia (Bassen-Kornzweig syndrome), and hypolipoproteinemia.

D. | **Degenerative diseases of white matter.** These diseases commonly start with loss of motor function accompanied by **spasticity** and **visual impairment**. Dementia and, occasionally, seizures appear as late manifestations. No cure is available for this group of disorders. Many of these diseases were formerly classified as sudanophilic leukodystrophies. However, as specific etiologies have been determined, the older term is used less frequently.

1. **Metachromatic leukodystrophy (sulfatide lipidosis)** is an autosomal recessive disease caused by a **deficiency of arylsulfatase A,** the enzyme that participates in the catabolism of myelin.
   a. **Clinical features.** Three forms of this disorder exist.
      (1) The most common—the **infantile form**—starts in the second year of life and presents initially as gait disturbance and spasticity, and then as dementia. Unexplained bouts of fever and severe abdominal pain develop as well. This form is invariably fatal by 5 or 6 years of age.
      (2) In the **juvenile form,** similar symptoms begin between 6 and 10 years of age.
      (3) In the **adult form,** dementia precedes the gait disturbance.
   b. **Diagnosis.** Metachromatic granules in the urine suggest the diagnosis and a deficiency of arylsulfatase A in the white cells establishes it.

2. **Adrenoleukodystrophy** is an X-linked disease that usually develops in children 5–8 years of age. The spastic gait disorder and dementia are accompanied by adrenal insufficiency. An MRI scan shows the degeneration of the white matter. Serum analysis shows an abnormal ratio of the C26–C22 fatty acids. The patients usually die within 2–5 years.

3. **Other diseases of white matter**
   a. **Pelizaeus-Merzbacher disease** is a slowly progressive X-linked disorder that begins in infancy. An initial diagnosis of cerebral palsy might be considered, but careful observation determines that the patient's problem is progressive (see IV D 3).

b. **Canavan disease** is a severe, progressive autosomal recessive disorder with increasing macrocephaly, blindness, hypotonia, and spasticity.

c. **Alexander disease** is a rare, apparently sporadic disorder characterized by macrocephaly and mental retardation.

d. **Krabbe disease** (cerebroside lipidosis, globoid leukodystrophy) is a severe, progressive autosomal recessive disorder with diffuse lack of myelin, which causes rigidity, dysphagia, blindness, deafness, mental deterioration, quadriplegia, and death.

E. **Degenerative diseases primarily affecting gray matter.** Many of these diseases are **neuronal storage diseases,** in which a lipid (usually a ganglioside or other sphingolipid) accumulates in cerebral neurons. Patients with gray matter diseases typically present with **seizures** and **dementia.**

1. **Tay-Sachs disease,** an autosomal recessive disorder, is one of the best known of the gray matter diseases and the most common of the gangliosidoses. The neuronal accumulation of gangliosides is the result of **hexosaminidase A deficiency.**

   a. **Clinical features.** Symptoms develop in patients at 3–10 months of age. A loss of alertness and excessive reaction to noise (**hyperacusis**) are the presenting complaints. Myoclonic and akinetic seizures follow 1–3 months later. Patients die by 3 or 4 years of age.

   b. **Diagnosis.** A cherry-red spot on the macula is noted in 75% of cases. This spot, caused by deterioration of the retina, can sometimes be seen in other gray matter diseases (e.g., Niemann-Pick disease, generalized gangliosidosis). The absence of hexosaminidase A in white cells, serum, or other tissue establishes the diagnosis.

   c. **Therapy.** Replacement therapy with a modified form of glucocerebrosidase by intravenous infusion is under investigation.

2. **Gaucher disease** occurs in three forms: infantile, juvenile, and adult. In all types, a **deficiency of glucocerebrosidase** causes an accumulation of glucoceramide in various tissues.

   a. **Clinical features.** Hepatosplenomegaly is seen in all patients.

      (1) The **infantile form** is most severe, with delayed development and signs of bulbar palsy by 6 months of age and death by 1–2 years of age.

      (2) The **juvenile form** commonly starts with dementia in late childhood and is characterized by progressive dementia.

      (3) With **adult onset,** neurologic involvement may be minimal, and in some adults, no neurologic abnormalities occur.

   b. **Diagnosis** is suggested by the finding of large foam cells (Gaucher cells) in the bone marrow and confirmed by enzyme analysis of white cells.

   c. **No treatment** is available for cases with neurologic involvement.

3. **Niemann-Pick disease** results from an accumulation of sphingomyelin in the reticuloendothelial system due to a **lack of sphingomyelinase.** There are at least five types, which vary in age at onset and rate of progression, and not all types show CNS involvement. All are autosomal recessive disorders associated with a limited life expectancy.

   a. **Clinical features.** Loss of alertness associated with an enlarged liver and spleen are the initial findings in the infantile form with CNS involvement. In juvenile types, neurologic symptoms begin as gait disturbances and learning difficulties.

   b. **Diagnosis** is suggested by the finding of vacuolated histiocytes (Niemann-Pick cells) in the bone marrow. An absence of sphingomyelinase in skin fibroblasts establishes the diagnosis.

4. **Other diseases affecting neurons** primarily include the following.

   a. **Neuronal ceroid lipofuscinoses** (a group of autosomal recessive disorders) are characterized by refractory seizures, loss of vision, ataxia, and dementia.

   b. **Generalized gangliosidosis** (a severe disorder, probably autosomal recessive) causes death before 2 years of age.

   c. **Fabry disease** (an X-linked glycolipid disorder) causes a burning, painful neuropathy, angiokeratomas, and renal and cardiac disorders; female carriers may show some symptoms.

    d. Menkes kinky hair disease (an X-linked defect in copper absorption) causes seizures, profound neurologic deficits, and death before 2 years of age.

    e. Rett syndrome is a progressive disease presenting as dementia and ataxia in girls. Autistic behavior, microcephaly, and a peculiar wringing motion of the hands are hallmarks of this disease. No inheritance pattern, enzymatic deficiency, or metabolic explanation has been identified.

XII. DISORDERS OF THE MOTOR UNIT (NEUROMUSCULAR DISORDERS).

Common to all patients with motor unit diseases are **weak muscles**. Most of the diseases in this category are progressive, and many are genetic.

A. Anterior horn cell diseases

1. **Spinal muscular atrophies** are autosomal recessive diseases primarily, although rare autosomal dominant and X-linked types have been described. Amyotrophic lateral sclerosis (involves the corticospinal tract as well) typically affects adults, although juvenile and familial forms have been described.

    a. Clinical features

      (1) In **Werdnig-Hoffmann disease** (infantile spinal muscular atrophy, or **type I**), the weakness is apparent at birth or shortly thereafter. However, some patients may be able to sit independently when placed, thereby placing them into the type II category.

      (2) In a second group of patients (**type II**), the muscle weakness may not appear until after 4–8 months of age, when sitting skills have normally been developed.

      (3) In **Kugelberg-Welander disease** (juvenile spinal muscular atrophy, or **type III**), the onset of weakness occurs after walking has been established, in some cases not until adolescence.

    b. Diagnosis in all three types of spinal muscular atrophy is established by the history and physical examination in association with denervation in a muscle biopsy.

    c. Therapy. A physical therapy program is combined with appropriate orthopedic intervention.

    d. Prognosis. All patients with spinal muscular atrophy lose function over time. Type I is often fatal before 2 years of age. The prognosis is best for patients with type III disease; life expectancy may be "normal."

2. **Arthrogryposis multiplex congenita** is a nonprogressive disease characterized by muscle weakness and contractures of at least two joints. Although the clinical findings are present at birth, the condition seldom is familial.

    a. Etiology. A viral or toxic etiology primarily affecting the anterior horn cells is suspected in most cases. In others, a uterine problem (e.g., amniotic bands) is suspected.

    b. Diagnosis is established by physical examination.

    c. Therapy and prognosis. The extent of the contractures determines how disabled the patient will be and how amenable the problem will be to surgical correction.

3. **Poliomyelitis** is rarely seen but must be considered in the differential diagnosis of muscle weakness secondary to anterior horn cell disease.

B. Peripheral neuropathies. Trauma, infections, postinfectious states, toxins (e.g., lead), and genetic factors all may affect the axon, the myelin (via the Schwann cell), or both.

1. **Hereditary sensory and motor neuropathy (HSMN)** is the current nomenclature for a group of inherited neuropathies that are differentiated by electrophysiologic criteria and by the associated problems (e.g., ataxia, retinitis, deafness). The most common of this group is **Charcot-Marie-Tooth disease (peroneal muscular atrophy)**.

    a. Clinical features. In HSMN, weakness begins in the foot muscles starting in the first decade of life; eventually, the hand muscles are affected. Mild sensory loss may accompany the motor disability.

     b. Diagnosis. In most types of HSMN, the EMG demonstrates denervation, and nerve con-
duction times are delayed. Rarely is a nerve biopsy needed for diagnosis. A trinucleotide repeat on chromosome 17 has been identified as the abnormality in HSMN 1.

     c. Therapy. A rehabilitation program, including physical and occupational therapy, is
indicated and should be devised by a knowledgeable physician, such as an orthopedist or a physiatrist. Vocational counseling also is important.

     d. Prognosis. Most diseases in this category are mild, and life expectancy is normal.
However, some patients become significantly physically handicapped, becoming
confined to a wheelchair by the fourth or fifth decade of life.

2. Guillain-Barré syndrome and other postinfectious, presumably autoimmune, neuropathies are discussed in XIII E. **Peripheral nerve injuries** are discussed in VIII C.

3. Other peripheral neuropathies are less common and include brachial and lumbar
plexus neuropathies, hereditary sensory neuropathies, giant cell neuropathy, Leber
optic atrophy, and neuroaxonal dystrophy.

C. **Diseases of the neuromuscular junction—myasthenia gravis**

1. Etiology. Myasthenia gravis usually is a sporadic disease, although familial cases have
been described. It is an autoimmune disease in which antibodies develop against the
acetylcholine receptor protein at the motor end-plate.

2. Clinical features
     a. Clinical forms. The disease may present at different ages.
       (1) Neonatal myasthenia. One in seven mothers with myasthenia gravis transmits
antibodies to the fetus transplacentally. The infant develops transient myasthenia,
starting during the first week of life and lasting less than 2 months.
       (2) Congenital myasthenia. Anti-acetylcholine antibodies are not detectable in the
patient's serum in this form of myasthenia. Ptosis, usually the first symptom, is
noted by 2 years of age; swallowing difficulties and truncal weakness may follow.
       (3) Juvenile myasthenia. This form is similar to the adult form, except it starts late in
the first decade or in the second decade of life.
     b. Associated diseases, including rheumatoid arthritis, thyroiditis, thymoma, and dia-
betes mellitus, occasionally may occur.

3. Diagnosis. Patients with myasthenia gravis show normal muscle strength after receiving
2–10 mg of edrophonium chloride; the involved muscles weaken 1–5 minutes later.
Occasionally, a repetitive nerve stimulation test, causing rapid muscle fatigue, helps to
establish the diagnosis.

4. Therapy. Pyridostigmine, an anticholinesterase agent, is helpful in more than 50% of
patients. Immunosuppressant therapy with corticosteroids may be necessary. Plasmapheresis and thymectomy may benefit some patients.

5. Prognosis. If the muscle weakness of congenital or juvenile myasthenia remains limited
to ocular muscles for more than 2 years, the progression of the disease is limited.

D. **Diseases of muscle.** Discussed here are the more common of the **hereditary myopathies**
(see Chapter 9 for inflammatory myopathies). The classification of the hereditary muscle
diseases is based on the clinical presentation, histology, and, more recently, by gene deletion and gene duplication findings.

1. Muscular dystrophies. These progressive genetic diseases are linked historically
because of similar histologic appearances.
     a. Duchenne (pseudohypertrophic) muscular dystrophy, the most common, is an X-linked
disease characterized by progressive muscle weakness seen first in the proximal muscles.
       (1) Clinical features. Symptoms typically begin at 2–4 years of age. Independent walk-
ing may be delayed; affected children never run normally and never walk up stairs
using alternating feet. The patients are wheelchair-bound by 12 years of age and
die, usually from congestive heart failure or pneumonia, before 25 years of age.

(2) Diagnosis

    (a) The muscle weakness may be difficult to detect on physical examination because children younger than 5 years of age have difficulty cooperating with a formal muscle evaluation. A positive Gowers sign (Figure 18-1) indicates weakness of the lower back and pelvic girdle muscles.

    (b) The serum creatine phosphokinase level is 10–20 times normal.

    (c) The EMG, usually an unnecessary study, is consistent with a myopathy; muscle biopsy is consistent with a dystrophy. The muscle tissue must be tested for the presence or absence of dystrophin.

    (d) The missing gene and gene product have been identified. The **lack of dystrophin** (the gene product) in the external muscle membrane is considered to be diagnostic of Duchenne muscular dystrophy. DNA testing shows the deletion in 65% of patients.

(3) Therapy. In addition to orthotic and orthopedic intervention, genetic counseling is extremely important. The latter is the reason that early diagnosis is so important. Steroid therapy may prolong ambulation. Gene therapy is under investigation.

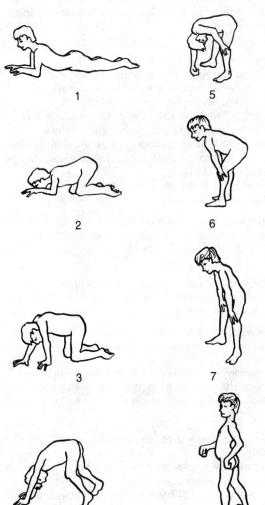

FIGURE 18-1. Gowers sign. A patient with mild hip weakness uses this maneuver to arise from the floor. Rather than assuming a squatting position, the patient first pushes off the floor (*1, 2, 3*), forming an arch with buttocks at apex (*4*), then pushes against the knee with the nonfloor hand (*5*), and then "walks" the hands up the legs (*6, 7*) to assume the standing position (*8*).

b. Other genetic muscular dystrophies include:

   (1) Becker dystrophy is a later-appearing, more benign form of Duchenne muscular dystrophy; dystrophin is quantitatively or qualitatively abnormal in the muscle tissue. The patients live into the fourth decade.

   (2) Landouzy-Dejerine dystrophy (facioscapulohumeral)

   (3) Leyden-Möbius dystrophy (limb-girdle, scapulohumeral; typically becomes clinically evident in the second decade of life)

   (4) Myotonic muscular dystrophies (see XII D 2)

2. Myotonic muscle disorders. Myotonia is the failure of voluntary muscles to relax after a contracture. The examiner can demonstrate myotonia by percussing the patient's tongue or thenar eminence.

   a. Myotonic muscular dystrophy (Steinert disease) is an autosomal dominant disorder that presents during the second decade of life. The patient initially complains of cramps or weakness. Cataracts and cardiac arrhythmias develop over the next 20 years in 60%–70% of the patients. In the asymptomatic or minimally involved patient, the diagnosis can be established by finding the trinucleotide repeat of the myotonic gene on chromosome 15.

   b. Congenital myotonic muscular dystrophy occurs only when the mother is the affected parent. It presents in the neonate as "floppiness" and a typical "fish-mouth" appearance. In addition to the dystrophy, mental retardation is present. The patient gradually becomes stronger and usually starts to walk by about 3 years of age. The diagnosis is established by examining the mother for evidence of the disorder.

   c. Myotonia congenita (Thomsen disease) is an autosomal dominant disorder of delayed muscle relaxation. The patient experiences muscle cramps, which can be relieved with phenytoin. The disease is not progressive and is not associated with weakness. A recessive form exists with a later onset and with more severe myotonia.

3. Metabolic myopathies. Several genetic abnormalities in carbohydrate or lipid metabolism cause identifiable myopathic syndromes; the underlying enzyme deficiencies have been elucidated in many of these disorders.

   a. Glycogen storage diseases (GSDs; see also Chapter 8). **GSD type II** (Pompe disease), **GSD type V** (McArdle disease), and **GSD type VII** (Tarui disease) affect the muscles. They can be diagnosed by finding glycogen inside the muscle cells or by ischemic exercise tests. Clinically, the patients complain of cramps and decreased muscle strength.

   b. Lipid storage myopathies, including carnitine deficiency and carnitine palmityl-transferase deficiency, are diagnosed by finding abnormal lipids in the muscle biopsy. Clinical findings include cramps, muscle weakness, and episodes of hepatic failure.

   c. Myopathy with abnormal mitochondria commonly presents as weakness and ophthalmoplegias in addition to CNS signs (e.g., dementia, intermittent coma).

   d. Familial periodic paralysis causes episodic muscle weakness in association with hypokalemia or hyperkalemia. Symptoms may start in the nursery or may not begin until the second decade of life. Acetazolamide may prevent or moderate attacks.

4. Congenital myopathies. Several disorders present as hypotonia in the newborn period and, therefore, must be considered in the differential diagnosis of the "floppy infant" syndrome. Specific disorders, usually named for the histologic findings, include **central core disease, nemaline myopathy** (rod disease), and **myotubular myopathy**.

   a. Clinical features. The congenital myopathies all are very similar. The patients are floppy at birth and have facial muscle weakness. Most of the diseases are static or improve with time. Scoliosis, manifesting during the teenage years, is common.

   b. Diagnosis is established by muscle biopsy because these disorders differ histologically.

   c. Therapy. Respiratory support and nasogastric feeding may be necessary during the first few months of life. Later, orthopedic intervention, orthoses, and physical and occupational therapy may be required.

XIII. POSTINFECTIOUS, PRESUMED AUTOIMMUNE NEUROLOGIC DISORDERS (see Chapter 10 for acute CNS infections). The neurologic disorders discussed in this section are presumed to have an immunologic basis. Many are clearly preceded by an infectious (usually viral) disease, and the infectious agent is presumed to initiate a cell-mediated autoimmune reaction. In some diseases, the immune response occurs shortly after the original infection, and in other diseases it does not occur until years later. In some of the disorders discussed here, no preceding infection has been identified, but clinicopathologic evidence strongly suggests an autoimmune, postinfectious etiology.

A. **Slow virus infections** are characterized by a lapse of months to years between the initial viral infection of the host and the appearance of a progressive CNS disease involving primarily dementia, seizures, and motor deficits.

1. **Subacute sclerosing panencephalitis (SSPE)** is caused by the measles virus or a measles-like virus that has been isolated from the brain.
   a. **Clinical features.** The disease starts 5–15 years after a natural measles infection or, uncommonly, after immunization with live measles vaccine. Changes in personality and other cognitive functions develop initially, followed by myoclonic seizures, and, ultimately, by dementia and choreoathetoid movements. Death within 2 years of onset is the usual outcome, but the patient's condition may plateau and remain static for several years.
   b. **Diagnosis.** The EEG shows bursts of spike and slow-wave activity, followed by suppression of the background rhythms. The measles antibody titer is elevated in both the CSF and the serum, differentiating SSPE from the hereditary lipidoses and from progressive rubella panencephalitis.

2. **Progressive rubella panencephalitis** is a syndrome resembling SSPE that develops at 10–20 years of age in some patients born with congenital rubella. The rubella antibody titer is elevated in both the CSF and the serum, and rubella virus can be recovered from brain tissue. The EEG does not show the pattern seen in SSPE.

B. **Acute disseminated (parainfectious) encephalomyelitis** occurs several days after certain viral infections (e.g., measles, chickenpox, and—rarely—influenza, rubella, or mumps) or after smallpox, rabies, or influenza vaccinations. A cell-mediated autoimmune reaction to myelin basic protein is the presumed etiology.

1. **Clinical features and diagnosis.** The patient becomes irritable and lethargic, even comatose. The CSF commonly shows a slight increase in lymphocytes and an increase in protein.

2. **Prognosis.** Many patients recover completely, but mental retardation, seizures, or even death can ensue.

3. **Post-pertussis vaccination encephalopathy** is controversial and deserves special comment. Within hours to a few days after a pertussis vaccination, approximately 1 in 300,000 patients may develop encephalopathy that, if not fatal, leaves the patient with mental retardation and a severe seizure disorder. Nevertheless, the argument for pertussis vaccination of infants is quite strong because the complications of pertussis itself are more common in this age-group than are the reactions to the vaccine (see also Table 1-5). Furthermore, recent research has suggested that the incidence of postvaccine encephalopathy may be much lower than previously thought.

C. **Presumed autoimmune diseases affecting the cerebellum**

1. **Acute cerebellar ataxia** occurs in young children 1–2 weeks after a nonspecific respiratory infection. A brain tumor, intoxications, and an occult neuroblastoma must be excluded as causes. The disease is self-limited, with recovery occurring in two thirds of patients within 6 months.

2. **Myoclonic encephalopathy (Kinsbourne syndrome)** usually starts by 6 months of age and causes irregular, rapid eye movements (opsoclonus) as well as polymyoclonus and ataxia. In some cases, the cause has been a neuroblastoma or a tumor of the brain stem or cerebellum. ACTH, usually needed for several years, has been helpful in suppressing the symptoms. Approximately half of the children who are afflicted are mildly retarded.

D. **Other presumed autoimmune postinfectious CNS diseases**

1. **Reye syndrome** (see Chapter 11)

2. **Multiple sclerosis** currently is thought to be the result of an autoimmune reaction to an infectious agent that occurs in genetically susceptible people. It is primarily a disease of young adults, but has been diagnosed as early as 2 years of age. A demyelinating disease noted for its exacerbations and remissions, multiple sclerosis in children manifests as ataxia, spasticity, and visual disturbances. MRI scan will demonstrate areas of demyelination, and abnormal immunoglobulins can be detected in CSF.

3. **Diffuse cerebral sclerosis (Schilder disease)** is a rare, acute, progressive demyelinating condition that histologically resembles multiple sclerosis. It occurs sporadically between 5 and 12 years of age and has an unremitting, fatal outcome. The cause is not known but is presumed to be autoimmune or infectious.

4. **Transverse myelitis (transverse myelopathy)** is a presumed autoimmune disease that affects the spinal cord, causing sudden back pain followed by rapidly progressing weakness and loss of sensation below the level of the lesion. Determining a sensory level on neurologic examination as well as loss of bladder and bowel function distinguishes this disorder from Guillain-Barré syndrome; a space-occupying lesion is ruled out by CT or MRI scan.

E. **Presumed autoimmune, postinfectious diseases of peripheral nerves**

1. **Guillain-Barré syndrome,** the most common of these disorders in children, is a postinfectious demyelinating polyneuropathy. Lymphocytes sensitized to the basic protein of myelin have been identified in this disease, supporting the presumed autoimmune pathogenesis.
   a. **Clinical features**
      (1) Typically, 2 weeks after a viral infection or an immunization, weakness insidiously begins to develop in the distal muscles of the lower extremities, occasionally with accompanying paresthesias.
      (2) The weakness progresses upward and centrally over a period of 2–4 weeks, so that the diaphragm and the cranial nerve musculature may eventually become involved. A plateau lasting about 4 weeks then develops, followed by gradual recovery, which may take up to 1 year.
      (3) At the height of the clinical manifestations, the CSF shows an elevated protein level without an elevation in the cell count.
   b. **Therapy** is supportive, until the patient loses ambulation, at which time plasmapheresis is indicated. Respiratory difficulties may require assisted respiration. Steroid therapy, plasmapheresis, or intravenous gamma globulin is recommended for patients whose condition is chronically progressive (worsening 4–6 weeks after onset) or relapsing.
   c. **Prognosis.** Approximately 10%–15% of patients have residual deficits, such as weakness of the distal muscles of the feet necessitating orthoses (e.g., special shoes, braces). Another 10% have a relapse, usually within the first year after recovery. Fatalities are rare, but can occur.

2. **Other presumably autoimmune, postinfectious neuropathies** include **Bell palsy** (facial nerve palsy) and **sixth nerve palsy**. **Gradenigo syndrome** (sixth nerve palsy associated with pain in the distribution of the fifth cranial nerve) is secondary to osteomyelitis of the petrous ridge of the sphenoid bone. Brachial plexus neuropathies have been associated with influenza vaccination.

BIBLIOGRAPHY

Fenichel GM: *Clinical Pediatric Neurology: A Signs and Symptoms Approach,* 2nd ed. Philadelphia, WB Saunders, 1992.

Holmes G: *Diagnosis and Management of Seizures in Children.* Philadelphia, WB Saunders, 1987.

Menkes J: *Textbook of Child Neurology,* 4th ed. Philadelphia, Lea & Febiger, 1990.

Swaiman K: *Pediatric Neurology Principles and Practice.* St. Louis, CV Mosby, 1989.

STUDY QUESTIONS

DIRECTIONS: Each of the numbered items or incomplete statements in this section is followed by answers or by completions of the statement. Select the ONE lettered answer or completion that is BEST in each case.

1. A 2-year-old boy is evaluated for macrocephaly and delayed development. His mother reports that he has been healthy and that his perinatal course was unremarkable. His head has always been large. He has just recently learned to walk, and he says only two or three words. He can feed himself with his fingers but not with a spoon. On examination, his head circumference is 52.5 cm (> 98%). He has several café-au-lait spots on his trunk and extremities. Examination of the axilla reveals freckling. The most likely diagnosis in this case is

(A) neurofibromatosis
(B) hydrocephalus
(C) Duchenne muscular dystrophy
(D) Tay-Sachs disease

2. A 4-month-old male infant presents with marked floppiness. His parents felt that he was normal until 2 months of age, when they were concerned by his failure to support his head. On examination, he is alert and tracks readily. He has a social smile. Facial grimace is normal but there are fasciculations of the tongue. His motor examination shows truncal weakness with slip-through on vertical suspension, and decreased movement in the lower extremities. No deep tendon reflexes are appreciated. The anatomic site most likely affected in this child is

(A) upper motor neuron
(B) anterior horn cell
(C) peripheral nerve
(D) neuromuscular junction
(E) muscle

3. The parents of a 3-year-old girl report that she has occasional nocturnal episodes consisting of sudden screaming and crying as though terrified. Her eyes will be open but she does not fixate or seem aware of her parents. This can last for 15–20 minutes, and then she resumes deep sleep. If awakened, she cannot recall a nightmare or discomfort. These episodes are most consistent with

(A) nightmares
(B) night terrors
(C) temper tantrums
(D) seizure

4. A 7-year-old child is seen in the clinic for evaluation of motor delay. The examination reveals limited voluntary movements as well as slow, writhing, continuous movements of the arms and legs whenever the patient initiates a motor movement. At rest, these movements are not seen. These movements are best characterized as

(A) spasticity
(B) athetosis
(C) dystonia
(D) ataxia
(E) hypotonia

5. While recovering from varicella, a 4-year-old boy manifests gait ataxia. When examined, he is alert and afebrile, with no meningismus or complaint of headache. He has no diplopia or facial weakness, but does have difficulty reaching for objects because of an intention tremor. Deep tendon reflexes are normal and plantar responses are flexor. He walks with a wide-based gait, and sways while standing still. The most likely diagnosis in this child is

(A) Guillain-Barré syndrome
(B) varicella encephalitis
(C) acute cerebellar ataxia
(D) ataxia–telangiectasia
(E) Reye syndrome

6. An 8-month-old girl is noted to have asymmetric use of her arms. The right arm is held in a flexed position, with the hand in a fist. The neurologic examination also reveals increased tone in the right ankle and hyperreflexia on the right side. The past history is significant for premature delivery at 28 weeks' gestation. The most likely diagnosis for this child is

(A) Duchenne muscular dystrophy
(B) spinal muscular atrophy
(C) brachial palsy
(D) cerebral palsy

DIRECTIONS: Each of the numbered items or incomplete statements in this section is negatively phrased, as indicated by a capitalized word such as NOT, LEAST, or EXCEPT. Select the ONE lettered answer or completion that is BEST in each case.

7. All of the following are characteristics of Rett syndrome EXCEPT

(A) autistic behavior
(B) microcephaly
(C) peculiar wringing motion of the hands
(D) autosomal recessive inheritance
(E) dementia

8. All of the following are problems commonly associated with cerebral palsy EXCEPT

(A) epilepsy
(B) mental retardation
(C) blindness
(D) emotional problems
(E) strabismus

9. All of the following statements about spina bifida cystica are true EXCEPT

(A) it is often associated with hydrocephalus
(B) it is fatal if not treated within 24 hours
(C) it may be diagnosed in utero with ultra-sonography
(D) it can cause urologic problems
(E) it requires orthopedic management

DIRECTIONS: The set of matching questions in this section consists of a list of four to twenty-six lettered options (some of which may be in figures) followed by several numbered items. For each numbered item, select the ONE lettered option that is most closely associated with it. To avoid spending too much time on matching sets with large numbers of options, it is generally advisable to begin each set by reading the list of options. Then, for each item in the set, try to generate the correct answer and locate it in the option list, rather than evaluating each option individually. Each lettered option may be selected once, more than once, or not at all.

Questions 10–12

For each set of clinical findings, select the appropriate diagnosis.

(A) Sturge-Weber syndrome
(B) Neurofibromatosis
(C) Tuberous sclerosis
(D) Ataxia–telangiectasia

10. An 11-month-old child with a capillary hemangioma involving the left forehead, who presents with right-sided seizures.

11. A 7-year-old with axillary freckles, multi-ple café-au-lait spots, and learning disabilities.

12. A 10-year-old with an ataxic gait and telangiectasias of the sclera.

ANSWERS AND EXPLANATIONS

1. The answer is A *[X A 1]*. Neurofibromatosis often presents with nonspecific developmental delay in the young child. Macrocephaly and the presence of café-au-lait spots and axillary freckling are clues to the diagnosis. Hydrocephalus is usually associated with signs of increased intracranial pressure, such as ataxia or vomiting. Duchenne muscular dystrophy may present with a delay in motor skill acquisition but not with macrocephaly and skin lesions. Children with Tay-Sachs disease may have developmental abnormalities and macrocephaly, but also have visual difficulties, seizures, and loss of milestones.

2. The answer is B *[XII A 1]*. This child has spinal muscular atrophy, with characteristic weakness, areflexia, and fasciculations of the tongue. The anterior horn cell is the site of the abnormality. This disorder is slowly progressive, leading ultimately to respiratory compromise.

3. The answer is B *[VI B 1]*. The episode is a sleep disturbance, night terrors, which occurs in stage 4 sleep. The patient gives the appearance of being awake and terrified during the event but cannot recall any dream content afterward, as would be expected in a nightmare that occurs in rapid eye movement sleep. Night terrors are distinguished from seizures by the description of the episode. An electroencephalogram also may be helpful at times.

4. The answer is B *[Table 18-4]*. Athetosis refers to slow, writhing, continuous movements in the extremities, which are seen in many diseases, but most commonly in patients with cerebral palsy. Chorea, athetosis, spasticity, dystonia, ataxia, and hypotonia are physiologic classifications for the abnormal muscle tone or movement disorders commonly seen in children with cerebral palsy. When classifying a patient's disorder, both the anatomic location of the abnormality and the physiologic characteristic of the abnormality are considered.

5. The answer is C *[XIII C 1]*. Acute cerebellar ataxia is a postinfectious encephalomyelitis that often presents with primarily cerebellar dysfunction. Other symptoms such as cranial neuropathies, confusion, or pyramidal tract weakness can also be seen. Guillain-Barré syndrome is a demyelinating neuropathy; clinically, areflexia and ascending limb weakness are noted. Varicella encephalitis is usually seen during the acute phase of the illness and is associated with fever and, often, seizures. Reye syndrome may occur with varicella, but presents with signs of acute increased intracranial pressure and confusion. Ataxia–telangiectasia is a slowly progressive disorder.

6. The answer is D *[IV A, B, D; Table 18-4]*. This child has evidence of a right hemiparesis, probably related to her prematurity. This lesion represents an insult to the developing brain, resulting in abnormal motor function. Assuming that this is not a progressive disease, the child has cerebral palsy.

7. The answer is D *[XI E 4 e]*. The genetics of Rett syndrome has not yet been determined. Although it is thought to be a genetic syndrome, no inheritance pattern and no enzymatic deficiency or other metabolic explanation has been established for Rett syndrome. The other characteristics (autistic behavior, microcephaly, peculiar wringing motion of the hand, dementia) are common in patients with this disorder.

8. The answer is C *[IV C 2]*. Rarely is blindness a complication of cerebral palsy. However, strabismus occurs in approximately 40% of patients with cerebral palsy, mental retardation or learning disabilities in approximately 40%–50%, behavior problems in at least 20%, and epilepsy in approximately 30%.

9. The answer is B *[III B 1 a]*. When a child is born with spina bifida cystica marked by either a meningomyelocele or a meningocele, early surgical closure of the defect is not necessary for survival, but it is indicated to prevent infection. Children with these defects commonly have hydrocephalus and require urologic care because the bladder is not under normal control and is prone to infection. Orthopedic care also is necessary because kyphoscoliosis and hip dislocation are common complications.

10–12. The answers are: 10-A *[X C]*,
11-B *[X A]*, **12-D** *[X E]*. Sturge-Weber syndrome is characterized by meningeal angiomatosis, often in the occipital region, and capillary hemangioma in the distribution of the upper division of the trigeminal nerve (port-wine stain). Seizures and local cerebral scarring can be associated with this vascular anomaly.

Neurofibromatosis is an autosomal dominant disorder with abnormalities of the skin, bones, and neural tissues. Epilepsy and cognitive difficulties can be associated with this disorder. Optic glioma, acoustic neuromata, and neurofibroma can also be seen in this disorder.

Ataxia–telangiectasia is a progressive, autosomal recessive disorder. Ataxia of gait is usually the initial symptom, with appearance of the characteristic scleral and conjunctival telangiectasias in the second half of the first decade. The disorder is associated with a defect in immunoglobulin A, which is associated with pulmonary infections.

CASE STUDIES IN CLINICAL DECISION MAKING

Case 1

An 18-month-old boy is brought to the pediatrician's office by his mother for a routine health supervision visit. A review of the record reveals that the child has had five episodes of acute otitis media since birth but has otherwise been well. The office nurse has obtained measurements and plotted them on the growth chart. The growth chart reveals that the child's length and weight have consistently tracked along the fiftieth percentile for age.

As the clinician opens the door to the examining room, she notes that water in the sink is running, children's books are scattered on the floor, and paper from the examination table is strewn all over the room. When the toddler notices the physician, he immediately runs to his very pregnant and tired-appearing mother, clutches onto her leg, and begins to cry.

QUESTIONS

- *Given this child's age and initial reaction, what techniques can the pediatrician use in an attempt to enhance the success of this encounter?*
- *List the important components of history taking for this visit.*

DISCUSSION

A health supervision visit for an older infant or young preschool-age child is a challenge to even the most seasoned clinician. Predictably, the patient demonstrates a high degree of motor activity and curiosity, along with obvious stranger anxiety. The effective clinician seeks to diminish the child's fears by allowing the child time and opportunity gradually to acquaint himself with physician, instruments, and procedures of the examination. To accomplish this, she enters the room slowly, seats herself in a chair across the room from the child and parent, avoids direct eye contact with the patient, and in a soft, friendly voice addresses the mother. Meanwhile, she covertly observes the patient's general appearance, interactions with the mother, speech patterns, and gait. As she begins to talk she lays down her stethoscope, reflex hammer, and tongue depressor on the table in front of the patient, along with a few small toys.

The physician asks a general opening question like, "How are things going?" to elicit the mother's concerns and general assessment of her child's health and behavior. After a general inquiry, she plans to pursue areas of parental concern and include age-related questions focused around the child's general health, daily functioning, and developmental progress. For this child, she plans to pay special attention to parental assessment of hearing, language development, and growth (because of the frequent episodes of otitis media), as well as plans for the birth of a new sibling.

In response to the physician's opening question, the mother appears as if she is about to cry. She says, "He's always sick with ear infections. And, even when he isn't sick, he's impossible to control. He won't eat anything that we want him to eat, he won't mind us when we tell him to stop doing something, and he's impossible to toilet train. We need help to fix things before the new baby comes."

QUESTION

- *To address the mother's concerns, what areas should further history taking focus on? To answer this question, begin by forming an initial problem list.*

DISCUSSION

The mother's concerns are:

1. Frequent episodes of illness
2. Poor eating habits
3. Behavior "out of control"
4. Difficulty in toilet training
5. Impact of child's behavior on arrival of new infant

Because of the mother's concerns, further history taking should include:

1. **Episodes of illness in addition to otitis media.** Although acute otitis media is very common in this age-group, it evokes a wide variety of concerns for parents. The clinician must seek to uncover specific parental anxieties and also confirm that the child does not have any other complicating or more serious medical problems. Potential hidden concerns may include permanent hearing problems or a more serious illness accounting for the frequent infections.
2. **Parental assessment of the child's growth, hearing, and language abilities.** These are particularly important in light of the history of otitis media.
3. **Typical daily diet.** The average 2-year-old requires a limited amount of food for growth. To respond to the mother's concerns about diet, it is important to obtain the actual diet history as well as review the growth chart.
4. **Parental expectations regarding feeding and behavior along with typical management strategies (including limit-setting) surrounding conflicts.** Before responding to parents' concerns, it is crucial that the clinician be knowledgeable about age-appropriate recommendations and normal behavior, but also determine what parents' expectations are.
5. **Parental management of toilet training up until now**
6. **Plans for the new infant** (including day-care arrangements, help at home, preparation of the household and child for a new sibling)

The mother responds to the clinician's inquiries. Meanwhile, the patient begins to roam around and wanders over to the table with the instruments and toys. He begins to handle them and play with them. Speaking softly, the pediatrician encourages him to continue his explorations.

History reveals that the child eats Cheerios and fruit for breakfast but refuses to be fed hot cereal. During lunch and dinner, the child "picks" at a wide variety of table foods eaten by the entire family. He prefers small pieces of fruit, cheese, and crackers. He drinks approximately two glasses of milk each day and eats a few ounces of chicken. At the beginning of a meal he eats eagerly while sitting in his high chair, and after about 20 minutes he cries until removed to the floor.

He has had six upper respiratory infections during the past year, complicated on four occasions by acute otitis media. Each infection resolved with antibiotic treatment. He has had no other illnesses. His mother states that his hearing is "too good." He says many words, uses three- and four-word sentences, and is not difficult for his parents to understand. "No" is his favorite expression.

He is "always on the go," seeming never to stop for a moment. He is "into everything," and throws frequent temper tantrums when disciplined. Access to household poisons is limited by locked cabinets, but there are many valuable small glass figurines which he "can't seem to keep away from." He requires constant supervision because of his high activity level, high level of curiosity, and inability to stay "out of trouble." He has had multiple forehead abrasions from falls while running. Parents find themselves constantly "yelling" and occasionally "spanking" without any resulting "improvement in behavior." Toilet training was begun at 16 months with introduction of a "potty chair" in which he has not demonstrated any interest thus far.

A bedroom for the new infant is being set up. Parents had planned to toilet train this child and move him out of his crib into a new bed shortly before the mother's due date.

QUESTION

- With the information you have obtained thus far, what aspects of the physical examination should you focus on?

DISCUSSION

A full physical examination should be performed with the child seated on the parent's lap. For this patient, extra emphasis is placed on:

1. Review of the growth chart
2. Parent–child interactions, with particular attention to observing reaction to negative behaviors
3. Subjective assessment of child's hearing
4. Observations about the clarity and content of the child's speech
5. Tympanic membranes
6. Other aspects of the physical examination that would be helpful in ruling out occult reasons for infection, including a careful head and neck examination, palpation of lymph nodes, chest auscultation, determination of liver and spleen size, and a survey of the skin
7. Observation for age-appropriate developmental milestones

The physical examination is entirely normal, including assessment of hearing, speech, developmental milestones, and age-appropriate behavior. The mother frequently admonishes the child to "stop crying" and "stay still for the doctor."

QUESTION

- Given the data thus far, what key aspects of anticipatory guidance is it important for the clinician to focus on now?

DISCUSSION

1. **Nutritional concerns.** The parent should be reassured about the child's growth by reviewing the growth chart and discussing the limited nutritional needs of this age-group. In addition, given the child's limited attention span, high degree of motor activity, and determination to feed himself, parents should be guided as to appropriate mealtime expectations. These include allowing the child to feed himself with finger foods, not expecting him to sit at the table for more than 15 or 20 minutes at a time, and keeping "battles" over food to a minimum by offering reasonable, small quantities and avoiding between-meal snacks.
2. **Frequent episodes of otitis media.** Although this child does have frequent episodes of upper respiratory infection and acute otitis media, there is no evidence of prolonged serous otitis, hearing loss, language delay, interference with growth, or other underlying illness. Antibiotic prophylaxis to reduce the frequency of acute otitis media may be offered at this point.
3. **"Out of control" behavior**
4. **Toilet training "failure"**
5. **Preparation for the new sibling**

To address concerns 3, 4, and 5, it is appropriate to review normal age-related developmental issues. A brief discussion of the 18-month-old's struggle between dependence and independence and resulting "negative" behaviors (e.g., food refusal, temper tantrums), combined with the child's highly active, curious, "motor-minded" temperament is an appropriate prologue to guiding parents toward more reasonable expectations for behavior and behavior management. Recommendations might include:

1. **Structuring the environment toward both child safety and child friendliness,** which might include putting away or out of reach all fragile objects. This would avoid the necessity for frequent admonitions to "stay away from that."

2. **Recognizing the child's abilities and structuring limits accordingly.** This child in particular will benefit from having toys that are not easily broken and encourage gross motor movement. Activities should be structured to allow exploration and rough-and-tumble play. If feasible, providing plenty of outdoor time would allow the child to "run off" extra energy. Allowing the child a reasonable degree of freedom and autonomy within a safe environment will diminish the number of conflicts with parents.

3. **Parental discussion and agreement on reasonable rules** based on their child's behavior style and age. Reminding them to "save your battles for the big ones" may avoid many potential conflicts.

4. **Suitable strategies for dealing with intolerable behaviors** (e.g., dangerous acts or deliberate physical antagonism toward another person). These include the use of "time out," and positive reinforcement for good behavior (e.g., "catch him when he's good").

5. **Deferring toilet training** until the child shows signs of interest, is past the peak of autonomy and independence struggles, and the household has begun to adjust to the new infant.

6. **Anticipating a deterioration of behavior when the new infant is born** and attempting to diminish sibling rivalry. Strategies include reading books with their child about a new brother or sister, visiting the hospital before and after the sibling is born, encouraging a limited number of "big brother" helper activities that are realistic and age-appropriate, providing special one-on-one time with each parent each day (without the infant), maintaining as many "before-baby" activities and rules as possible after the new child is born, and deferring a move out of the crib until the household has settled after the birth. It is especially important to remind these parents to "never leave the child alone with the new baby even for a minute."

7. **Encouragement to the mother to seek baby-sitting assistance and time away** from this active, demanding child can be offered as a "prescription" from the pediatrician. Diminishing guilt and validating the difficulties of parenting are two extremely important aspects of the pediatrician's role in health supervision.

Case 2

An 18-year-old woman presents to her physician with right upper quadrant abdominal pain of 4 day's duration. She had been in good health before the onset of this pain. She works full time in a day-care program for young children as a summer job. She graduated from high school this past spring and plans to attend college in the fall.

She denies any vomiting or diarrhea. Food does not make the pain any better or worse. She has had no black or red stools. She does add that over the past day she has felt some right shoulder pain, although she does not remember doing anything that may have caused the shoulder pain.

Past medical history is negative for any hospitalizations or major illness. She has no known allergies, and her only medication is birth-control pills, which she has been taking regularly for the past 2 years. She lives at home with both parents and a younger sister. She gets along well with her family but tends to talk about her personal issues with her friends.

She denies using cigarettes, drugs, or alcohol, although she has drunk some wine and beer on special family occasions. When asked if she has a special boyfriend or is going out with anyone, she becomes very quiet. After a couple of minutes, she is able to add that she had broken up with someone 3 weeks ago. She had been going out with him for 3 months, although she had known him for over 1 year. At this point, tears come to her eyes. When asked what happened, she adds that he had forced her to have sex with him. No condom was used. She had not been able to discuss this with anyone up to this point. She really did not want anyone else to know. She is able to confirm that this episode has made her feel quite depressed, and she has been spending most of her time on her own, but she denies any suicidal ideation.

Further review of systems is essentially negative, except that she had a normal menstrual period 2 weeks ago and subsequently developed a vaginal discharge that now leaves yellow stains on her underwear. She has never had any vaginal infections or sexually transmitted disease (STD). Her last visit to the family planning clinic was 2 months ago, when she had her annual Pap smear and was told that all her tests were normal or negative.

Her vital signs are stable, and she is afebrile. While she is changing for the physical examination, the physician has a chance to collect his thoughts and call his colleague at the family planning clinic to find that the patient had a normal Pap smear and negative gonorrhea and *Chlamydia* studies.

QUESTION

- *What is the physician's problem list to this point?*

DISCUSSION

This case illustrates that the presenting complaint may only be the tip of the iceberg. Adolescents often come for help with one issue but actually have something else much more important on their minds. The problem list should include the following:

1. **Health maintenance**
2. **Reproductive health care.** The patient has a good method of pregnancy prevention with the use of birth-control pills. It is important to review the method used for STD protection.
3. **Date rape.** This is a common problem that often goes unreported. As a health care provider, the physician needs to explore this problem and is obligated to report it to the appropriate authorities.
4. **Abdominal pain.** The patient's pain is not associated with gastrointestinal symptoms or food. There is no alcohol or drug abuse, which may be associated with inflammation of the pancreas. Use of birth-control pills has been associated with gallbladder disease.
5. **Right shoulder pain.** The pain in this situation is not associated with trauma or activity. It may be related to phrenic nerve irritation from the source of the abdominal pain.
6. **Vaginal discharge.** The discharge is purulent in nature by the patient's description, although she tested negative for the common STDs 2 months earlier. Sexual intercourse occurred without the protection of a condom.

Physical examination reveals the following findings:

1. **Diffuse right upper quadrant abdominal pain without rebound. No liver enlargement or other masses appreciated. Good bowel sounds.**
2. **Moderate yellow vaginal discharge without cervical motion tenderness but with some discomfort on movement of the uterus. A normal saline preparation of the vaginal discharge showed sheets of white blood cells, and not *Trichomonas*.**
3. **No swelling, erythema, or point tenderness over the right shoulder but clear associated pain in that area. No other significant findings on the physical examination.**

QUESTIONS

- *What modifications should the physician make to the problem list at this point?*
- *What laboratory tests should the physician order?*
- *What should be the physician's treatment plan?*

DISCUSSION

The finding on the normal saline preparation from the vaginal discharge is very suggestive of an STD. This scenario correlates well with the history of the discharge appearing after unprotected sexual intercourse and becoming more prominent after a menstrual period. The abdominal and shoulder pain may be related to perihepatic spread of the infection, resulting in a Fitz-Hugh Curtis syndrome–like presentation. Initial laboratory studies could include a complete blood count and an erythrocyte sedimentation rate (ESR), gonorrhea, and *Chlamydia* studies from the cervix, blood test for syphilis, liver function studies, and evaluation of amylase levels. An ultrasound of the gallbladder and liver would also be helpful.

Because the most likely diagnosis is a pelvic infection with perihepatitis, the patient should be admitted to the hospital for intravenous management of the infection with antibiotics. This plan will also give additional time to explore the date rape and initiate appropriate counseling. Laboratory studies would probably show an elevated white blood cell count and ESR, as well as a positive gonorrhea or *Chlamydia* study. Liver function studies and amylase evaluation are usually negative, as is the ultrasound. Hospitalization is continued until the symptoms subside. A total 2-week course of treatment can be completed on an ambulatory basis with oral antibiotics. Follow-up studies for the identified STD need to be performed after the end of the course of therapy. Efforts should be made to make sure that the partner is also treated.

Case 3

A 3-month-old infant is brought to the emergency department by her parents. She was well until 24 hours earlier, when she began to have emesis, followed shortly thereafter by profuse diarrhea. Initially, she took her formula eagerly, but her intake has decreased over the last 12 hours, and she has become less arousable. Her parents are uncertain whether she has urinated in the past 12 hours, because the diarrhea is so watery.

QUESTIONS

- *What are your immediate concerns about this patient?*
- *What is the most likely source of this child's unresponsiveness?*

DISCUSSION

This child has had profuse emesis and diarrhea without significant oral intake. Infants have a larger surface area per unit weight than do adults, causing them to require relatively larger maintenance volumes of fluid. For this reason, even simple gastroenteritis can produce hypovolemic shock, if the infant's intake is limited, as seen here.

Your first concern should be to see if this child is in shock, and if so, whether it is early or late shock. The decreased arousability raises your concern that this is relatively advanced shock. A rapid cardiopulmonary assessment should be performed, with particular attention to capillary refill, peripheral pulses, skin temperature, and blood pressure.

Physical examination reveals a lethargic, pale infant, breathing 50 times per minute, but without retractions. Her distal extremities are cool, distal pulses are not appreciated, and her capillary refill time is 7 seconds. Heart rate is 190 and blood pressure is 60/45. Auscultation of the chest reveals good air entry, no pathologic airway sounds, and no murmurs or gallops. There is no hepatosplenomegaly, and bowel sounds are present. During the examination you note a profuse, watery stool.

QUESTIONS

- *What is this child's physiologic status?*
- *What should be your initial sequence of interventions?*

DISCUSSION

This child is in late shock, indicated by her poor peripheral perfusion, decreased level of consciousness, tachycardia, tachypnea without increased work of breathing, and her low blood pressure. Blood pressure does not fall in infants until circulating blood volume has been decreased by more than 40%. This shock is likely hypovolemic in origin because there is no liver enlargement or pulmonary crackles indicating congestive heart failure, and the history also is suggestive of hypovolemia. This child requires emergency rehydration to restore her circulating volume to adequate levels. The initial intervention should be to establish vascular access rapidly. If venous access is difficult to obtain—a likely situation—an intraosseous needle should be placed to administer boluses of crystalloid. The emergency phase of the rehydration should be as rapid as possible, until perfusion, pulses, heart rate, and end-organ function return toward normal levels.

Laboratory tests should include bedside glucose and electrolyte measurement. The bladder should be cannulated so that urine output can be quantified; this is an excellent indicator of cardiac output. Frequent reassessments prevent shock from reappearing unnoticed, because the diarrhea may continue for some hours after initiation of therapy.

One hundred milliliters (20 ml/kg) of 0.9 normal saline is administered by intraosseous needle. Reassessment shows heart rate of 180, thready distal pulses, capillary refill time of 5 seconds, and blood pressure of 70/55. The glucose value is < 40 mg/dl.

QUESTIONS

- *What is the child's current status?*
- *What is your next intervention, if any?*

DISCUSSION

Although the intervention is showing results, the child is still in shock; the blood pressure is now (barely) in the normal range for age. She requires additional emergency rehydration. In addition, her glucose level is low, and glucose should also be provided.

Another 100 ml of 0.9 normal saline is given by bolus. Ten milliliters of D25W is given, also by bolus. The child becomes more alert, heart rate drops to 160, capillary refill time is 2 seconds, and peripheral pulses are full. Urine is beginning to come from the bladder catheter. The infant is admitted to the hospital, and a schedule of slower rehydration is instituted. As her physiologic status continues to normalize, she will be started on an oral rehydration formula, which will help to decrease her stool losses.

Case 4

A 13-year-old boy is brought to his pediatrician with the complaint of abdominal pain that has been present for the past year. He states that it was intermittent at first, but more recently it has been occurring on a daily basis and occasionally awakens him from sleep. The pain is primarily in the lower abdominal quadrants and is sometimes relieved by defecation. His stools have varied between loose and normal. He denies rectal bleeding. There has been some fatigue, his appetite has decreased, and he has lost 3 pounds. The remainder of his review of systems is negative. His mother has Crohn disease.

QUESTIONS

- What is the definition of recurrent abdominal pain (RAP) in children and adolescents?
- How common is the complaint of RAP?
- What distinguishes "organic" causes of abdominal pain from "functional" causes?

DISCUSSION

RAP has been classically defined as three episodes of abdominal pain that are severe enough to affect activity and that occur over a period of 3 months. It has been estimated that up to 15% of school-age children experience RAP. The literature on RAP suggests that despite extensive evaluation, an organic cause of RAP can be discovered in only 10% of cases. Organic causes would include disorders such as inflammatory bowel disease and peptic ulcer disease. Functional bowel disease is probably better labeled as dysfunctional bowel disease and would include disorders such as irritable bowel syndrome (which may be a disorder of intestinal motility) and lactose intolerance (which results from insufficient intestinal mucosal lactase activity). There also exists a small subgroup of children whose abdominal pain appears to be psychogenic in origin.

QUESTIONS

- What is the differential diagnosis for RAP?
- What are worrisome characteristics of the patient with RAP?

DISCUSSION

Whereas a very large differential diagnosis exists for the child with RAP, most affected children have one of five disorders. These include irritable bowel syndrome, carbohydrate malabsorption, peptic ulcer disease, inflammatory bowel disease, and urinary tract infection. Pancreatic, hepatobiliary, gynecologic, metabolic, and collagen vascular disorders are much less common. The presence of an infectious process, such as giardiasis, may be more common in certain geographic locations than others. A thorough history and physical examination usually direct the caretaker to the correct diagnosis. Most patients with irritable bowel syndrome state that their pain is in the lower quadrants, relieved by defecation, and often accompanied by a sense of incomplete evacuation and bloating. Stool habit may range from constipation to diarrhea to a variable pattern. Peptic ulcer disease often tends to present with epigastric discomfort, which is frequently burning in nature and often accompanied by vomiting.

Certain features of the patient with RAP should prompt the clinician to pursue more aggressively a diagnostic evaluation for organic disease. Weight loss, diarrhea, rectal bleeding, vomiting, nocturnal pain, fever, rash, and arthritis are all worrisome signs. A family history of inflammatory bowel disease or peptic ulcer disease should be sought.

Physical examination reveals a thin boy with normal vital signs. His weight is below the fifth percentile for his age; his height is in the tenth percentile. No rashes are noted. A superficial ulcer is noted in the right buccal mucosa. Heart and lungs are normal. Abdominal examination reveals mild tenderness in the lower quadrants, especially on the right. There is no perirectal disease, and stool is free of occult blood. Pubertal development is delayed. There is mild clubbing.

QUESTION

- *What features of the physical examination are particularly helpful in the evaluation of the patient with RAP?*

DISCUSSION

An evaluation of growth parameters should be included in the evaluation of the patient with RAP. Growth percentiles should be examined in comparison to previous data for that patient, and the patient's growth should be evaluated in the context of parental values as well. A falling-off in growth velocity should alert the clinician to the possibility of more serious disorders, such as inflammatory bowel disease.

Skin abnormalities such as erythema nodosum and pyoderma gangrenosum, inflamed joints, stomatitis, and clubbing may indicate the presence of inflammatory bowel disease. A rectal examination should be performed in all patients with RAP, with careful note made of the presence of perirectal inflammation (fissures, fistula, skin tags), and a stool guaiac test should be performed.

The pediatrician decides to perform some screening laboratory tests, including a complete blood count, erythrocyte sedimentation rate (ESR), chemistry profile, and urinalysis. Data obtained include hematocrit of 32%, white blood cell count of 11,300 cells/mm³, platelet count of 650,000/mm³, ESR of 54, albumin 3.1 g/dl, and normal electrolytes, blood urea nitrogen, and creatinine.

QUESTION

- *What is the role of a screening evaluation in the patient with RAP?*

DISCUSSION

The evaluation of a patient with RAP does not mandate screening hematologic and biochemical studies. In the presence of a convincing history for disorders such as irritable bowel syndrome and carbohydrate malabsorption, specific therapy can safely antedate further evaluation. In consideration of inflammatory disorders, such as ulcerative colitis and Crohn disease, certain studies can be very helpful. Hypochromic, microcytic anemia is common in patients with both disorders. The ESR is elevated in about 80% of subjects with Crohn disease at presentation, compared to less than 50% of those with ulcerative colitis. The platelet count is often elevated, which reflects its role as an acute-phase reactant. Hypoalbuminemia may reflect poor nutrition or, more likely, indicates the presence of protein-losing enteropathy.

Based on the history, physical examination, and the screening laboratory data, the physician determines that further evaluation is warranted.

QUESTIONS

- *What is the role of radiographic evaluation of the patient with RAP or suspected inflammatory bowel disease?*
- *What is the role of endoscopy in the evaluation of the patient with RAP or suspected inflammatory bowel disease?*

DISCUSSION

Radiologic studies are often performed in the evaluation of the patient with RAP. When considering the presence of peptic ulcer disease, an upper gastrointestinal series (UGI) may be ordered. Unfortunately, the yield of radiographic studies in detecting peptic ulcer disease is very low in children. This likely reflects the presence of superficial mucosal peptic inflammation, which is present more often than deeper ulceration. UGI with small bowel follow-through is the procedure of choice for the detection of Crohn disease that affects the small bowel. Barium enema has no role in the evaluation of a child with RAP. Ultrasound examination may be helpful if hepatobiliary disease or renal disease is suspected.

Endoscopic evaluation may be helpful in several situations, especially in the diagnosis of peptic ulcer disease. Mucosal biopsy as well as gross inspection at the time of the procedure is important. Detection of *Helicobacter pylori* in the presence of gastric inflammation may guide therapy. Lower gastrointestinal endoscopy (flexible sigmoidoscopy or colonoscopy) should be the first procedure performed if ulcerative colitis is suspected. Colonic involvement in patients with Crohn disease is best detected with colonoscopy. More unusual disorders, such as collagenous colitis and lymphocytic colitis, may also be detected at colonoscopy with the use of mucosal biopsies.

Contrast radiography reveals nodularity of the terminal ileum and deformity of the cecum and ascending colon. Colonoscopy reveals a normal rectum, sigmoid, and left colon, but aphthoid lesions in the ascending and transverse colon.

QUESTIONS

- *What is the final diagnosis?*
- *How should this patient be managed?*

DISCUSSION

A diagnosis of Crohn disease affecting the terminal ileum and colon is made. Ileocolonic involvement is seen in about 60% of pediatric patients with Crohn disease, isolated small bowel disease in 30%, and involvement limited to the colon in only 10%.

Treatment of Crohn disease is directed toward decreasing bowel inflammation, ensuring adequate nutrition and growth, and anticipating possible psychological difficulties emanating from being affected by a chronic illness. Initial medical therapy may include 5-aminosalicylic acid (mesalamine), which has antiinflammatory activity in both the distal small bowel and colon. Alternatively, corticosteroids may be used in more severe cases, with initial therapy given on a daily basis (1–2 mg/kg) and then gradually tapered to alternate-day therapy. More refractory cases may mandate the addition of another agent, such as 6-mercaptopurine. Surgical therapy may be required for intractable corticosteroid-resistant disease, obstruction, severe bleeding, or complications of refractory fistulas. Because the most important factor in growth delay in children with Crohn disease appears to be inadequate nutrition, dietary counseling with the provision of high-calorie foods and oral supplements is essential. Nocturnal nasogastric tube feedings or, more rarely, parenteral hyperalimentation, may be needed to improve growth parameters. Frank discussions with the patient and family may address many unwarranted fears about the disease. Age-appropriate support groups are very helpful.

Case 5

You are asked to evaluate an 18-hour-old infant who was found to be cyanotic in the nursery. The infant was born at term, after a normal pregnancy and delivery and without risk factors for sepsis.

QUESTION

- *What are the causes of cyanosis in the newborn?*

DISCUSSION

The more common causes of cyanosis in the newborn include sepsis, persistent pulmonary hypertension of the newborn, cyanotic congenital heart disease, pulmonary disease, and hypoventilation secondary to central nervous system disease or upper airway obstruction. Less common causes include hypoglycemia, hypocalcemia, polycythemia, and the hemoglobinopathies.

On examination the infant is vigorous, mildly tachypneic, but not in respiratory distress. There is moderate cyanosis of the mucous membranes and skin. The lungs are clear, peripheral pulses are strong, the precordium is active, S_2 is single, and there are no heart murmurs. The liver is not enlarged. A bedside evaluation of blood glucose determines levels of 80–120 mg/dl.

QUESTIONS

- *How does the physical examination narrow the focus of the differential diagnosis?*
- *What is the significance of the active precordium?*
- *How would you proceed in your evaluation?*

DISCUSSION

The mild tachypnea without distress and clear lung fields make it unlikely that the cause of the cyanosis is lung disease. The presence of an active precordium suggests right ventricular enlargement. Absence of splitting of S_2 is not helpful because splitting is often difficult to hear in the newborn. Your next step should be to verify the cyanosis by measuring an oxygen saturation by pulse oximetry or arterial blood gas analysis while the infant is breathing room air and 100% oxygen.

An arterial sample of blood shows the P_{O_2} to be 38 mm Hg (saturation of 70%) in room air and 40 mm Hg (saturation of 75%) while the infant is breathing 100% oxygen. Blood samples are sent to the laboratory for a complete blood count and culture.

QUESTION

- *How does the very slight response to oxygen help your differential diagnosis? How do you proceed?*

DISCUSSION

Raising the ambient oxygen environment should significantly raise the Pa_{O_2} and saturation if the right-to-left shunt is variable (due to hypoventilation, for example, or lung disease), but not if it is fixed (due to heart disease). The very slight response (from a saturation of 70% to 75%) verifies that the right-to-left shunt is fixed and therefore of cardiac origin. The absence of a significant heart murmur suggests that there is no turbulence. A chest x-ray to evaluate heart size and pulmonary vascularity would be of help in the differential diagnosis and in confirming the absence of pulmonary causes of the cyanosis.

A chest x-ray demonstrates a normal heart size. The lungs are expanded bilaterally, and there is no infiltrate, but the pulmonary vascularity is diminished.

QUESTION

- *What is the differential diagnosis of cyanosis of the newborn with diminished pulmonary blood flow?*

DISCUSSION

Diminished vascularity in a cyanotic newborn rules out the presence of transposition of the great arteries and total anomalous pulmonary venous return. The diagnoses compatible with diminished pulmonary blood flow are those that have right ventricular outflow obstruction, including tricuspid atresia, pulmonary valve atresia with or without a ventricular septal defect (VSD), tetralogy of Fallot, and truncus arteriosus with small pulmonary arteries.

QUESTION

- *How does the absence of a murmur in this infant help in the differential diagnosis?*

DISCUSSION

The fact that there is no turbulence (absent heart murmur) makes it unlikely that this infant has a tetralogy of Fallot or truncus arteriosus with small pulmonary arteries. Infants with pulmonary atresia with an intact septum usually have a murmur of tricuspid regurgitation, and those with tricuspid valve atresia usually have a murmur of a VSD, unless the right ventricle is essentially nonexistent.

QUESTION

- *Would an electrocardiogram (ECG) help in the differential diagnosis?*

DISCUSSION

An ECG would be helpful in diagnosing tricuspid valve atresia because it is one of a few cyanotic congenital heart abnormalities in which the frontal plane axis is leftward. It might also help in determining the presence of right atrial and right ventricular enlargement. However, all of this information would be more accurately determined with an echocardiogram, which will in any case need to be performed for diagnosis.

QUESTION

- *What should be your next step?*

DISCUSSION

This infant has cyanotic congenital heart disease with diminished pulmonary blood flow that must be ductus dependent. Before proceeding with further diagnostic procedures, you should start a prostaglandin (PGE$_1$) drip to open the ductus arteriosus. This should be done before echocardiography, unless the latter is immediately available.

The infant is started on a PGE$_1$ drip with a response within 15 minutes; the oxygen saturation rises into the mid-80s. Echocardiography is then performed that shows the infant to have pulmonary valve atresia with a VSD and pulmonary arteries supplied by a ductus. Cardiac catheterization confirms the diagnosis, demonstrating small pulmonary arteries and normal aortic arch anatomy. The following day, a modified Blalock-Taussig shunt is performed, PGE$_1$ is discontinued, and the ductus allowed to close. The infant goes home after a few days. Correction of the abnormality is planned in the future.

Case 6

A previously well 3-year-old boy presents with a 2-week history of irritability, decreased appetite, brief nosebleeds, bruising of his arms, legs, and trunk, and leg pain that has progressively worsened so that he refuses to run or to climb stairs. For the last 2 days, he has felt warm and has had an oral temperature of 39.4°C. The only medication he has received has been acetaminophen, which has lowered his temperature and produced a modest decrease in his leg pain. On physical examination, his vital signs are normal except for temperature of 38.8°C. He is pale, has scattered petechiae and ecchymoses on his extremities and torso, discrete, nontender, anterior cervical lymph nodes that are 1–2 cm in diameter, a grade II/VI short systolic ejection murmur at the upper left sternal border, and a spleen palpable 2 cm below the left costal margin. Examination of the extremities and neurologic examination are negative.

QUESTIONS

- *What type of disease is suggested by this history and physical examination?*
- *What is the first test that should be ordered?*

DISCUSSION

This patient's history and physical examination suggest a serious blood dyscrasia affecting all aspects of bone marrow function. The history of epistaxis and bruising and his petechiae and ecchymoses indicate that he may be thrombocytopenic. His anorexia, irritability, and pallor suggest anemia, and the fever could result from infection in a child with a paucity of neutrophils. The bone pain, lymphadenopathy, and splenomegaly all raise the possibility of infiltrative disease.

The first test should be a complete blood count (CBC), with a differential white blood cell count (WBC), platelet count, and reticulocyte count. All of these parameters are useful indicators of bone marrow function.

The patient's CBC values are hemoglobin 5 g/dl, hematocrit 15%, WBC 3800/mm³ with 4% polymorphonuclear leukocytes, 1% bands, 2% monocytes, 89% lymphocytes, and 4% blasts, platelets 11,000/mm³, and reticulocyte count 2.4%. On peripheral smear, the red blood cell morphology is normal and the blasts have scant cytoplasm, fine nuclear chromatin, and a small, inconspicuous nucleolus.

QUESTIONS

- *What do these findings suggest?*
- *What test must be done to evaluate them further?*

DISCUSSION

The normochromic and normocytic anemia is a hypoproliferative anemia because the reticulo-cyte index (corrected reticulocyte count) is low. This type of anemia is caused by the marrow's inability to produce adequate numbers of red cells, due either to aplasia or to infiltration by abnormal cells. The mild leukopenia, more severe neutropenia, and very severe thrombocyto-penia also suggest that the bone marrow has failed to produce blood cells normally. The blasts in the peripheral blood indicate that this most likely results from marrow replacement by immature cells rather than from bone marrow aplasia.

A bone marrow aspiration must be performed.

The bone marrow aspirate is hypercellular, and the normal hematopoietic elements are almost totally replaced by lymphoblasts that have scant cytoplasm and a small, inconspicuous nucleolus. They correspond to L1 cells of the French-American-British (FAB) classification. They are termi-nal deoxynucleotidyl transferase (TdT) positive and peroxidase and nonspecific esterase negative.

The cells lack T-cell antigens, including the sheep erythrocyte receptor, and are negative for surface immunoglobulin heavy and light chains and for cytoplasmic immunoglobulin heavy chains. They do express common acute lymphocytic leukemia antigen (CALLA). On cytoge-netic analysis, the cells are hyperdiploid and contain 53 chromosomes. No translocations are identified. Analysis of DNA for antigen receptor gene rearrangements demonstrates a clonal rearrangement of the immunoglobulin heavy chain genes and a clonal rearrangement of the genes for the delta chain T-cell receptor.

QUESTION

• *What do these findings indicate?*

DISCUSSION

The findings are typical for the lymphoblasts of childhood acute lymphoblastic leukemia (ALL), which usually have L1 morphology and are TdT positive and lack enzymes expressed by granu-locyte and monocyte precursors. Their immunophenotypic characteristics are also typical for early pre–B-cell ALL, which is the most common type of childhood ALL. The cells have matured only to the point where they express CALLA, but not further along the pathways of B-cell differ-entiation (synthesis of cytoplasmic heavy chains or of complete surface immunoglobulin mole-cules) or along the pathways of T-cell differentiation, where they express various T-cell antigens. The incomplete pattern of antigen receptor gene rearrangements is typical for this type of ALL, and its clonality indicates that all the cells are the progeny of a single abnormal precursor cell. Hyperdiploidy and the absence of chromosomal translocations are also characteristics of CALLA-positive early pre–B-cell ALL.

QUESTIONS

• *What is this child's prognosis?*
• *What factors determine his prognosis?*

DISCUSSION

His prognosis is good.

His age places him in a good prognostic category because he is between 1 and 10 years old. However, he must also have a WBC less than 50,000/mm³, a favorable immunophenotype, and no adverse cytogenetic features. He meets all these criteria. He has non–T, non–B-cell ALL rather than either T- or B-cell ALL, a low WBC, and hyperdiploidy without any translocations.

QUESTIONS

- *What other areas of the body should be evaluated?*
- *How should they be evaluated?*

DISCUSSION

The sanctuary areas, the testes, and central nervous system (CNS) must be evaluated. The chest should also be evaluated for an anterior mediastinal mass, and because he is febrile, for pneumonia.

The testes are evaluated by direct examination and are normal. The CNS is evaluated by examination of the optic fundi and by examination of cerebrospinal fluid (CSF) obtained by lumbar puncture. The optic fundi are normal, and the CSF is also normal. The chest is evaluated by chest radiograph, which is negative and demonstrates neither a mediastinal mass nor an infiltrate.

QUESTIONS

- *What other tests should be done before starting chemotherapy?*
- *What therapies need to be instituted before beginning chemotherapy?*

DISCUSSION

Blood urea nitrogen, creatinine, electrolytes, and uric acid should be measured. Dying leukemic cells release purines that are catabolized to uric acid, which must be excreted in the urine. Uric acid can precipitate in the renal tubules, causing obstructive uropathy with renal insufficiency and inability to clear electrolytes such as potassium. The patient is neutropenic and febrile and at risk for serious bacterial infection. Cultures of blood and urine should be obtained.

As soon as cultures have been obtained, broad-spectrum intravenous antibiotic therapy should be instituted as treatment for a possible serious bacterial infection as the cause of the fever. The patient should also receive transfusions of packed red blood cells and platelets to correct the anemia and thrombocytopenia. Because he will soon commence immunosuppressive chemotherapy, the blood products should be irradiated to kill any viable lymphocytes in them, which could mount a transfusion-induced graft-versus-host disease. This patient with a low WBC has a low risk for uric acid nephropathy. To prevent it from developing, allopurinol should be administered to block uric acid production and intravenous hydration begun to ensure a good urine output. These measures are even more important in patients with a high WBC or bulky collections of leukemic cells, such as a large anterior mediastinal mass, who are at high risk for uric acid nephropathy. At the time of diagnostic lumbar puncture, chemotherapy is also administered intrathecally as prophylaxis against development of meningeal leukemia.

QUESTIONS

- *How would you treat this boy?*
- *What are the phases of this treatment?*
- *When would you consider treatment with bone marrow transplantation?*
- *Which type of transplant would have the best outcome?*

DISCUSSION

This child should be treated with chemotherapy, which is administered in a number of distinct phases. The first phase is remission induction, which lasts for 4 weeks and is followed by consolidation, during which CNS prophylaxis is given. This child's prognosis is good, and CNS prophylaxis will consist entirely of intrathecal chemotherapy. He will be spared potentially neurotoxic cranial radiation. He will then receive a prolonged maintenance phase of therapy, which will last approximately 2 years. Early during the maintenance phase, he may undergo a brief period of more intensive therapy designed to eradicate any remaining leukemic cells that escaped destruction during the earlier phases of therapy. Eradication of these cells is more easily accomplished when they are few in number, as is the case after successful remission induction and consolidation therapy.

This child's chances of cure with chemotherapy are excellent. Bone marrow transplantation would be considered only if he suffered bone marrow relapse, especially while still on chemotherapy or within 12 months of its discontinuation. The most efficacious type of transplantation would involve a human leukocyte antigen (HLA)-matched allogeneic transplant from a relative, usually a sibling. If there were no HLA match within the family, an autologous transplant could be considered. The patient's marrow, collected in second remission and purged with antibody to CALLA, could be used for this procedure. An autologous transplant eliminates the risk of graft-versus-host disease, which can complicate an allogeneic transplant, but it is associated with a higher relapse rate than an HLA-matched allogeneic transplant from a related donor. If neither of the above transplants were possible, either a partially HLA-matched transplant from a relative or an HLA-matched transplant from an unrelated donor could also be considered. Both of these transplants are associated with a greater risk of death from severe graft-versus-host disease.

COMPREHENSIVE EXAM

QUESTIONS

DIRECTIONS: Each of the numbered items or incomplete statements in this section is followed by answers or by completions of the statement. Select the ONE lettered answer or completion that is BEST in each case.

1. The most common explanation for colic in an infant is

(A) formula intolerance
(B) otitis media
(C) constipation
(D) teething
(E) none of the above

2. Which of the following bacteria is a common cause of infective endocarditis in adults but a rare cause of this infection in children?

(A) Enterococcus
(B) *Staphylococcus aureus*
(C) *Staphylococcus epidermidis*
(D) Viridans streptococcus (α-hemolytic streptococcus)

3. A 2-year-old child is brought to your office because of recent onset of pallor and icterus. He had been in good health except for a mild febrile illness. Complete blood count is as follows: hemoglobin 5 g/dl, hematocrit 16%, white blood cell count 5300/mm³ (normal differential), platelets 300,000/mm³. Microspherocytes and polychromatophilia are noted on peripheral blood smear. Reticulocyte count is 20%. Direct Coombs' test is strongly positive. The most likely explanation for his anemia is

(A) autoimmune hemolytic anemia
(B) isoimmune hemolytic anemia
(C) congenital spherocytosis
(D) pyruvate kinase deficiency

4. A 4-year-old boy is brought to a pediatrician's office by a nursery school worker because of concerns about evidence of injury to the child. Of the following injuries that a pediatrician might discover, which would most likely suggest child abuse?

(A) Forehead swelling with an underlying linear skull fracture
(B) Multiple bruises of the extensor surfaces of the lower legs
(C) Unilateral periorbital bruising ("black-eye")
(D) Linear bruises over the back
(E) Multiple infected excoriated lesions over the arms and legs

5. Acute rheumatic fever may cause which of the following disorders?

(A) Chronic joint disease
(B) Isolated pericarditis
(C) Pulmonary valve insufficiency
(D) Prolonged low-grade fever
(E) Aortic or mitral valvulitis

6. A 5-year-old has 1 day of cola-colored urine with red blood cell casts. Two weeks ago, he had a culture-positive streptococcal tonsillitis. To diagnose acute poststreptococcal glomerulonephritis (APSGN), the single best evidence would be

(A) blood pressure above the 95th percentile for age
(B) positive streptozyme test
(C) mildly elevated blood urea nitrogen and creatinine
(D) negative antinuclear antibody, hepatitis profile, and human immunodeficiency virus
(E) a low C3

7. A 4-month-old female infant has petechiae, pallor, and hepatosplenomegaly. Her complete blood count values are hemoglobin 7 g /dl, white blood cell count 178,000/mm³ with 2% polymorphonuclear, 3% lymphocytes, and 95% blasts, and platelets 31,000/mm³. Her blasts are terminal deoxynucleotidyl transferase (TdT)-positive and common acute lymphocytic leukemia antigen (CALLA)-, myeloperoxidase-, and nonspecific esterase–negative. The most likely diagnosis is

(A) acute nonlymphoblastic leukemia (ANLL)
(B) stage IVS neuroblastoma
(C) Letterer-Siwe disease
(D) acute lymphoblastic leukemia (ALL)

8. The best initial treatment for scald burns is to

(A) debride the wound
(B) apply cool water
(C) apply butter or margarine
(D) cover the wound with a bandage
(E) apply pressure to the site of the burn

Questions 9–10

A fourth-year medical student attends what is expected to be a normal delivery, and the child—a boy—is born with a unilateral cleft lip and palate.

9. What is the most important evaluation to be performed to determine the cause of the cleft lip and palate?

(A) Physical examination
(B) Computed tomography (CT) scan of the head
(C) Serum alcohol level
(D) Urine toxic screen
(E) Amino acid analysis

10. Evaluation of the newborn boy and his parents suggests a diagnosis of isolated cleft lip and palate. What is the most likely form of inheritance of this defect?

(A) Autosomal recessive
(B) Autosomal dominant
(C) X-linked
(D) Multifactorial
(E) Nongenetic (sporadic)

11. A 2-year-old child presents to the emergency room with lethargy after a period of unobserved play. The child was previously healthy with normal development. The family history is significant for a sibling who has epilepsy and takes phenobarbital. The examination reveals an afebrile, lethargic child who opens his eyes briefly to noxious stimuli. There are no signs of trauma or focal abnormality. Pupils are small, but reactive. The most likely etiology for the child's lethargy is

(A) unobserved seizure
(B) intoxication
(C) intracranial hemorrhage
(D) unobserved head injury

12. The mother of a 16-year-old who came home 3 hours late from a dance is concerned. The daughter says that she forgot to call because she was having such a good time. The mother considers grounding her or maybe taking away her phone privileges for a week. The mother remembers the anticipatory guidance talk that she had with her daughter's physician. What is the central issue during midadolescence?

(A) Peer support
(B) Pubertal development
(C) Adult role models
(D) Separation

13. A positive human immunodeficiency virus (HIV) culture confirms the diagnosis of HIV infection in a 6-month-old girl. She has had the following problems: one episode of pneumococcal bacteremia, several episodes of otitis, chronic thrush, poor weight gain, and anemia. Her CD4 T-cell count is 2100/μl, which is 22% of total T cells. Which of the following is appropriate therapy for this child?

(A) Trimethoprim–sulfamethoxazole (TMP-SMX) for prophylaxis against *Pneumocystis carinii* pneumonia
(B) Monthly administration of intravenous gamma globulin (IVIG) to prevent further bacterial infections
(C) Zidovudine (ZDV, AZT)
(D) No therapy is needed because the child has a normal CD4 T-cell count for age
(E) Amoxicillin for prophylaxis against recurrent otitis media

14. A mother is referred to a perinatologist for intrauterine growth failure. An ultrasound examination reveals that there is asymmetric growth retardation. A urinalysis reveals proteinuria. The most likely cause of the growth failure is

(A) trisomy 21
(B) trisomy 18
(C) preeclampsia
(D) cytomegalovirus infection
(E) fetal alcohol syndrome

15. A 7-year-old boy with hereditary spherocytosis has a high fever and is brought to the emergency room in a state of circulatory collapse. He has had no medical problems and has taken no medications since splenectomy was performed at 6 years of age. What is the most likely cause of his current condition?

(A) *Pseudomonas* sepsis
(B) Acute hemorrhage from splenic vessels
(C) *Haemophilus influenzae* meningitis
(D) Pneumococcal sepsis

16. An 18-month-old child is found to have dental decay in the upper central and lateral incisors. This is most suggestive of

(A) excessive fluoride ingestion
(B) milk-bottle caries
(C) tetracycline exposure
(D) insufficient fluoride intake
(E) failure to brush the child's teeth properly

17. Occasionally, early adolescent girls with familial tall stature may be treated to reduce predicted adult stature. This treatment usually consists of which one of the following agents?

(A) Glucocorticoid
(B) Thyroid hormone
(C) Estrogen
(D) Gonadotropin-releasing hormone (GnRH)
(E) Progesterone

18. A 9-year-old girl develops urticaria 2 months after a viral syndrome. The urticaria is still present more than 6 weeks after onset. All laboratory tests are normal. The most likely explanation for her urticaria is

(A) food allergy
(B) connective tissue disease
(C) drug allergy
(D) idiopathic etiology

19. A 31-month-old boy presents with an 8-month history of loose stools. His mother states that he has 3–5 watery stools daily, often containing undigested food particles. He is quite gassy and complains of abdominal pain. He is consuming an age-appropriate diet, although his physician suggests that he is given increased fluids to prevent dehydration. Previous evaluation has shown a normal complete blood count, negative stool examination for enteric pathogens as well as ova and parasites, and a normal urinalysis. Appropriate initial dietary intervention would include

(A) restriction of fatty foods
(B) restriction of lactose-containing products
(C) restriction of fluids, especially fruit juices
(D) increased dietary fiber
(E) restriction of gluten-containing products

20. A 6-year-old girl experiences staring spells once or twice a day. They last only 15–30 seconds. During these spells, she will stare, breaking off in midsentence at times. Eyeblinking and lipsmacking are sometimes seen. After the spell, she will either continue talking or she may look momentarily puzzled. She has no other neurologic symptoms, and her schoolwork has not deteriorated. The episodes described are most consistent with

(A) major motor seizures
(B) partial complex seizures
(C) absence (petit mal) seizures
(D) daydreaming

21. A 12-year-old boy wants to try out for a soccer team. On physical examination, a constant ejection click and a harsh systolic ejection murmur characteristic of aortic valve stenosis are heard. Which of the following is the best statement regarding aortic valve stenosis?

(A) The patient should be restricted from competitive sports
(B) The patient does not need endocarditis prophylaxis
(C) The electrocardiogram demonstrates right ventricular hypertrophy
(D) The aortic valve is probably calcified

22. A 7-month-old boy presents with oral candidiasis and *Pneumocystis carinii* pneumonia. Which of the following is the best screening test for evaluating this child's immune system?

(A) Quantitative serum immunoglobulins
(B) Delayed hypersensitivity skin testing to recall antigens
(C) Total hemolytic complement (CH_{50})
(D) Nitroblue tetrazolium test

23. While riding his bike, a 14-year-old boy crashes into a parked car. He falls forward and has the "wind knocked out of him." There is no head trauma, and several minutes later he is feeling fine. The next day, following breakfast, he complains of periumbilical and epigastric abdominal pain and vomits. The pain worsens over the next several hours and he becomes febrile to 38°C. The most likely diagnosis is

(A) duodenal hematoma
(B) appendicitis
(C) mesenteric avulsion
(D) pancreatitis
(E) volvulus

24. A 10-year-old boy presents with a history of recurrent abdominal pain. There is a past history of bronchitis but no history of pneumonia. On physical examination, there has been no significant increase in weight over the past 3 years, with flattening of the growth curve. Trace digital clubbing is noted. Which of the following is the most appropriate test to be ordered at this time?

(A) Pulmonary function tests
(B) Sweat test
(C) Chest x-ray
(D) Abdominal x-ray
(E) IgE level

25. A healthy 3-year-old girl presents with the acute onset of petechiae, purpura, and epistaxis. Her complete blood count is as follows: hemoglobin 12 g/dl, white blood cell count 5550/mm³, differential normal, platelet count 2000/mm³. The most likely diagnosis is

(A) idiopathic thrombocytopenic purpura (ITP)
(B) acute lymphocytic leukemia
(C) aplastic anemia
(D) disseminated intravascular coagulation (DIC)

26. Which of the following conditions has a better prognosis if it occurs in a child younger than 1 year of age?

(A) Neuroblastoma
(B) Acute lymphoblastic leukemia (ALL)
(C) Medulloblastoma
(D) Histiocytosis X
(E) Juvenile chronic myelogenous leukemia (CML)

27. In a child who is poisoned, the most effective way to remove gastric contents is by the use of

(A) saline lavage with a wide-bore nasogastric tube
(B) tartar emetic
(C) syrup of ipecac
(D) manual induction of vomiting
(E) citrate of magnesia

Questions 28–30

A 12-year-old boy is hit by a car while riding his bicycle without a helmet. On arrival at a pediatric trauma center, he is unconscious, apneic, hypotensive, and tachycardic.

28. Priorities for care in the first 10 minutes after arrival include all of the following EXCEPT

(A) intubation or tracheotomy
(B) establishment of large-bore vascular access
(C) stabilization of the cervical spine until after an adequate cervical radiographic series has been performed and cleared
(D) head and abdominal computed tomography (CT) scans
(E) infusion of isotonic crystalloid, colloid, or blood

29. After initial treatment and stabilization, a computed tomography (CT) scan reveals severe cerebral edema without other significant injuries. Which of the following modalities of therapy will be LEAST effective in controlling this patient's increased intracranial pressure?

(A) Mannitol
(B) Hyperventilation
(C) Removal of cerebrospinal fluid (CSF) by ventriculostomy
(D) Pentobarbital infusion
(E) Fluid restriction

30. Despite aggressive management, the patient deteriorates and a brain death evaluation is begun. Which of the following statements about this state is true in this case?

(A) Brain death can be documented if the patient has a Glasgow Coma Score of 3
(B) Brain death can be documented without an isoelectric electroencephalogram (EEG)
(C) A four-vessel cerebral angiogram must be performed before the diagnosis of cerebral death is made
(D) Use of barbiturate medications will not affect the ability to diagnose brain death
(E) Decerebrate posturing is compatible with a diagnosis of brain death

31. A previously well 4-year-old girl presents with a 2-week history of morning headaches, vomiting, and unsteadiness of gait. A computed tomography scan shows a lesion in the cerebellar vermis. The most likely diagnosis is

(A) brain abscess
(B) medulloblastoma
(C) glioblastoma multiforme
(D) central nervous system leukemia

32. Parents who already have two biologic children bring their newly adopted 2-year-old Korean child to their pediatrician's office for her first visit. To the best of the adoptive parents' knowledge, there are no special risk factors in the child's biologic family's history. Which of the following sets of tests would be best to order or perform?

(A) Bayley scales of infant development, early language milestone scale, hearing test
(B) Complete blood cell count (CBC); screening for electrolyte, blood urea nitrogen (BUN), and creatinine levels; urinalysis; liver and thyroid function tests
(C) Tine test, chest x-ray
(D) Hepatitis B profile, purified protein derivative test, stool screening for ova and parasites
(E) Pediatric behavioral checklist

33. Physiologic jaundice in term newborns is best characterized by

(A) the onset of clinical jaundice by 12 hours of age
(B) persistence of clinical jaundice for at least 1 week
(C) equal elevation of direct and indirect serum bilirubin values
(D) a decrease in serum bilirubin level after discontinuation of breast-feeding
(E) a rise in serum bilirubin concentration of less than 5 mg/dl/day.

34. A 5-year-old child presents with coarse facial features, hepatosplenomegaly, and progressive loss of developmental milestones. In considering this clinical picture, the most likely cause is

(A) mucopolysaccharidosis
(B) carbohydrate metabolism disorder
(C) aminoaciduria
(D) urea cycle enzyme deficiency
(E) hereditary fructose intolerance

35. An infant with atopic eczema will most likely present with which of the following clinical manifestations?

(A) An erythematous, papulovesicular, exudative rash
(B) Lichenified lesions on the flexural surfaces
(C) Urticaria
(D) Posterior subcapsular cataracts

36. Which is the correct pattern of coagulation test results for a patient with vitamin K deficiency?

| | Partial | | |
Prothrombin Time (PT)	Thromboplastin Time	Factor VIII	Factor IX
(A) Prolonged	Prolonged	Low	Low
(B) Prolonged	Normal	Normal	Normal
(C) Normal	Prolonged	Low	Low
(D) Prolonged	Prolonged	Normal	Low

37. A 2-year-old boy is brought to the emergency room after his mother noted him passing several grossly bloody stools. There is no accompanying abdominal pain, fever, or vomiting. Family history is positive for colonic cancer in several paternal uncles. On admission, his hematocrit is 26%. The most likely diagnosis is

(A) colonic polyp
(B) intussusception
(C) ulcerative colitis
(D) lymphonodular hyperplasia
(E) Meckel diverticulum

38. A 6-year-old child presents to a pediatrician with headaches, fever, and pain over the left maxillary sinus. A sinus x-ray shows an air-fluid level in the left maxillary sinus. The two most likely bacterial causes of this illness are

(A) *Streptococcus pyogenes* and *Staphylococcus aureus*
(B) *Haemophilus influenzae* and *S. aureus*
(C) *H. influenzae* and *Streptococcus pneumoniae*
(D) *S. pyogenes* and *S. pneumoniae*
(E) *Moraxella catarrhalis* and anaerobic bacteria

39. A 4-month-old boy is brought to the emergency room. His parents report that the child stopped breathing at home, turned blue around his lips, and felt limp. After vigorous shaking of the infant and several mouth-to-mouth breaths, the boy's color returned to normal, and he resumed breathing. The infant's condition is best described as

(A) obstructive apnea
(B) central apnea
(C) apparent life-threatening event (ALTE)
(D) pneumonia
(E) congestive heart failure

40. A 5-year-old child is brought to the emergency room after a fall onto a concrete floor. The diagnosis of concussion is established by which of the following findings?

(A) Pupillary constriction
(B) Nausea and vomiting
(C) Brief loss of consciousness and amnesia for the event
(D) A positive Babinski reflex

41. A 4-month-old boy develops a temperature of 101°F and is irritable for 2 hours after immunization with diphtheria–tetanus–pertussis (DTP) vaccine. What is the appropriate procedure when this boy is seen at 6 months of age?

(A) Defer immunization with the pertussis vaccine, and instead administer diphtheria and tetanus toxoid vaccine
(B) Defer immunization with the pertussis vaccine, and instead administer tetanus toxoid and reduced-dose diphtheria toxoid vaccine
(C) Administer half the usual dose (i.e., split dose) of the DTP vaccine
(D) Defer all immunizations until the infant is 12 months old
(E) Administer the DTP vaccine with instructions for fever control

42. A 15-year-old boy with asthma is allergic to cats. He went to a friend's house after school who has a pet cat. Later that evening (6 hours after exposure) he starts to wheeze. Which of the following drugs should have been administered in the afternoon to prevent his symptoms?

(A) Theophylline
(B) Cromolyn sodium
(C) Antihistamine
(D) Albuterol

43. A 9-month-old infant presents with extreme irritability alternating with lethargy. His parents note that he had an upper respiratory illness several days ago and for the past 24 hours has been screaming or sleepy. He vomited once earlier in the day. He passed one stool four hours ago, which was loose and not bloody. He has a temperature of 38°C. On examination he is lethargic but arousable to painful stimuli. Abdominal examination shows diffuse tenderness and a mass in the right upper quadrant. The next, most appropriate diagnostic test would be

(A) computed tomographic scan of the head
(B) lumbar puncture
(C) barium enema
(D) upper gastrointestinal series with small bowel follow-through
(E) abdominal ultrasound

44. A 2-year-old girl presents with poor weight gain and slow growth. She has episodes of vomiting and dehydration. Evaluation reveals hyperchloremic metabolic acidosis, normal creatinine, and a persistently alkaline urine. Therapy indicated is

(A) high-caloric nutritional supplements
(B) institution of antiesophageal reflux precautions
(C) alkalinizing agents sufficient to normalize the serum CO_2
(D) pancreatic enzymes for probable cystic fibrosis
(E) acetazolamide (carbonic hydrase inhibitor)

45. A 16-year-old boy presents with shortness of breath. Chest radiography reveals a large anterior mediastinal mass, and a moderate right-sided pleural effusion. The pleural fluid contains numerous lymphoblasts that are terminal deoxynucleotidyl transferase (TdT)-positive, and express the sheep red blood receptor and other T-cell antigens. On bone marrow aspiration, lymphoblasts with identical characteristics comprise 12% of the total cells. The diagnosis is

(A) Hodgkin disease
(B) T-cell acute lymphoblastic leukemia
(C) Burkitt lymphoma
(D) lymphoblastic lymphoma

46. A 10-year-old girl presents with a 2-week history of rectal bleeding. She states that she was well until 1 month ago, at which time her stools became looser and more frequent. Two weeks ago she noted blood streaking of the stool, and for the past 3 days her stools have been grossly bloody. There has been mild lower abdominal cramping during defecation. She denies vomiting, fever, arthritis, weight loss, or rash. There has been no antibiotic exposure or recent travel. Laboratory examination shows a hematocrit of 38%, erythrocyte sedimentation rate of 15 mm/hr, serum albumin of 4.3 g/dl, and normal serum aminotransferases. The most likely diagnosis is

(A) colonic polyp
(B) Crohn disease
(C) hemorrhoid
(D) ulcerative colitis
(E) Meckel diverticulum

47. An infant of a mother with insulin-dependent diabetes has a hematocrit of 68%. On day 3 of life, he suddenly manifests gross hematuria and a flank mass on the left. The most likely diagnosis is

(A) meconium plug
(B) neuroblastoma
(C) renal venous thrombosis
(D) ureteropelvic junction obstruction
(E) adrenal hemorrhage

48. A child who displays loss of developmental milestones, or regression, should be investigated for

(A) dysmorphic syndrome
(B) neuronal storage disorder
(C) chromosomal translocation
(D) teratogenic exposure during fetal development

49. A 7-year-old boy with leukemia in remission develops a fever, vesicular rash, and cough. A Tzanck test is positive, and a chest x-ray shows a small left lower lobe infiltrate. The boy's mother is uncertain whether he has had chickenpox. What is the most appropriate initial course of action?

(A) Administer herpes zoster immune globulin
(B) Administer antibiotics based on Gram stain from bronchoscopic washings
(C) Administer intravenous acyclovir and ceftriaxone
(D) Admit patient to the hospital and observe closely

50. A 3-year-old boy experiences the death of his paternal grandfather, who helped care for him because both parents work. The parents seek the advice of their pediatrician about the child's attending the grandfather's wake. Which of the following statements is the most accurate regarding the child's potential attendance?

(A) Because of his young age, what the child says he wants to do has little bearing on his likely reaction to the wake
(B) The father should be assigned the task of taking the child home if the child becomes upset or disruptive during the wake
(C) Expressed indifference, even cheerfulness, at the wake would be a sign of insecure attachment to the grandfather
(D) Because of his age, there will be little upset for the child if he attends the wake
(E) The reaction of the child may be affected by viewing the grandfather's body or by the emotional state of the surviving family

51. A 5-year-old boy is seen for the evaluation of clumsiness. His kindergarten teacher noticed that he tended to fall easily and had an awkward gait. Examination reveals a healthy-appearing boy with prominent calf muscles. He waddles slightly when walking and demonstrates a mild lumbar lordosis. When asked to stand up from a sitting position on the floor, he uses his hands to push himself up. Deep tendon reflexes are normal, except at the ankles, where they are decreased. The most likely diagnosis in this case is

(A) cerebral palsy
(B) spinal muscular dystrophy
(C) Charcot-Marie-Tooth disease
(D) myasthenia gravis
(E) Duchenne muscular dystrophy

52. A 3-month-old infant has suffered recurrent episodes of fever, skin pustules, and pneumonia since the first week of life. Repeated blood counts have shown absolute neutrophil count (ANC) to be less than 500/mm³, whereas hemoglobin and platelet count are normal. The most likely diagnosis is

(A) aplastic anemia
(B) congenital leukemia
(C) Kostmann disease
(D) cyclic neutropenia

53. A 15-year-old boy presents with a large anterior mediastinal mass. Laboratory findings include a white blood cell count of 180,000/mm³, with 97% blasts on differential; the blasts are positive for terminal deoxynucleotidyl transferase (TdT). The most likely diagnosis is

(A) juvenile chronic myelogenous leukemia (CML)
(B) adult CML
(C) T-cell non-Hodgkin lymphoma
(D) acute nonlymphocytic leukemia (ANLL)
(E) T-cell acute lymphoblastic leukemia (ALL)

54. The group A β-hemolytic streptococcus may trigger an attack of acute rheumatic fever when it

(A) spreads via the bloodstream
(B) causes an upper respiratory infection
(C) lodges in the myocardium
(D) invades the joints
(E) enters through a skin infection

55. At 11 weeks' gestation, a pregnant woman undergoes ultrasonography and is discovered to have quadruplets. She is electively hospitalized at 21 week's gestation to prevent this most common complication of a multiple-gestation pregnancy.

(A) Premature birth
(B) Maternal hypertension
(C) Maternal anemia
(D) Hyperemesis

56. An 18-month-old girl is brought to a pediatrician by her parents, who say she has had a fever of 104°F and has refused to walk since she awoke that morning. The pediatrician obtains a hip x-ray, which shows a subtle widening of the left hip joint space. The most appropriate initial course of action is

(A) close observation in the hospital or at home if the parents are reliable
(B) administration of intravenous ceftriaxone
(C) surgical drainage of the hip joint
(D) administration of intravenous oxacillin

57. A 6-year-old boy with hemophilia A (factor VIII level 10%) strikes his elbow and subsequently has swelling and tenderness at the site of trauma. The proper treatment of this is

(A) infusion of cryoprecipitate
(B) infusion of desmopressin (dDAVP)
(C) infusion of fresh frozen plasma
(D) infusion of factor VIII concentrate

58. Hemoglobin Bart's is found in which of the following disorders?

(A) Homozygous β thalassemia
(B) Thalassemic hemoglobinopathy
(C) Homozygous α thalassemia
(D) Double heterozygote α and β thalassemia

59. Which of the following patients with acute lymphoblastic leukemia (ALL) has a good prognosis?

(A) A 14-year-old with a white blood cell count (WBC) of 2000/mm^3 and hyperdiploid, common acute lymphocytic leukemia antigen (CALLA)-positive pre-B cells
(B) A 7-year-old with a WBC of 79,000/mm^3 and CALLA-negative B cells that have a t(8;14) on cytogenetic analysis
(C) A 4-year-old with a WBC of 7000/mm^3 and hyperdiploid, CALLA-positive early pre-B cells
(D) A 7-year-old with a WBC of 4000/mm^3 and CALLA-positive early pre-B cells that have t(9;22) on cytogenetic analysis

60. The parents of a 4-month-old girl phone the pediatrician's office complaining that their daughter has a persistent diaper rash. The rash has been present for a week and has not responded to frequent diaper changes, exposing the diaper area to air, or an over-the-counter cream. Because of the rash's persistence, the parents are instructed to bring their daughter to the office for examination. On examination in the office, the pediatrician notes that there are satellite lesions and bright red erosions involving the deep skin folds. This diaper dermatitis is most likely

(A) candidal
(B) infantile seborrheic
(C) generic
(D) intertrigo
(E) staphylococcal

61. A full-term male infant is noted to have circumoral cyanosis and twitching of his left hand at 12 hours of age. On physical examination, he is found to have absent pupillary response to light and a small penis. The most likely diagnosis is

(A) hypocalcemia
(B) hypoglycemia
(C) congenital hypothyroidism
(D) congenital heart disease
(E) idiopathic epilepsy

62. Starting mid-May and lasting through June, a 6-year-old boy complains of itchy eyes, a watery nose, and sneezing. The safest and most direct approach to the treatment of this child is with

(A) antihistamines
(B) avoidance of the offending allergen
(C) desensitization therapy
(D) topical steroids
(E) antibiotics

63. A patient with newly diagnosed acute nonlymphocytic leukemia (ANLL) who presents with neutropenia and a temperature of 40°C should be managed by

(A) prompt institution of chemotherapy because the fever is most likely due to leukemia
(B) prompt procurement of cultures and initiation of broad-spectrum parenteral antibiotics
(C) administration of granulocyte transfusions to correct the neutropenia
(D) extensive search for an underlying infection and withholding antibiotics until one is found
(E) vigorous antipyretic therapy with aspirin to lower the temperature

64. A developmentally delayed 10-month-old girl is referred to a pediatrician for evaluation of small size for age, unusual facial features, abnormal palmar creases, and a heart defect. Which of the following is the LEAST likely etiology for this infant's condition?

(A) A sporadic syndrome
(B) A single gene abnormality
(C) A chromosome anomaly
(D) A multifactorial disorder
(E) A teratogenic exposure

65. A 12-year-old boy presents with an erythematous, sandpaper-like rash, a temperature of 103°F, and an infected laceration of the leg. A rapid streptococcal test performed on the purulent discharge is positive for group A β-hemolytic streptococcus. The most likely diagnosis is

(A) rheumatic fever
(B) scarlet fever
(C) erysipelas
(D) impetigo
(E) erythema infectiosum

66. During fetal life, oxygen saturation is highest in organs that cannot sustain prolonged anaerobic metabolism without injury. In which blood vessel is the oxygen saturation likely to be the highest during normal and stressful periods?

(A) Carotid
(B) Renal
(C) Mesenteric
(D) Pulmonary
(E) Femoral

67. An 18-month-old girl with a 4-month history of no significant weight gain has failed to gain weight on a prescribed high-calorie diet. A thorough medical and psychosocial history, physical examination, and routine laboratory testing have revealed no cause. Referral to a dietician has also been unsuccessful. Which of the following would be the best next step?

(A) Repeat of routine laboratory tests, including stool culture to screen for ova and parasites
(B) Referral to a pediatric gastroenterologist
(C) Hospital admission
(D) Diagnostic imaging, including computed tomography scan of the head and abdomen
(E) Referral of the family for psychological and social service evaluation

68. A 6-year-old child presents with her second episode of meningococcal meningitis. The most likely immunodeficiency disorder in this child is

(A) neutrophil dysfunction
(B) deficiency of complement component C3
(C) deficiency of carboxypeptidase N
(D) deficiency of complement component C6
(E) deficiency of T cells

69. A healthy, 2-day-old, full-term infant has generalized petechiae and is found to have a platelet count of 15,000/mm³. Her mother has no history of prior illnesses and has a normal complete blood count. The most likely diagnosis is

(A) consumption coagulopathy
(B) passively acquired idiopathic thrombocytopenic purpura
(C) von Willebrand disease
(D) isoimmune thrombocytopenia

70. A 7-month-old boy previously diagnosed with tetralogy of Fallot is seen in the emergency room because of irritability, hyperpnea, increasing cyanosis, and episodic loss of consciousness. Which of the following is the best course of management for this patient?

(A) Administration of digoxin
(B) Administration of supplemental oxygen and morphine sulfate
(C) Administration of epinephrine
(D) Administration of bronchodilators

71. A neonatologist is called to attend the delivery of an infant whose fetal heart tracing is suggestive of fetal distress. It is likely that the infant will require resuscitation. The primary goal of resuscitation of the newborn is to

(A) establish spontaneous breathing
(B) improve the heart rate
(C) reoxygenate the central nervous system (CNS)
(D) improve the infant's color
(E) make the infant cry spontaneously

72. A 2-year-old boy presents with fever, weight loss, pain in the legs, proptosis of the right eye, ecchymoses around the right eye, and a large left flank mass. The most likely diagnosis is

(A) orbital rhabdomyosarcoma
(B) Hand-Schüller-Christian disease
(C) metastatic neuroblastoma
(D) Wilms tumor

73. An anaphylactoid reaction can be caused by

(A) pollen
(B) bee venom
(C) aspirin
(D) peanuts

74. A 5-year-old boy with insulin-dependent diabetes on a single morning dose of insulin has begun to have nightly enuresis. His fasting blood glucose level generally is 200–250 mg/dl, and his blood glucose level before supper generally is 75–150 mg/dl. The most likely cause of this patient's enuresis is

(A) glucosuria from under-insulinization overnight
(B) stress of chronic disease
(C) urinary tract infection
(D) Somogyi phenomenon
(E) hypoglycemia

75. A 3-year-old girl with sickle cell anemia presents with pallor, tachycardia, hypotension, and massive splenomegaly. The most likely explanation is

(A) hemorrhagic shock
(B) splenic sequestration
(C) septic shock
(D) cardiogenic shock

76. In late summer, a 2-year-old boy presents with a 2-day history of painful, ulcerative lesions of the mouth and a 1-day history of fever to a temperature of 103°F. He refuses to eat. On physical examination he is irritable, has a temperature of 102°F, and has numerous erythematous, ulcerative lesions on the buccal mucosa, gums, and tongue. The most likely diagnosis is

(A) herpangina
(B) aphthous stomatitis
(C) candidal gingivostomatitis
(D) herpetic gingivostomatitis
(E) necrotizing ulcerative gingivitis

77. Purpuric skin lesions and oozing from the gums develop in a 3-month-old male infant with congenital biliary atresia. Complete blood count (including platelet count) is normal, whereas both prothrombin time (PT) and partial thromboplastin time (PTT) are prolonged. The most likely explanation for this hemorrhagic diathesis is

(A) hemophilia A
(B) hemophilia B
(C) vitamin K deficiency
(D) disseminated intravascular coagulation (DIC)

78. The best indicator of cystic fibrosis is

(A) a positive family history of cystic fibrosis
(B) the presence of digital clubbing
(C) a sweat test with a chloride concentration of 70 mEq/L
(D) bronchiectasis on a chest x-ray

79. Which of the following statements best characterizes the diagnosis of urinary tract infection in children?

(A) The presence of fever localizes the infection to the renal parenchyma
(B) The diagnosis is likely if there is pyuria with more than 10 white blood cells per high-power field
(C) The diagnosis is likely if a clean-catch specimen shows 10^5 organisms of a single species
(D) Diagnosis is difficult because the typical causative organisms grow poorly in culture
(E) Vesicoureteral reflux localizes the infection to the lower urinary tract

DIRECTIONS: Each of the numbered items or incomplete statements in this section is negatively phrased, as indicated by a capitalized word such as NOT, LEAST, or EXCEPT. Select the ONE lettered answer or completion that is BEST in each case.

80. A 12-year-old boy comes in for a physical for basketball camp. The physician has followed his health care since he was a baby. On physical examination, the physician notes that his testicular volume and pubic hair are consistent with stage 2 of pubertal development. During the discussion after the physical examination, he asks the physician how tall he is going to be. All of the following statements about pubertal growth spurt are true EXCEPT

(A) it is early in boys and late in girls
(B) it is associated with muscle development in boys
(C) it is the last of three growth spurts during childhood
(D) it is associated with fat deposition in girls
(E) its average duration is approximately 3 years

81. A 12-year-old presents to a physician with the signs and symptoms of seasonal allergic rhinitis. In discussions with the child's mother, the physician explains that all of the following conditions are associated with hay fever EXCEPT

(A) nosebleeds
(B) nasal congestion
(C) loss of smell and taste
(D) thick, yellow nasal discharge

82. During a private consultation with their pediatrician, the parents of a 5-year-old child reveal that they are about to be divorced. They would like to optimize custody arrangements and seek the pediatrician's advice. In considering what would be "in the best interest of the child," which of the following should the pediatrician tell the parents is LEAST important?

(A) Daily contact between the divorced parents to discuss the child and other issues
(B) Minimizing changes in school, friends, and life routines for the child
(C) Assuring as much financial security for the child as possible
(D) Maintaining as much contact between the child and each parent as is possible and safe for the child

83. In a child receiving chemotherapy for T-cell leukemia, the tumor lysis syndrome with acute renal failure develops. All of the following laboratory results might be expected EXCEPT

(A) elevated serum potassium
(B) elevated serum bicarbonate
(C) decreased serum sodium
(D) elevated serum phosphate
(E) increased serum uric acid

84. A chlamydial genital infection can result in all of the following EXCEPT

(A) lower abdominal pain
(B) infertility
(C) epididymitis
(D) right shoulder pain
(E) arthritis

85. A 2-week-old female infant has a head circumference of 40 cm (> 98%), with a large, tense fontanelle and downward deviation of the eyes. She has been vomiting her formula and she is irritable. Common causes of her symptoms include all of the following EXCEPT

(A) intraventricular hemorrhage
(B) brain tumor
(C) meningitis
(D) aqueductal stenosis
(E) Arnold-Chiari malformation

86. All of the following tests would be indicated in the evaluation of a 2-year-old child with x-ray documentation of recurrent pneumonia EXCEPT

(A) immunoglobulin analysis
(B) complete blood count
(C) sweat test
(D) sputum culture
(E) pulmonary function tests

87. All of the following statements about the epidemiology of childhood injuries are true EXCEPT

(A) injuries are responsible for a greater percentage of hospital admissions among children than among adults
(B) death is the least likely outcome of childhood injuries
(C) respiratory diseases cause more deaths in children than do injuries
(D) most childhood injuries are treated at home
(E) "loss of working years of life" is a powerful measure of injury outcome

88. An infant has been diagnosed with a tracheoesophageal fistula. All of the following statements about the management and anatomic defects of an infant with a tracheoesophageal fistula are true EXCEPT

(A) the fistula most commonly is found between the distal esophagus and trachea
(B) the proximal esophagus sometimes ends in a blind pouch
(C) the goal of initial management is to keep the airway clear of secretions
(D) a contrast study of the esophagus should have been performed to establish the diagnosis
(E) definitive therapy consists of surgical repair of the fistula and reanastomosis of the proximal and distal portions of the esophagus

89. A 5-year-old boy presents with indications of significant developmental delay or mental retardation. All of the following evaluations are indicated for this patient EXCEPT

(A) chromosome analysis
(B) fragile X study
(C) urinalysis for aminoaciduria
(D) serum α-fetoprotein (AFP) testing
(E) pedigree analysis

90. All of the following findings may occur in juvenile rheumatoid arthritis (JRA) EXCEPT

(A) uveitis
(B) high, spiking fever
(C) erythema marginatum
(D) enlargement of the spleen
(E) lymphadenopathy

91. Bone marrow transplantation is a potential therapeutic option for each of the following patients EXCEPT

(A) a 4-year-old girl with stage IV neuroblastoma with metastases to bone cortex and bone marrow
(B) a 6-year-old boy with acute nonlymphocytic leukemia (ANLL) in first remission who has a human leukocyte antigen (HLA)-matched sibling
(C) a 2-year-old boy with good prognosis acute lymphoblastic leukemia (ALL) who relapses during the first year of maintenance therapy
(D) a 7-year-old boy with good prognosis ALL in first remission who is on the second year of maintenance therapy

92. An infant is born at term and weighs 1600 grams. The infant's weight, length, and head circumference are all less than the fifth percentile. Which of the following is NOT a cause of the growth retardation?

(A) Congenital infection
(B) Chromosomal defects
(C) Cell toxins
(D) Preeclampsia
(E) Fetal alcohol syndrome

93. During an obstetrics rotation, a third-year medical student has the opportunity to follow a 17-year-old pregnant adolescent. Which of the following is LEAST likely to be a complication of her pregnancy?

(A) Anemia
(B) Pelvic complication
(C) Toxemia
(D) Low–birth-weight infant
(E) Infant mortality

94. A 24-month-old child who has not begun to speak is brought to the pediatrician's office. All of the following conditions should be considered in the differential diagnosis EXCEPT

(A) autism
(B) developmental delay
(C) hearing impairment
(D) severe parental neglect
(E) childhood schizophrenia

95. A healthy, 14-year-old black girl experiences the sudden onset of gross hematuria, which persists for 2 days. All of the following are reasonable immediate steps in the evaluation of this patient EXCEPT

(A) hemoglobin electrophoresis to exclude hemoglobin S
(B) cystoscopy to establish the site of bleeding
(C) blood urea nitrogen and serum creatinine measurement
(D) urine culture
(E) renal ultrasonography to assess renal anatomy

96. A pediatrician volunteers to be a consultant for a local foster care agency. In making a case for more funding, all of the following statements about foster care are true EXCEPT

(A) foster children have no greater risk for behavioral and psychiatric problems than their non-foster, age-matched peers
(B) families of foster children frequently have histories of psychological dysfunction, substance abuse, or both, requiring significant resources for rehabilitation
(C) twenty-five percent of children placed in foster care have multiple placements before a permanent resolution
(D) foster children are less likely to have defined primary medical care providers
(E) foster children have a high incidence of failure to thrive

97. A physician is asked to examine a 3-month-old infant. The infant should display all of the following reflexes EXCEPT

(A) parachute reflex
(B) tonic neck reflex
(C) rooting reflex
(D) Moro reflex

98. Oral contraceptives prevent pregnancy by all of the following mechanisms EXCEPT

(A) blocking sperm
(B) changing the cervical mucus
(C) decreasing implantation
(D) suppressing ovulation

99. Hyperbilirubinemia is diagnosed in a 2-day-old infant whose serum bilirubin concentrations are 17.5 mg/dl (indirect fraction) and 0.2 mg/dl (direct fraction). All of the following statements concerning the evaluation and management of this infant are true EXCEPT

(A) the indirect and direct bilirubin concentrations are consistent with a physiologic jaundice
(B) the initial evaluation should include a complete blood count with reticulocyte count, maternal and infant blood types, and Coombs' test
(C) breast-feeding may have contributed to the elevated bilirubin concentration
(D) phototherapy should be administered

100. A 14-year-old girl is taken to her pediatrician because she has not begun to menstruate. On physical examination, she is noted to be in less than the fifth percentile for height and weight. She has no breast development. The remainder of the history and physical examination are normal. Possible conditions responsible for this patient's presentation include all of the following EXCEPT

(A) Turner syndrome
(B) 21-hydroxylase deficiency
(C) hypothyroidism
(D) constitutional delay of growth and puberty
(E) anorexia nervosa

101. A 16-year-old woman is brought in by her parents for evaluation of her weight loss. They claim that over the past year she has gradually dropped from 115 to 95 pounds. She does well at school and is very concerned about how she looks, often exercising several hours a day. To be able to make the diagnosis of anorexia nervosa, the physician needs to find all of the following factors EXCEPT

(A) weight loss to at least 15% less than expected for height
(B) obsessive and overachieving personality traits
(C) disturbed body image
(D) fear of gaining weight or being fat
(E) absence of at least three consecutive menstrual cycles

102. All of the following studies are helpful in the evaluation of an infant with bronchopulmonary dysplasia EXCEPT

(A) sleeping respiratory rate
(B) oxygen saturation
(C) chest x-ray
(D) sweat test
(E) electrocardiogram

103. A young, married, professional couple meets with their physician for a prenatal visit and to discuss their concerns about child care. The wife plans to return to work when the baby is approximately 2–3 months of age. The couple is ambivalent about this arrangement but is resigned to enrolling the baby in a center-based child care facility at the wife's place of employment. Which of the following statements about the effects of early child care is LEAST likely to be true?

(A) High-quality child care carries no greater risk for the emotional development of the child than being at home
(B) Children from deprived, at-risk environments can benefit the most both socially and emotionally from day-care enrollment
(C) Children placed early in day care often suffer from emotional withdrawal, exaggerated shyness, shallow relationships, and passivity later in life
(D) Cognitive gains seen with early placement in high-quality child care are most evident in socially at-risk and deprived children
(E) Persistence of the positive social and cognitive effects of high-quality child care on at-risk children depends on later school quality and continued improvement of the home environment

104. A nurse believes that a 12-hour-old infant has experienced a seizure lasting 2 minutes. Labor history includes rupture of the fetal membranes 24 hours before delivery and a difficult delivery with forceps. The Apgar score was 7 at 1 minute and 8 at 5 minutes. The nurse reports that the infant had been feeding poorly and was lethargic before the seizure. The differential diagnosis includes all of the following EXCEPT

(A) asphyxia
(B) meningitis
(C) kernicterus
(D) intracranial hemorrhage

105. A 6-year-old boy is shorter than all of his classmates. Diagnostic testing supports a diagnosis of idiopathic isolated growth hormone (GH) deficiency. All of the following are expected clinical findings in this patient EXCEPT

(A) normal body proportions
(B) a growth velocity of 3 cm/yr
(C) mild truncal obesity
(D) hypertension
(E) delayed skeletal maturation

106. A mother calls the family physician frantically stating that her daughter has seemed sick since the morning. The daughter has been on her menstrual cycle for several days, and she uses tampons to help absorb the blood. She has been away from home for the past 36 hours participating in various high school graduation activities. Toxic shock syndrome (TSS) comes to the physician's mind as a potential diagnosis. This diagnosis is associated with all the following findings EXCEPT

(A) vomiting and diarrhea
(B) disorientation
(C) increased platelet count
(D) elevated liver function tests
(E) elevated blood urea nitrogen

DIRECTIONS: Each set of matching questions in this section consists of a list of four to twenty-six lettered options (some of which may be in figures) followed by several numbered items. For each numbered item, select the ONE lettered option that is most closely associated with it. To avoid spending too much time on matching sets with large numbers of options, it is generally advisable to begin each set by reading the list of options. Then, for each item in the set, try to generate the correct answer and locate it in the option list, rather than evaluating each option individually. Each lettered option may be selected once, more than once, or not at all.

Questions 107–111

For each developmental issue listed below, select the behavior pattern with which it is associated.

(A) Synchrony
(B) Temperament
(C) Attachment
(D) Autonomy/independence
(E) State organization

107. The markedly irregular sleeping and feeding schedules of a 3-week-old infant

108. The night awakening and night crying of an 8-month-old infant

109. The temper tantrum of a 15-month-old toddler who is not allowed to climb on a chair

110. A 2-year-old's resistance to toilet training

111. The quiet, subdued classroom behavior of a "slow-to-warm-up" child in early September

Questions 112–115

For each pregnant patient described below, select the optimal first test to offer the patient for prenatal diagnosis.

(A) Level II (specialized) fetal ultrasound
(B) Amniocentesis or chorionic villus sampling (CVS)
(C) Maternal serum α-fetoprotein (AFP)
(D) Percutaneous umbilical blood sampling (PUBS) or fetoscopy

112. A 27-year-old woman in her eighteenth week of pregnancy; both the patient and her husband are heterozygous for the sickle cell gene.

113. A 30-year-old woman with negative family history for birth defects and genetic disorders who is 16 weeks' pregnant.

114. A 29-year-old woman who previously had a child with microcephaly.

115. A 22-year-old woman in her tenth week of pregnancy whose husband is a carrier of a familial balanced translocation.

Questions 116–120

Match each of the following allergens with the time of year it is most likely to cause symptoms of allergic rhinoconjunctivitis in the North Atlantic region of the United States.

(A) Late summer, early fall
(B) Late fall, winter
(C) Early spring
(D) Spring, early summer
(E) Spring through fall

116. Grass pollens

117. Ragweed pollen

118. *Alternaria* mold

119. House dust mite

120. Tree pollens

Questions 121–125

Match each congenital heart defect with the chest x-ray finding that is most suggestive of that deformity.

(A) "Snowman" sign
(B) Egg-shaped heart
(C) "3" sign
(D) Convex left heart border
(E) Boot-shaped heart

121. Coarctation of the aorta

122. Tetralogy of Fallot

123. D-Transposition of the great arteries

124. L-Transposition of the great arteries

125. Total anomalous pulmonary venous return

Questions 126–128

For each renal disorder, select the laboratory finding with which it is most likely to be associated.

(A) Hypocomplementemia
(B) Chronic hepatitis B antigenemia
(C) Microangiopathic anemia and thrombocytopenia
(D) Vesicoureteral reflux
(E) Elevated thyroxine and thyroid-stimulating hormone levels

126. Hemolytic–uremic syndrome

127. Poststreptococcal glomerulonephritis

128. Recurrent pyelonephritis

Questions 129–131

For each set of clinical characteristics listed below, select the birth defect with which it is most likely to be associated.

(A) Platybasia
(B) Syringomyelia
(C) Arnold-Chiari malformation
(D) Klippel-Feil syndrome
(E) Agenesis of the corpus callosum

129. An 18-year-old patient with loss of pinprick and temperature sensation over her shoulders and upper arms. Magnetic resonance imaging scan of the spinal cord reveals a fluid-filled cystic cavity in the cervicothoracic cord

130. A newborn infant with meningomyelocele who has progressive enlargement of the head after birth

131. A 6-month-old infant with infantile spasms and delayed development

ANSWERS AND EXPLANATIONS

1. The answer is E *[Chapter 1 V F 4]*. Many infants display intermittent, unexplained crying, typically beginning in the first month of life and occurring during the late afternoon and evening hours. Formula intolerance, constipation, teething, or illness usually do not account for such episodes. Spontaneous resolution by 3 months of age usually occurs.

2. The answer is A *[Chapter 10 IX A 1 c]*. Enterococcus, which is a common cause of infective endocarditis in adults, is a rare cause of endocarditis in children. The reasons for this are unknown. Viridans streptococcus causes many cases of endocarditis in children and adults but has decreased in importance since the introduction of antimicrobial therapy. *Staphylococcus aureus* and *Staphylococcus epidermidis* have become progressively more important causes of infective endocarditis in patients of all ages, especially hospitalized patients.

3. The answer is A *[Chapter 15 III D 4]*. The presence of jaundice, polychromatophilia, and reticulocytosis indicates that the patient has a hemolytic anemia. The positive direct Coombs' test confirms the presence of either complement components or antibody molecules on the surface of the patient's red blood cells (RBC), thereby establishing the diagnosis of autoimmune hemolytic anemia. Because the patient is not a newborn and has not recently received blood products, this cannot be an isoimmune hemolytic anemia with anti-RBC membrane antibodies acquired passively. The microspherocytes seen in this patient's blood smear are generated by membrane damage resulting from removal of membrane components by reticuloendothelial macrophages; a patient with congenital spherocytosis would not have a positive direct Coombs' test.

4. The answer is D *[Chapter 3 III D, F 1]*. When considering the possibility that an injury is the result of child abuse, it is important for the pediatrician to determine if the injury could have some other plausible cause (e.g., an accidental fall). It is critical to determine if the explanation given for the child's injury is consistent with the physical findings and feasible given the child's likely development. Soft tissue injuries to the forehead are commonly the result of accidental falls, and linear skull fractures may occur with such

accidents. Similarly, unilateral bruising around the eye could feasibly be owed to a fall or accidental blow to the face. Multiple bruises on the lower legs are common in active, young preschoolers as are impetiginous lesions on the extremities. However, linear bruise marks, especially over the back, are difficult to explain as being caused by an accidental injury, and are suggestive of intentional injury via whipping.

5. The answer is E *[Chapter 9 V A 4]*. The joint manifestations of rheumatic fever have no long-term sequelae. Rheumatic fever may cause pericarditis, but only in association with myocarditis or valvulitis. The pulmonary valve rarely, if ever, is affected, in contrast to the mitral and aortic valves. Prolonged fever of unknown origin does not usually emerge as rheumatic fever.

6. The answer is E *[Chapter 14 IV A 1 a (2)]*. Most children with acute poststreptococcal glomerulonephritis (APSGN) have a reduced C3. Although complement activation and a low C3 can occur in several other glomerulopathies, the clinical picture suggests APSGN. A follow-up complement to document return to normal is indicated in 6 to 8 weeks. Although blood pressure elevation and mild renal insufficiency may frequently occur in the course of APSGN, there is nothing specific about either. The negative antinuclear antibody, hepatitis profile, and human immunodeficiency virus may be important to rule out other causes of glomerulonephritis, but their exclusion does not diagnose APSGN. The positive streptozyme test is evidence for a recent streptococcal infection but does not add any more information than to confirm the previously culture-documented streptococcal infection.

7. The answer is D *[Chapter 16; Table 16-3]*. This is a characteristic presentation of acute lymphoblastic leukemia (ALL) in a young infant. The lymphoblasts are usually common acute lymphocytic leukemia antigen (CALLA)-negative and the infants often have high white blood cell counts and organomegaly. Acute nonlymphoblastic leukemia (ANLL) could present in a similar manner, and the blasts would also be CALLA-negative. However, they would also be terminal deoxynucleotidyl transferase (TdT)-negative and positive for myeloperoxidase or nonspecific esterase, or both. Stage IVS neuroblastoma may present with hepatomegaly and marrow infiltration, but not with circulating blasts and splenomegaly. Letterer-Siwe disease may present with hepatosplenomegaly, but not with blasts in the circulation.

8. The answer is B [Chapter 2 VII B 2]. Immediate application of cool water to a scald burn decreases the thermal injury to tissue. For many years, it was taught that warm water should be applied; warm water, however, helps in frostbite but not in scald burns. The application of butter or margarine, a home remedy, is of no help. A large burn from which skin has sloughed should be covered with saline-soaked gauze, but only as a second response after cooling. Pressure, although helpful for controlling bleeding, can increase tissue damage after a burn.

9–10. The answers are: 9-A, 10-D [Chapter 8 V C 1 b]. Cleft lip with or without cleft palate can result from teratogenic exposure; it can be part of the fetal alcohol syndrome; it can be inherited as a multifactorial disorder; or it can be part of an autosomal dominant, autosomal recessive, or X-linked condition. In all, more than 50 syndromes are associated with cleft lip with or without cleft palate. Physical examination reveals whether there are any dysmorphic features or malformations suggestive of such a syndrome. Computed tomography (CT) scan of the head, serum alcohol level, and urine toxic screen might be helpful in specific situations, depending on the physical examination and history. Cleft lip with or without cleft palate is not associated with amino acid disorders. When isolated, cleft lip with or without cleft palate is considered a multifactorial disorder, resulting from the effects of genes contributed by both parents (genetic liability) and some nongenetic (environmental) factors, which often cannot be identified.

11. The answer is B [Chapter 18 II C; Table 18-3]. The most common cause of acute onset of obtundation in a toddler is intoxication. The presence of potential intoxicants in the home is an important historical feature. Pupillary constriction also suggests intoxication, and the lack of signs of trauma or focal abnormality makes trauma or hemorrhage less likely.

12. The answer is A [Chapter 5 II B; Table 5-1]. The central issue during midadolescence is peer support. These adolescents no longer

consider themselves to be children, yet they also have not received full recognition as adults. Hence, their peer group serves as their buffer. This is also why adolescents often develop their own music, dress, and language as ways of signalling their uniqueness and separate identity. By grounding or taking phone privileges away, the parent separates the adolescent from her peer support. This often leads to further acting out and anger on the part of the adolescent. Most of pubertal development usually takes place during early adolescence. Adolescents seek out adult role models throughout their teens, but most often during early adolescence when they are taking initial steps toward independence. Separation usually occurs during late adolescence when it is time to leave home.

13. The answer is C [Chapter 9 II E 6 a]. This child has symptomatic human immunodeficiency virus (HIV) infection, but she does not have severe immunodeficiency. Because her CD4 T-cell count is normal for age, prophylaxis for *Pneumocystis carinii* pneumonia is not indicated. However, because she has symptomatic HIV infection, she should be treated with the antiretroviral drug zidovudine (ZDV, AZT). Intravenous gamma globulin (IVIG) has not been shown to have sufficient benefit in preventing common bacterial infections in HIV-positive infants to justify its use in this case. Amoxicillin has limited usefulness for prophylaxis against recurrent otitis media.

14. The answer is C [Chapter 6 I C 1 b]. Asymmetric growth retardation occurs as a result of an insult late in gestation; cell number is normal, but cell size is decreased. Asymmetric growth retardation is associated with factors that decrease uterine, placental, or umbilical blood flow and transfer of nutrients to the fetus, as occurs with preeclampsia. Chromosomal defects (e.g., trisomy 18 and 21), congenital infection (e.g., with cytomegalovirus), and maternal use of drugs (e.g., alcohol) are factors that adversely affect fetal growth early in gestation, causing symmetric growth retardation.

15. The answer is D [Chapter 15 III D 6 e, 10 d (1) (c) (ii)]. In the absence of a functioning spleen, encapsulated organisms (e.g., pneumococci, *Haemophilus influenzae*) are not filtered from the bloodstream and may cause septicemia. To protect the asplenic patient from this complication, he or she should be immunized with pneumococcal and *H. influenzae* vaccines before splenectomy and placed on prophylactic penicillin indefinitely after surgery. Patients with congenital agammaglobulinemia are also at increased risk for pneumococcal or *H. influenzae* sepsis, whereas gram-negative sepsis is seen more commonly as a complication of severe neutropenia.

16. The answer is B *[Chapter 1 VI C 3 c].* Inappropriate bedtime practices may result in several problems. The child who falls asleep with a propped bottle in his mouth may be predisposed to otitis media caused by reflux through the eustachian tube. The bathing of teeth in milk while the child sleeps causes decay. The upper central and lateral incisors are particularly susceptible because the lower teeth are protected by the tongue.

17. The answer is C *[Chapter 16 VIII C 1].* High-dose estrogen treatment may induce premature epiphyseal fusion and a reduction of final adult stature. The growth-suppressing effects of corticosteroids are accompanied by severe side effects. Thyroid hormone promotes linear growth in prepubertal children. Gonadotropin-releasing hormone (GnRH) agonists will initially stimulate gonadotropin release. However, continued administration will actually suppress gonadotropin, making GnRH agonists useful in treating precocious puberty. Progesterone has no role in accelerating skeletal maturation.

18. The answer is D *[Chapter 9 IV F 2 c].* In 70% of patients with chronic urticaria, an underlying etiology cannot be elucidated (idiopathic etiology). The most common cause of acute urticaria, particularly in children, is viral infections. Urticaria can also be caused by or associated with food allergies, connective tissue disease, or drug allergy.

19. The answer is C *[Chapter 11 V D 4 a–c].* This child has chronic nonspecific diarrhea. Usually seen in otherwise healthy children, it appears to be associated with rapid intestinal transit. Undigested food in the stool, particularly vegetables, is common. Large amounts of fluids, particularly fruit juices containing sorbitol and fructose, often exacerbate symptoms. In many children, the restriction of these fluids will often markedly decrease stool frequency and improve consistency. Restriction of fatty foods may exacerbate symptoms because fat

slows transit through the gastrointestinal tract. Lactose malabsorption may be seen in some children and at this age is always secondary to a process that damages small intestinal mucosa. Restriction of lactose may be attempted but usually not as the first step in an otherwise healthy child. Gluten restriction should not be attempted unless a diagnosis of celiac disease has been established. Increasing dietary fiber may be helpful in some patients with chronic nonspecific diarrhea who do not respond to fluid restriction.

20. The answer is C *[Chapter 18 V B 1 b (1), C 2].* The spells described are brief seizures, associated with sudden onset and cessation with no apparent postictal state. This is consistent with absence seizures, and given the age of the child and her negative neurologic examination, suggests the epileptic syndrome of absence seizures of childhood. The lack of convulsive motor activity and postictal state excludes major motor seizures. Partial complex seizures usually last longer than 30 seconds, and are associated with postictal confusion. Daydreaming is usually more variable in duration, and rarely occurs in midsentence.

21. The answer is A *[Chapter 12 IV H 5 a].* Patients with aortic valve stenosis have an increased risk for sudden death during exercise due to myocardial ischemia and arrhythmias secondary to increased myocardial work with less blood supply. In all cases except mild aortic stenosis, restriction from athletics is recommended. Patients with aortic valve stenosis are at risk for endocarditis, and therefore prophylaxis is recommended. The electrocardiogram may show left ventricular hypertrophy due to the increased left ventricular mass, but not right ventricular hypertrophy. The aortic valve usually has fused commissures, a thickened valve, or both; calcification of the valve is usually not present until adulthood.

22. The answer is B *[Chapter 9; Table 9-4].* Several laboratory tests are available to evaluate T-cell immune competence, including lymphocyte proliferative responses to antigens or mitogens and flow cytometry for T-cell subsets. However, the best screening test for T-cell deficiency, which is available in any office or clinic setting, is delayed skin reactivity to recall antigens (e.g., *Candida,* tetanus) The total hemolytic complement (CH_{50}) is important in diagnosing congenital complement deficiencies. The nitroblue tetrazolium test is important in the diagnosis of chronic granulomatous disease.

23. The answer is D *[Chapter 11 X B 1].* Trauma is a common cause of pancreatitis in children. The pancreas is situated in front of the hard vertebral column and is prone to injury when blunt force strikes the mid-abdomen. The onset of pancreatitis may range from several hours to days or weeks following the injury. Serum amylase and lipase should be measured. Duodenal hematoma may also follow blunt abdominal injury and may be difficult to distinguish clinically from pancreatitis, although the onset of symptoms is generally more rapid and obstructive symptoms more common. Mesenteric avulsion is uncommon and presents as an acute abdomen with guarding and rebound. Appendicitis would be consistent with this boy's clinical history, although the history of trauma is important in suggesting pancreatitis rather than appendicitis. Volvulus is in the differential diagnosis and should be initially evaluated with a plain radiograph of the abdomen.

24. The answer is B *[Chapter 13 I C 2 d (1); IV D 5].* The most common cause of digital clubbing in children, other than cyanotic congenital heart disease, is cystic fibrosis. The history of bronchitis and of abdominal pain (probably secondary to malabsorption) is compatible with this diagnosis. Therefore, a sweat test is the best test to order. Pulmonary function tests are not diagnostic but may suggest obstructive pulmonary disease; a chest x-ray may show chronic changes; an abdominal x-ray may show dilated loops of filled bowel; and an IgE level may demonstrate allergies as the etiology of the bronchitis. Only the sweat test is diagnostic.

25. The answer is A *[Chapter 15 VI C 1 b].* Idiopathic thrombocytopenic purpura (ITP) is most commonly seen in previously healthy children, who may have encountered a recent viral infection. Because the pathogenesis involves peripheral destruction of platelets, the bone marrow appears normal and other hemic lineages are not affected (unlike the case for acute leukemia or aplastic anemia). In contrast to the patient with ITP, the child with disseminated intravascular coagulation (DIC) usually is extremely ill.

26. The answer is A *[Chapter 16 V F 1].* Age younger than 1 year is a favorable prognostic indicator in neuroblastoma. Histiocytosis X in an infant is much more likely to present as Letterer-Siwe disease, which often has a fatal outcome. Infants with acute lymphocytic leukemia (ALL) do particularly poorly, and children with medulloblastoma who are younger than 4 years of age do not do as well as older children. Children with juvenile chronic myelogenous leukemia (CML) do poorly at any age.

27. The answer is C *[Chapter 2 XI D 1 a].* Syrup of ipecac has been demonstrated to be a safe, efficient method to remove stomach contents in children. Nasogastric lavage is less apt to remove large pill fragments, given the limitations on tube diameter in small children. In addition, many children vomit, with incomplete stomach evacuation, during attempts to place the tube. Nasogastric lavage is the method of choice, however, in unconscious patients. Manual induction of vomiting is an inefficient method. Citrate of magnesia is a good choice for catharsis, but not for emesis.

28. The answer is D *[Chapter 7 VI B, C].* Initial priorities in the treatment of the severely traumatized patient include assurance of airway, breathing, and circulatory sufficiency. The cervical spine should be protected until it has been certified as uninjured. Hypotension is treated by isotonic crystalloid, colloid, or blood infusions. Although this child may well benefit from the diagnostic power of head and abdominal computed tomography (CT) scans, these should not be done until hypoxia and hypotension have been treated.

29. The answer is C *[Chapter 7 V A 4 b].* Ventriculostomy is unlikely to be helpful in controlling intracranial pressure in this patient; the ventricles are quite small owing to compression by the interstitial fluid and compensatory shunting of cerebrospinal fluid (CSF) into the spinal canal. Mannitol, hyperventilation, and pentobarbital may all be beneficial in controlling increased intracranial pressure in this setting. Fluid restriction may contribute to vasoconstriction of the cerebral vasculature, which will help to control cerebral blood flow in the absence of autoregulation.

30. The answer is B *[Chapter 7 V B 1–3].* Brain death is a state in which there is complete and irreversible failure of cortical and brain stem function. Electroencephalography (EEG) and physical examinations for determination of brain death are not reliable in the presence of significant levels of barbiturates. In children older than 1 year of age who have a known etiology for their neurologic status, brain death may be diagnosed without EEG, based on physical findings alone. The Glasgow Coma Score is a prognostic score, and does not assess cranial nerve functions such as pupillary response. Decerebrate posturing indicates some function, although abnormal, of the brain stem. Four-vessel angiography is a highly sensitive but very invasive diagnostic technique. It is not required for the determination of brain death.

31. The answer is B [Chapter 16 IX B 2 b (1)]. The patient's presentation and computed tomography scan findings are characteristic of medulloblastoma. Brain abscess would be unusual in this location, and absence of fever also makes a brain abscess unlikely. Glioblastoma multiforme arises above rather than below the tentorium and would therefore be expected to arise in the cerebral hemispheres rather than in the cerebellum. It also is a less common tumor in children than medulloblastoma. Central nervous system leukemia causes signs and symptoms of increased intracranial pressure, but is rarely the initial manifestation of leukemia, and it is associated with diffuse meningeal infiltration rather than a discrete intracranial mass.

32. The answer is D [Chapter 3 V G 2]. Because the child is an international adoptee and is from Korea, testing for hepatitis B and tuberculosis would be most important. The tine test is an inaccurate screening tool for tuberculosis; the purified protein derivative test is indicated for a child at risk for tuberculosis. Because of the overall high incidence of parasitic infestation among international adoptees (less for Korean children), screening for parasites is also indicated. The circumstances of the child's birth and subsequent decision to place the child for adoption may suggest risk factors for the child's development and long-term psychological outcome. If there were specific risk factors in this child's background (e.g., known substance abuse, extreme prematurity with central nervous system complications, or adoption later in childhood), then concern about behavioral problems or development may warrant screening in those areas. Because there was no such history and the child is presumably doing well so far, the pediatrician should focus on less overt medical problems. A complete blood cell count (CBC); screening for electrolyte, blood urea nitrogen (BUN), and creatinine levels; urinalysis; and liver and thyroid function tests are fairly broad and non-specific, and they are not indicated by this child's history.

33. The answer is E [Chapter 1 III E 4]. Physiologic jaundice in term newborns is characterized by the appearance of clinical jaundice after 24 hours, an increase in bilirubin concentration of less than 5 mg/dl/day, total serum bilirubin concentrations of less than 13 mg/dl, direct serum bilirubin levels of less than 1.5–2 mg/dl, and the resolution of jaundice by the age of 1 week. Jaundice related to breast-feeding is termed breast-feeding jaundice, which typically responds to temporary discontinuation of breast-feeding.

34. The answer is A [Chapter 8 III B 3 e]. Mucopolysaccharidoses are a group of disorders caused by an inability to catabolize the molecules that make up the intracellular substance. Therefore, mucopolysaccharides accumulate in the skin (causing coarse features), internal organs (causing hepatosplenomegaly), and the brain (causing progressive intellectual impairment). Disorders of carbohydrate metabolism, amino acid metabolism, and the urea cycle and hereditary fructose intolerance are not associated with storage of metabolites.

35. The answer is A [Chapter 9 IV E 2 b (1)]. Infantile eczema is characterized by a rash that is erythematous, papulovesicular, and, occasionally, exudative. In infants, the rash involves the facial and extensor surfaces. Older children or adults have lesions on the flexural surfaces, which become lichenified. Urticaria is not part of atopic eczema, but is a separate atopic disorder. Posterior subcapsular cataracts take a number of years to develop and, therefore, would not be found in infants, but rather in older children or adults.

36. The answer is D [Chapter 15 VI D 3]. The vitamin K-dependent factors are involved in maintaining integrity of the intrinsic (factor IX), extrinsic (factor VII), and common (factors II, X) pathways of coagulation. Thus, both prothrombin time (PT) and partial thromboplastin time (PTT) will be prolonged in vitamin K deficiency. Factor VIII is not vitamin K–dependent, and, therefore, its level will be normal.

37. The answer is E [Chapter 11 IV A; Table 11-3]. Meckel diverticulum usually presents with painless rectal bleeding in the first 3 years of life. The blood may range from bright red to maroon to dark red. The volume of bleeding is variable but may be large. Colonic polyps are common in the first several years of life but rarely cause massive bleeding or anemia. Intussusception is usually associated with crampy abdominal pain and vomiting. Ulcerative colitis is unusual in a child this age and usually has a more insidious onset. Lymphonodular hyperplasia is believed to be an unusual cause of rectal bleeding and is associated with small amounts of blood mixed with the stool.

38. The answer is C *[Chapter 10 V C 3 a].*
Air-fluid level on sinus x-ray is strong evidence of acute sinusitis in this 6-year-old child. Sinusitis is inflammation of the mucous membrane lining the paranasal sinuses, which may be acute or chronic. Common features in children older than 5 years of age include fever, facial pain, and headache. The predominant microorganisms in acute sinusitis are *Streptococcus pneumoniae,* unencapsulated strains of *Haemophilus influenzae,* and *Moraxella catarrhalis.*

39. The answer is C *[Chapter 13 VI A 2, B].*
An apparent life-threatening event (ALTE) is an episode of apnea associated with marked change in color and muscle tone, such that an observer typically believes the infant will die without vigorous stimulation or resuscitation. Central apnea is cessation of breathing without respiratory effort, whereas obstructive apnea is cessation of airflow at the mouth and nose with continued respiratory effort. Apnea may be a symptom of many diseases in infants and should be labeled an ALTE only if no cause can be found. Sudden infant death syndrome (SIDS) is the death of an infant without adequate explanation by history or autopsy examination. Less than 10% of infants who die of SIDS have had a prior ALTE.

40. The answer is C *[Chapter 18 VIII A 1].*
The diagnosis of concussion is based on a history of a transient loss of consciousness lasting less than 20 minutes; the patient is amnesic for the event, and may not recall the events leading up to the trauma. Nausea and vomiting are commonly associated with concussion, but are not diagnostic. Abnormalities in the neurologic examination suggest the possibility of a more serious lesion.

41. The answer is E *[Chapter 1; Table 1-5].*
A history of encephalopathy within 7 days of diphtheria–tetanus–pertussis (DTP) immunization unexplained by another cause is a con-

traindication to repeat administration. Other severe reactions (including seizures, extreme irritability, and high fever) are considered precautions against repeating pertussis immunization, mandating individual case-by-case weighing of the potential risks of immunization versus risks of contracting the disease. Low-grade fever and brief fussiness are considered to be mild reactions and are not contraindications to repeat administration. If the child developed a high fever and had a prolonged period of extreme irritability, administration of the diphtheria and tetanus toxoid vaccine with elimination of the pertussis component would be a reasonable approach at the age of 6 months. Split doses should never be used because their efficacy is uncertain.

42. The answer is B *[Chapter 9 IV A 1 e].*
Corticosteroids and cromolyn sodium are important pharmacologic agents useful in the treatment of late-phase allergic reactions, which occur 6–8 hours after exposure to an allergen. Theophylline, albuterol, and antihistamines are useful for the early or immediate allergic phase of an IgE-mediated hypersensitivity reaction, but not for the late-phase allergic response.

43. The answer is C *[Chapter 11 VII A 3 c (2)].*
This infant has a classic history and physical examination for intussusception. Lethargy may be a prominent feature of intussusception and may occur in the absence of obvious gastrointestinal symptoms, leading to initial diagnostic studies aimed at the central nervous system. Following a plain radiograph of the abdomen to exclude the possibility of perforation, a barium enema will not only establish a diagnosis of intussusception but may also be therapeutic in facilitating its reduction. Abdominal ultrasound may be used in the diagnosis of intussusception but will not facilitate its reduction.

44. The answer is C *[Chapter 14 IX C 2 c].* This child probably has renal tubular acidosis, and bicarbonate therapy should restore good clinical health and normal growth. Although nutritional supplements may provide extra calories, the child will continue to grow poorly unless the acidosis is corrected. If the acidosis is corrected, the extra caloric supplementation will probably not be required. The child is slightly old for esophageal reflux, but even so, children with reflux uncommonly fail to gain weight normally and may be overweight. Furthermore, the electrolyte picture this child presents is not compatible with chronic vomiting. If cystic fibrosis is suspected, a sweat test is indicated, and not empiric therapy. Furthermore, children with cystic fibrosis usually do not have metabolic acidosis. The use of the agent acetazolamide produces metabolic acidosis through inhibition of carbonic anhydrase, and would not be used to treat it.

45. The answer is D *[Chapter 16 III B 1 a, 2 a, C 1]*. Lymphoblastic lymphoma usually presents with an anterior mediastinal mass and characteristically develops in older children and male adolescents. The immunophenotype is also typical and indicates the cells are immature T cells. Lymphoblastic lymphoma also spreads to the marrow. However, a diagnosis of T-cell acute lymphoblastic leukemia cannot be made in this case because of the limited degree of marrow involvement. To diagnose leukemia, the marrow must contain at least 25% lymphoblasts, and in most cases lymphoblasts are the predominant cell in the marrow. Hodgkin disease can present with a mediastinal mass and pleural effusion, but the mass is often in the middle mediastinum and the effusion would not contain lymphoblasts. Lymphoblasts also would not be seen in the marrow. Burkitt lymphoma usually presents in older male children and adolescents, but the mass is usually in the abdomen rather than in the chest. In addition, the malignant cells would have a B-cell immunophenotype if this were Burkitt lymphoma.

46. The answer is D *[Chapter 11 VI; Table 11-5; Table 11-6]*. Ulcerative colitis most commonly presents with loose stools that turn bloody. Abdominal cramping is usually mild at first and often relieved by defecation. Laboratory studies are frequently normal at diagnosis, especially in mild cases. Crohn disease affecting the colon may present in a similar fashion, although the erythrocyte sedimentation rate more frequently is elevated (approximately 80% of cases). Colonoscopy or flexible sigmoidoscopy with mucosal biopsies may be needed to differentiate between the two disorders. Colonic polyps usually present with painless rectal bleeding in the presence of formed stools. Hemorrhoids generally present with anal discomfort and blood on the outside of the stool or on the toilet tissue. Meckel diverticulum, unusual at this age, often presents with abrupt onset bleeding of greater magnitude.

47. The answer is C *[Chapter 14 II C 3]*. Renal venous thrombosis in the newborn period commonly presents with gross hematuria and a flank mass. Infants of diabetic mothers by virtue of polycythemia are at slightly increased risk for this condition. A meconium plug may cause abdominal distention, but probably would not cause a discrete flank mass and would not lead to gross hematuria. A neuroblastoma would not produce hematuria nor grow so fast as to suddenly produce a flank mass. A ureteropelvic junction obstruction is usually not associated with hematuria and should have been palpable at the time of birth. An adrenal hemorrhage may present as a sizeable mass but would not be associated with gross hematuria.

48. The answer is B *[Chapter 8 VIII C 3]*. Loss of previously attained developmental progress is seen in neurodegenerative disorders, most of which are genetic. These include, among others, neuronal storage disorders, mucopolysaccharidoses, demyelinating conditions, dementing disorders (e.g., Huntington disease), and uncontrollable seizure disorders. Dysmorphic syndromes and chromosomal translocations usually do not cause regression. The effects of teratogens occur prenatally.

49. The answer is C *[Chapter 10 VII E 4 b]*. Immunocompromised children who have not had varicella and who are exposed to the disease are at increased risk for such complications as meningoencephalitis, pneumonia, and hepatitis. The mortality rate in such cases is approximately 20%. Because of this danger, susceptible immunocompromised children (e.g., those with leukemia) should receive varicella-zoster immune globulin within 48 hours of exposure for maximal effectiveness (and no later than 96 hours after exposure) and be closely observed. Those who develop signs of disseminated varicella (as in this case) or herpes zoster should be treated with acyclovir or vidarabine. Because there is evidence of possible bacterial pneumonia, antibiotic therapy also should be provided for this patient.

50. The answer is E *[Chapter 3 VIII E 3]*. The pediatrician who has established an ongoing primary care relationship with the child and family can have a very important consulting role when the child loses a close family member. Although children (and adults) vary in their particular patterns of reaction to bereavement, some general conclusions can be drawn based on developmental principles. The overall anxiety of the young child, often a reaction to the emotional environment around him, may lead to the child expressing a strong desire not to attend the funeral or wake. This wish should be heeded if at all possible. If the young child does attend, an adult who is close to the child, but who is less likely to be overwhelmed by the loss, may be helpful in comforting the child or taking the child home if he desires. Apparent indifference of younger children to death can be a reflection of their stage of cognitive development and their relative egocentrism and not of their relationship to the deceased. It is difficult to predict the actual behavior of a given child attending a funeral or wake. However, children's fears, specifically of distorted human images, may cause a negative reaction to the viewing of a corpse. In addition, young children are more likely to react negatively to the highly emotional environment of grieving adult family members than their own internal sense of grief.

51. The answer is E *[Chapter 18 XII D 1 a].* Duchenne muscular dystrophy is an X-linked disease of muscle caused by an absence of dystrophin in the muscle. The symptoms consist of progressive weakness and motor disability, culminating in respiratory and, occasionally, cardiac failure. Clues to the diagnosis include prominent calf muscles, progressive loss of proximal muscle strength (e.g., difficulty climbing stairs, getting up from a chair), and the presence of a positive Gowers sign.

52. The answer is C *[Chapter 15 V B 2].* The patient has a severe congenital cytopenia that is limited to the neutrophil lineage; thus, aplastic anemia and acute leukemia, which affect all hemic lineages, are very unlikely. Cyclic neutropenia is characterized by a periodicity in absolute neutrophil count (ANC) rather than a constant lowering of ANC. The use of granulocyte colony-stimulating factor to stimulate neutrophil production has markedly improved the prognosis for patients with both Kostmann agranulocytosis and cyclic neutropenia.

53. The answer is E *[Chapter 16 II B 3 b (3)].* A teenage boy with a high white blood cell count acute lymphoblastic leukemia (ALL) most likely has T-cell disease. Both the presence of the mediastinal mass and the terminal deoxynucleotidyl transferase (TdT) in the blasts are much more suggestive of T-cell ALL than of acute nonlymphocytic leukemia (ANLL); TdT is found in almost all lymphoblasts of patients with ALL, whereas it is rare in ANLL. Chronic myelogenous leukemia (CML) of either the adult or juvenile type would be

unlikely because of the predominance of blasts in the blood, and juvenile CML would also be unlikely owing to the patient's age. The presence of many circulating blasts indicates a leukemia rather than a lymphoma.

54. The answer is B *[Chapter 9 V A].* For reasons that are unclear, the upper respiratory tract is the only site of streptococcal infection preceding an attack of rheumatic fever. Skin infections caused by this organism are common and may lead to nephritis but apparently not to rheumatic fever. Streptococci are not present in the heart, joints, or bloodstream in rheumatic fever.

55. The answer is A *[Chapter 6 V I 4 e].* Multiple-gestation pregnancies are fraught with problems for both the mother and the fetuses (infants). The most common problem is premature birth. Other problems include maternal hypertension, anemia, hyperemesis, and growth disturbances in the fetuses.

56. The answer is C *[Chapter 10 X B 3 a, 4 b].* This patient most likely has septic arthritis of the hip. Signs and symptoms associated with septic arthritis of the hip often are subtle and may be limited to a limp or refusal to walk. X-ray frequently shows a widening of the joint space. Septic arthritis of the hip requires immediate surgical drainage, because the blood supply to the femoral head may be compromised, causing permanent destruction to the joint. Drainage may be performed by needle aspiration or surgical excision. Gram stain and culture of the synovial fluid should be obtained and appropriate antibiotic therapy begun.

57. The answer is B *[Chapter 15 VI D 1 b (4)].* With a factor VIII level of 10%, the patient has mild hemophilia A. In the absence of a life-threatening bleed (e.g., intracranial) or major surgery, such patients may be managed with desmopressin (dDAVP), which will raise the factor VIII level within the therapeutic range without exposing the patient to the risk of blood-borne viruses. Although recently developed recombinant factor VIII products are also free of viral contaminants, they are much more expensive than dDAVP.

58. The answer is C *[Chapter 15 III B 5 c; Table 15-3].* Hemoglobin Bart's (Hb Bart's) is a tetramer composed of four γ chains that is found in fetuses with homozygous α thalassemia whose red blood cells lack the ability to produce α chains, which would normally combine with the γ chains to form fetal hemoglobin (Hb F). Hb Bart's is an unstable molecule that binds oxygen avidly and releases it poorly to the tissues; the precipitation of Hb Bart's leads to a severe hypochromic microcytic anemia and ineffective erythropoiesis. The condition leads to death in utero. Unlike the α chains, β chains are not a major component of the hemoglobin tetramer until late in gestation. Thus, the infant with β thalassemia major or mixed heterozygosity for α and β thalassemia does not have significant anemia until he or she is several months of age.

59. The answer is C *[Chapter 16 II B 4; Table 16-6]*. This child has all the prerequisites for a good prognosis: age 1 through 9 years, non-T, non-B immunophenotype, and white blood cell count (WBC) less than 50,000/mm³. Hyperdiploidy is also associated with a good prognosis. In (A), the child's age precludes a good prognosis. In (B), the WBC greater than 50,000/mm³ and the B-cell immunophenotype are associated with a poor prognosis. The t(8;14) in this case is characteristic for this type of leukemia. In (D), the presence of t(9;22) [the Philadelphia chromosome] automatically confers a poor prognosis.

60. The answer is A *[Chapter 1 V F 3]*. Both candidal and intertrigo dermatitis involve the deep skin folds. Candidal diaper rash has bright red erosions that spread peripherally by satellite lesions to involve the genitalia, lower abdomen, thighs, and buttocks. Intertrigo is characterized by moderate erythema and a white or yellow exudate. Generic diaper dermatitis, the most common variety of diaper rash, is characterized by erythema involving the lower abdomen, thighs, scrotum, and labia. This rash usually spares the deep skin folds and produces dryness and wrinkling of the skin. Infantile seborrheic dermatitis often begins in the diaper area and appears as a beefy red, sharply circumscribed rash with satellite lesions. The rash frequently spreads to other areas of the body. Common sites of involvement include the flexural creases, cheeks, scalp, and extremities. Staphylococcal diaper rash is characterized by superficial erythematous pustules and bullae.

61. The answer is B *[Chapter 16 I B 3]*. The cyanosis and focal seizures in this infant are due to hypoglycemia related to congenital hypopituitarism. The physical findings of microphallus and lack of light response suggest the syndrome of septooptic dysplasia, which frequently is associated with deficiency of growth hormone (GH), adrenocorticotropic hormone (ACTH), thyroid-stimulating hormone (TSH), and arginine vasopressin [antidiuretic hormone (ADH)]. Hypoglycemia should be anticipated in infants with these findings. Low cortisol and GH levels during hypoglycemia confirm the diagnosis of congenital hypopituitarism. Hypoglycemia resolves with appropriate hormone replacement. Hypocalcemia is a cause of neonatal seizures but would not explain the other findings. Seizures are not characteristic of congenital hypothyroidism. Congenital heart disease may result in cyanosis but would not explain the other findings. Idiopathic epilepsy is an unlikely etiology for neonatal seizures and would similarly not account for the other findings.

62. The answer is A *[Chapter 9 IV C 5]*. Although topical steroids and desensitization therapy may be useful in the treatment of allergic rhinitis, the safest and most direct approach to therapy in a patient with allergies to pollens (grass pollen in this child) is with antihistamines. Avoiding allergens can also be helpful if feasible. For example, someone who is allergic to animal dander should avoid contact with pets; this includes the removal of pets from the home. However, allergies to pollens are difficult to avoid, but partial avoidance measures can still be instituted (e.g., the use of air conditioning and electrostatic filters).

63. The answer is B *[Chapter 16 II A 5 a (2)]*. Prompt treatment of the febrile, neutropenic patient with acute nonlymphocytic leukemia (ANLL) is essential and lifesaving. Appropriate cultures should be obtained to identify the responsible microorganism, but extensive evaluation in lieu of treatment places the patient in jeopardy of overwhelming sepsis. Because fever most likely is the result of infection rather than leukemia, institution of antibiotic therapy takes precedence over antileukemic therapy, which can begin once antibiotic treatment has commenced. Granulocyte transfusions are not indicated at this point but may be considered if the patient's infection does not respond to antibiotics. Vigorous antipyretic therapy should certainly not be the initial approach. Should antipyretics be needed subsequently for comfort, aspirin, which interferes with platelet function, must be specifically avoided in the patient who is potentially thrombocytopenic as well as neutropenic.

64. The answer is D *[Chapter 8 I D 2, 3; VIII C 2].* When several dysmorphic, functional, and structural abnormalities are seen together, they often form a syndrome (a recognizable pattern of malformations). Syndromes may be sporadic or may be caused by a single gene or chromosome abnormality. Teratogenic agents also can cause a recognizable pattern of anomalies. All of these possibilities should be investigated through the use of family history analysis and chromosome analysis. With very few exceptions, syndromes of dysmorphic features and malformations are not associated with multifactorial inheritance.

65. The answer is B *[Chapter 10 VII F 1–2].* The most likely diagnosis for this 12-year-old boy is scarlet fever. Scarlet fever is an acute illness characterized by fever, an erythematous rash, and in most cases, pharyngitis. Scarlet fever is caused by infection with group A streptococcal strains that produce erythrogenic toxin. Although the disease most often is associated with pharyngeal infection, it rarely may follow streptococcal infection at other sites (e.g., cellulitis, impetigo). The cutaneous manifestations of other streptococcal infections such as erysipelas, rheumatic fever, and impetigo are quite different. Erythema infectiosum is caused by a parvovirus.

66. The answer is A *[Chapter 6 I B 1 a (1)].* Highly saturated blood returns to the fetus via the umbilical vein, ductus venosus, and inferior vena cava. This blood is preferentially shunted across the foramen ovale to the left side of the heart to supply the coronary and cerebral circulation. Desaturated blood from the head and rest of the body returns to the right ventricle, is pumped out to the pulmonary artery, and is shunted across the ductus arteriosus to the descending aorta. Therefore, apart from umbilical vein blood, the most highly saturated blood is preductal, and the postductal blood is relatively desaturated. Therefore, the carotid artery is the correct choice. The coronary artery also contains highly saturated blood.

67. The answer is C *[Chapter 3 II C, D].* A thorough review of studies of failure to thrive concludes what astute clinicians have long known, that expensive and complicated testing rarely results in a definitive medical diagnosis when the history or physical exam does not point to a specific organic cause. Although it is usually found that such infants

and families have interactive problems, close evaluation and observation in a hospital allow a multidisciplinary team to identify specific areas that are deficient. This allows for directed treatment of both family psychological problems and the particular pattern of aberrant feeding behavior.

68. The answer is D *[Chapter 9 II A 3].* A deficiency of one of the late-acting complement components (i.e., C5, C6, C7, and C8) results in recurrent *Neisseria* infections, especially recurrent meningococcal meningitis and gonococcal septicemia. Deficiency of the complement component C3 results in bacterial infections, particularly with gram-negative bacteria. Neutrophil dysfunction usually results in infection with gram-positive organisms. T-cell immunodeficiencies result in viral, parasitic, and fungal infections. Carboxypeptidase N deficiency is associated with recurrent angioedema.

69. The answer is D *[Chapter 15 VI C 1 c].* Isoimmune thrombocytopenia results from the passive acquisition of maternal antibodies directed against a platelet membrane antigen of the fetus that the mother's platelets lack. The diagnosis should be suspected in a healthy, thrombocytopenic infant whose mother has a normal platelet count (and no prior history of idiopathic thrombocytopenic purpura or splenectomy). Consumption coagulopathy, on the other hand, usually complicates the course of an extremely ill patient.

70. The answer is B *[Chapter 12 IV F 5 a (2)].* Hypoxemic spells (Tet spells) are treated by placing the child in the knee-chest position, providing supplemental oxygen, and administering morphine sulfate to depress the respiratory center. Phenylephrine hydrochloride can be used to increase systemic vascular resistance and increase pulmonary blood flow. Epinephrine increases myocardial contractility and can increase right ventricular outflow obstruction, resulting in increased cyanosis. Bronchodilators will not affect oxygenation and may increase heart rate, myocardial contractility, and right ventricular outflow obstruction, resulting in increased cyanosis. Tetralogy of Fallot does not result in congestive heart failure; digoxin plays no role in the management of this case.

71. The answer is C *[Chapter 6 III E].* The primary goal of resuscitation of anyone—infant, child, or adult—is to reoxygenate the central nervous system (CNS). This is achieved by providing adequate oxygen and ventilation and by establishing adequate cardiac output. Improvement in heart rate and color and spontaneous respiration are signs that the goal is being achieved.

72. The answer is C *[Chapter 16 V B 1, 2].* The diagnosis is metastatic neuroblastoma. This tumor often occurs in young children and metastasizes widely before diagnosis. With metastases, systemic symptoms of fever and weight loss are common. The leg pain and the proptosis with periorbital ecchymoses reflect spread to the cortex of the long bones of the lower extremities and to the soft tissues of the right orbit, respectively. The large left flank mass is caused by the primary tumor, which most likely arose in the medulla of the left adrenal gland. Orbital rhabdomyosarcoma often presents with proptosis, but it is usually localized to the orbit and metastasizes late. It would also not be associated with a flank mass. Hand-Schüller-Christian disease can present with unilateral proptosis and with bone pain from multifocal eosinophilic granulomas. The flank mass and systemic symptoms make this diagnosis unlikely. Wilms tumor is common at this age and certainly presents as a flank mass and may occasionally present with fever. However, orbital and bony metastases are not characteristic of Wilms tumor.

73. The answer is C *[Chapter 9 IV I 2 b].* Reactions caused by pollen, bee venom, and peanuts all are IgE-mediated. In contrast, reactions to aspirin or aspirin-like compounds are believed to be mediated by perturbations of the arachidonic acid pathway, not IgE. These reactions are called anaphylactoid reactions because they produce the same signs and symptoms as are seen in anaphylaxis, but they are not IgE-mediated.

74. The answer is A *[Chapter 16 I A 1 e].* The development of enuresis in this child not previously enuretic is most likely related to hyperglycemia and resultant increased urine volume due to osmotic diuresis. During the day, this may present as increased frequency of urination (polyuria). At night, in some children, it presents as bedwetting (enuresis). Most children require a split-dose (every 12 hours) of insulin to maintain good glycemic control. Emotional stress of chronic disease is an unlikely cause of enuresis. A urinary tract infection typically presents as other signs and symptoms, such as unexplained fever and abdominal complaints. If an evening dosage of insulin is too high, hypoglycemia (without obvious signs or symptoms) may occur during sleep, resulting in the release of counter-regulatory hormones and an elevated blood sugar in the morning. These events, termed the Somogyi phenomenon, are unlikely to cause enuresis. Hypoglycemia may be associated with early morning lethargy, pallor, sweating, and a seizure. Enuresis is not a feature.

75. The answer is B *[Chapter 15 III D 10 d (1) (c) (i)].* The key physical finding is the massively enlarged spleen. The sudden engorgement of the spleen with red blood cells can sequester a significant portion of the blood volume, leading to hypotension. Aggressive volume replacement with colloid or crystalloid products is essential to stabilize the patient's condition until the spleen releases the trapped red blood cells.

76. The answer is D *[Chapter 10 V D 3].* This patient most likely has herpetic gingivostomatitis, the most common type of gingivostomatitis in children. Herpetic gingivostomatitis is characterized by painful, erythematous, edematous, and ulcerative lesions that occur on the buccal mucosa, gums, and, occasionally, the hard palate and tongue. There usually is a fever, which may be quite high. Herpetic gingivostomatitis may be so severe that a child refuses to eat or drink. Although herpangina occurs during the summer and is associated with fever, the oral lesions of herpangina are located in the posterior pharynx. The oral lesions of aphthous stomatitis may appear anywhere on the oral mucosa but are localized as a single, shallow ulcer or a small cluster of ulcers and are not associated with fever. Candidal gingivostomatitis can cause widespread oral involvement, as in this child, but the lesions are grayish-white, usually are not associated with fever, and are uncommon after 3 months of age. Necrotizing ulcerative gingivitis consists of necrosis and ulceration of the interdental papillae.

77. The answer is C *[Chapter 15 VI D 3].* Vitamin K is a fat-soluble vitamin whose absorption is compromised in the absence of bile acids. The consequent decline in vitamin K–dependent coagulation factors (II, VII, IX, X) impairs the intrinsic, extrinsic, and common pathways of coagulation, leading to prolongation of both the partial thromboplastin time (PTT) and prothrombin time (PT). Disseminated intravascular coagulation (DIC) also involves multiple coagulation factors (platelets, II, V, VIII, fibrinogen) resulting in prolongation of PT and PTT, but rarely occurs in a healthy infant. Both hemophilia A (factor VIII deficiency) and hemophilia B (factor IX deficiency) are congenital X-linked disorders, but they rarely present with hemorrhagic manifestations until late in the first year of life; furthermore, because the defects involve only the intrinsic pathway of coagulation, the PTT is prolonged whereas the PT is normal.

78. The answer is C *[Chapter 13 I C 3 d (2); IV D].* A positive sweat test (i.e., a sweat chloride level greater than 60 mEq/L) is diagnostic of cystic fibrosis. Children without cystic fibrosis have values less than 40 mEq/L. Although a positive family history of cystic fibrosis, the presence of digital clubbing, and evidence of bronchiectasis by chest x-ray may suggest cystic fibrosis, the sweat test is diagnostic.

79. The answer is C *[Chapter 14 VI E 1].* A colony count of 10⁵ for a single organism usually is accepted as proof of urinary tract infection. Although urine obtained for culture by suprapubic aspiration or catheterization is less likely to be contaminated, clean-catch specimens are very reliable in diagnosing urinary tract infection if collected properly. There is no practical, accurate way to localize the site of infection to the renal parenchyma or the lower urinary tract. The presence of fever or of vesicoureteral reflux is certainly not a differentiating symptom because either may occur with cystitis. High fever, however, usually occurs only in pyelonephritis, and reflux definitely increases the risk of parenchymal involvement. Pyuria may occur in children without a urinary tract infection who have acute illnesses, especially those with fever and dehydration. Pyuria also may occur in any form of interstitial nephritis. Most urinary tract infections in children are caused by coliform bacteria, which grow regularly on standard culture media.

80. The answer is A *[Chapter 5 II C 2; Figure 5-3].* The pubertal growth spurt is late in boys and early in girls. It is associated with muscle development in boys and fat deposit in girls. It is the final growth spurt in humans, and usually lasts approximately 3 years.

81. The answer is D *[Chapter 9 IV C 2 a].* Nosebleeds, nasal congestion, and loss of smell and taste are all characteristic findings in seasonal allergic rhinitis. However, the nasal discharge is usually thin, watery mucus and not a yellow discharge. A thick yellow or green nasal discharge suggests sinusitis.

82. The answer is A *[Chapter 3 VII C 2, E 4].* Excessively frequent contact between the divorced parents themselves, especially if parental hostility continues, may contribute to further discord between the parents, which subsequently is associated with poor psychological outcome for the child. A number of factors are associated with better long-term psychological outcomes for children of divorce. Among these factors are the maintenance of a familiar physical and psychological environment, including school, friends, and daily life routines, in addition to as much contact as feasible with the noncustodial parent. As much financial security for the child as possible is also helpful.

83. The answer is B *[Chapter 14 X B 2].* The expected acid–base disturbance in acute renal failure is metabolic acidosis. The acidosis is the result of increased endogenous acid load, volume expansion, defective hydrogen ion secretion, decreased excretion of titratable acid, and diminished ammonia production. Hyperkalemia, hyperphosphatemia, and hyperuricemia all are expected consequences of increased renal load and decreased renal excretion. The tumor lysis syndrome also increases the serum uric acid levels.

84. The answer is E *[Chapter 5 IV A 1 a, E 1; Table 5-5].* Joint involvement is not a characteristic of chlamydial infection, although it is a possible outcome of gonorrhea. Chlamydial infection may spread to cause lower abdominal pain, infertility, epididymitis, and right shoulder pain. Lower abdominal pain is the result of a pelvic infection; infertility is caused by scarring of the fallopian tubes from infection; epididymitis may result from an untreated chlamydial urethritis; and right shoulder pain is caused by irritation of the phrenic nerve from perihepatitis as a result of infection.

85. The answer is B *[Chapter 18 III D 2].* The common causes of hydrocephalus in neonates are intraventricular hemorrhage, infection, and congenital malformations (e.g., aqueductal stenosis, Arnold-Chiari malformation). Brain tumors rarely occur in the first year of life, and if present at this age, they are most likely to be supratentorial. When tumors occur infratentorially, hydrocephalus may be present.

86. The answer is E *[Chapter 13 I C 3 b (1) (b)].* Sweat testing, immunoglobulin analysis, complete blood count, and sputum culture are helpful in evaluating children with suspected lung disease. Pulmonary function tests require a child to cooperate by taking a deep breath to total lung capacity and then exhaling completely; therefore, these tests cannot be successfully performed on a 2-year-old child. These tests can sometimes be performed on a research basis using a different technology.

87. The answer is C *[Chapter 2 I B 1–3].* Before the mid-1940s, respiratory disease was the most common cause of death; however, the widespread use of antibiotics has dramatically decreased childhood mortality due to pneumonia. Since the mid-1940s, injuries have consistently been the most common cause of death in childhood, resulting in four times the number of childhood deaths due to any disease. Although children are responsible for a larger percentage of hospital admissions due to injury than are adults, most childhood injuries are treated at home and have death as their least likely outcome. "Loss of working years of life" is a powerful measure of injury outcome because it measures the loss to society.

88. The answer is D *[Chapter 6 V A 2 a].* The diagnosis of esophageal atresia with tracheoesophageal fistula is established by the inability to pass a nasogastric tube into the stomach and the observation on chest radiograph that the tube is coiled up in the esophageal pouch. Although the fistula between the trachea and distal esophagus may be seen on a lateral chest radiograph as a column of air between the stomach and trachea, special studies usually are not necessary because the fistula almost always starts at the level of the carina and connects to the superior aspect of the distal esophagus. Contrast studies of the esophageal pouch may result in aspiration, and should not be undertaken.

89. The answer is D *[Chapter 8 I F 1; VIII D 1].* Serum α-fetoprotein (AFP) testing is used only for prenatal screening or screening for cancer. Mental retardation can be associated with chromosome abnormalities, including the fragile X syndrome, metabolic disorders, and heritable syndromes.

90. The answer is C *[Chapter 9 V B 2].* Erythema marginatum is the hallmark skin lesion of rheumatic fever. It differs from the maculopapular rashes seen in systemic juvenile rheumatoid arthritis (JRA). Other features of systemic JRA include high, spiking fever, lymphadenopathy, and hepatosplenomegaly. Children with pauciarticular JRA are at risk for uveitis.

91. The answer is D *[Chapter 16 II B 5, 6, C 3 b (2); V E 4].* This boy has an approximately 80% chance of cure with current chemotherapy regimens and certainly need not be subject to the risks of bone marrow transplantation. However, patient (C), who has relapsed during initial therapy, is unlikely to be salvaged without transplant. The most efficacious transplant for this patient would be an allogeneic transplant from a fully human leukocyte antigen (HLA)-matched family donor. Patient (B) would also benefit from this type of transplant, because children with acute nonlymphocytic leukemia (ANLL) have a better survival if they receive an HLA-matched family donor transplant in first remission than if they are treated with chemotherapy alone. Patient (A)'s chances of survival may also be better with transplant. Provided the neuroblasts can be eliminated or markedly reduced from the marrow, this patient could be offered a purged autologous transplant and spared the risk of graft-versus-host disease, which often complicates allogeneic transplants.

92. The answer is D *[Chapter 6 I C 1].* Early fetal growth is due to cellular hyperplasia. Congenital infection, chromosomal defects, cell toxins, and maternal alcohol use all affect the fetus during early gestation and result in a decrease in both the total cell number and the growth of all organs. This is termed symmetric growth retardation. Preeclampsia, a complication that occurs in the last trimester, results in fetal malnutrition, which primarily reduces birth weight but does not affect the brain (head circumference) or linear growth. This is termed asymmetric growth retardation.

93. The answer is B *[Chapter 5 V B 2].* Pelvic complications resulting from incomplete pelvic development are likely to occur in women who are younger than 15 years of age. By 16 or 17 years of age, most women have completed their pubertal development and the pelvic bones are fully formed.

94. The answer is E *[Chapter 4 VII B 1 b].* Childhood schizophrenia usually does not present until after 7 years of age. Autism develops by 30 months of age and is associated with gross defects in language. Children with developmental delay also can present with limited language. Extreme parental neglect has been reported to cause delays in language acquisition and to cause depression, which can lead to elective mutism.

95. The answer is B *[Chapter 14 I C 1 b].* Cystoscopy is an invasive procedure that has a role in the evaluation of persistent hematuria, although not immediately. More important to the initial evaluation of gross hematuria in this 14-year-old black girl is to establish that there are normal renal function, infection-free urine, the absence of sickle cell trait, and the absence of major renal anomalies (e.g., cysts, stones, tumor). In this patient, hematuria associated with sickle cell trait is quite possible.

96. The answer is A *[Chapter 3 IV D 4, F, G].* Under optimal circumstances, foster placement may be helpful in protecting a socially at-risk child in addition to providing a potential means of remediation for the family. However, given the problems of resource availability and the underlying pathology of the family, foster children remain at risk for poor medical and psychological outcome in spite of placement. Twenty-five percent of foster children face multiple placements in their lives. They are less likely to have a defined, continuous, and coordinated source of primary medical care and have a high incidence of medical problems, including failure to thrive. Families of foster children often have such marked social pathology that they may require major interventive services, thereby taxing available social service agencies. All of these and other factors contribute to foster children being at significantly higher risk for behavioral and psychiatric problems than their non-foster peers.

97. The answer is A *[Chapter 18; Table 18-1].* The Moro reflex, rooting reflex, and tonic neck reflex are all developmental reflexes present within the first 3–6 months of life. The parachute reflex appears only at 6–8 months.

98. The answer is A *[Chapter 5 V A 1 a].* The hormones of oral contraceptives essentially turn off the ovulatory function of the ovaries. The uterine lining is not vascularized as extensively and, hence, is not as able to receive a fertilized egg. The cervical mucus becomes more hostile to sperm, making it less likely that sperm enter the uterus.

99. The answer is A *[Chapter 6 V C].* In physiologic jaundice, the maximum bilirubin concentration should not exceed 12–15 mg/dl. The initial investigation should include tests that evaluate for the presence of hemolytic disease, the most common cause of hyperbilirubinemia aside from decreased glucuronyl transferase activity (physiologic jaundice). Appropriate tests include a complete blood count with reticulocyte count, determination of maternal and infant blood types, Coombs' test, and indirect and direct bilirubin concentrations. Initiation of phototherapy is appropriate in this infant. As long as the infant is well hydrated, breast-feeding should be encouraged.

100. The answer is B *[Chapter 16 V A 1 a (2)].* All of the conditions noted in the question, except 21-hydroxylase deficiency, may present as short stature and delayed puberty. 21-Hydroxylase deficiency may present as signs of virilization with accelerated growth in childhood secondary to excessive adrenal androgens. Girls with Turner syndrome may not have the physical stigmata associated with the syndrome. Likewise, physical findings in acquired hypothyroidism may be quite subtle. Although Turner syndrome and hypothyroidism should be considered, the most likely diagnosis is constitutional delay of growth and development. A history of weight loss, compulsive exercise, and abnormal eating behavior might indicate anorexia nervosa.

101. The answer is B *[Chapter 5 VI D 1 a, c].* Although most people with anorexia nervosa do display obsessive and overachieving personality traits, these traits are not a part of the definition of this disease. Weight loss to at least 15% less than expected for height, a disturbed body image, fear of gaining weight or being fat, and an absence of at least three consecutive menstrual cycles are all traits associated with anorexia nervosa.

102. The answer is D *[Chapter 13 V E].* The sweat test is used in the diagnosis of cystic fibrosis but is not helpful in assessing children with bronchopulmonary dysplasia. In the evaluation of children with bronchopulmonary dysplasia, the sleeping respiratory rate, oxygen saturation (obtained by oximetry), and chest x-ray all provide valuable information. The severity of the lung disease also is assessed by the rate of growth and the number of calories needed to produce good growth. The electrocardiogram is helpful when looking for signs of right ventricular hypertrophy secondary to pulmonary hypertension from chronic hypoxemia.

103. The answer is C *[Chapter 3 VI D].* In general, there is no substantial evidence that child care outside of the home by providers other than the parents results in harm to the child. In fact, if the specific child care arrangement is of high quality, not only is there no greater risk for poor emotional outcome, but a number of beneficial effects may be realized. Children from psychosocially at-risk environments may show major benefits from high-quality day care in both cognitive and emotional areas; however, these benefits are likely to persist only if later school quality and stabilization of the home environment are ensured.

104. The answer is C *[Chapter 6 V F 1 b (2), G 3; Chapter 18; Table 18-5].* The two important points in the history described in the question are the length of time between the rupture of the fetal membranes and delivery, which increases the risk for infection, and the use of forceps, which is associated with intracranial trauma and hemorrhage. Although asphyxia is a major cause of seizures during the first day of life, there is nothing in the history to suggest its occurrence (i.e., there has been no history of abnormal fetal heart tracing or meconium-stained fluid, and the Apgar score was normal). Clinical signs of kernicterus are not seen at 12 hours of age.

105. The answer is D *[Chapter 16 IV A 1 b; V A 3 b].* Idiopathic growth hormone (GH) deficiency accounts for most cases of GH deficiency. Typical features include short stature, slow growth velocity (< 5 cm/yr in older children), mild truncal adiposity, and delayed skeletal maturation. Body proportions are normal, in contrast to the immature proportions seen in congenital hypothyroidism. Hypertension is not associated with idiopathic GH deficiency, although it is a common feature of Cushing syndrome, another cause of slow growth during childhood.

106. The answer is C *[Chapter 5 IV C 1].* Toxic shock syndrome (TSS) is a total body response to the release of endotoxin from a *Staphylococcus aureus* infection. The platelet count decreases to less than 100,000/mm^3. Treatment requires the removal of the causative agent, such as a tampon or a diaphragm, and treatment with systemic antibiotics. Prevention

requires the limited and careful use of diaphragms and tampons and the recognition of the symptoms associated with TSS.

107–111. The answers are: 107-E *[Chapter 1 III F 6 a],* **108-C** *[Chapter 1 VI E 7 c, F 2],* **109-D** *[Chapter 1 VI E 7 a, F 1],* **110-D** *[Chapter 1 VI E 4; VII E 8 a],* **111-B** *[Chapter 1 VII E 8 c].* The state organization of the newborn is characterized by "predictable unpredictability." Thus, irregular feeding and sleeping schedules are to be expected. By 2 months of age, the infant's demands should become more regular.

Night awakening reflects the continuing importance of attachment. Reinforcing the awakening by holding or feeding the infant should be avoided. The behavior will resolve normally within several weeks if parents provide only brief, positive interaction and lovingly, but firmly, indicate that the child must sleep.

By 15–18 months of age, a child's negativism and resistant behavior dramatically reflect the struggle for autonomy, typified by temper tantrums. The child continually explores the limits of the environment, while remaining dependent on adults. Distracting the child or ignoring her behavior (having first ensured her safety) is a reasonable approach to temper tantrums. Toilet training can also provide a forum for the struggle for independence. Toilet training is most successful when it is child oriented. Attempts at toilet training should, therefore, be deferred until the child's negativism and resistance behavior subside.

The consistency of a child's style of behavior, or temperament, is predictive of the child's responses to certain situations. Slow adjustment to new situations, people, and places is typical of the "slow-to-warm-up" child. Entering school may pose particular difficulties for this child until he becomes more comfortable on repeated exposure.

112–115. The answers are: 112-B *[Chapter 8 I F 3 b; Table 8-4],* **113-C** *[Chapter 8 I F 1 a, b],* **114-A** *[Chapter 8 I F 2],* **115-B** *[Chapter 8 I F 3, 4; Table 8-4].* Amniocentesis is a procedure performed as early as 12 weeks' gestation for various analyses of amniotic fluid, including the study of specific cell or fluid biochemical or DNA markers. Chorionic villus sampling (CVS) is performed at 8–11 weeks' gestation and can provide fetal cells for biochemical or DNA analysis; amniotic fluid is not available by this technique. Sickle cell disease is an autosomal recessive disorder for which a DNA probe is available. When both parents are heterozygotes, their child has a 25% chance of being affected. Amniocentesis and CVS provide material containing fetal DNA that can be analyzed for the sickle cell gene.

The American College of Obstetricians and Gynecologists now recommends that maternal serum α-fetoprotein (AFP) testing be considered in every pregnancy because it carries no risk and can raise suspicion that the fetus has an open defect, such as a neural tube defect, if it is elevated, or a chromosomal aneuploidy if it is low.

Microcephaly can be genetic and may be diagnosed in utero, where accurate head measurements can be obtained by ultrasound, because norms exist for head size at each gestational age.

A familial balanced translocation predisposes the couple to having chromosomally unbalanced and, therefore, abnormal offspring. Amniocentesis or CVS allows determination of fetal chromosome constitution. Percutaneous umbilical blood sampling (PUBS) will also detect a chromosomal alteration, but carries a higher risk.

116–120. The answers are: 116-D, 117-A, 118-E, 119-B, 120-C *[Chapter 9 IV C 3 a–c].* The clinical symptoms of allergic diseases such as allergic rhinitis should correlate with the time of year in which certain trees, grasses, or weeds pollinate. In the North Atlantic region of the United States, grasses pollinate in spring and early summer, and ragweed pollinates in late summer and early fall. *Alternaria* spores are present from spring through fall, and they are especially related to the fallen leaves from trees during autumn. Trees pollinate in early spring. Identification of the inhalant allergens causing symptoms in a particular patient is helpful in formulating a suitable treatment plan. For example, the onset of symptoms of allergic rhinitis in late October or November, as the weather gets cold and the heat is turned on in a house, may suggest a hypersensitivity to house dust mites. Simple measures of environmental dust control may significantly help a patient with a dust mite allergy.

121–125. The answers are: 121-C *[Chapter 12 IV I 4 b (1); Figure 12-6],* **122-E** *[Chapter 12 IV F 4 b (1)],* **123-B** *[Chapter 12 IV K 4 b (1)],* **124-D** *[Chapter 12 IV L 4 b (1)],* **125-A** *[Chapter 12 IV M 1 d (2) (a)].* The chest x-ray may give clues to the type of congenital

heart defect present. In coarctation of the aorta, the "3" sign is produced by soft tissue densities consisting of the aortic knob and the dilated descending aorta. In tetralogy of Fallot, the apex of the heart is upturned and the base, where the pulmonary artery would have been, is convex, producing a boot-shaped heart. In D-transposition of the great arteries, the anterior–posterior arrangement of the great arteries produces a narrow base and the heart resembles an egg on its side. In L-transposition of the great arteries, the ascending aorta produces convexity of the left heart border as it emerges from the right ventricle on the left side of the heart. In supracardiac total anomalous pulmonary venous return, the cardinal veins above the heart produce a double shadow resembling a snowman or a "figure 8" as they drain into the superior vena cava.

126–128. The answers are: 126-C *[Chapter 14 X C 1],* **127-A** *[Chapter 14 IV A 1 a (2)],* **128-D** *[Chapter 14 VI C 2].* Hemolytic–uremic syndrome is characterized by the triad of microangiopathic hemolytic anemia, thrombocytopenia, and azotemia. Although these features may vary in severity, they usually all occur together. Approximately 85% of cases of poststreptococcal glomerulonephritis show decreased serum levels of complement component C3. Levels return to normal within 8 weeks of the onset of disease. Vesicoureteral reflux is present in about 35% of children with urinary tract infection and in a much higher percentage of those in whom pyelonephritis develops.

129–131. The answers are: 129-B *[Chapter 18 III B 1 c (3)],* **130-C** *[Chapter 18 III B 1 b],* **131-E** *[Chapter 18 III C 1].* Syringomyelia is a cyst in the spinal cord, most commonly in the cervical or thoracic area. Patients present with loss of sensation to pinprick and cold because the crossing fibers in the spinal cord are affected initially. Eventually, the corticospinal tract is involved, leading to spasticity of the lower extremities.

In the Arnold-Chiari malformation, downward displacement of the cerebellar tonsils and kinking of the medulla lead to hydrocephalus. This anomaly commonly is associated with meningomyelocele.

Agenesis of the corpus callosum is often associated with epilepsy and mental retardation. This disorder may be suspected if there is abnormal midfacial development such as hypertelorism (widening of the orbital fissures).

Index

Note: Page numbers in *italic* indicate illustrations; those followed by (t) indicate tables. Q and A denote questions and answers. C denotes case studies.